Concepts in Hand Rehabilitation

Contemporary Perspectives in Rehabilitation

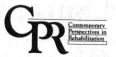

Steven L. Wolf, PhD, FAPTA
Editor-in-Chief

PUBLISHED VOLUMES

The Biomechanics of the Foot and Ankle
Robert Donatelli, MA, PT

Pharmacology in Rehabilitation
Charles D. Ciccone, PhD, PT

Wound Healing: Alternatives in Management
Luther C. Kloth, MS, PT, Joseph M. McCulloch, PhD, PT, and
Jeffrey A. Feedar, BS, PT

Thermal Agents in Rehabilitation, 2nd Edition
Susan L. Michlovitz, MS, PT

Electrotherapy in Rehabilitation
Meryl R. Gersh, MS, PT

Understanding the Dynamics of Human Biologic Tissue
Dean P. Currier, PhD, PT, and Roger M. Nelson, PhD, PT

Cardiopulmonary Rehabilitation: Basic Theory and Application,
2nd Edition
Frances J. Brannon, PhD, Julie Starr, MS, PT, Margaret Wiley Foley,
MSN, and Mary J. Geyer Black, MS, PT

Concepts in Hand Rehabilitation

Barbara G. Stanley, PT
Capital District Hand Therapy Center
Schenectady, New York

Susan M. Tribuzi, OTR
Director, Hand Therapy
Hand Surgery Specialists, Ltd.
Richmond, Virginia

 F. A. DAVIS COMPANY • **Philadelphia**

Printed in the United States of America

Last digit indicates print number: 10 9 8 7 6 5 4 3 2 1

acquisitions editor: Jean-François Vilain
developmental editor: Ralph Zickgraf
production editor: Gail Shapiro

As new scientific information becomes available through basic and clinical research, recommended treatments and drug therapies undergo changes. The author(s) and publisher have done everything possible to make this book accurate, up to date, and in accord with accepted standards at the time of publication. The authors, editors, and publisher are not responsible for errors or omissions or for consequences from application of the book, and make no warranty, expressed or implied, in regard to the contents of the book. Any practice described in this book should be applied by the reader in accordance with professional standards of care used in regard to the unique circumstances that may apply in each situation. The reader is advised always to check product information (package inserts) for changes and new information regarding dose and contraindications before administering any drug. Caution is especially urged when using new or infrequently ordered drugs.

Library of Congress Cataloging–in–Publication Data

Concepts in hand rehabilitation / [edited by] Barbara G. Stanley,
Susan M. Tribuzi.
      p. cm. — (Contemporary perspectives in rehabilitation)
   Includes bibliographical references and index.
   ISBN 0-8036-8092-9 (hardbound : alk. paper)
   1. Hand—Surgery—Patients—Rehabilitation. 2. Hand—Diseases-
Patients—Rehabilitation. 3. Hand—Wounds and injuries—Patients-
Rehabilitation. 4. Hand—Wounds and injuries—Physical therapy.
5. Hand—Diseases—Physical therapy. I. Stanley, Barbara G., 1958-
   II. Tribuzi, Susan M., 1957- . III. Series.
   [DNLM: 1. Hand Injuries—physiopathology. 2. Hand Injuries—
   rehabilitation. WE 830 C744]
   RD559. C665 1992
   617.5'7506—dc20
   DNLM/DLC
   for Library of Congress   92-49865
                                                                   CIP

Dedication

To our husbands, Tom and Scot, for all their patience, support, understanding, and love.

Foreword

The editors of *Concepts in Hand Rehabilitation* are to be congratulated for the excellent work they have accomplished with this latest book in the *Contemporary Perspectives in Rehabilitation* series. As contributors they have attracted fine professionals who have excelled in their speciality of upper-extremity trauma and disability.

Each contributing author is recognized within the field as an accomplished clinician. All contributors have shared their skills by presenting the theoretical information and medical base for each topic along with the specific therapeutic management protocols. They have presented the rationale for each approach, followed by evaluations, modalities, splint requirements, and precautions. This is truly a gem of a reference book.

Susan Tribuzi, OTR, and Barbara Stanley, PT, are both practicing hand therapists who have spent untold days refining and editing the chapters so that they represent a balanced and coordinated presentation, the state of the art in therapeutic management of hand injuries. This text is an excellent training tool and reference for the entry-level therapist as well as the experienced clinician. This book deserves a prominent, easy-to-reach place on every therapist's library shelf.

Maude H. Malick, OTR, ASHT

Foreword

Our primary tools for manipulating the environment are our hands. With only one, an individual is significantly limited. Loss of both hands necessitates the use of prostheses, which can only partially compensate for the incredible proficiency of the machinery controlling the hands' intrinsic and extrinsic musculature. To manage the rehabilitation of patients whose hands have suffered injury due to trauma or diseases of metabolic, joint, or connective tissue requires the combined efforts of talented clinicians from many disciplines. Barbara Stanley, PT and Susan Tribuzi, OTR have recruited physicians, occupational therapists, and physical therapists to present their combined expertise in an exceptionally comprehensive text.

In *Concepts in Hand Rehabilitation,* unlike other books on this subject, each contributor has painstakingly addressed a single area of specialization. Equally important is the fact that each topic has been developed along the theme of the entire *Contemporary Perspectives in Rehabilitation* series; that is, with exhaustive, up-to-date references and thought-provoking challenges in problem solving. The latter are designed to tax the thinking processes and call on the learning experiences of all readers — from beginning students to experienced clinicians.

We have chosen to divide this text into four sections: I, Fundamentals in Hand Therapy; II, Evaluation of the Hand; III, Concepts in Clinical Treatment; and IV, Clinical Treatment by Diagnosis. This arrangement allows the reader to progress from an anatomic review of structures composing the hand and the physiology of wound healing to the evaluation process. Coverage of this process includes a method for clinical measurement, very comprehensively covered and progresses to sensibility testing and functional assessment. Allied health students will find both of these sections very helpful, whereas experienced clinicians might wish to begin their reading with the evaluation section.

In either case, Sections I and II are appropriate precursors to the problem-solving activities in Sections III and IV. The chapters on hand treatment procedures address wound management, therapeutic exercise, and the use of thermal agents and electrical stimulation. Section IV uses a thought-provoking approach to clinical problems; its nine chapters showcase the problem-solving skills and clinical experience of their authors. The presentations on skeletal injury, nerve and tendon injuries, rheumatoid arthritis, cumulative and acute trauma, crush injuries and amputations, and reflex sympathetic dystrophy are state-of-the-art discourses that will enlighten both student and clinician.

The chapter on returning the patient with a hand injury to work is particularly relevant to all readers. The concepts of job analysis, work capacity, and effort assessment are thoroughly discussed; moreover, astute readers will see the relevance of this

ix

presentation as a model for work-return programs for patients with problems other than hand injuries.

The text concludes with appendices on methods of measuring hand volume, joint range of motion, and finger strength. We hope that the reader will appreciate the comprehensive nature of this text and recognize its contribution to the knowledge base of hand rehabilitation. It is our belief that after digesting its contents the student or clinician will view this book as an indispensable companion in the treatment of hand patients.

Steven L. Wolf, PhD, FAPTA
Series Editor, Contemporary
Perspectives in Rehabilitation

Preface

Concepts in Hand Rehabilitation is intended, as part of the series *Contemporary Perspectives in Rehabilitation*, to promote an understanding of hand therapy and to challenge the clinical thinking processes of its readers. With this purpose in mind, the more than 20 distinguished contributors wrote their chapters from a clinical decision-making perspective. As a result, each chapter in Sections II through IV, in addition to providing the relevant facts, emphasizes the reasoning process necessary to develop an effective rehabilitation program.

As editors, we have organized *Concepts in Hand Rehabilitation* in accordance with the focus on clinical decision making. The book consists of four sections, designed together to present an integrated picture of the state of the art of hand rehabilitation.

In Section I, Fundamentals in Hand Therapy, Chapter 1 covers the functional anatomy of the hand and Chapter 2 discusses the wound healing processes as they apply to skin, bone, tendon, and nerve.

Section II, Evaluation of the Hand, includes material on the many forms and tools of evaluation relevant to hand therapy. Chapter 3, "Clinical Evaluation," discusses evaluation techniques common to most hand injuries, including evaluation of range of motion, strength, edema, and pain, with an emphasis on standardized evaluation techniques. Chapter 4 addresses the increasingly complex subject of sensibility evaluation. Topics covered include indications for testing, testing techniques, and interpretation. Chapter 5 deals with the frequently overlooked issue of functional evaluation; as well as describing such techniques as the interview, questionnaires, and observation, the author provides a comprehensive review of standardized tests for functional evaluation.

Section III, Concepts in Clinical Treatment, covers in detail such "tools of the trade" as wound management (Chapter 6), therapeutic exercise (Chapter 7), modalities (Chapter 8), and splinting (Chapter 9). In addition to discussing care of the open wound, for instance, Chapter 6 deals with edema control and scar management, two factors that must be considered in all hand injuries. Unique to *Concepts in Hand Rehabilitation* is Chapter 7, which imparts the basic rationale for selection of therapeutic exercises to maintain and restore hand mobility. Chapter 8 reviews the theory and application in hand rehabilitation of thermal and electrical modalities. Chapter 9 presents in dialectic format the decision-making process of designing and fabricating a splint.

Section IV, Clinical Treatment by Diagnosis, combines the knowledge and skills imparted in the preceding sections and shows how they are applied to a variety of diagnoses: skeletal, nerve, and tendon injuries (Chapters 10, 11, and 12); rheumatoid arthritis (Chapter 13); cumulative trauma (Chapter 14); reflex sympathetic dystrophy (Chapter 15); and crush injuries and partial hand amputations (Chapter 16). In Chapter

17, Section IV ends with a consideration of the ultimate goal of every therapy program: returning the injured patient to work.

Finally, four appendices provide detailed information on hand volumetry, goniometry, strength testing, and equipment suppliers.

It has been our goal and remains our strong hope that *Concepts in Hand Rehabilitation* will provide students and practitioners alike a clear, detailed introduction to and a valuable reference for the practice of hand injury therapy.

Barbara G. Stanley, PT
Susan M. Tribuzi, OTR

Acknowledgments

Undertaking a project of this magnitude would be impossible without the hard work and dedication of many. We are indebted to the following people for their enthusiasm, patience, and willingness to share their time and expertise:

- Each contributor
- Maude Malick, for her constructive comments and moral support
- Tom Mack, Richard Goodwyn, and Cheryl Rilee for their photographic assistance
- Jean-François Vilain of F. A. Davis, for just the right combination of passion, forbearance, and, of course, laughter
- Ralph Zickgraf and the F. A. Davis staff for their skillful preparation of the manuscript for production
- Our families for encouragement and support
- Paulette R. Miller for her secretarial assistance

- The many distinguished and perceptive reviewers, from several disciplines, whose criticisms and encouragement were of equal importance:

Mallory Anthony, MMSc, RPT, Curtis Hand Center, Union Memorial Hospital, Baltimore, Maryland

Paula Bohr, MS, OTR, FAOTA, Department of Occupational Therapy, College of Allied Health, University of Oklahoma Health Science Center, Oklahoma City, Oklahoma

Ann D. Callahan, MS, OTR/L, Hand Rehabilitation Center, Philadelphia, Pennsylvania

Nancy M. Cannon, OTR, Director, The Hand Rehabilitation Center of Indiana, Indianapolis, Indiana

Margaret Carter-Wilson, OTR, Director, Hand Rehabilitation Unit, Hand Surgery Association, Phoenix, Arizona

Rhea Cohn, MS, PT, Editorial Consultant, Silver Spring, Maryland

Dale Eckhaus, OTR, CHT, Curtis Hand Center, Union Memorial Hospital, Baltimore, Maryland

Roslyn B. Evans, OTR/L, Director, American Society of Hand Therapists, Indian River Hand Rehabilitation, Inc., Vero Beach, Florida

Kenneth R. Flowers, LPT, Valley Forge Hand Rehabilitation Service, Phoenixville Hospital, Phoenixville, Pennsylvania

Russell Foley, MS, PT, Fayette Medical Center, Fayetteville, Georgia

Carlos A. Garcia-Moral, MD, Oklahoma Hand Surgery Center, Oklahoma City, Oklahoma

Sigita Duda Hays, PT, CHT, Clinical Specialist, Victoria Hospital, London, Ontario, Canada

Paula Kader, PT, Hand Rehabilitation Center, Philadelphia, Pennsylvania

Kim Kovac, MS, PT, Department of Hand Therapy, Hand Surgery Specialists, Ltd., Richmond, Virginia

Evelyn J. Mackin, PT, Hand Rehabilitation Center, Philadelphia, Pennsylvania

Maude H. Malick, Vice President, Specialty Programs, Harmarville Rehabilitation Center, Pittsburgh, Pennsylvania

Joseph McCullough, PhD, PT, Associate Professor and Head, Rehabilitation Services, School of Medicine in Shreveport, Louisiana State University Medical Center, Shreveport, Louisiana

Christine Moran, MS, PT, CHT, Director, Richmond Upper Extremity Center, Richmond, Virginia

Rod Schlegel, PT, ECS, Curtis Hand Center, Union Memorial Hospital, Baltimore, Maryland

Lauren Valdata Eddington, RPT, CHT, Curtis Hand Center, Union Memorial Hospital, Baltimore, Maryland

Diana A. Williams, OTR/L, Supervisor, Hand Rehabilitation Service, Geisinger Medical Center, Danville, Pennsylvania

Heidi Hermann Wright, MBA, OTR, CHT, Helping Hands Work, Indianapolis, Indiana

Contributors

SUSAN M. BLACKMORE, MS, OTR, CHT

Assistant Chief, Occupational Therapy
Director of Hand Rehabilitation
The New York Hospital
Cornell Medical Center
New York, New York

WILLIAM H. BOWERS, MS, MD

Chief, Hand and Upper Extremity Service
Childrens Hospital
Richmond, Virginia
    and
Associate Professor of Orthopedics and Plastic Surgery (Hand)
Medical College of Virginia
Richmond, Virginia

LAURA BRUENING-REILLY, OTR/L

Hand Center of Western New York
Buffalo, New York

SHARON FLINN-WAGNER, MEd, OTR/L, CVE

Center for Work Enhancement
Cleveland, Ohio

JAMES W. KING, MA, OTR, CHT

Waco Rehabilitation Institute
Waco, Texas

SUSAN L. MANNARINO, OTR, CHT

Director of Hand Therapy
Hand Surgery of Southwestern Michigan
Kalamazoo, Michigan

HELEN MARX, OTR, CHT

Therapist, Hand Surgery Associates
Phoenix, Arizona

xv

SUSAN MICHLOVITZ, MS, PT

Clinical Associate Professor
Hahnemann University Programs in Physical Therapy
Philadelphia, Pennsylvania

PATRICIA A. TAYLOR MULLINS, RPT, CHT

Director, Hand Rehabilitation Services of Oklahoma
Oklahoma City, Oklahoma

ELAINE MUNTZER, PT, CHT

Partner, Hand and Orthopedic Rehabilitation Services
Levittown, Pennsylvania

BETH NICHOLSON, OTR, CHT

Owner, Center for Occupational Rehabilitation and Evaluation, Inc.
Birmingham, Alabama

VERONICA PENNEY, OTR/L

Senior Therapist, The Hand Center, Inc.
Scranton, Pennsylvania

PATRICIA BAXTER PETRALIA, MS, OTR/L

Adjunct Instructor of Orthopaedic Surgery
Jefferson Medical College
Thomas Jefferson University
Philadelphia, Pennsylvania

KAREN SCHULTZ-JOHNSON, MS, OTR, CVE, CHT

Owner/Director, Rocky Mountain Hand Therapy
    and
Director of Occupational Therapy, Valley View Hospital
Glenwood Springs, Colorado

LAURA R. SEGAL, PT

Director, Franklintowne Hand and Rehabilitation Center
Philadelphia, Pennsylvania

TERRI SKIRVEN, OTR/L, CHT

Director, Hand Therapy Program
Department of Occupational Therapy
University of Pennsylvania Medical Center
Philadelphia, Pennsylvania

KEVIN L. SMITH, MD

Charlotte Plastic Surgery Center
Charlotte, North Carolina

BARBARA G. STANLEY, PT

Capital District Hand Therapy Center
Schenectady, New York

KAREN M. STEWART, MS, OTR, CHT

Assistant Director of Hand Therapy, New York Group for Plastic Surgery
   and Rehabilitation
Monroe, New York

ANNA MAE TAN, OTR, CVE, CHT

Hand Rehabilitation Center
University of California San Diego Medical Center
San Diego, California

PATRICIA A. TOTTEN, OTR/L, CHT

Department of Occupational Therapy
Cooper Hospital University Medical Center
Camden, New Jersey

SUSAN M. TRIBUZI, OTR

Director, Hand Therapy
Hand Surgery Specialists, Ltd.
Richmond, Virginia

MARK WALSH, MS, PT, CHT

Adjunct Instructor, Philadelphia College of Pharmacy and Science
Philadelphia, Pennsylvania
      and
Partner, Hand and Orthopedic Rehabilitation Services
Levittown, Pennsylvania

Contents

Fundamentals in Hand Therapy

CHAPTER 1

Functional Anatomy

William H. Bowers, MD
Susan M. Tribuzi, OTR

The human hand is a delicate and complicated multisystem organization that provides sensory information and precise motor execution. Hand function is dependent on 27 bones, 30 joints, 33 muscles, innervation from three peripheral nerves, an intricate vascular system, and a variety of support structures.

An understanding of the functional anatomy of the hand is a necessary transitional step from classic anatomy to anatomy as a clinical tool in hand reconstruction and rehabilitation. As clinicians we must first recognize normal stasis structure and anatomy before we can address factors that produce deformity and therefore impede function.

The objectives of this chapter are to (1) review the anatomic systems in the hand including the cutaneous covering, connective tissue, skeletal, muscular, nerve, and vascular systems; (2) provide the reader with an understanding of the functional components of hand anatomy; and (3) discuss the clinical significance of the anatomy. The anatomy of the hand is extensive, with entire books devoted to discussing the topic. The intent of this chapter is to provide the reader with an overview of the critical concepts on which to base clinical decisions in hand rehabilitation.

CUTANEOUS COVERING

The skin is the protective covering of the hand. The unique qualities of the volar and dorsal skin facilitate hand function. The skin on the dorsum of the hand is fine, supple, and mobile and can easily be separated from the deep fascia. These characteristics contribute to the dorsal skin's ability to adjust to the extremes of finger flexion and extension. Hair follicles present in the dorsal skin serve to protect as well as to activate touch receptors when the hair is slightly deformed. The dorsal skin terminates into the specialized keratinized appendages of the skin known as the fingernails. The fingernails are composed of the nail matrix, nail bed, hyponychium, nail plate, and eponychium. On the average, nails grow 0.5 mm a week, although rates may vary with fingernails growing faster than toenails. In the lower primates fingernails functioned as claws; in humans, however, they are used for scratching, pinching, and providing external stability to the finger pulp to assist in prehension.

Unlike the dorsal skin, the volar skin is thick, hairless, inelastic, rich in sensory receptors, and supplied with sweat glands. The volar skin is firmly attached to the palmar aponeurosis, which prevents slippage when grasping an object. The volar and dorsal skin is impregnated with skin lines or creases. Riordan[8] classifies these skin lines into three groups: course lines, papillary ridges, and Langer's lines. The course lines are the flexion folds or skin joints. These course lines are located where the skin adheres to the deeper fascia and permit the hand to close without the skin bunching up into folds. The papillary ridges are located on the volar pulps of the digits, and over the thenar and hypothenar eminences. The papillary ridges provide friction to increase the efficiency of the hand during grip and also serve as the "eyes of the hand" with their rich sensory nerve endings. The papillary ridges in the finger pulps, also referred to as the friction ridges, are more commonly known as fingerprints, which are always individually distinct. Langer's lines or tension lines are distributed throughout the hand in different directions and are determined by the functional requirements of the particular area. Figure 1–1*A* identifies the common volar skin creases, and Figure 1–1*B* demonstrates the relationship of these creases to the underlying skeleton.

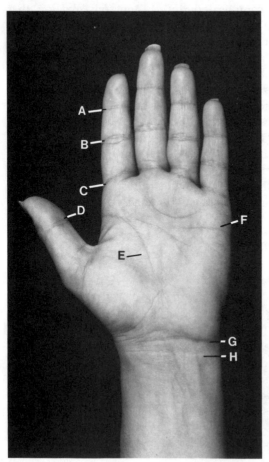

FIGURE 1–1. Palmar creases and surface landmarks of the left hand of a 28-year-old woman. *A*, Distal interphalangeal crease. *B*, Proximal interphalangeal crease. *C*, Palmar digital crease. *D*, Interphalangeal crease. *E*, Thenar crease. *F*, Distal palmar crease. *G*, Distal wrist crease. *H*, Proximal wrist crease.

CONNECTIVE TISSUE

Every muscle, tendon, nerve, and vessel is surrounded by connective tissue that separates or connects these structures from adjacent structures.[11] Connective tissues are divided into ordinary and special types. Components of connective tissue are the cells and extracellular matrix. The matrix is composed of fibrous elements: collagen, elastin and reticulin, and ground substance. Classification of connective tissue is dependent on the predominance of cells, the type concentration and arrangement of fibers, and the nature of the ground substance. Ordinary connective tissue includes dense and loose types and comprises structures such as ligaments, tendons, synovial membrane, fascia, and fibrous joint capsules.[4,5] The connective tissue discussion focuses on the primary characteristics and function of the fascia, ligaments, retinaculum, and fibrous tendon sheaths in the hand.

Fascia

"Fascia is elastocollagenous connective tissue through which muscles, nerves, blood vessels, lymph vessels and bones course."[13] Fascia is generally divided into superficial and deep layers, with the superficial layer being deep to the skin. In the hand, superficial and deep layers of fascia are present on both the dorsum and palmar surfaces. The fascia on the dorsum of the hand is thin and less developed than the palmar surface.

The superficial palmar fascia or aponeurosis shown in Figure 1–2 (classified as aponeurosis for its flattened characteristic) is a strong fibrous sheet that consists of central, lateral, and medial zones. The central zone is considered by some to be the most important anatomically and pathologically. The central zone is strong with its apex being a continuation of the distal margin of the flexor retinaculum (transverse carpal ligament) and the tendon of the palmaris longus. Distally, the superficial palmar aponeurosis divides into slips, which extend to each finger. This central palmar aponeurosis provides cover to the flexor tendons of the flexor digitorum superficialis and profundus, the terminal part of the median nerve, and the superficial branch of the ulnar nerve. The medial (hypothenar aponeuroses) and lateral (thenar aponeuroses) zones of the superficial palmar aponeuroses are the coverings of the hypothenar and thenar eminences. These zones are continuous with the central zone, as well as the dorsal fascia covering the interosseous muscles.

The deep palmar aponeurosis is the covering of the floor of the palm, between the thenar and hypothenar eminences. This fascia covers the anterior aspect of the interosseous muscles and metacarpals. Distally, the fascia merges with the deep transverse metacarpal ligament and proximally with the fascia of the anterior surface of the pronator quadratus.

The dorsal aponeurosis, like the palmar aponeurosis, has superficial and deep layers. The superficial dorsal fascia lines the superficial aspect of the extensor tendons and merges proximally with the extensor retinaculum. The deep dorsal fascia lines the dorsal aspect of the metacarpals and interosseous muscles.

The palmar and dorsal fascia functions to protect, cushion, restrain, conform, and maintain the concavity of the palm. Clinically, the palmar fascia proliferates in Dupuytren's disease, in which the fascia becomes diseased resulting in shortening and thickening of the fibrous bands that extend to the digits.

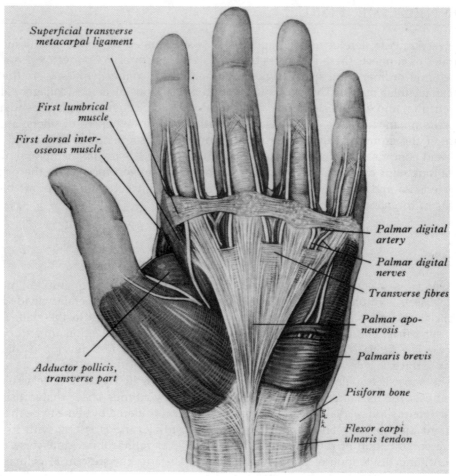

FIGURE 1-2. Palmar aponeurosis. (From Williams, P and Warwick, R: Gray's Anatomy, ed 36 [British]. Churchill Livingstone, Edinburgh, 1980, p 585, with permission.)

Ligament

Ligaments are dense connective tissue thickenings and extensions of the joint capsule. Ligaments that are part of the capsule are referred to as *intrinsic ligaments*, whereas those that pass between bones but are separate from the capsule are called *extrinsic ligaments*. Ligaments provide stability, connection, coordination, tendon guidance, and restraint.

The ligamentous system in the hand is intricate. Table 1-1 summarizes the most commonly referred to ligaments in the hand, their location, function, and (when known) their clinical significance.

Retinaculum

As the tendons of the extrinsic flexor and extensor muscles enter the hand they are held into position by the flexor and extensor retinacula. The flexor retinaculum (Fig. 1-3) (transverse carpal ligament) is a thick fibrous band that attaches to the palmar

TABLE 1–1 Ligamentous Structures of the Hand

Ligament	Location	Function	Clinical Significance
Cleland's ligament	Originates edge of osseous flexor tendon gutter at PIP, inserts into digital fascia	Retention	Dorsal fibers taut when the PIP joint is flexed; volar fibers taut when PIP joint is extended
Grayson's ligament	Originates volar aspect of flexor tendon sheath, inserts into skin	Holds neurovascular bundle in place, preventing "bowstringing" when the finger is flexed	
Transverse retinacular ligament	Originates edge of flexor tendon sheath at PIP, inserts into lateral edges of conjoined lateral bands	Prevents excessive dorsal shift of the lateral bands	Taut when the finger is flexed
Oblique retinacular ligament (Landsmeer's ligament)	Originates volar lateral crest of proximal phalanx, inserts into lateral terminal extensor tendon	Extends DIPs when PIPs are extended	Taut when PIP joint is extended, relaxed when PIP joint is flexed; tightness of this ligament may limit DIP flexion
Triangular ligament	Transversely directed fascia bounded proximally by the insertion of the central tendon laterally by lateral bands, distally by terminal extensor tendon	Prevents excessive volar shift of lateral bands	Taut when PIP joint is flexed, relaxed when PIP joint extended
Sagittal bands	Originates from central tendon inserts volar periosteum of proximal phalanx and borders of volar plate	Stabilizes extensor tendons at midline, prevents dorsal "bowstringing," limits excursion of extensor communis tendon	
Collateral ligaments MCP joints	Obliquely from dorsolateral aspect of the metacarpal head to palmar lateral aspect of the base of proximal phalanx	Joint stability	Taut in MCP flexion, relaxed in MCP extension. Contractures of this ligament are a contributing factor to limited MP flexion

(continued)

TABLE 1–1 (*continued*)

Ligament	Location	Function	Clinical Significance
Proper collateral ligament IP joints	Originates on the proximal condyle inserts onto the phalanx	Provides stable linkage for transmission of force across the joint, resists lateral displacement in grip and pinch	Taut at 25° of IP flexion
Accessory collateral ligaments	Originates with proper collateral ligament inserts onto the volar plate	Works with volar plate to stabilize joint to lateral stress in extension	
Volar plate	Volar side of MP, PIP, and DIP joints	Prevents interphalangeal hyperextension and maintains proper function of extensor mechanism, improves efficiency of the flexors	Stronger at the PIP joints than the DIP joints, involved in swan neck and boutonnière deformities
Transverse carpal ligament (flexor retinaculum)	Transverse from the scaphoid and crest of trapezium to the pisiform and hamate	Provides the pulley mechanism of the flexor tendon sheath	Forms the roof of the carpal tunnel
Deep transverse metacarpal ligament	Transverse from volar plate to volar plate at the MP joints	Stabilizes the volar plates	

aponeurosis. Medially, the flexor retinaculum attaches to the pisiform and the hook of the hamate and laterally to the scaphoid and trapezium and on occasion to the styloid process of the radius. The flexor retinaculum forms the roof of the carpal tunnel through which course the long extrinsic flexor tendons and the median nerve. The flexor retinaculum maintains the carpal arch, acts as a pulley for the flexor tendons, and provides protection for the median nerve.

The extensor retinaculum (Fig. 1–3) is a strong fibrous band under which the extensor tendons travel. This retinaculum is formed by superficial and deep layers. Medially, the extensor retinaculum is attached to the styloid process of the ulna, triquetrum, and pisiform and laterally to the lateral margin of the radius. Absence of these retinacula results in "bowstringing" of the tendons at the wrist level.

Tendon Sheaths and Pulleys

As the extrinsic flexor and extensor tendons descend through the wrist into the hand, they are encased in synovial sheaths. The sheaths are responsible for the nourishment of the tendons. They also serve as a friction abatement system.

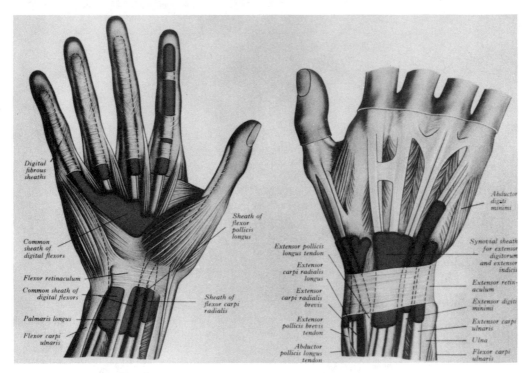

FIGURE 1–3. Flexor retinaculum *(left)* and extensor retinaculum *(right)*. (From Williams, P and Warwick, R: Gray's Anatomy, ed 36 [British]. Churchill Livingstone, Edinburgh, 1980, p 584, with permission.)

The extensor tendon sheaths are localized at the wrist, extending approximately 1 cm distal to the extensor retinaculum and to the bases of the metacarpals. The extensor tendons pass through six tendon compartments, with separate synovial sheaths. From radial to ulnar, these compartments house the following extensor tendons:

First dorsal wrist compartment: Abductor pollicis longus, extensor pollicis brevis
Second dorsal wrist compartment: Extensor carpi radialis longus, extensor carpi radialis brevis
Third dorsal wrist compartment: Extensor pollicis longus
Fourth dorsal wrist compartment: Extensor digitorium communis, extensor indicis proprius
Fifth dorsal wrist compartment: Extensor digiti minimi
Sixth dorsal wrist compartment: Extensor carpi ulnaris

These compartments are illustrated in Figure 1–4. Ariyan[27] simplifies remembering the distribution of these extensor tendons by remembering "221211."

The flexor tendon sheaths are more complex and intricate than those of its extensor counterpart. In the palm, the flexor tendons are encased in two synovial sheaths: the common flexor tendon sheath (ulna bursa or palmocarpal synovial sac) and the tendon sheath of the flexor pollicis longus (radial bursa). The flexor tendon sheaths are depicted in Figure 1–5. The common flexor tendon sheath contains the tendons of the flexor digitorum superficialis and profundus. The tendons to the index, long, and ring fingers are without tendon sheaths for a short distance in the middle of the palm. They then

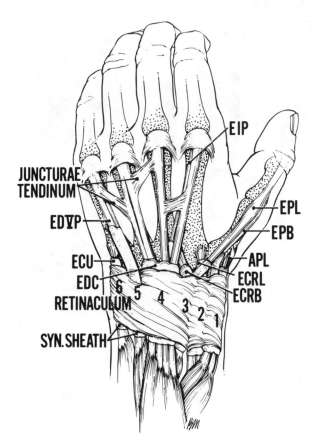

FIGURE 1–4. The extensor tendons pass through six compartments under the extensor retinaculum, which prevents the tendons from "bowstringing." (Illustration by Elizabeth Roselius, © 1988. Reprinted with permission from Green, DP: Operative Hand Surgery, 2nd ed. Churchill Livingstone, New York, 1988.)

have individual digital sheaths extending from the metacarpal heads to the terminal phalanges. However, the small finger sheath is continuous to the wrist.

These digital sheaths are composed of synovial and retinacular or pulley components. The retinacular portion overlies the synovial portion and constitutes the palmar aponeurosis pulley, five annular (A) pulleys and three cruciform (C) pulleys. Figure 1–6 illustrates these annular and cruciform pulleys (with the exception of the A5 pulley). The retinacular system holds the flexor tendons close to the bone, prevents "bowstringing," and promotes efficient flexor tendon excursion, which produces maximum digital flexion.

SKELETAL SYSTEM

The skeletal system of the hand is a complex series of short bones connected by joints, as shown in Figure 1–7. The skeleton of the hand and wrist consists of 27 bones. These are divided into five digital rays, each constituting a polyarticular chain. These digital rays are then arranged in a group of integrated arches, the concavities of which face volarly forming the hand into a cup. The depth of the cup is varied by the adjustment of each arch. The stable focus of the arch complex is the rigid base of the second and third metacarpal pillars. The other end, the second and third metacarpophalangeal (MCP) joints, form the keystone of the two major mobile arch systems, the

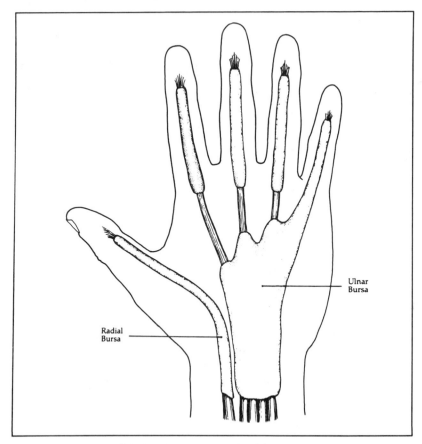

FIGURE 1–5. Flexor synovial sheaths. (From Schneider, L: Flexor Tendon Injuries. Little, Brown & Co, Boston, 1985, p 8, with permission.)

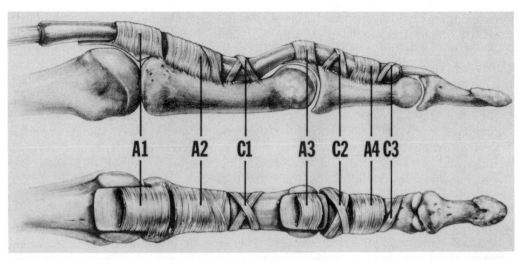

FIGURE 1–6. The four annular and three cruciform pulleys of the finger. (Illustration by Elizabeth Roselius, © 1988. Reprinted with permission from Green, DP: Operative Hand Surgery, 2nd ed. Churchill Livingstone, New York, 1988.)

A   B

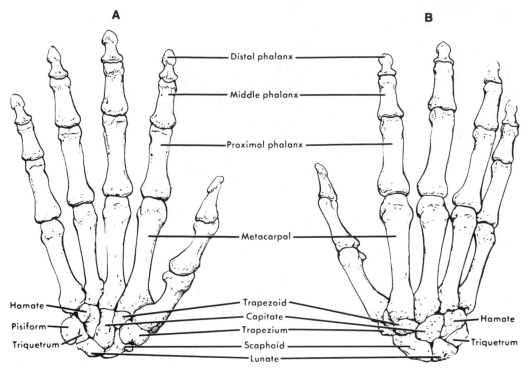

— Distal phalanx —

— Middle phalanx —

— Proximal phalanx —

— Metacarpal —

Hamate —   — Trapezoid —
                            — Capitate —   — Hamate
Pisiform —   — Trapezium —
                            — Scaphoid —   — Triquetrum
Triquetrum —   — Lunate —

FIGURE 1–7. Bones of the right hand. *A*, Palmar surface. *B*, Dorsal surface. (From Fess, E and Philips, C: Hand Splinting Principles and Methods, ed 2, CV Mosby, St Louis, 1987, p 4, with permission.)

distal transverse and longitudinal arches. Figure 1–8 illustrates these arches. The distal transverse arch gains most of its flexibility by mobility inherent in the first ray and, to a lesser degree, in the fourth and fifth rays. The skeletal basis for this mobility is the thumb carpometacarpal joint and the four or five carpometacarpal joints, which allow a corresponding ray to be depressed and elevated in relation to the stable second and third metacarpal rays. This capability changes the radius of the transverse arch. The adjustment of this arch allows the palm to adapt to various-shaped objects. The proximal transverse arch is stable and permanent in shape, unless altered by a carpal tunnel release or other volar wrist surgery involving transection of the transverse carpal ligament. The mobile longitudinal arches are the five digital rays. These rays are more mobile than the transverse arch and can alter their shape individually in response to demands of grasp. The flexion arc of the digital ray follows a strict mathematic pattern known as the equiangular spiral, seen in nature in the accretive shell of the chambered nautilus and in the common egg. This spiral is multiplaned and describes the sweep of the digital tips from extension and abduction to flexion, adduction, and rotation. This spiral allows for the hand's limitless grasp adaptability. The equiangular spiral was described by Descartes in 1638 and is constructed by a series of isosceles triangles with apical angles of 36°.[4,5] The structural length, joint configuration, and range determine individual patterns of digital movement. The extrinsic and intrinsic muscles of the forearm and hand are responsible for gross and refined action, respectively. Without balanced joint forces, the transverse and longitudinal equiangular curves are broken and hand adaptability is lost. Despite the elegance of the normal pattern, the congenitally or traumatically disabled hand has an exceptional degree of adaptability in many coura-

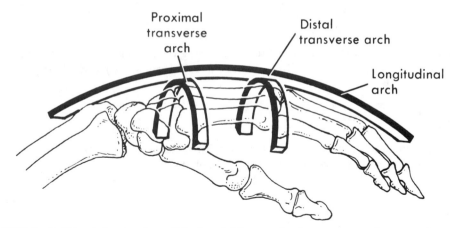

FIGURE 1–8. The skeletal arches of the hand. The proximal transverse arch passes through the distal carpus. The distal transverse arch passes through the metacarpal heads. The longitudinal arch passes through the four distal rays and the carpus. (From Fess, E and Philips, C: Hand Splinting Principles and Methods, ed 2. CV Mosby, St Louis, 1987, p 5, with permission.)

geous and admirably motivated people. The perfect balance of distribution of forces in the equiangular spiral can be illustrated by the grasp of an egg by the human hand (Fig. 1–9). Here the hand adapts perfectly to the dual curvature of the egg in both the longitudinal and transverse planes. The distribution of forces is so perfect that even the most powerful grasp is unable to crush it.

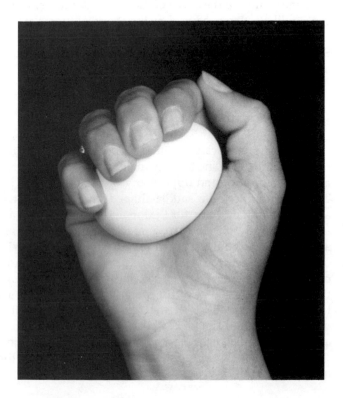

FIGURE 1–9. The perfect balance of the distribution of forces in the equiangular spiral is apparent in how the hand grasps an egg.

JOINTS

All the joints have basic anatomic forms favoring flexion. However, joint configuration and ligamentous apparatus differ in the interphalangeal (IP) and MCP joints.

Interphalangeal Joints

The IP joints are simple hinge joints with joint surfaces that travel on the same arch through their entire range of movement. The collateral ligaments, therefore, provide constant stability because there is some degree of tension on them in any position of the joint. Stability is greatly increased by the dynamic support of the flexor-extensor apparatus running over the joint.

Metacarpophalangeal Joints

The MCP joint, on the other hand, must provide mobility in two planes and its mechanism is therefore correspondingly more complicated. The collateral ligaments are slack with the joint in extension, thereby allowing lateral movement. Strength and stability of the extended joint are provided by the dynamic tone of the extrinsic muscles and the interosseous muscles. As the joint moves into flexion, the base of the proximal phalanx becomes firmly seated on the metacarpal head. This security is produced by a tightening of the collateral ligaments. The ligaments are fixed to the metacarpal necks and become tight in two planes as the joint flexes. This tightness is maximum in 70° of flexion. The ligaments tighten in the longitudinal direction because they arise eccentrically in relation to the curve of the upper portion of the metacarpal head and because of the camlike action produced by the shape of the volar portion of the metacarpal head. In the transverse direction, the ligaments tighten over the bulging sides of the condyles. Should the injured joint be splinted in extension, the collateral ligaments would tighten and thereby limit flexion.

Carpometacarpal Joint

The carpometacarpal joint is responsible for the greater part of the border mobility of the thumb, allowing this ray to become widely separated from the palm and to swing around in front of and oppose any of the digits. The joint is almost universal in type. The joint surfaces are saddle-shaped and movement takes place through two main axes — a radioulnar axis for flexion and extension and a dorsopalmar axis for abduction and adduction. With the proximal joint in midposition, the capsular structures are slack and rotation around the longitudinal axis can occur. When the thumb is fully abducted or fully adducted the joint surfaces are congruous and held closely together by tense capsular and ligament structures. The rotational component is eliminated, thus forming the two stable positions of function of the joint. The fourth and fifth common carpometacarpal articulations with the hamate provide for flexion and extension and some degree of rotation similar to those of the thumb carpometacarpal joint. The abduction and adduction degrees of freedom noted in the thumb joint, however, are unavailable in the fourth and fifth carpometacarpal joints owing to the presence of distal transverse intermetacarpal ligaments.

The mobility of the border rays (in relation to the stable second and third metacarpal rays), coupled with the equiangular multiplane spiral of the converging digital tips, provides for rotation of the border digits as they converge to the long axis of the third metacarpal. This metacarpal is the only ray that lies in its own longitudinal axis. The topical landmark for convergence of the digital tips is the scaphoid tubercle, which is a clinical landmark for realignment of rays in traumatic injuries. Table 1–2 summarizes the characteristics of the MCP, IP, and carpometacarpal joints of the hand.

MUSCULATURE

The muscles of the hand rarely act alone, but rather function as an integral part of a group. All movements require precise integration of a group of muscles functioning as the prime mover, antagonist, synergist, and stabilizer. Movements of the hand are accomplished through the precise integration and dynamic balance of the extrinsic and intrinsic muscles. These muscles, their innervation, functions, and clinical significance are summarized in Tables 1–3 and 1–4.

The nine muscles that contribute to thumb motion allow the thumb greater mobility than the other digits. The thumb extrinsic muscles are the abductor pollicis longus, extensor pollicis longus, extensor pollicis brevis, and the flexor pollicis longus. The intrinsic thumb muscles include the flexor pollicis brevis, opponens pollicis, abductor pollicis brevis, adductor pollicis (thenar muscles), and the first dorsal interosseous muscle.

The 20 muscles that contribute to finger motion and permit independent motion of each digit are also composed of extrinsic and intrinsic muscles. The extrinsic muscles include the flexor digitorum superficialis, flexor digitorum profundus, extensor digitorum communis, extensor indicis proprius, and extensor digiti minimi. The intrinsic counterparts include the four lumbrical muscles, the eight interosseous muscles, flexor digiti minimi, adductor digiti minimi, and opponens digiti minimi.

NERVE SUPPLY

The brachial plexus (Fig. 1–10) gives origin to the median, radial, and ulnar nerves, which supply the upper extremity (Figs. 1–11, 1–12, 1–13). Each of these nerves has a unique course from origin to termination. As these nerves course distally they pass through various anatomic structures, and the potential for entrapment and injury exists. Uninterrupted innervation of the median, radial, and ulnar nerves is necessary for normal hand functioning.

Median Nerve

The median nerve is formed by the union of the lateral and medial cords of the brachial plexus and therefore contains fibers from C5, C6, C7, C8, and T1. The median nerve was named from its position in the middle of the forearm. The nerve enters the forearm between the two heads of the pronator teres. The first branch then courses in the middle of the forearm between the flexor digitorum superficialis and profundus. In the forearm the nerve also innervates the palmaris longus, flexor carpi radialis, and flexor digitorum superficialis. Shortly after entering the forearm, the median nerve gives

TABLE 1-2 Joints of the Hand

Joint	Abbreviation	Joint Classification	Joint Movements	Supporting Structures	Clinical Significance
Carpometacarpal	CMC	Sellar saddle-shaped	Flexion/extension, abduction/adduction, rotation	Fibrous capsule; anterior oblique carpometacarpal, posterior oblique carpometacarpal, radial carpometacarpal, intermetacarpal ligaments; abductor pollicis longus; extensor pollicis brevis, extensor pollicis longus, thenar muscles	Capsule of the joint is thin and lax, which facilitates the thumb's most important movement of opposition; during prehension the thumb provides the stability for grip by opposing to the digits
Metacarpophalangeal (thumb)	MP	Condyloid	Flexion/extension, abduction/adduction, rotation, circumduction	Fibrous capsule; collateral, intersesmoid ligaments	Provides additional range to the thumb pad in opposition, permits the thumb to grasp and contour objects
Interphalangeal (thumb)	IP	Hinge	Flexion/extension	Fibrous capsule; collateral ligaments	The "epicenter" of the hand and hand surgery

Metacarpophalangeal (digits)	MCP	Condyloid	Flexion/extension, abduction/rotation circumduction	Fibrous capsule; collateral, assessory collateral, volar plate, deep transverse metacarpal ligaments; sagittal bands; interossei, extensor tendons	Determines position of distal joints, governing joint of the finger; normal prehension—MCP flexes last, extends first; stable in flexion, mobile in extension
Proximal interphalangeal (fingers)	PIP	Hinge	Flexion/extension	Fibrous capsule; collateral, accessory collateral, volar plate, retinacular ligaments of Landsmeer and Cleland; middle extensor, fibrous flexor sheath, flexor digitorum superficialis muscles	Important in control of flexion/extension of entire finger, stable in all positions; greater range of motion than the distal phalangeal joint
Distal interphalangeal (fingers)	DIP	Hinge	Flexion/extension	Fibrous capsule; collateral, accessory collateral, volar plate, Cleland's ligaments; fibrous flexor sheath, flexor digitorum profundus muscles; terminal extensor tendon	Places terminal pulp of the finger in optimum position for tactile gnosis, precision, manipulation

TABLE 1-3 Extrinsic Muscles of the Hand

Muscle	Abbreviation	Innervation	Primary Action	Secondary Action(s)	Clinical Significance
Dorsal					
Abductor pollicis longus	APL	Posterior interosseous branch of radial nerve C7–C8	Abducts, extends thumb at CMC joint	Assists in wrist flexion and radial deviation	Without it, the thumb cannot be drawn away from the palm
Extensor pollicis brevis	EPB	Posterior interosseous branch of radial nerve C7–C8	Extends thumb at CMC and MP joints; abducts the CMC	Assists in radial deviation at the wrist	When absent, MP joint rests in a flexion stance
Extensor pollicis longus	EPL	Posterior interosseous branch of radial nerve C7–C8	Extends the thumb IP joint, extends and adducts the thumb MP and CMC joints, supinator of the thumb metacarpal	Extends and radially deviates the wrist	Used to pull the thumb back when a flat open hand is needed (i.e., for clapping, slapping, or pushing)
Extensor digitorum communis	EDC	Posterior interosseous branch of radial nerve C7–C8	Extends the MP joints	Extends the PIP and DIP joints; assists in abduction of the index, ring, and little fingers; assists in wrist extension	Rarely used as a tendon transfer; powerful extensor
Extensor indicis proprius	EIP	Posterior interosseous branch of radial nerve C7–C8	Extends the index finger and permits isolated extension of the index finger	Extends the wrist; adducts the index finger	Allows extension of the index finger for pointing while all other fingers are in a fist; one of the most used muscles for tendon transfer

18

					Useful muscle for tendon transfer
Extensor digit quinti or minimi	EDQ EDM	Posterior interosseous branch of radial nerve C7–C8	Extends the little finger; permits isolated extension of the little finger	Assists in abduction of the little finger	

Volar

Flexor pollicis longus	FPL	Anterior interosseous branch of the median nerve C8–T1	Flexes IP joints of the thumb	Flexes the MP and CMC joints of the thumb; assists in flexion of the wrist	The only muscle to flex the thumb IP joint
Flexor digitorum superficialis	FDS	Median nerve C7–C8, T1	Flexes just the middle then proximal phalanges and PIP joints of index, long, ring, and little fingers	Flexes the MP joints; assists in wrist flexion	Important in power grip; frequently used in tendon transfers
Flexor digitorum profundus	FDP	Medial portion by the ulnar nerve C8–T1; lateral portion by the anterior interosseous branch of the median nerve C8–T1	Flexes the distal phalanges	Flexes the MP and PIP joints; assists in wrist flexion	The only muscle to flex the distal phalanges, rarely used for tendon transfers

TABLE 1–4 Intrinsic Muscles of the Hand

Muscle	Abbreviation	Innervation	Primary Action	Secondary Action(s)	Clinical Significance
Interossei	IO				
Dorsal interossei	DI	Deep branch ulnar nerve C8–T1	Abducts index, middle, ring fingers	1st dorsal interossei adducts thumb; flexes digits at MP joint, extends IP joint	Important movements in typing, piano playing, writing
Volar interossei (palmar)	VI	Deep branch ulnar nerve C8–T1	Adducts thumb, index, ring, and little fingers	Flexes digits at MP joints, extends IP joints	
Lumbricals	L	1st and 2nd median nerve C8–T1; 3rd and 4th deep branch ulnar nerve C8–T1	Flexes digits at the MP joints, extends IP joints simultaneously; extends IP joints with MP joints in extension	Radial deviates MP joints	Places the fingers in writing or billiard cue position
Thenar Muscles					
Abductor pollicis brevis	APB	Recurrent branch of median nerve C8–T1	Abducts the thumb; flexes thumb at MP and CMC joint	Draws thumb forward at a right angle to palm, rotates it medially	Works with opponens to "post up" the thumb
Oppones pollicis	OP	Recurrent branch of median nerve C8–T1	Flexes thumb MP, bends thumb medially across palm, and rotates thumb medially (opposition)		Opposition the most important function of the thumb

Muscle	Abbreviation	Nerve supply	Action	Secondary action	Function
Flexor pollicis brevis	FPB	Superficial head of recurrent branch of median nerve; deep head of deep branch of ulnar nerve C8–T1	Flexes proximal phalanx thumb; flexes thumb MP CMC joints	Assists in opposition and adduction	Important in the group of muscles which position the thumb
Adductor pollicis	ADD.P	Deep branch of ulnar nerve C8–T1	Approximates (adducts) thumb to the palm		Gives power to grasp

Hypothenar Muscles

Muscle	Abbreviation	Nerve supply	Action	Secondary action	Function
Abductor digiti minimi (quinti)	ADQ ADM	Deep branch of ulnar nerve C8–T1	Abducts little finger; flexes MP joint of little finger	May assist in extension of interphalangeal joints	Enable 5th digit to abduct, increasing span of grasp; produces hypothenar eminence
Flexor digiti minimi (quinti)	FDQ FDM	Deep branch of ulnar nerve C8–T1	Flexes little finger at MP joint	Assists in opposition of the little finger to thumb	Produces hypothenar eminence
Oppones digiti minimi (quinti)	ODQ ODM	Deep branch of ulnar nerve C8–T1	Draws 5th metacarpal anteriorly and rotates laterally for opposition with the thumb	Stabilization of the 5th carpal bone	Produces hypothenar eminence
Palmaris brevis	PB	Superficial branch of ulnar nerve C8–T1	Wrinkles the skin on the ulnar side of the palm		Deepens hollow of palm, aiding in grip; covers and protects ulnar nerve and artery

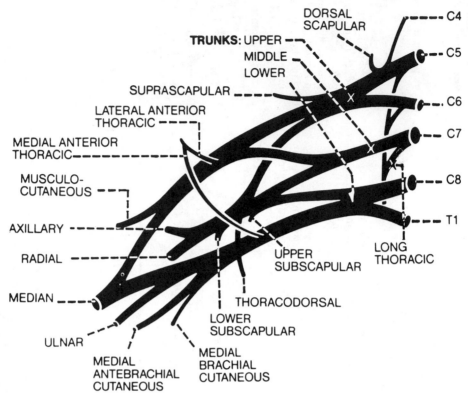

FIGURE 1-10. The brachial plexus. (From Engelberg, A [ed]: The extremities [Supplement, Chap 3]. In Guides to the Evaluation of Permanent Impairment, ed 3 [revised]. American Medical Association, Chicago, 1988, p 34, with permission.)

off the anterior interosseous branch, which is predominantly a motor nerve, innervating the flexor pollicis longus, the radial segment of the flexor digitorum profundus, and the pronator quadratus. The median nerve enters the hand through a passage at the carpal tunnel, where it is accompanied by the flexor tendons (Fig. 1-14). The median nerve is the most superficial structure in the carpal tunnel. For surface anatomy, the median nerve is located in the middle of the volar wrist, medial to the flexor carpi radialis tendon and lateral to the palmaris longus tendon. Proximal or through the transverse carpal ligament, the palmar cutaneous branch of the median nerve supplies cutaneous sensation to the volar wrist, thenar eminence, and radial palm. At the distal border of the transverse carpal ligament, the palmar cutaneous branch divides into the terminal branches of the median nerve. These branches are referred to as the radial or lateral branch and the ulnar or medial branch.

The radial branch further branches to give off the recurrent branch, the proper digital nerve to the radial side of the thumb, and the first common digital nerve. The recurrent branch is the motor branch to the abductor pollicis brevis, opponens pollicis brevis, and the short head of the flexor pollicis brevis. The proper digital nerve supplies the pulp of the thumb, the dorsal subungual area, and MCP and IP joints. The first common digital nerve branches into the proper digital nerve to the ulnar thumb and the proper digital nerve to the radial index. The proper digital nerve to the ulnar thumb supplies the MCP and IP joints as well as the subungual area. The proper digital nerve

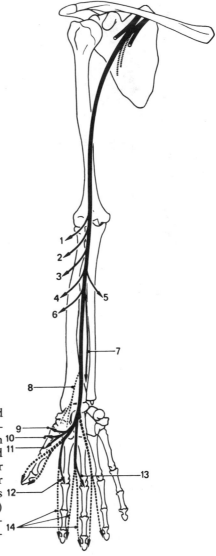

FIGURE 1–11. The median nerve: muscles supplied and cutaneous distribution. (1) Pronator teres; (2) palmaris longus; (3) palmaris brevis; (4) flexor digitorum superficialis; (5) flexor digitorum profundis to the second and third digits; (6) flexor pollicis longus; (7) pronator quadratus; (8) palmar cutaneous branch; (9) abductor pollicis brevis; (10) superficial branch to flexor pollicis brevis; (11) opponens pollicis; (12) first lumbrical; (13) second lumbrical; (14) digital sensory nerves. The sensory branches are represented as dotted lines. (From Tubiana,[2] p 201, with permission.)

to the radial index provides branches to the first lumbrical muscle, the index MCP and IP joints, the skin on the palm, the radial volar aspect of the index finger, and the dorsal radial aspect of the index finger over the middle and distal phalanges.

The ulnar branch gives off branches to two common digital nerves which further branch into two proper digital nerves. The first of the two common digital nerves divides at the second intermetacarpal space, giving off a branch to the second lumbrical muscle; it then branches into the proper digital nerve to the ulnar side of the index and the proper digital nerve to the radial side of the long finger. These proper digital nerves supply the MCP and IP joints, the dorsal subungual regions, the volar aspect of the respective sides of the digit, and the dorsal area over the middle and distal phalanges. The latter of the two common digital nerves branches at the third intermetacarpal space, and, in turn, also branches into the proper digital nerve to the ulnar side of the long

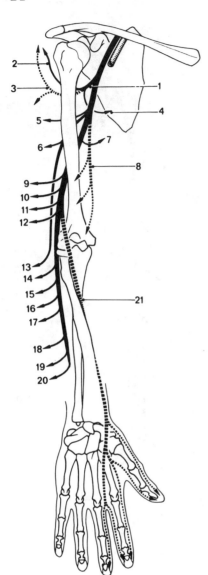

FIGURE 1–12. The radial and axillary nerves: muscles supplied and cutaneous distribution. (The forearm in this illustration is pronated.) (1) Axillary nerve; (2) deltoid; (3) cutaneous branch to the shoulder; (4) teres minor; (5) triceps (long); (6) triceps (lateral); (7) triceps (medial); (8) medial cutaneous branch; (9) brachioradialis; (10) extensor carpi radialis longus; (11) extensor carpi radialis brevis; (12) supinator; (13) anconeus; (14) extensor digitorum communis; (15) extensor digitorum to the fifth finger; (16) extensor carpi ulnaris; (17) abductor pollicis longus; (18) extensor pollicis brevis; (19) extensor pollicis longus; (20) extensor indicis proprius; (21) anterior sensory branch. The sensory branches are represented as dotted lines. (From Tubiana,[2] p 196, with permission.)

finger and the proper digital nerve to the radial ring finger. These proper digital nerves, like those previously mentioned, supply the volar aspects of the respective sides, the dorsal area over the middle and distal phalanges, the dorsal subungual regions, and the MCP and IP joints.

The median nerve can functionally be identified as the precision manipulator of the hand. Common compression neuropathies that involve the median nerve include carpal tunnel syndrome, pronator syndrome, and anterior interosseous syndrome.

Radial Nerve

The radial nerve is the largest branch of the brachial plexus, arising from the posterior cord, with contributions from C5, C6, C7, C8, and T1. The radial nerve enters the radial tunnel at the radial head, having supplied the brachioradialis, the extensor

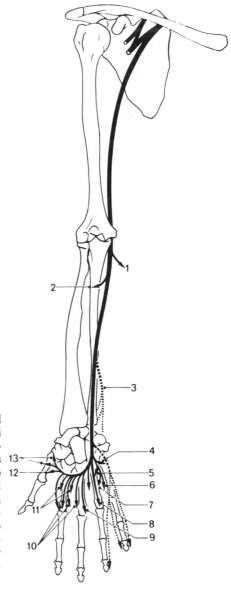

FIGURE 1-13. The ulnar nerve: muscles supplied and cutaneous distribution. (1) Branch to flexor carpi ulnaris; (2) branch to flexor digitorum profundus supplying the fourth and fifth digits; (3) dorsal cutaneous branch; (4) palmar cutaneous branch; (5) branch to abductor digiti minimi; (6) branch to opponens digiti minimi; (7) branch to flexor digiti minimi; (8) fourth lumbrical branch; (9) third lumbrical branch; (10) branch to palmar interosseous muscles; (12) deep branch to flexor pollicis brevis; (13) branch to adductor pollicis. The sensor branches are represented by dotted lines. (From Tubiana,[2] p 203, with permission.)

carpi radialis longus, and the extensor carpi radialis brevis above the elbow. The radial nerve then divides into the deep and superficial branches. The deep branch is muscular and articular. The deep branch supplies the supinator before emerging into the posterior compartment where it becomes the posterior interosseous nerve.

The posterior interosseous nerve passes under the arcade of Frosche and terminates on the dorsum on the wrist. The posterior interosseous nerve supplies the extensor digitorum communis, extensor digiti minim, extensor carpi ulnaris via its short branch, and the abductor pollicis longus, extensor pollicis brevis, and extensor indicis proprius via its long branch. The terminal portion of the interosseous nerve supplies the ligaments and articulations of the radiocarpal, carpal, and carpometacarpal joints.

The superficial branch of the radial nerve is the smaller of the two terminal branches. At the wrist this branch divides into four to five digital branches, which are

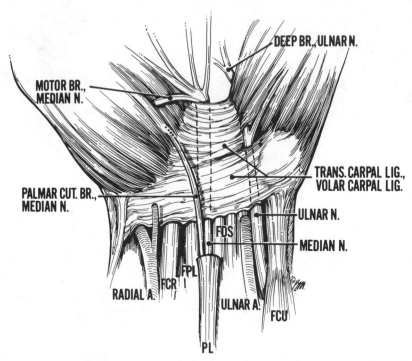

FIGURE 1–14. The median nerve and the long flexor tendons course through the carpal tunnel, lying beneath the transverse carpal ligament. (Illustration by Elizabeth Roselius, © 1988. Reprinted with permission from Green, DP: Operative Hand Surgery, 2nd ed. Churchill Livingstone, New York, 1988.)

cutaneous and articular innervations. The cutaneous innervation includes the lateral two thirds of the dorsum of the hand and the dorsal lateral 2½ fingers to the proximal phalanx.

The radial nerve can be considered preparatory in function, in that it prepares the hand for motion. Common compression neuropathies involving the radial nerve are radial tunnel syndrome, posterior interosseous syndrome, and superficial radial nerve syndrome (Wartenberg's symptom).

Ulnar Nerve

The ulnar nerve is the largest branch of the medial cord from the brachial plexus, with contributions from C8 and T1. The ulnar nerve has multiple branches including muscular, articular, palmar cutaneous, dorsal cutaneous, and the superficial and deep terminal branches.

The nerve enters the forearm below the elbow, coursing between the medial epicondyle and the olecranon. The nerve is subcutaneous and easily palpated at this point. The ulnar nerve passes between the two heads of the flexor carpi ulnaris and then proceeds distally to the hand. Innervation to the flexor carpi ulnaris and medial half of the flexor digitorum profundus is provided by the ulnar nerve in the forearm. Two branches arise distal in the midforearm: (1) the palmar cutaneous branch, which supplies a portion of the skin over the hypothenar eminence and occasionally the palmaris brevis; and (2) the dorsal cutaneous branch. The dorsal cutaneous branch courses along the medial side of the dorsum of the wrist and hand and terminates into digital branches, which supply sensation to the dorsal mid-middle phalanx of the ring and little fingers.

In the palm the ulnar nerve passes through the canal of Guyon at the wrist, where it divides into its superficial and deep terminal branches. The superficial branch, which is primarily sensory with the exception of its innervation of the palmaris brevis, divides into three branches. The first of these three branches is a sensory branch to the ulnar aspect of the little finger; the second, a sensory branch to the central ulnar palmar area. The third (referred to as the common digital nerve) innervates the fourth intermetacarpal space. The common digital nerve further divides into two proper digital nerves supplying the ulnar portion of the ring finger and the radial portion of the little finger.

Unlike the superficial branch, the deep terminal branch of the ulnar nerve is a motor branch supplying innervation to the hypothenar muscles, the volar and dorsal interossei, and the adductor pollicis, before terminating in the deep head of the flexor pollicis brevis. In addition to muscular innervations, the deep branch has articular branches to the intercarpal, carpometacarpal, and intermetacarpal joints.

The ulnar nerve has been referred to as the nerve of fine movements because it innervates muscles responsible for fine movements in the hand. The motor component of the ulnar nerve is important for power and grasp. Common compression neuropathies that involve the ulnar nerve include compression at the cubital tunnel at the elbow and Guyon's canal at the wrist.

Figure 1–15 reviews the segmental and peripheral distribution of the volar and dorsal surfaces of the hand.

VASCULAR SYSTEM

Arterial System

The main arterial supply to the hand is from the radial and ulnar arteries, both terminal branches of the brachial artery. These arteries anastomose into a complex arterial arch system consisting primarily of the superficial and deep palmar arches (Fig. 1–16).

The radial artery, the smaller of the two terminal branches of the brachial artery, can be palpated proximal to the radial styloid, anteriomedial to the tendons of the abductor pollicis longus (APL) and extensor pollicis brevis (EPB) muscles; its deep branch can be felt in the floor of the anatomic snuff box. The radial artery gives off a superficial palmar branch, which anastomoses with the ulnar artery to form the superficial palmar arch and also with the deep branch of the ulnar artery at the base of the fifth metacarpal to complete the deep palmar arch.

The ulnar artery is the primary arterial contribution to the hand. This artery is larger than the radial artery and enters the hand behind the expansion of the tendon of the flexor carpi ulnaris (FCU) muscle, lateral to the ulnar nerve and pisiform bone yet superficial to the flexor retinaculum. The ulnar artery can be palpated lateral to the pisiform bone. The ulnar artery continues across the palm to join the superficial branch of the radial artery and thus complete the superficial palmar arch. The deep palmar branch of the ulnar artery anastomoses with the radial artery to form the deep palmar arch.

Segmental Distribution

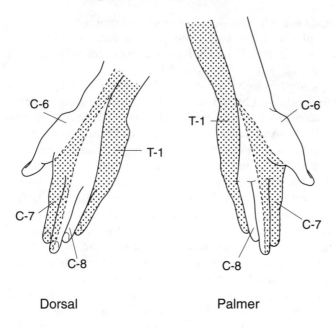

Dorsal

Palmer

A

Peripheral Distribution

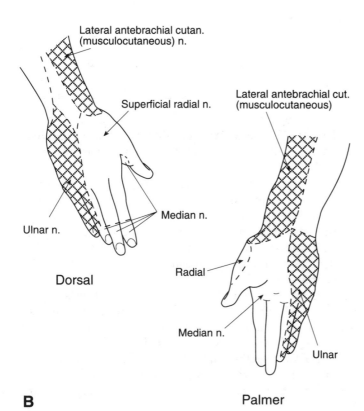

Dorsal

Palmer

B

FIGURE 1–15. *A*, Segmental distribution of the dorsal and palmar surfaces of the hand. *B*, Peripheral distribution of the dorsal and palmar surfaces of the hand.

28

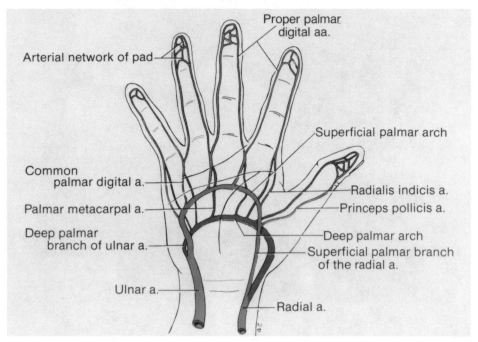

FIGURE 1–16. The palmar and arterial arches of the hand and their branches. The superficial palmar arterial arch is the larger of the two palmar arches. The deep palmar arch is proximal to the superficial palmar arch and at a deeper plane. (From Moore,[12] p 752, with permission.)

ARCHES

The arterial arch system in the hand provides a generous collateral blood supply. This system is composed of the superficial and deep palmar arches, which are separated by the extrinsic flexor tendons. The superficial palmar arch is larger and relatively more important than the deep palmar arch.

The superficial palmar arch is formed primarily from the ulnar artery and is located distal to the deep palmar arch. This arch is convex toward the fingers at the approximate level of the proximal transverse crease. The superficial palmar arch branches into three common digital arteries, which in turn anastomose with the palmar metacarpal arteries from the deep palmar arch. These common digital arteries further branch into proper palmar digital arteries or phalangeal branches, which course the sides to the index, middle, ring, and little fingers.

The deep palmar arch formed mainly by the radial artery is proximal and deeper than the superficial palmar arch. This arch gives off three palmar metacarpal arteries, which join the common digital arteries from the superficial palmar arch.

Venous System

The venous system in the hand consists of superficial and deep veins, which, as in the arterial system, form a system of arches. The superficial veins are located under the skin in the superficial fascia, whereas the deep veins accompany the arteries. The superficial veins become distended and more apparent when the hand is held down at

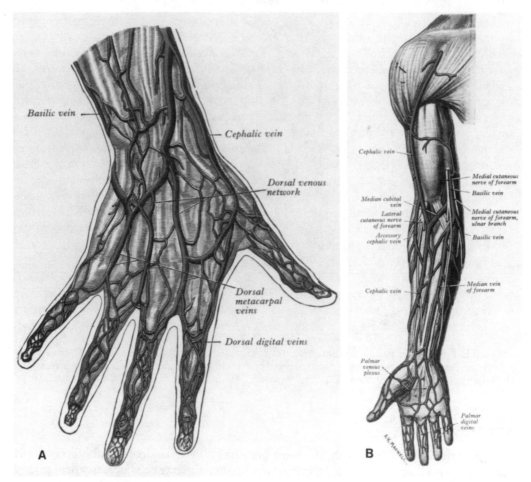

FIGURE 1–17. *A*, The venous system of the dorsal hand. *B*, The venous system of the palmar hand. (From Williams, P and Warwick, R: Gray's Anatomy, ed 36 [British]. Churchill Livingstone, Edinburgh, 1980, p 752, with permission.)

the side. These superficial veins are larger and more important than the deep veins and are accompanied by the finger and hand lymphatics. Figure 1–17 illustrates the dorsal and palmar venous systems.

PATTERNS OF USE

All patterns of use in the normal hand are based on the mobility of the integrated arch system. Stability of the arch system, however, is necessary for effective force transmission of power across the skeletal link system. Van der Meurlen has suggested that the longitudinal arch is a set of two biarticular-bimuscular systems.[6] The proximal system includes the metacarpal, proximal phalanx, and middle phalanx, whereas the distal system includes the three phalanges. The proximal interphalangeal (PIP) joint is the link joint. If a single system of three bones and two joints is controlled by two muscles, one joint in the terminal position must seek static stability, causing collapse. A third muscle force can establish dynamic equilibrium in this system, thereby balancing the unequal force in the extrinsic flexor-extensor system. The intrinsics constitute the third force. This balance of power is delicate and totally dependent on the skeletal-ligamentous stability of the joints and the skeletal beams between each joint. Rupture of extrinsic flexor or extensor tendons will produce a gross, obvious disturbance of function. Less initially obvious but none the less important are disturbances of the intrinsics by nerve injury, rheumatic or ischemic disease or injury to the static support structures such as a volar plate rupture or capsular ligament attenuation. Synovitis can alter the direction of pull and angle of attachment of tendons crossing the joint and thereby alter their function. Swan neck and boutonnière deformities are digital flexion plain zigzag collapse deformities (which have lateral components also, owing to the equiangular spiral course of the flexing digit). These deformities are predictable, as the third force balance is lost and the digits return to a bimuscular-biarticular system with strong extrinsics pulling across an unstable arch. Fractures may evoke this imbalance by diminishing stability in a more obvious way. As collapse begins, the grasp weakens, and the unwitting patient responds by exerting increased force through the extrinsic flexors. This valiant effort is what is so destructive to the weakening arch system of the hand. The extrinsic flexors and extensors do not take direct routes to their insertion. Where the line of pull is altered, pulley systems are required and are subjected to large forces in hand function. An example is the dislocating force normally exerted on the MCP joint, keystone of the longitudinal arch in patients with rheumatoid arthritis. A 1-g digital force requires 6 g longitudinal pull with a 3-g vectored force palmarly at the MCP joint.

THE HAND IN USE

Proper grasp is impossible without adequate sensory input. One fourth of all pacinian corpuscles in the body are present in the pulp and skin of digits. Brand[7] has suggested that power of grasp is governed by sensation of pressure on palmar skin and not by muscle spindles in the forearm muscles and tendons. The derangement and misjudged power application in nerve injury patients with compressive neuropathies will obviously have a disturbing effect on arch balance in the "blind" hand.

The hand is used in two functional ways. The less common and completely unspecialized form of usage is as a fixed object on a mobile base with the hand simply being a passive transmitter of force. Examples would include a clenched fist, a flattened palm, a weight, or a hook. This form comprises approximately 20 percent of usage patterns. The more common skilled use is as a mobile organ on a mobile limb (80 percent). The three functional applications of the hand in this way are (1) slow to rapid movement with controlled rate, intensity, and direction (e.g., playing the guitar, writing, or sewing); (2) ballistic, or rapid repetitive, movement (e.g., typing or piano playing); and (3), the most specialized use, fixation of the digits including co-contractions yielding prehension.

In prehensile use, the hand is considered to have two parts, the thumb and the rest of the digits. Most activity combines thumb and finger prehension. Three patterns of prehension occur most frequently are (1) *tip grip*, (2) *lateral grip*, and (3) *palmar grip* (Fig. 1–18). For the first and last of these types, thumb opposition is critical. The most common prehensile movements are the picking up of an object and its handling in use. In these movements, palmar grip is used predominantly (from 50 to 80 percent of the time). This overriding importance of palmar prehension must be appreciated with splinting of the injured hand and in reconstructive surgery. The functional patterns of prehension at work can be described qualitatively as power and precision activities.

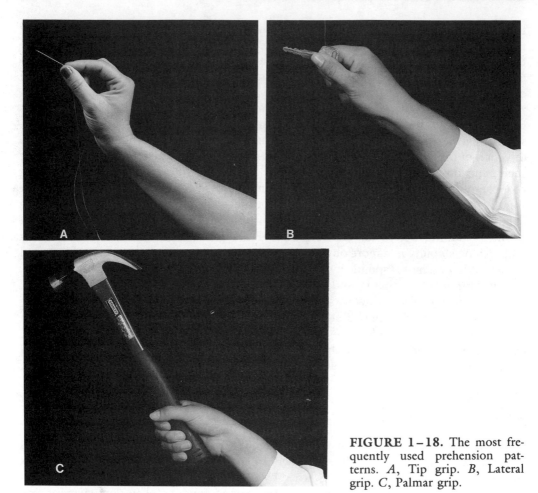

FIGURE 1–18. The most frequently used prehension patterns. *A,* Tip grip. *B,* Lateral grip. *C,* Palmar grip.

In precision activities, the fingers are both flexed and held abducted away from the palm. The object is held lightly at the digital tips and manipulated by the fingers. This posturing is most aptly called *precision handling.* The basic position of the MCP joint is flexion and abduction, with a significant degree of opposition between the digits. Movements are flexion, rotation, and ulnar deviation and the number of digits involved depends on the size of the object. Small objects require only the use of the radial digits (the smallest only the index and thumb), whereas larger objects require all of the digits. The second qualitative description of prehension at work is *power grip.* Here the fingers flex, rotate, and ulnar deviate to point to the thenar eminence, compressing the object against the thumb buttress as this ray is stabilized in abduction.

Occasionally the two functions overlap, as in tying a knot or in using a light hammer. In both grip movements, the radial hand provides precision, the ulnar hand power and stability.

Along with speech, the hand in use is a mode of human expression that deserves admiration from all of us. For those who would treat its infirmities, its dynamics should be the subject of continued investigation.

SUMMARY

The hand is a delicate organ with an intricate anatomy. A knowledge of this anatomy is necessary to understand hand function and therefore to provide a basis for clinical decision making. This chapter has summarized the cutaneous coverings, connective tissue, skeletal system, musculature, innervation, and arterial system in the hand and has provided the reader with clinical application.

REFERENCES

1. Riordan, D: Functional anatomy of the hand and forearm. Ortho Clin North Am 5:199, 1971.
2. Bishop, T: Fascia: A literature review. Physical Therapy Forum 4:1, 1985.
3. Ariyan, S: The Hand Book. McGraw-Hill, New York, 1989.
4. Littler, JW: The hand and upper extremity. In Converse, JM (ed): Reconstructive Plastic Surgery, ed 2, Vol 6. WB Saunders, Philadelphia, 1977.
5. Littler, JW: On the adaptability of man's hand. Hand 5:187, 1973.
6. Flatt, AE: The Care of the Rheumatoid Hand, ed 3. CV Mosby, St. Louis, 1974.
7. Brand, P: Clinical Mechanics of the Hand. CV Mosby, St. Louis, 1985.

BIBLIOGRAPHY

American Society for Surgery of the Hand: The Hand, Examination and Diagnosis, ed 2. Churchill Livingstone, New York, 1983.

Ariyan, S: The Hand Book. McGraw-Hill, New York, 1989.

Backhouse, KM: Innervation and vascularization. In Tubiana, R: The Hand, Vol 1. WB Saunders, Philadelphia, 1981.

Barron, JN: The structures and function of the skin of the hand. Hand 2:93, 1970.

Basmajian, JV: Muscles Alive: Their Function Revealed by Electromyography. Williams & Wilkins, Baltimore, 1962.

Bendz, P: The functional significance of the oblique retinacular ligament of Landsmeer: A review and new proposals. J Hand Surg 10B:25, 1985.

Bishop, T: Fascia: A literature review. Physical Therapy Forum 4:1, 1985.

Bowers, W: The Interphalangeal Joints, Vol 1, The Hand and Upper Limb. Churchill Livingstone, New York, 1987.

Boyes, JH: Bunnell's Surgery of the Hand, ed 5. JB Lippincott, Philadelphia, 1970.

Brand, P: Clinical Mechanics of the Hand. CV Mosby, St. Louis, 1985.

Chukuka, E: Anatomy and Applied Anatomy of the Forearm and the Hand. 10th Annual Conference, American Society of Hand Therapists, San Antonio, Texas, 1987.

Cleland, J: On the cutaneous ligaments of the phalanges. J Anat Physiol 12:526, 1878.

Donatelli, R: Effects of immobilization on the extensibility of periarticular connective tissue. Journal of Orthopaedic and Sports Physical Therapy 3:67, 1981.

Doyle, J: Anatomy of the finger flexor tendon sheath and pulley system. J Hand Surg 13A:473, 1988.

Dubousset, JF: The digital joints. In Tubiana, R: The Hand, Vol 1. WB Saunders, Philadelphia, 1981.

Eaton, R and Littler, W: Joint Injuries of the Hand. Charles C Thomas, Springfield, Il, 1971.

Flatt, AE: The Care of the Rheumatoid Hand, ed 3. CV Mosby, St. Louis, 1974.

Gray, H: Anatomy of the Human Body, ed 30 (American). Carmine Clemente (ed). Lea & Febiger, Philadelphia, 1985.

Grayson, J: The cutaneous ligaments of the digits. J Anat 75:164, 1941.

Green, D: Operative Hand Surgery. Churchill Livingstone, New York, 1982.

Green, D: Operative Hand Surgery. Churchill Livingstone, New York, 1988.

Hamilton, WJ: Textbook of Human Anatomy. CV Mosby, St. Louis, 1976.

Harty, M: The hand of man. Phys Ther 51:777, 1971.

Ioanis, P and Kuczynski, K: The distal interphalangeal joints of the human fingers. J Hand Surg 7:176, 1982.

Jones, FW: The Principles of Anatomy as Seen in the Hand. Bailliere, Tindall & Cox, London, 1941.

Kapandji, IA: The Physiology of the Joints, Vol 1, The Upper Limb. Churchill Livingstone, New York, 1982.

Keil-Hunt, J: Basic Hand Splinting: A Pattern-Designing Approach. Little, Brown & Co, Boston, 1983, pp 1–23.

Kendall, H, Kendall, F, and Wadsworth, G: Muscles, Testing and Function. Williams & Wilkins, Baltimore, 1971.

Kuczynski, E: Less-known aspects of the proximal interphalangeal joints of the human hand. Hand 7:31, 1975.

Landsmeer, JMF: The anatomy of the dorsal aponeurosis of the human finger and its functional significance. Anat Rec 103:31, 1949.

Littler, JW: The physiology and dynamic function of the hand. Surg Clin North Am 40:259, 1960.

Littler, JW: The finger extensor mechanism. Surg Clin North Am 47:415, 1967.

Long, C: Intrinsic-extrinsic muscle control of the fingers. J Bone Joint Surg 50A:973, 1968.

Long, C: Intrinsic-extrinsic muscle control of the hand in power grip and precision handling. J Bone Joint Surg 52A:853, 1970.

Mackinnon, S and Dellon, L: Surgery of the Peripheral Nerve. Thieme Medical Publishers, New York, 1988.

Milford, L: The retaining ligaments of the digits and hand. In Tubiana, R: The Hand, Vol 1. WB Saunders, Philadelphia, 1981.

Minami, A, et al: Ligament stability of the metacarpophalangeal joint, a biomechanical study. J Hand Surg 10A:255, 1985.

Moore, K: Clinically Oriented Anatomy, ed 2. Williams & Wilkins, Baltimore, 1985.

Napier, JR: The form and function of the carpometacarpal joint of the thumb. J Anat 89:362, 1955.

Napier, JR: The prehensile movements of the human hand. J Bone Joint Surg 38:902, 1956.

Regional Review Course in Hand Surgery. American Society for Surgery of the Hand, Philadelphia, 1988.

Riordan, D: Functional anatomy of the hand and forearm. Ortho Clin North Am 5:199, 1971.

Schneider, L: Flexor Tendon Injuries. Little, Brown & Co, Boston, 1985.

Shrewsbury, M and Johnson, R: Form, function and evolution of the distal phalanx. J Hand Surg 8:475, 1983.

Smith, R: Balance and kinetics of the fingers under normal and pathologic conditions. Clin Orthop 104:92, 1974.

Spinner, M: Kaplan's Functional and Surgical Anatomy of the Hand, ed 3. JB Lippincott, Philadelphia, 1984.

Staubesand, J (ed): Sobatta Atlas of Human Anatomy, ed 11 (English). Vol 1, Head, Neck, Upper Limb, Skin. Urban & Schwarzenberg, Baltimore, 1990.

Sunderland, S: Nerves and Nerve Injuries. Churchill Livingstone, Edinburgh, 1978.

Tortora, G and Anagnostakos, N: Principles of Anatomy and Physiology, ed 6. Harper & Row, New York, 1990.

Tubiana, R: The Hand, Vol 3. WB Saunders, Philadelphia, 1988.

Tubiana, R: Anatomic and physiologic basis for surgical treatment of paralyses of the hand. J Bone Joint Surg 31A:643, 1969.

Tubiana, R, Thomine, JM, and Mackin, E: Examination of the Hand and Upper Limb. WB Saunders, Philadelphia, 1984.

Tubiana, R: The Hand, Vol 1, WB Saunders, Philadelphia, 1981.

Valentin, P: Extrinsic muscles of the hand and wrist, an introduction. In Tubiana, R: The Hand, Vol 1, WB Saunders, Philadelphia, 1981.

Van DeGraaff, KM: Human Anatomy. Wm C Brown, Dubuque, 1984.

Wadsworth, C: Clinical anatomy and mechanics of the wrist and hand. Journal of Orthopaedic and Sports Physical Therapy 4:206, 1983.

Walton, H (ed): Surgical Anatomy of the Hand. Ciba Pharmaceutical, Medical Education Div, Summit, NJ, 1969.

Williams, P and Warwick, R: Gray's Anatomy, ed 36. WB Saunders, Philadelphia, 1980.

CHAPTER 2

Wound Healing

Kevin L. Smith, MD

The process of wound healing is an important function of the human organism, essential for the maintenance of life. Despite centuries of observation and experimentation, we are still limited in our ability to exert a positive influence on the wound healing process. Lost along the ladder of human evolution is the ability to regenerate all structures; therefore, wounds in higher animals must heal by fibrous tissue proliferation (scar formation) that can only *approximate* the normal anatomy. The capacity for wounds to heal is remarkable. Regardless of the severity of injury, most wounds will heal with minimal therapeutic intervention, given enough time and adequate nutrition. In structures as delicately balanced as the hand, however, uncontrolled healing can be devastating (Fig. 2–1).

The hand serves as an interface with the environment. Through it, one receives sensory input and manipulates the environment. These functions are accomplished by the ability to position the hand in space and to change its configuration. Movement of the hand is achieved by alterations in the balance between opposing muscle forces transmitted by gliding tendons to movable bones which glide on articular surfaces. The unique anatomy of the hand allows it to be both stable and movable, and it is the goal of the surgeon and hand therapist to restore these characteristics to the injured hand and help prevent uncontrolled healing that would interfere with function.

Wound healing has paradoxical features. Since scar tissue is not as strong as the normal structures it replaces; scar strength is directly proportional to scar volume. Generally, when there is a heavy scar—especially one that traverses gliding planes— scar volume is inversely proportional to motion.

The patient with a post-traumatic or postoperative hand wound faces unique problems of healing. For most wounds, an optimum environment for healing requires immobilization, but total immobility can counteract the successful maintenance of gliding surfaces.

The objectives of this chapter are to, (1) present a historic perspective of wound healing; (2) discuss the three phases of wound healing: inflammatory, fibroplastic, and scar maturation; (3) present the biologic processes involved in the healing of specialized tissues: skin, tendon, bone, and nerve; and (4) discuss the therapist's role in influencing the healing process.

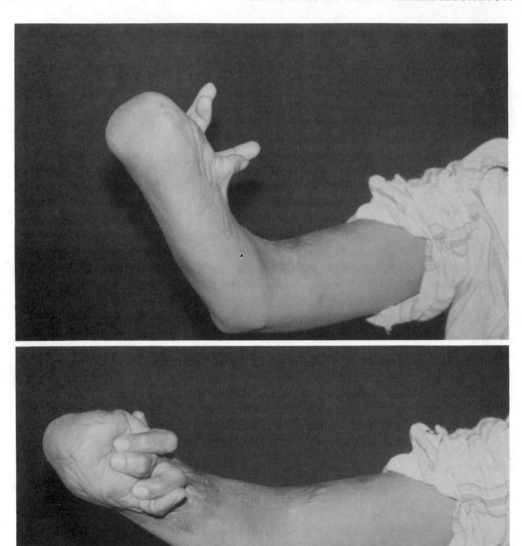

FIGURE 2–1. *Top* and *bottom*. The hand of a young woman burned as a child. Though healed, this is an example of uncontrolled healing which has led to irreversible contracture and a functionless hand.

HISTORICAL PERSPECTIVE

The facilitation of wound healing has been of foremost interest to human beings since the beginning of time. Wound care has figured prominently in daily life, religion, and ritual, and people have treated wounds with potions and poisons or bound and manipulated wounds to influence the natural process of wound healing. In the Edwin Smith papyrus (1700 BC), one of the earliest examples of medical literature, 7 of the 48 presented cases dealt with wound management.[1] The ancient civilizations developed gentle wound handling techniques, applied poultices and dressings, and demonstrated primary healing of clean wounds approximated by rudimentary suture techniques.[2]

Following the ancient Egyptian, Greek, Indian, and Chinese civilizations most of the lessons learned were forgotten and the "dark ages" of wound care were entered. Attempting to accelerate wound healing, surgeons manipulated wounds using such things as boiling oil, hot cautery, and caustic salves. On the battlefield in 1545, Ambrose Paré rediscovered gentle tissue handling techniques almost by serendipity. When his supply of hot oil was depleted, Paré was forced to use simple soap and water and gentle dressing methods for his wounded soldiers. To his credit, he recognized that these wounds went on to heal much more quickly than the cauterized wounds and without the presence of "laudable pus."[1] Through his observations, Paré made the first step toward the recognition that the surgeon could control wound healing by minimizing impediments to normal healing.

In the mid-18th century, John Hunter (1728–1793) appreciated the beneficial effects of inflammation on wound healing. He recognized the differences between wound contraction and contracture and appreciated the multiple causes of delay of normal wound healing.[3] Lord Lister (1827–1912) began the era of antiseptic surgery when he linked contamination and infection with delay of wound healing. These tenets were built upon by William Stewart Halsted (1852–1922), who demonstrated that minimizing tissue injury by careful tissue handling techniques, hemostasis, and aseptic surgery further decreased wound complications and hastened wound healing.

In 1960, Marcy[4] published a summation of the attitude regarding wound healing at the time. He stated that wound healing, being as physiologically perfect as possible, could not be accelerated in a healthy animal. Marcy felt that impediments to wound healing could be avoided by:

1. Debridement and accurate approximation of the wound margins.
2. Application of Lister's principles of antisepsis.
3. The Halstedian tenets of gentle tissue handling and meticulous technique.[5]

Today, wound healing is recognized as a series of biochemical events. The future holds the ability to affect changes in wound healing and even accelerate the process of healing by manipulation of both intracellular and extracellular biochemical events. As more endogenous growth factors are described, we come closer to finding the "switches" that will turn the wound healing process on and off and we may find the key to controlling the character of the scar within the healed wound.

THE BIOLOGIC PROCESS OF WOUND HEALING

Wound healing is a coordinated dynamic event involving cell multiplication and active migration. Cells are stimulated to increase intracellular synthetic activity and produce substrate for extracellular biochemical events. The entire sequence of events of wound healing is geared to produce new collagenous tissue to replace that which was destroyed. Through the understanding of the process of collagen synthesis and degradation, as well as the process of collagen organization into different higher-order structures such as tendons, ligaments, joint capsules, and bone, we will be able to affect alterations in collagen structure (i.e., wound healing) by both physical and chemical means.

Whether a wound is incised or excised and regardless of the amount of tissue lost, wound healing proceeds in three recognizable phases: inflammation, fibroplasia, and scar maturation. These are not necessarily sequential phases but meld into a single physiologic process with parts of each occurring simultaneously.

Phase 1: Inflammation

The inflammatory phase is the vascular and cellular response to wounding that clears the wound of devitalized tissue, debris, and foreign materials. This cleansing effect is mediated by the following: (1) dilution through vascular dilation and subsequent edema, (2) chemical neutralization with the release of proteolytic and collagenolytic enzymes, (3) the precipitation of toxins, and (4) a cellular response leading to the phagocytosis of debris and invading bacteria by polymorphonuclear leukocytes and macrophages.[1,3,6,7]

As healing during the inflammatory phase progresses, enzymatic breakdown of cellular debris causes increased osmolarity of the local tissue fluid, which attracts more water by osmosis, resulting in further swelling. Within the increased interstitial space, there is a high concentration of fibronectin-glycoprotein produced as components of the initial fibrin clot. This protein complex promotes cell to cell and cell to collagen matrix adherence and also acts as a chemoattractant for the cells of reconstruction: neutrophils, monocytes, fibroblasts, and epithelial cells. The inflammatory cells also release many growth factors and other proteins that are known to stimulate fibroblast proliferation and collagen production.[8] By this mechanism, the inflammation phase provides the wound with cells essential for debridement, the elimination of bacteria and the mediation of repair.

Within a clean wound (i.e., little debris) there is minimal work to be done; therefore, the inflammatory phase is usually over in 5 days. Conversely, a dirty wound in which there is considerable debris requires a longer inflammatory phase to clean up this debris, resulting in a delay in the fibroplasia phase of wound healing. A prolonged inflammatory phase can also result from severe tissue trauma at the time of injury, rough tissue handling during surgery, and overly aggressive therapy. Steroid administration and chronic debilitation are other factors that decrease both the quality and quantity of the cellular participation during the inflammatory phase and thereby prolong wound healing.[9]

Phase 2: Fibroplasia

The fibroplastic phase of wound healing lasts from 2 to 6 weeks depending on the extent of the wound. This phase, beginning 3 to 5 days after wounding, consists of fibroplastic proliferation, which is accompanied by the endothelial budding of new capillary growth. On a framework of fibrin and fibronectin, the fibroblasts begin to produce glycosaminoglycans, (the ground substance "gel") and collagen. Together, the collagen matrix and vascular endothelial cells form granulation tissue.

Collagen has a very complex structure consisting of three polypeptide chains wound together in a left-handed helix. This helix then joins with two others to form a three-chain right-handed coil, making the basic collagen unit. Covalent intermolecular bonds join the basic building blocks, forming filaments which then join to become fibrils. Multiple fibrils join to become fibers, the structural elements of soft tissue (Fig. 2–2).

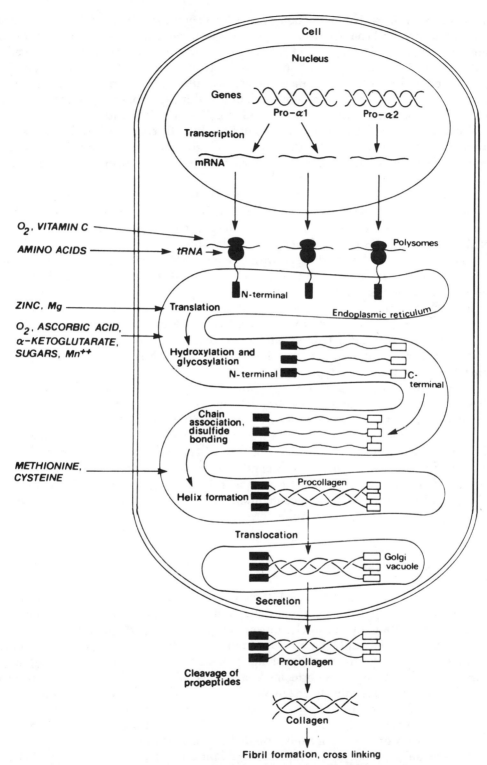

FIGURE 2–2. Collagen synthesis. (Adapted from Kloth, LC, McCulloch, JM, and Feedar, JA: Wound Healing: Alternatives in Management. FA Davis, Philadelphia, 1990, p 35, with permission.)

There are at least five identifiable types of collagen that differ by their amino acid makeup and physical characteristics. *Type I*, or *adult, collagen* makes up the majority of bone, tendon, skin, ligaments, and fascia. *Type II collagen* is predominant in hyaline cartilage. *Type III collagen* is found in skin and arteries, and *type IV collagen* is found in high concentration in basement membranes. In acute wounds, the principal collagen found is type IV. High concentrations are found within skin appendages and at sites of proliferation epithelium. Later, type IV and V collagens are found within the wound blood clot and by 24 hours following wounding, type III collagen is detectable at the wound margin. By 48 hours type III collagen is in high concentration and type I collagen begins to form. At 60 hours after the appearance of any collagen, type I collagen is predominant.[3]

Collagen types I through IV are present in both normal and wounded skin. The ratio between types I and III collagen in normal skin is 4 to 1; however, in hypertrophied and immature scars the ratio of type I to III collagen may be as low as 2 to 1.[10] Perhaps learning to control this ratio will allow us to alter the character of the scar.

Replacement of all injured tissue with immature collagen that is devoid of "architectural memory" interferes with the regeneration of adjacent structures and the reestablishment of gliding surfaces. Currently, there is no mechanism that will prevent a wound from healing in an amalgamated fashion, "melting" together tissue planes and creating "one wound – one scar." In other words, wounds involving the skin, subcutaneous tissue, tendon sheath, tendon, and bone heal normally as a continuous mass without differentiating into the preinjury architecture, thus destroying the gliding planes between each tissue type.[6]

During the fibroplasia phase of wound healing, immobilization helps prevent collagen fiber disruption and consequent delay in the increase in tensile strength of the wound.[6,11] There is an increase in tensile strength during this phase that parallels the increase in collagen content for about 3 weeks. Then the collagen accumulation reaches a plateau in which collagen synthesis becomes balanced by collagen degradation.[12] When this plateau is reached, tensile strength is approximately 15 percent of normal and continues to increase linearly for at least 3 months. During this period intramolecular and intermolecular bonding and reconfiguration alter tensile strength without quantitative changes in the collagen amount.

Phase 3: Scar Maturation

The last phase of wound healing is the *maturation* or *remodeling phase*, which begins as the fibroblastic activity decreases and may last for years. At this time the amount of collagen decreases and the wound becomes stronger.[12] In the early maturation phase the immature scar is bulky and is composed of random configurations of collagen bundles. As remodeling proceeds, fibers orient along the lines of tension and become increasingly compact. The collagen fibers form more intermolecular cross-linkages, the collagen becomes both less susceptible to enzymatic breakdown by collagenases and structurally stronger. The fibers do not physically move to orient themselves along the lines of tension, but the structural change is accomplished by the degradation of random fibrils and the synthesis of more uniformly oriented collagen bundles.[3]

As remodeling proceeds, its rate is dependent on many factors. Because this is a cellular and biochemical process, an optimum environment is required. This environment includes a good blood supply with sufficient oxygen tension, minimal edema and no ongoing inflammatory process (such as produced by infection or too aggressive therapy). Age is another factor. Younger patients have a greater rate of collagen turnover; therefore, there is more rapid wound maturation. In patients who are nutritionally depleted, wound healing and scar maturation will be slowed, owing to lack of the necessary substrates and vitamins for biochemical reactions.

Tensile strength progressively increases with approximately 50 percent of normal tensile strength of skin regained by 6 weeks,[11,13] as suggested in Figure 2-3. Early, the new scar is red, raised, thick, rigid, and pruritic. As scar maturation proceeds, the scar will soften, becoming more pliable and thin.

During the maturation phase, the newly formed scar shrinks in all dimensions, squeezing water out of the extracellular spaces within the scar and making the collagen more dense. As the collagen fibers increase cross-linkage, the resultant scar becomes more insoluble and less susceptible to collagenolysis.[3] Any scar becomes more compact in the process of maturation. Any scarred structure therefore has a tendency to shorten

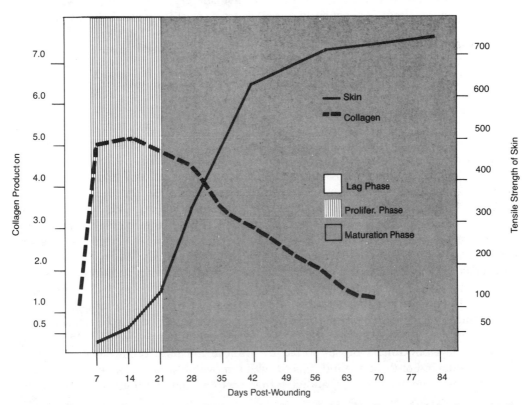

FIGURE 2-3. Relationship of collagen production and skin tensile strength in the rat in the context of the classic phases of wound healing. Note that in the classic phases of wound healing there are varying degrees of collagen deposition and with this a direct effect on the strength of the healing skin. During the lag phase, when the wound is held together by the strength of the fibrin in the blood clot, essentially no collagen is being produced and the skin has very little strength. With the beginning of the proliferative phase, or the phase of fibroplasia, increased numbers of fibroblasts synthesize collagen. Thus, collagen production now achieves its greatest rise and with this skin strength begins to increase. The period of maturation relates to the cross-linking of the collagen that has already been produced; collagen synthesis therefore decreases while the wound continues to gain in strength. (From Dellon,[13] p 553, with permission.)

during the maturation phase unless subjected to therapeutic stretching. Circumferential scars, such as those around nerve repair vessels or tendon sheaths, have a tendency to constrict and impede conduction, flow, or motion.

SKIN WOUND HEALING

The healing of a surgically closed skin wound is perhaps the best understood healing mechanism. In elective surgery of the hand, the surgeon exercises the greatest control over the wound healing process by the choice of incision placement and by the technical expertise with which he or she reapproximates the wound. Care demonstrated in these two aspects greatly reduces the need for concern on the part of the therapist, as these wounds generally heal without difficulty. More importantly, well-planned and repaired wounds heal without disruption when moved, and the resultant scar does not restrict range of motion when healed.

Hand wounds are not all the result of elective surgery, nor are they always clean and able to be repaired. Consequently, three strategies exist for wound closure that take into account the nature of the wound, the amount of tissue loss, the degree of contamination, and the exposure of underlying structures: (1) primary closure, (2) delayed primary closure, and (3) secondary intention healing.

Primary Closure

A surgically clean wound, free of bacterial contamination and having minimal debris, is amenable to direct suture approximation. When done within the first 2 to 3 days following wounding, this approach is termed *primary closure* and re-epithelialization seals the wound by 48 hours.[1] The basal layer of epithelial cells is responsible for the basic steps of epithelialization in the surgically closed wound. This basal cell layer responds to local injury by *mobilization*, causing the cells to flatten, enlarge, and break their intercellular links. Next, the cells undergo *migration* and move across the collagen-fibronectin scaffolding that is formed between the wound edges. When they meet the basal cells migrating from the opposite side of the wound, their motion is abruptly stopped through contact inhibition. The cell population throughout this process is increased by mitosis, and once the wound gap is crossed, normal cellular *differentiation* begins and the progression of cell maturation reproduces the skin architecture.[1,14]

During the time that the wound is healing and while the wound develops tensile strength, the wound must be supported by artificial means. Commonly this support involves sutures. For those wounds closed with removable sutures, leave the sutures in place for approximately 14 days, allowing therapy to proceed without worry of wound rupture.

Delayed Primary Closure

Occasionally, the therapist will be faced with a wound that the surgeon has deemed too grossly contaminated to close primarily. With sterile dressings intact, the therapist can proceed with initial hand therapy. After 2 to 3 days have elapsed, during which time dressings and the inflammatory processes of wound healing have cleansed the wound and lessened the chance of infection, delayed primary closure can be performed. This wound is then treated by the therapist, just as a wound that has been closed primarily.

Secondary Intention Healing

A third type of healing wound is one that has been allowed to close by secondary intention. These wounds have associated soft tissue or skin loss, and contraction plays the primary role and epithelialization the secondary role in the healing of these wounds. In a wound in the palm of the hand, for example, where the dermis is relatively immobile, the wound will fill with a bed of granulation tissue, then epithelialization will occur on top of this granulating wound to effect skin closure. If dermal apposition cannot be achieved by contraction, the remaining wound, covered only by a layer of epithelial cells, is marginal in both strength and stability and requires careful protection.

CONTRACTION

In a full-thickness skin wound that is not primarily closed (by suture approximation, skin graft, or flap) healing occurs by the process just described of contraction and epithelialization. The size of the wound progressively decreases by the centripetal migration of the skin edges until they achieve apposition. If the skin edges cannot be drawn together by contraction, the remaining gap is filled with granulation tissue — collagen matrix, fibroblasts, and capillary buds. The epithelium then migrates across this fertile field to achieve closure.

The contraction of secondary intention healing is usually not a problem for most areas of the body in which there is sufficient surrounding loose skin, but in the hand (or around any joint) the result of contraction can be limited motion or fixed flexion deformity. This situation is termed *contracture*.

Contraction is an active cellular process that may be caused by cells resembling smooth muscle, the myofibroblasts.[15] Smooth muscle antagonist drugs have yet to become clinically helpful.[16] The only reliable and effective method to prevent wound contraction is by the replacement of the missing tissue by the application of a flap or skin graft.[17] Timely coverage combined with mechanical splinting has proven to be the most effective method for the prevention of wound contracture.[18] With an effective mechanical splinting and therapy program,[19] it may be feasible to allow wound contraction to expand tissue, stretching the surrounding skin and ultimately overcome a minimal tissue deficit without problematic contraction. For example, Figure 2–4 illustrates an open treatment of Dupuytren's contracture.

Open Wounds with Tissue Loss

Very few wounds of the hand should be allowed to go on to complete healing by secondary intention. Large open wounds are best treated by skin grafting or flap closure. When a flap procedure is performed on a hand, the wound can usually be considered to have been closed primarily and hand therapy can proceed under the surgeon's guidance. For skin-grafted wounds, however, a short period of time must be allowed before the therapist can begin therapy, lest the skin graft be lost.

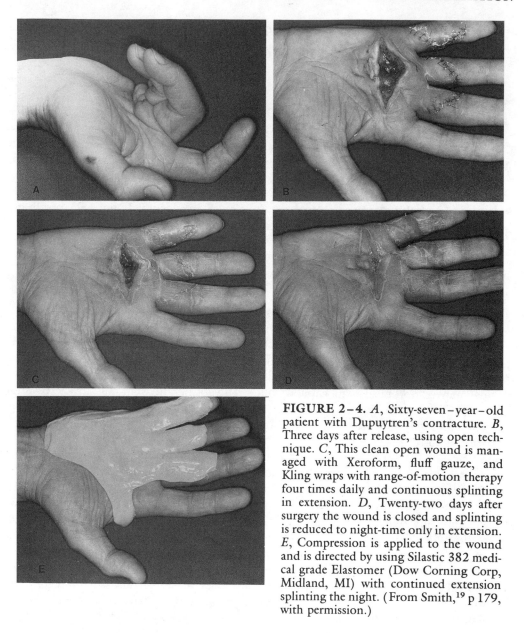

FIGURE 2–4. *A*, Sixty-seven–year–old patient with Dupuytren's contracture. *B*, Three days after release, using open technique. *C*, This clean open wound is managed with Xeroform, fluff gauze, and Kling wraps with range-of-motion therapy four times daily and continuous splinting in extension. *D*, Twenty-two days after surgery the wound is closed and splinting is reduced to night-time only in extension. *E*, Compression is applied to the wound and is directed by using Silastic 382 medical grade Elastomer (Dow Corning Corp, Midland, MI) with continued extension splinting the night. (From Smith,[19] p 179, with permission.)

SKIN GRAFTS

The healing of skin grafts, whether full-thickness or split-thickness, involves the same process. When a skin graft is placed on a suitably vascular bed, it is immediately nourished by plasmatic imbibition, the absorption of the plasmalike fluid from the recipient bed. This occurrence helps nourish the graft for the first 48 hours until inosculation of blood vessels has begun. Inosculation is the process by which blood vessels from the vascular recipient bed join the existing blood vessels within the transplanted dermis and reestablish flow. This provides vascular supply to the skin graft, and by 4 or 5 days true circulation has occurred.[20]

THERAPY AFTER SKIN GRAFTING

During the first days after skin-graft application, adequate contact must be maintained between the graft and the recipient bed. Depending on the surgeon's preference, many techniques of graft fixation can be used, but regardless of the technique, the therapist working with the freshly skin-grafted hand must be careful not to produce increased edema or any motion of the graft on its bed, thereby shearing the fragile attachments and often causing loss of the graft.

When very mobile areas of the hand are skin grafted, these grafts are generally left undisturbed for 4 to 5 days. The graft can be examined as early as after 2 days but therapy should not be instituted until the graft has begun to stabilize. For less mobile areas such as the palm or dorsum of the hand, a good graft "take" is apparent by 2 or 3 days, and therapy can usually be instituted at this time if it is absolutely necessary. Obviously no pressure should be placed on the graft site, as this can cause shear. Therapy should usually be done without dressings. Once a graft has shown to have a satisfactory take by 4 or 5 days, there is usually no prohibition to hydrotherapy. Other direct modalities should be avoided for at least 7 to 10 days.

TENDON HEALING

Over the years, the literature reviewing tendon healing has been contradictory and quite controversial. Arguments about a tendon's ability to heal following injury without extratendinous cellular participation (intrinsic healing) seem to be as valid as those that state a tendon is dependent on surrounding tissues for healing (extrinsic healing). The healing tendon is a complex biologic system within which both the intrinsic and extrinsic healing mechanisms play a part. Tenocytes within the tendon as well as fibroblasts from the surrounding perivascular tissues all probably play a role in the healing of tendons. Diffusion from synovial fluid and intrinsic blood supply offer parallel nutrition systems, each of which provides nutrition during healing. Clinically separating the intrinsic and extrinsic components of the healing process is probably impossible and is irrelevant in the clinical situation, because one healing system cannot be separated from the other.

A tendon is a highly specialized cellular and connective tissue network that is longitudinally unyielding. Three fibrous proteins—collagen, elastin, and reticulin—provide its strength and structure. Collagen, mostly type I, constitutes 86 percent of the total weight of the tendon and, with so much collagen in tendon, replacing the tendon bundles with scar (i.e., collagen) renders the healed tendon almost normal microscopically.[21] The first two phases of tendon wound healing, inflammation and fibroplasia, share the same characteristics as healing of other tissues. The third phase, scar maturation, is unique as it applies to tendons, because this tissue can achieve a state of repair that is akin to regeneration.

Phase 1: Inflammation

In the inflammatory phase of healing, the repaired tendon undergoes proliferation of the cells on the outer edge of the tendon bundles during the first 4 days. By day 7, these cells begin to migrate into the substance of the tendon.[22] This migration is accompanied by intense vascular proliferation within the tendon[23] and, together, are the bases for the intrinsic healing mechanism.

The situation is clouded by the healing response of the immediately adjacent tissues, which participate in the tendon healing by providing collagen-producing fibroblasts and blood vessels (extrinsic repair).[22] This fibrovascular tissue, infiltrating from the peritendinous structures, can become the future adhesions that will prevent tendon excursion if allowed to mature under conditions of immobility.

Phase 2: Fibroplasia

By 7 days, collagen synthesis is proceeding. In areas where there was a technically good repair without a gap between the tendon ends, collagen is seen to bridge the repair.[24] Initially, the collagen fibers and fibroblasts are oriented perpendicular to the long axis of the tendon,[25] but by 10 days the new collagen fibers begin to align parallel to the old longitudinal collagen bundles of the tendon stumps.[22]

Phase 3: Scar Maturation

Collagen synthesis reaches a maximum after 4 weeks but continues to be active at a rate of three to four times normal even after 3 to 4 months, reflecting active remodeling.[3] This active collagen synthesis continues for a longer time than in skin or muscle; hence, the maturation phase is more lengthy in tendon.[6] Fortunately, tendon strength increases after repair in a predictable fashion. This fact allows the surgeon and therapist to design therapeutic protocols that need only vary slightly among patients.

First pointed out by Mason and Allen[26] in 1941, the tensile strength of a repaired tendon is solely a function of the suture material and surgical technique at the time of repair and strength progressively falls over the next 5 days as collaginase, elaborated during the inflammatory process, softens the tendon. By day 9, the holding power of the repair has increased enough to equal the initial strength of the suture and then continues to increase. When early restricted range of motion is allowed, producing stress on the tendon, the resistence to rupture of the tendon repair increases much faster. Subjected to controlled testing by Gelberman and colleagues,[27] tensile load values of repaired tendons were shown to be greater in those tendons subjected to early mobilization. At 3 weeks following repair, mobilized tendons achieved twice the strength of immobilized tendons and continued to be twice as strong throughout the 12-week duration of the study. At 12 weeks, immobilized tendons possessed only 20 percent of the strength of a normal tendon but the mobilized tendon had achieved almost 50 percent of normal strength. Because stress on the collagen biopolymer is known to produce a change in the electrical potential of the tendon surface (piezoelectric effect), the resultant electrical field may help facilitate realignment of the collagen bundles. This fact may help explain the more rapid increase in tensile strength in the mobilized tendon.[28]

Characteristics and Control of Adhesions

Ideally, if tendons could be made to heal by intrinsic means alone, near-normal functional results could be expected following tendon repair. Unfortunately, participation in the tendon healing process by peritendinous tissues frequently creates restricted gliding. This is because of unyielding adhesions to less movable structures surrounding the tendon. Despite preinjury architectural separation, the trauma of injury and the mechanism of wound healing produces healing as one mass without differentiation of the preexisting tissue planes, especially when immobilized.

The greater the tissue damage, the greater is the likelihood that there will be significant scar limiting tendon excursion. Also, when the tendon is rendered ischemic by tight suturing or by aggressive mobilization, there is a stimulus for increased amounts of fibrovascular tissue to form around the tendon juncture. Increased tendon adhesions also occur with immobilization. The key to the differentiation of the collagen bundles within the tendon and those in the peritendinous structures remains unknown. In cases when a repaired tendon achieves limited excursion due to very thick unyielding adhesions, these adhesions are histologically similar to the tendon itself. In some cases, the adhesions are thin and elongated and do not restrict motion. What is it that causes the peritendinous collagen scar to be nonrestrictive in some cases but restrictive in others?

Tendon adhesions are currently considered a part of the normal tendon healing process. The surgical goal is to minimize factors that create adhesions during phase 1 and phase 2 healing. This goal is accomplished by gentle atraumatic technique and accurate tendon repair with care taken not to devascularize the tendon stumps. There is no statistical evidence that closure (or reconstruction) of the tendon sheath improves the results of tendon repair following hand therapy if early motion is used.[29] The goal in hand therapy is to minimize the amount of restrictive adhesions by maximizing gliding. When adhesions occur, we rely on the remodeling process to lengthen adhesions over time as well as to weaken and/or break adhesions allowing them to form as a more elongated structure. This gradual process of scar remodeling by continuous degradation and deposition of collagen allows us, through therapy, to elongate scar adhesions progressively and to improve motion through exercise and splinting.

BONE HEALING

Because bony stability is one of the prerequisites for initiation of hand therapy, the understanding of bone healing is essential. While bone has the capacity for limited regeneration, the quality of healing and the rapidity of the process is largely dependent on the methods of fixation and the length and adequacy of immobilization. The bones of the hand are morphologically like the other long bones of the body, in that they are composed of a hard shell of cortical bone that surrounds the medullary cavity, composed of cancellous or trabecular bone. All nonarticular surfaces of bone are covered by a two-layer periosteum that provides a rich blood supply to the bone. The outer layer is a thick fibrous tissue and the deeper layer (cambium) contains cells that are osteogenic.[30]

The process of bone healing follows the phases similar to the healing of other tissues—inflammation, fibroplasia, and scar maturation. Most of the cells that participate in the bone healing process are already present within the periosteum or endosteum that lines the inside of the cortical layer. Inflammation and edema immediately follow the fracture, and the subsequent gap between the fracture fragments fills with a hematoma. Fibroblast and periosteal osteogenic cells proliferate and migrate to the area of injury and then elaborate a ground substance and collagen matrix around the bone fragments, which is termed *callus*. Within a few days, the fractured bone is surrounded by a ring of callus, the thickness of which is directly proportional to the amount of injury and the motion at the fracture site.

Primary Healing

Stable, anatomically precise rigid fixation yields little callus, and in this situation the bone undergoes primary healing, with little scar, in much the same fashion as a carefully reapproximated skin wound. Primary bone healing is achieved when the fracture fragments are held in close approximation by rigid fixation leading to contact healing by the union of cortex to cortex.[6,31,32] Rigid fixation is advantageous in hand fractures not only because it accelerates healing and reduces scar but also because it allows gentle hand therapy within days to promote the maintenance of gliding surfaces.

Secondary Healing

When techniques other than rigid internal fixation are used, bony union is achieved by secondary healing. The temporal course of secondary fracture healing spans the average of 7 or more weeks, depending on the location and the kind of fracture. During the first 12 hours, the fracture hematoma forms and cell proliferation begins. For the next 12 hours, active periosteal, endosteal, and parosteal (tissues adjacent to bone) cell mobilization and proliferation occurs, beginning the catabolic period that leads to peak cellular proliferation by 48 hours. At this time, synthesis of glycosaminoglycans begins, forming the osteoid matrix that, by 3 days, becomes filled with collagen, thereby forming the fibrous callus. Osteogenic cells within the callus are pleuripotential and their differentiation depends on the oxygen tension (i.e., vascularity of the callus). Vascular areas stimulate the differentiation to osteoblasts, and avascular areas produce chondrocytes. During the avascular phase of the callus formation, the healing callus is cartilaginous as a result of the production of chondrocytes.

Intense vascularization then begins by 4 days and, as it proceeds, bone is laid down in the cartilaginous callus. Within the medullary cavity of the bone, debris and dead bone at the fracture site are removed by phagocytes and simultaneously immature trabecular bone is laid down.

Over the next 10 days maximum collagen synthesis is reached and the fracture callus is metabolically very active. Synthesis exceeds degradation, and further ossification yields greater stability. From 3 to 6 weeks, intense bony metabolism fills in the trabecular bone with lamellar bone and callus resorption begins the extensive remodeling about the fracture site. During the following several months, the preinjury architecture is progressively restored, yielding healed bone that is indistinguishable from normal cortical compact bone.[20,31,32] The timing of therapy following fracture depends on the adequacy of fixation. Therefore, the therapeutic plan is designed with close cooperation between the surgeon and therapist.

When evaluating fracture-healing clinically, the absence of pain on palpation of the fracture site and on gentle stress of the involved bone usually denotes sufficient healing for resisted range-of-motion exercises. These clinical findings precede radiographic evidence of bony union. Nonunion, except in segmental bone loss is uncommon, but delayed union is more common and should probably be treated aggressively by the surgeon with bone graft and internal fixation as early as 4 months to prevent increased stiffness from further immobilization.[33]

Nerve Healing

As a consequence of any severe nerve injury, there is a predictable sequence of distal (wallerian) and proximal axonal degeneration. If the injury does not lead to nerve cell death, the peripheral "arm" of the nerve cell—the axon—will regenerate.[32] This regeneration does, however, require nerve repair if the nerve is severed. The goal of the surgeon is to provide optimal conditions for nerve regeneration. These include accurate microcoaptation of adequately debrided nerve stumps under minimal tension, accomplished by proximal or distal nerve transposition, release, or interposition grafting.

The severity of the injury to the nerve, as well as associated injuries, is of considerable importance if one is to estimate the regenerative capacity of the nerve. These considerations also may dictate the timing and method of nerve repair. Not only is a poorer prognosis associated with more severe injuries, but also the condition of the associated tissues (skin, bone, joint, and vascular system) must be addressed before nerve repair. Nerve reconstruction or repair should not be done in a limb unless good skin cover, adequate vascularity, and skeletal stability with supple joints can be ensured.[34]

Nerve regeneration occurs by outgrowth of the proximal stump and not by autoregeneration of the degenerated distal nerve.[34,35] After a latent period of up to 24 hours the cut axon tip bulges into a growth cone. Anterograde growth occurs by advancement of the tip in conjunction with the sprouting of collaterals from the growth cone, as well as from the nodes of Ranvier up to several segments proximal to the axon tip.[36] By the end of 24 hours a few sprouts have reached the area of injury and penetration of the developing scar at the site of microcoaptation proceeds from the second or third day. Accompanying the axonal sprouts out of the proximal stump are Schwann cells derived from the replication of the terminal satellite cells.[34,37] At the time of injury, the distal axon begins to undergo wallerian degeneration. The resulting fragmented axonal debris and myelin is degraded by the remaining Schwann cells, which have become phagocytotic. They also proliferate within the basal lamina tubes of the distal nerve.[38] As they proliferate, the Schwann cells become densely packed in longitudinal rows, ready to accept the axon buds and remyelinate the advancing regenerating axons.[39] The regenerating axons do not penetrate the old Schwann cell tubes but create new tubes as they grow through the longitudinal rows of Schwann cells (Fig. 2–5).

In nerve regeneration, outgrowth of the axon is only the first step in a series of developments leading to the restoration of a mature functional system. After bridging the site of nerve injury or repair (by 4 or 5 days) the axonal sprouts grow down the distal nerve at a rate inversely proportional to the distance from the cell body as observed by a progressing Tinel's sign.[40] Reported rates of growth are 8.5 mm or more per day at the proximal arm and 1 to 1.5 mm per day in the hand.[41] When the growing axon reaches the end organ (if it is of the appropriate type), connectivity occurs and maturation follows.

Important information that the surgeon must share with the therapist is the degree of tension on the microcoaptation and the amount of motion that will be allowed in the initial postoperative period. With today's more liberal approach to nerve grafting which allows tension-free microcoaptation in neutral or extended extremity positions, surgeons are less likely to require that the nerve-injured extremity be kept in an exaggerated, usually flexed position until healing has progressed to the point that a functional position can be restored. Tension-free repairs, therefore, have improved the results of nerve reconstruction not only by providing more ideal healing but also by lessening the chance of iatrogenic contracture.[34]

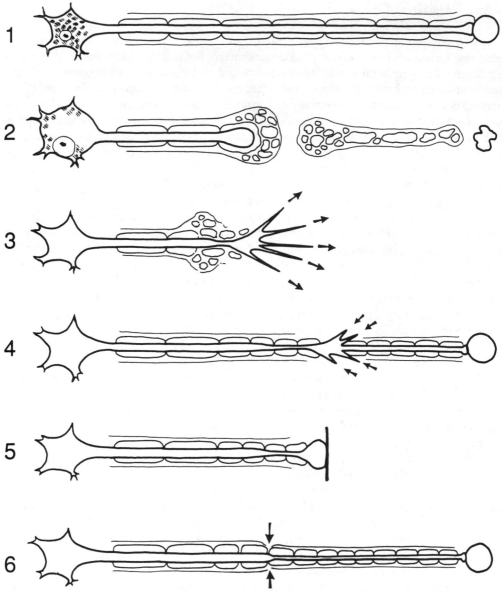

FIGURE 2–5. Axon regeneration. 1. Normal neuron with soma and myelinated axon. 2. Following injury, the proximal axon has undergone retrograde reaction with somal chromatolysis, nuclear migration, and nuclear enlargement. The distal axon has undergone Wallerian degeneration with axonal fragmentation and phagocytosis. The end organ has begun degenerative changes. 3. The proximal axon has begun to sprout filopodia from the growth cone to begin axonal regeneration. 4. Upon successful connectivity of one axonal sprout, redundant sprouts undergo the dying-back process. 5. A terminal bulb is created by damming up axonal contents if an insurmountable obstruction is encountered. 6. If scar produces an annular constriction around a regenerating axon (arrows), the resulting axonal caliber will never return to normal. (From Terzis and Smith,[34] p 74, with permission.)

THE THERAPIST AND WOUND HEALING

Unchecked, the natural process of wound healing may yield the results desired following injury to the hand, but, as we better understand the process of wound healing, we are learning ways to modify connective tissue scar to the patient's advantage. Hand therapy is a very important component of the rehabilitation of the injured hand and is directed toward the restoration of function by the manipulation of healing tissues in such a way as to promote differential healing of tissues and to approximate regeneration. To do so, the therapist and surgeon must consider each tissue type and its condition and then individualize each patient's therapy program. Some injuries will benefit from therapeutic motion, others will not. Before each therapy plan is devised, the checklist shown in Table 2–1 should be reviewed.

Currently, there are many pharmacologic agents that affect alterations in the synthesis, deposition, degradation, and structure of scar tissue. None are safe or effective enough to be used routinely. Eventually, drugs will be used that will promote healing of bone, nerve, tendon, and skin and perhaps allow us to manipulate unfavorable scar. Until then, we must rely on conventional therapeutic modalities to influence wound healing.

The current tools of the therapist are motion, tension, pressure, heat, cold, ultrasound, electricity (electric fields, direct current application, iontophoresis), and education. The *science* of therapy dictates which modality is used; the *art* of therapy combines the modalities for a comprehensive and effective therapeutic plan.

TABLE 2–1 Designing a Therapy Program

Consider the **skin**:
  What is the condition?
  Is it stable? Will it break down during therapy or splinting?
  Can we expect contraction? Will it lead to contracture?
Consider the **bone**:
  Has there been a fracture? Is there bone loss?
  Is the fixation stable?
  What can be moved and still protect the involved bones?
Consider the **joints**:
  Are they stable? Do they need to be protected during therapy?
  How can they be protected?
  To what degree can they be moved?
  If they cannot be moved, are they in a "position of protection"?
Consider the **tendons**:
  Have any injuries occurred? What kind of repair? Where?
  How much can the repair be stressed during motion?
  How much motion is allowed? Through what range?
  What is necessary to protect the repair?
Consider the **nerve**:
  Is there altered sensibility?
  Has there been a nerve injury that has been repaired?
  Can full range of motion be performed without tension on the coaptation?
  Should sensory reeducation be included in the program?
Consider the **muscle**:
  Has there been an injury?
  Is it denervated?
  Is strengthening required?

Phases I and II: The Inflammatory/Fibroplasia Phase

Therapy during the initial healing phases following hand injury or surgery concentrates on *preservation* of function by *prevention* of edema and subsequent fibrosis, as well as *maintenance* of gliding surfaces. Edema is treated by elevation, compression, and massage, and gliding surfaces are maintained by motion. Whereas some modalities are contraindicated in the early period, depending on the individual situation, *there should never be a contraindication to elevation.* Educating the patient as to the importance of keeping the injured hand elevated is the first step toward involving the patient in the rehabilitation of his or her hand.

The condition of the skin is an obvious consideration in the early therapy of the hand. Most wound-s will allow gentle range of motion (except fresh skin grafts less than 4 or 5 days old). With proper suture technique and some attention to avoid overzealous stretch of a fresh wound, wound healing in a surgically closed wound is not adversely affected by careful hand therapy.

Motion is contraindicated when treatment of a fracture is by immobilization alone. In this instance, bony union is achieved in 4 to 6 weeks, after which time motion can be started. Fractures treated by rigid fixation are stable and therefore allow early motion (a distinct advantage of this technique). Nerves, when repaired with fine suture under no tension, must be protected until axons bud across the microcoaptation and the delicate repair is stented by the surrounding tissue. This event usually occurs by 5 to 6 days, at which time motion is allowed. Periarticular structures such as ligaments are usually immobilized from 1 to 3 weeks before the involved joint is vigorously moved.

Perhaps the greatest controversy surrounds the early postoperative care of the repaired tendon. In most cases, research has been directed toward the flexor tendon repair; however, extensor tendons heal in the same manner and essentially the same considerations apply. Research[6,42-44] has shown that the tendon that is subjected to motion and some tension during the healing phase not only achieves a greater excursion but also results in a repair that is mechanically stronger and microscopically more normal than one that was immobilized during healing. The motion seems to encourage tendon healing by *intrinsic* means, creating a gliding surface by shearing the tendon away from the attachments to the surrounding tissues (adhesions). Also, the tension created by motion has a positive effect on collagen synthesis, alignment, and cross-linkage.

Whether the program involves controlled active motion, passive motion, or both does not seem to be as important as the mere fact that the tendon in question is moving in relation to its surrounding tissues. Also, the alternate stress and relaxation that occurs when a tendon is moved induces a cellular response within the epitenon, which promotes cell differentiation and inhibits inflammatory cell ingrowth from the surrounding tissues.[44] Thus, controlled motion can partially overcome the biologic "one wound–one scar" scheme.

Unrestricted active motion does not yield the same outcome. The healing tendon is a delicate structure that is soft and susceptible to gaping at the repair or rupture during the initial phases of healing if subjected to too much stress. Because of the tendomalacia that occurs during the first 2 weeks of healing,[26] active motion is not instituted until 3 weeks following repair. This motion is *nonresistive* until 5 or 6 weeks at which time the tendon repair has achieved 20 percent normal strength.[27]

Early active exercise (3 to 4 weeks) is primarily of the "place/hold" variety which avoids stress on the tendon juncture by passively placing the finger in question into the fully flexed position and then asking the patient to hold it in that position by gentle muscle action.[44] By 12 weeks, tendon juncture strength is 50 percent of normal[27,45] and resistive exercises can be increased.

Phase III: Scar Maturation

The third phase of therapy begins with the maturation phase of wound healing (usually by 6 to 8 weeks) and relies on the prolonged metabolic turnover of scar collagen. During this phase the therapist can influence healing by the use of exercise, splinting, stretching, and the other therapeutic modalities. All collagen, whether it be scar, connective tissue, or higher-order structures such as tendon, consists of a visco-elastic material that exhibits a high resistance to rapidly applied tension but displays a plastic character when subjected to low-tension prolonged loads. In other words, whenever tissue is rapidly stretched by the application of high energy, it will resist this stretch and will tear. This tear would create further wounding, more inflammation, and eventually more scar. The patient in this instance feels pain and the therapeutic intervention has failed. When scar tissue is placed under low stress over a prolonged period, it responds by relaxation (or creep), and the eventual metabolic turnover will result in new collagen laid down in an elongated conformation.[47] This essential fact underlies the therapeutic maxim, the "inevitability of gradualness."[48]

Scar tissue, when left alone under no tension, does contract, which shortens the scar. This phenomenon is also used to therapeutic advantage and underlies the principle by which static splinting for a prolonged time will shorten a structure healed in an elongated position (e.g., mallet finger deformity).

The therapeutic modalities of dynamic traction, dynamic and static splinting, and serial casting take advantage of the metabolic characteristics of scar tissue and provide the prolonged low-tension stress that stimulates the cellular elements of the scar tissue to become metabolically active as well as to break and reform new collagen cross-linkages in elongated lower-tension states. Young scars are more susceptible to modification by conditions of stress—a principle that applies to both the age of the scar and the age of the patient. The actual mechanism that causes a scar to respond to stress is poorly understood but must in some way depend on the ability of cells within the scar matrix to translate the applied stress into biochemical action.[48]

TEMPERATURE

The physicochemical properties of connective tissue can be altered as well by temperature. As tissue temperature rises, the tissue extensibility increases and it becomes more plastic. Therefore, under high-temperature conditions elongation is achieved more easily than at body temperature and is more permanent. At 104°F there is a change induced in the microstructure of collagen, which enhances the viscous stress relaxation by a mechanism that is thought to be secondary to intermolecular bond destabilization. The stretch must be maintained during the cooling phase as this phase presumably allows the collagen microstructure to restabilize (form new cross-linkages) in the elongated position. Unloading the tissue before cooling encourages reformation of the original (shortened) structure.[49,50]

Clinically, modalities that provide therapeutic heat are hot packs, paraffin baths, whirlpool baths, and Fluidotherapy.[50] Also, part of the efficacy of ultrasound and diathermy may be due to the resultant deep-tissue temperature elevations.

ELECTRICAL STIMULATION

The therapist may also influence wound healing and maturation through other modalities. Electrical stimulation has long been shown to influence bone healing by the induction of osteogenesis and is frequently used in the treatment for nonunions.[51] Recent research indicates that the application of electrical current may also augment the healing of tendon[52] and nerve.[53] Certainly, functional electrical stimulation is efficacious to decrease muscle atrophy while reinnervation proceeds after nerve repair[54] and can maintain the excursion of the muscle-tendon unit during this period.

Electrical current is used also to deliver medications by the technique of iontophoresis and will undoubtedly serve a greater role in the future as we learn more about the wound healing process and discover more useful medications. Currently, iontophoresis is commonly used for the delivery of corticosteroids.

SUMMARY

Wound healing of all tissues follows a predictable sequence of events that can be influenced. Hand surgery and rehabilitation requires a team approach involving the surgeon, therapist, and patient if optimum results are to be realized. If the surgeon can carefully restore the anatomy of the injured hand using meticulous technique and in the process not create more injury, the hand wound will heal quickly with a minimum of scar. This sequence, however, does not ensure that the healed product will be functional. The work of the educated patient, done under the guidance of the therapist and surgeon, ensures that gliding planes are restored and tissues strengthened through an individually designed supervised therapy program. The careful application of therapeutic modalities alters healing tissues making them more susceptible to the patient's and therapist's efforts. The therapeutic modalities are chosen logically out of knowledge of their actions and knowledge of wound healing in all the tissues of the hand. The rehabilitation of the hand is based on a sound biologic knowledge of wound healing, how this knowledge relates to each tissue of the hand, and how healing can be optimized to achieve the best functional result after injury.

REFERENCES

1. Madden, JW: Wound healing: Biologic and clinical features. In Sabiston, DC (ed): Davis-Christopher Textbook of Surgery, ed 11. WB Saunders, Philadelphia, 1977, p 271.
2. Majno G: The Healing Hand. Man and Wound in the Ancient World. Harvard University Press, Cambridge, MA, 1975.
3. Mathes, SJ and Abouljoud, M: Wound healing. In Davis, JH (ed): Clinical Surgery. Vol I. CV Mosby, St Louis, 1987, p 461.
4. Marcy, R: Les methodes d'essai des "cictrisants." Therapie 15:534, 1960.
5. Howes, RM and Hoopes, JE: Current concepts of wound healing. Clin Plast Surg 4(2):173, 1977.
6. Peacock, EE: Wound Repair, ed 3. WB Saunders, Philadelphia, 1984.
7. Falcone, PA and Caldwell, MD: Wound metabolism. Clin Plast Surg 17(3):443, 1990.
8. Falcone, PA, et al: The effect of exogenous fibronectin on wound breaking strength. Plast Reconstr Surg 74(6):809, 1984.
9. Barbul, A: Immune aspects of wound repair. Clin Plast Surg 17(3):433, 1990.

10. Bailey, AJ, Robins, SP, and Balian, G: Biological significance of the intermolecular crosslinks of collagen. Nature 251:105, 1974.
11. Westaby, S: Fundamentals of wound healing. In Westaby, S (ed): Wound Care. William Heineman Medical Books, London, 1985, p 11.
12. Madden, JW and Peacock, EE: Studies on the biology of collagen during wound healing. III. Dynamic metabolism of scar collagen and remodeling of dermal wounds. Ann Surg 174:511, 1971.
13. Dellon, AL: Wound healing in nerve. Clin Plast Surg 17(3):545, 1990.
14. Montandon, D, D'Andiran, G, and Gabbiani, G: The mechanisms of wound contraction and epithelialization. Clinical and experimental studies. Clin Plast Surg 4(3):325, 1977.
15. Majno, G, et al: Contraction of granulation tissue: Similarity to smooth muscle. Science 173:548, 1971.
16. Madden, JW, Morton, DJR, and Peacock, EE: Contraction of experimental wound I. Inhibiting wound contraction by using topical smooth muscle antagonist. Surgery 76:8, 1974.
17. Frank, DH and Bonaldi, LC: Inhibition of wound contraction: Comparison of full thickness skin grafts, Biobrane and aspartate membranes. Ann Plast Surg 14(2):103, 1985.
18. Stone, P and Madden, JW: Effects of primary and delayed split skin grafting on wound contraction. Surg Forum 25:41, 1974.
19. Smith, KL: Wound care for the hand patient. In Hunter, JM, et al (eds): Rehabilitation of the Hand, Surgery and Therapy. CV Mosby, St Louis, 1990, p 172.
20. Grabb, WC: Basic techniques of plastic surgery. In Grabb, WC and Smith, JW (eds): Plastic Surgery, ed 3. Little, Brown & Co, Boston, 1979, p 3.
21. Van Der Meulen, JC and Leistikow, PA: Tendon healing. Clin Plast Surg 4(3):439, 1977.
22. Lindsay, WK: Cellular biology of flexor tendon healing. In Hunter, JM, Schneider, LH, and Mackin, EJ (eds): Tendon Surgery in the Hand. CV Mosby, St Louis, 1987, p 50.
23. De Klerk, AJ and Jouck, LM: Primary tendon healing: An experimental study. S Afr Med J 62(9):276, 1982.
24. Gelberman, RH, et al: The early stages of flexor tendon healing: A morphologic study of the first fourteen days. J Hand Surg 10A(6):776, 1985.
25. Strickland, JW: Flexor tendon injuries. Orthopaedic Review 15(10):21, 1986.
26. Mason, ML and Allen, HS: The rate of healing of tendons. Ann Surg 113(3):424, 1941.
27. Gelberman, RH, et al: Effects of early intermittent passive mobilization on healing canine flexor tendons. J Hand Surg 7(2):170, 1982.
28. Ketchum, LD: Tendon healing. In Fundamentals of Wound Management in Surgery. Selected Tissues. Chirurgecom, South Plainfield, NJ, 1977, p 121.
29. Saldana, MJ, et al: Flexor tendon repair and rehabilitation in Zone II. Open sheath versus closed sheath technique. J Hand Surg 12A(6):1110, 1987.
30. Snell, RS: Clinical Anatomy for Medical Students. Little, Brown, Boston, 1973.
31. Lindner, J: Bone healing. Clin Plast Surg 4(3):425, 1977.
32. Bryant, WM: Wound healing. Ciba Symposia 29(3):1, 1977.
33. O'Brien, ET: Fractures of the metacarpals and phalanges. In Green, DP (ed): Operative Hand Surgery, ed 2. Churchill Livingstone, New York, 1988, p 760.
34. Terzis, JK and Smith, KL: The Peripheral Nerve: Structure, Function and Reconstruction. Raven Press, New York, 1990.
35. Ramon-Y-Cajal, S: Degeneration and regeneration of the Nervous System. Vol I. Oxford University Press, London, 1928.
36. Grafstein, B, and McQuarrie, IG: Role of the nerve cell body in axonal regeneration. In Cotman, CW (ed): Neuronal Plasticity. Raven Press, New York, 1978, p 155.
37. Spencer, PS: Morphology of the injured peripheral nerve. In Daniel, RK and Terzis, JK (eds): Reconstructive Microsurgery. Little, Brown & Co, Boston, 1977, p 342.
38. Satinsky, D, Pepe FA, and Liu, CN: The neurilemma cell in peripheral nerve degeneration and regeneration. Exp Neurol 9:441, 1964.
39. Selzer, ME: Regeneration of the peripheral nerve. In Sumner, AJ (ed): The Physiology of Peripheral Nerve Disease. WB Saunders, Philadelphia, 1980, p 358.
40. Tinel, J: The sign of "tingling" in lesions of the peripheral nerves. J Presse Med 23:388, 1915. (Translated in Arch Neurol 24:574, 1971.)
41. Sunderland, S: Nerve and Nerve Injuries. E & S Livingstone, Edinburgh, 1968.
42. Strickland, JW and Glogovac, SV: Digital function following flexor tendon repair in Zone II: A comparison of immobilization and controlled passive motion techniques. J Hand Surg 5(6):537, 1980.
43. Lister, GD: Flexor tendon. In McCarthy, JG, May, JW, and Littler, JW (eds): Plastic Surgery. WB Saunders, Philadelphia, 1990, p 4516.
44. Schneider, LH and McEntee, P: Flexor tendon injuries. Treatment of the acute problem. Hand Clin 2(1):119, 1986.
45. Gelberman, RH and Manske, PR: Factors influencing flexor tendon adhesions. Hand Clin 1(1):35, 1985.
46. Kottke, FJ, Pauley, DL, and Ptak, RA: The rationale for prolonged stretching for correction of shortening of connective tissue. Arch Phys Med Rehab 47:345, 1966.
47. Brand, PW: Quoted in Bell, JA: Plaster cylinder casting for contractures of the interphalangeal joints. In

Hunter, JM, et al (eds): Rehabilitation of the Hand, Surgery and Therapy. CV Mosby, St Louis, 1990, p 875.

48. Arem, AJ and Madden, JW: Effects of stress on healing wound: I. Intermittent noncyclical tension. J Surg Res 20:93, 1976.
49. Sapega, AA, et al: Biophysical factors in range of motion exercise. The Physician and Sports Medicine 9(12):57, 1981.
50. Mullins, PAT: Use of therapeutic modalities in upper extremity rehabilitation. In Hunter, JM, et al (eds): Rehabilitation of the Hand, Surgery and Therapy, CV Mosby, St Louis, 1984, p 195.
51. Kennedy, MA: Changes in the mechanical and electrical environment and the effect on bone. Orthopaedics 10(5):789, 1987.
52. Nessler, JP and Mass, DP: Direct-current electrical stimulation of tendon healing in vitro. Clin Orthopaed 217:303, 1987.
53. Osterman, AL and Bora, FW: Electrical stimulation applied to bone and nerve injuries in the upper extremity. Orthopaed Clin North Am 17(3):353, 1986.
54. Pachter, BR, Eberstein, A, and Goodgold, J: Electrical stimulation effect on denervated skeletal myofibers in rats: A light and electron microscope study. Arch Phys Med Rehab 63:427, 1982.

Evaluation of the Hand

CHAPTER 3

Clinical Evaluation

Beth Nicholson, OTR, CHT

Evaluation is the cornerstone of sound clinical decision making. The clinician's evaluative skill is dependent on an in-depth understanding of structural and functional anatomy, the effects of injury and disease on tissue, wound healing concepts, and an appreciation of sociologic, psychologic, and spiritual influences. The integrity of the entire treatment process hinges on our ability to evaluate and assess patient signs and symptoms carefully and to use that assessment as the basis for care. As Feinstein[1-4] stated, "To advance the art and science in clinical exam, the equipment a clinician most needs to improve is himself."

The objectives of this chapter are to enable the reader to (1) identify the critical components of hand evaluation, (2) identify methods and techniques for measurement of limitations, and (3) understand analysis of clinical data and implications for treatment.

GENERAL CONSIDERATIONS

Evaluation

Rarely is a clinical entity purely subjective or objective; rather, it is a matter of degree. The terms subjective and objective may apply to the quality of a measurement or to the phenomenon being measured. The ideal is to obtain valid, objective measurements of subjective and objective phenomena.[5] In reality, clinical practice is not that simple. Clinical decisions have to be made within the parameters set by the limitations of our measurement tools.

Standardization

Few standardized instruments or procedures exist for many of the clinical entities we wish to measure. The degree of objectivity or reliability is reduced if the evaluation procedure is not standardized. Although an individual therapist can establish a baseline and measure change over time fairly effectively within the context of a given case and even within multiple cases, lack of standardization makes it difficult to compare information among therapists. The following information, although currently not all standardized and still subject to research scrutiny, represents those approaches and techniques generally accepted among hand specialists.

Standardized instruments and procedures that are available will be noted in specific sections of this chapter. The clear challenge for hand therapists is to research instruments and evaluation techniques to improve further the objectivity of the evaluation process and to enhance communication.

COMPONENTS OF HAND EVALUATION

Evaluation of the hand and upper extremity includes a detailed history and physical examination.

History

Relevant personal history and history of the primary complaint are both important. Personal history including the patient's age, sex, dominance, occupation and avocations, marital status, number of children and status of family and employer relationships may have an impact on the prognosis, the patient's participation in treatment, and the establishment of realistic, individualized goals.

History of the primary complaint should recreate the incident of onset and follow through to the day of the initial therapy visit. This portion of the evaluation relates to the patient's report and interpretation of signs and symptoms. Questions posed to the patient should advance from general to specific, and encourage answers that are as objective as possible without influencing the patient's report. Documentation by the patient of the location and type of symptoms provides the therapist with a wealth of information. Use of a numeric or visual analog scale provides a means for the patient to communicate perceived degree of pain.

Details such as the mechanism of injury may influence interpretation of the physical examination, subsequent treatment, and prognosis. For example, the therapist can expect a tendon laceration resulting from a crush injury to require more intense efforts to restore joint mobility and tendon excursion due to the extent of scarring and surrounding tissue adherence than a tendon laceration from a clean, sharp knife.[6-9]

The sources of information included in the patient's history, such as medical records or patient report, should also be identified, as there may be discrepancies between the patient's perception and the actual medical documentation. A suggested sequence of questioning relative to the primary complaint is outlined in Table 3–1.

Physical Examination

UPPER QUARTER SCREENING

The initial step in the physical examination is an upper quarter screening. The screening provides an overview of the extremity and direction for the more detailed

TABLE 3–1 History

I. Identification of the problem—what is the primary complaint that brought the patient to the therapist in the first place?
II. History of the primary complaint
  A. If sudden onset, etiology and date of injury or spontaneous onset; if gradual onset, when and what symptoms were first noticed
  B. Location, intensity, and type of symptoms such as stiffness, weakness, paresthesias, anesthesias, pain
  C. Behavior of symptoms as related to posture and activity
    1. Are symptoms constant or intermittent?
    2. What brings them on or makes them worse (e.g., certain positions, sustained posture, type or level of activity at home or work)?
    3. What relieves them?
    4. If not constant, how long do symptoms last?
    5. Do the symptoms specifically interfere with sleep and, if so, how?
    6. What are symptoms like first thing in morning versus later in day?
    7. Does pain radiate? Where?
    8. Are symptoms referred to other areas? Where?
  D. Have symptoms changed since onset?
  E. Prior types and dates of medical, surgical, and therapy treatment
  F. Current medications
  G. Previous test results (electromyogram, x-ray, and so on)
III. General health screen and medical history
  A. Family history for diabetes, stroke, cancer, heart disease, lung disease
  B. General health prior to injury
  C. Dates and reasons for previous hospitalizations, surgeries
  D. Previous injuries
  E. Frequency of caffeine, alcohol consumption, and smoking
  F. Any particular dietary or exercise habits?
  G. Any recent illnesses?
  H. Any of the following? High blood pressure, chest pain, shortness of breath, coughing or wheezing, urinary or bowel problems, ulcers, seizures, dizziness or fainting, headaches, blurred vision, hearing problems, balance problems, acquired immunodeficiency syndrome (AIDS), or any other problems
  I. Current resting blood pressure and heart rate
  J. Any psychologic or emotional problems?

aspects of the examination. This screening, along with the history, serves to focus the evaluator's time and attention on the specific problem areas.

The screening should include general observation of upper extremity and total body posture; willingness to move and the presence of protective positioning, guarding, or compensatory movement; presence of atrophy, swelling, or other deviations in comparison to the contralateral extremity; surface inspection for wounds, scars, grafts, amputations, or discoloration; cervical, shoulder, elbow, wrist, and digit range of motion; gross muscle strength for each joint motion and gross sensibility testing for light moving touch appreciation.

Muscle and sensibility screening relative to spinal and peripheral nerve distributions is outlined in Tables 3–2 and 3–3. Digital range of motion can be screened for by asking the patient to assume a "hook" position of finger metacarpophalangeal (MP) extension and interphalangeal (IP) flexion, full fist position of finger MP, proximal interphalangeal (PIP), and distal interphalangeal (DIP) simultaneous flexion, full finger extension and thumb radial abduction, palmar abduction, and flexion to the base of the little finger.

TABLE 3–2 Neurology of the Upper Extremity

Root	Reflex	Muscles	Sensation
C5	Biceps reflex	Deltoid, biceps	Lateral arm, axillary nerve
C6	Brachioradialis reflex (biceps reflex)	Wrist extensors	Lateral forearm, musculocutaneous nerve
C7	Triceps reflex	Wrist flexors, finger (MP) extensors, triceps	Middle finger
C8	—	Finger flexion	Medial forearm, medial antebrachial, cutaneous nerve
T1	—	Hand intrinsics	Medial arm, medial brachial, cutaneous nerve

Adapted from Hoppenfeld,[10] p 125.

Areas where no limitations are observed can simply be documented as "within normal limits" as opposed to any specific measurements. Detailed examination is indicated whenever limitations are noted by the examiner or symptoms are reproduced. A more detailed examination may also be indicated by the history to detect more subtle problems not revealed through the screening.

SPECIFIC COMPONENTS OF HAND EVALUATION

The more detailed aspects of the physical examination of the hand include inspection, measurement of edema, palpation, sensibility, range of motion, as well as differential diagnosis, strength, circulation, function, and other special tests. Sensibility and functional evaluation are addressed thoroughly in Chapters 4 and 5.

In addition to the direction provided by the history and upper-quarter screening, other points should be considered in planning for the detailed hand examination, including assessment of the patient's symptoms in regard to severity, irritability, and ease of exacerbation, and whether the condition requires caution in performing certain aspects of the examination.

As a specific example, surgical procedures performed before the therapist sees the patient necessitate a modified approach to the initial evaluation. The therapist must

TABLE 3–3 Major Peripheral Nerves

Nerve	Motor Screen	Sensation Screen
Radial nerve	Wrist extension, thumb extension	Dorsal thumb–index web space
Ulnar nerve	Abduction–little finger	Ulnar aspect–little finger
Median nerve	Thumb opposition, thumb abduction	Radial aspect–index finger
Axillary nerve	Deltoid	Lateral upper arm
Musculocutaneous nerve	Biceps	Lateral forearm

Adapted from Hoppenfeld,[10] p 125.

consider the specific information obtained in the history regarding the date, type, and technique of any surgical procedure. The therapist must also recognize that variations in surgical technique and surgeon philosophy regarding postoperative management have to be considered in addition to the therapist's perspective. Ideally, in the presence of a close working relationship between surgeon and therapist, patients will be seen as early as possible postoperatively. The primary goal at this stage is to protect tissue repairs that may be easily disrupted while avoiding the secondary complications associated with pain, swelling, and immobilization. In this case the evaluative focus depends on the current stage of wound healing of repaired structures, the presence of any related problems such as edema, and the degree of intervention and tissue mobilization that can be tolerated. Evaluative procedures that may be contraindicated initially can be integrated as the healing process tolerates.

Inspection

The therapist should initially inspect the appearance of the patient's hand for any discoloration; evidence of use or nonuse such as calluses and abrasions, or smooth skin with diminished creases; evidence of diminished sensibility such as burns, blisters, or loss of papillary ridges; and the presence of any wounds, incisions, or scars. Status of incisions and scars should be noted such as whether sutures are intact, whether incisions are healed, and whether scars are red, raised, sensitive, mobile, or adhered. Evaluation of wound status is discussed further in Chapter 6.

Edema

Currently, because there are no normal standards for hand volume or circumference, swelling must be considered relative to the uninvolved extremity and relative to change over time in response to activity or treatment. Although one hand may be normally larger than the other, comparison of the involved and uninvolved hands gives some indication of the initial degree of swelling. Subsequent measurements should also be made bilaterally to determine if changes in the involved hand are in response to treatment, activity level, or variables such as time of day and level of activity that normally affect the volume of both hands. The same tests and same techniques should be used before and during the course of treatment; when the measurements are recorded, the time should be noted and the patient's activities just prior to the evaluation documented in detail.

The location and type of edema such as pitting or hard brawny edema should also be noted. The therapist should be attuned to any associated signs of inflammation such as heat or redness that indicate swelling and may be related to overactivity. Localized swelling, redness, and tenderness may also be signs of infection and should be discussed with the physician.

Edema can be measured by water displacement or circumferential measurements or both. Several volumeters are commercially available and the evaluator should know the reliability of the instrument prior to use. Studies performed by Waylett-Rendall and Seibly[11] with the Brand-designed Volumeter[12] demonstrated intrarater accuracy within 1 percent with both normal and edematous hands on successive measures. Changes in

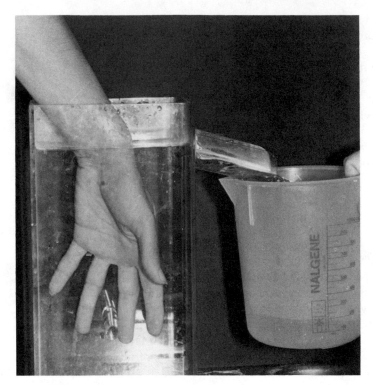

FIGURE 3–1. The volumeter measures edema by volume displacement. The patient submerges the hand until the dowel within the container rests in the web space between the third and fourth digits.

volume of edematous hands with the same examiner beyond 12 ml can therefore be considered significant.[11]

To obtain volumetric measurements with this volumeter, the patient submerges one hand at a time into the container until the web space between the third and fourth digits rests on a dowel within the container as illustrated in Figure 3–1. The displaced water flows out of a spout on the side of the container and is then measured in a graduated cylinder. Specific guidelines for test position and procedure are outlined in Appendix A.

Experience shows if only one digit or isolated joints are involved, the volumeter is not sensitive enough to monitor swelling. In addition, the volumeter does not measure volume proximal to the wrist. In this case, circumferential measurements using consistent and documented landmarks are more helpful. Standard tape measures may be used; tapes for measuring circumference are also commercially available.

Palpation

Relevant structures are palpated to determine variations in skin temperature and sweating; the consistency of subcutaneous tissue; the presence and location of hypersensitivity, muscle spasm, or trigger points; and any tenderness over tendons, tendon sheaths, tendon attachments, joint capsule, or fracture sites.

Range of Motion

MEASUREMENT METHODS

Range-of-motion measurements are based on a 0° position of the joint as a starting point in accordance with recommendations by the American Academy of Orthopaedic Surgeons (AAOS), in 1965.[13] The degree of motion is added in the direction the joint moves from this point and measured with a goniometer as an angle of extension and an angle of flexion. Flexion is recorded as a positive number; lack of extension, as a negative number. Extension of a digital joint beyond 0 is hyperextension and is recorded as a positive number.[14] For example, MP joint flexion of 75° and extension to 25° would be recorded as −25/75. MP joint flexion of 75° with hyperextension to 15° would be recorded as 15/75. A sample range-of-motion form is illustrated in Figure 3–2.

The method of assigning a plus or minus to angles representing lack of full extension or hyperextension has been somewhat controversial but the most recent revisions of the American Medical Association (AMA) Guide to the Evaluation of Permanent Impairment, with input from the American Society for Surgery of the Hand (ASSH), the American Society of Hand Therapists, and AAOS, recommend assigning a negative to lack of full extension and a positive to hyperextension. This approach will probably become the most accepted, consistent method.

INSTRUMENTS

The goniometer is not technically a standardized tool but it does provide reliable information for which norms have been established within a margin of error as small as 3° in the hands of the same evaluator following a standard procedure. Accuracy may be affected by the complexity of the joint being measured, active versus passive measurements, multiple examiners, and patient diagnosis.[15-25] Limited studies of various types of goniometers and lateral versus dorsal placement do not reveal any significant differences and are a matter of preference.[15] The critical point is that the goniometer axis should be in line with the joint axis and the arms parallel to the bones forming the joint and not influenced by bony prominences, swelling, or other interfering factors. Small metal goniometers with arms that have a broad, flat surface of contact are specifically designed for dorsal placement and are commercially available. Dorsal placement and the use of a small, clear plastic goniometer with the arms cut 1 to 2 in long for digital joints, and a larger goniometer for the wrist, with rounded ends is preferred by this author. The rounded ends fit the contour of the concave surface of the hand and forearm that is created when the wrist is dorsiflexed and allow dorsal placement of the goniometer. These goniometers can frequently be obtained as samples from pharmaceutic or therapy equipment companies, or they can be purchased from most therapy catalogs along with other types of goniometers.

ACTIVE RANGE OF MOTION

Active range of motion should be measured first as there is no need to measure passive joint mobility if active motion is within normal limits. Active motion reflects the presence and degree of joint irritability, the patient's willingness to move and the ability of the muscle-tendon unit to move the joint.

Right   **Left**   Name _____

Date	Active	Passive	Active	Passive	Active	Passive	Active	Passive	Active	Passive
SHLDR abd/flex										
ext/int rot										
ELBOW flex/ext										
WRIST flex/ext										
sup/pron										
rad/uln dev										
MPs Index										
Long										
Ring										
Little										
PIPs Index										
Long										
Ring										
Little										
DIPs Index										
Long										
Ring										
Little										
THUMB MP										
IP										
abd (°)										
ext (°)										
FWS (cm)										

		T	I	L	R	L	T	I	L	R	L	T	I	L	R	L	T	I	L	R	L	T	I	L	R	L
Distance	act																										
D.P.C.	pass																										
Intrinsic tightness																											
ORL tightness																											
Extr. flex. tightness																											
Extr. Ext. tightness																											
TAM	MP																										
	PIP																										
	DIP																										
Total																											
TPM	MP																										
	PIP																										
	DIP																										
Total																											

PS-6936

FIGURE 3–2. Sample range-of-motion form.

Active motion of the wrist in dorsiflexion, flexion, radial, and ulnar deviation and forearm pronation and supination is measured and recorded as described in Appendix B.

Range-of-motion measurements of the thumb should include the carpometacarpal (CMC), MP, and IP joints. Specific techniques are described in Appendix B. The CMC joint is measured in radial abduction, palmar abduction, and adduction, as described by the most recent edition of the AMA Guide to the Evaluation of Permanent Impairment and accepted by ASSH and AAOS. Another helpful measurement that is not standard is that of "functional web space,"[26] defined as the distance in centimeters between the radial border of the index proximal finger flexion crease and the ulnar border of the thumb IP flexion crease with the thumb moved actively away from the palm of the hand midway between palmar and radial abduction. This space is significant in that it is the available space that the patient has to get the hand around objects. Although not a structure-specific measurement, "web space" is a functional representation of the combined joint and soft tissue involved in achieving the position.

Active motion of each digital joint is measured as described in Appendix B. The proximal joints are supported at 0 to indicate the muscle-tendon's maximum ability to move the joint. Measurement of each individual joint but with all joints simultaneously flexed and then extended (composite motion) can also be measured as a more functional representation, as illustrated in Figure 3–3A,B. These two methods, which offer different information, may not be indicated for every patient. In the case of tendon adherence or muscle weakness, however, the differences noted in joint motion between these two methods may influence treatment decisions. For example, an adherent flexor digitorum profundus tendon just proximal to the MP joint may have adequate excursion to flex the DIP joint to 30° with the MP and PIP joints extended but may not have adequate excursion to flex the DIP joint to the same degree with the MP and PIP joints flexed. Treatment techniques in this case may involve specific positions of the MP and PIP joints for exercise or splinting to decrease the adherence of the tendon most effectively.

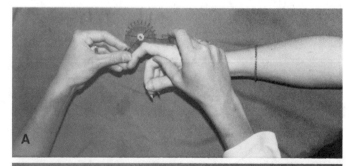
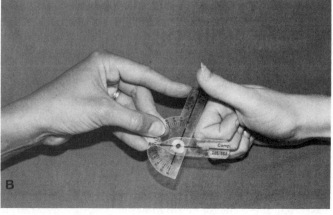

FIGURE 3–3. Active and passive range of motion can be measured with the proximal joints supported in 0° of extension (A) or with the joints simultaneously flexed and then extended (composite motion) (B).

PASSIVE RANGE OF MOTION

Passive motion, reflecting the maximum potential motion of the joint, is accomplished by positioning the adjacent joints to minimize any other soft tissue restrictions. A general rule is to support the proximal joints at 0 and to note any necessary deviations from this position. For example, in the presence of extrinsic extensor tightness maximum passive MP flexion may not be possible unless the wrist is dorsiflexed beyond the 0 position. To indicate the joint potential clearly in this case the wrist should be dorsiflexed, maximum MP joint flexion measured, and the position of wrist dorsiflexion also noted.

TOTAL ACTIVE MOTION/TOTAL PASSIVE MOTION

Full simultaneous flexion and extension of all digital joints as an indication of maximum muscle-tendon excursion is measured in terms of total active motion (TAM)

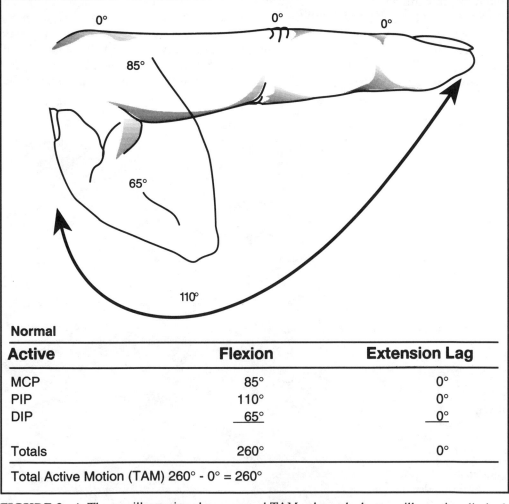

Normal

Active	Flexion	Extension Lag
MCP	85°	0°
PIP	110°	0°
DIP	65°	0°
Totals	260°	0°

Total Active Motion (TAM) 260° - 0° = 260°

FIGURE 3–4. The top illustration shows normal TAM values; the bottom illustration, limited TAM values.

and total passive motion (TPM) as recommended by the ASSH Clinical Assessment Committee, 1977.[27,28]

Total active motion is the sum of the angles formed by the MP, PIP, and DIP joints in simultaneous maximum active flexion, minus the total extension deficit at the MP, PIP, and DIP joints (including hyperextension at the IP joints) in maximum active extension. Hyperextension at the PIP or DIP joints is considered an abnormal value and is therefore included as a deficit (Fig. 3–4).

Total passive motion is the same as TAM but with passive force. A normal value for TAM and TPM in the absence of a normal contralateral digit for comparison is 260° based on 85° of MP motion, 110° of PIP motion, and 65° of DIP motion.

COMPARING ACTIVE AND PASSIVE MOTION

Comparison of active and passive motion indicates the efficiency of flexor and extensor excursion and/or degree of muscle strength within the available passive range

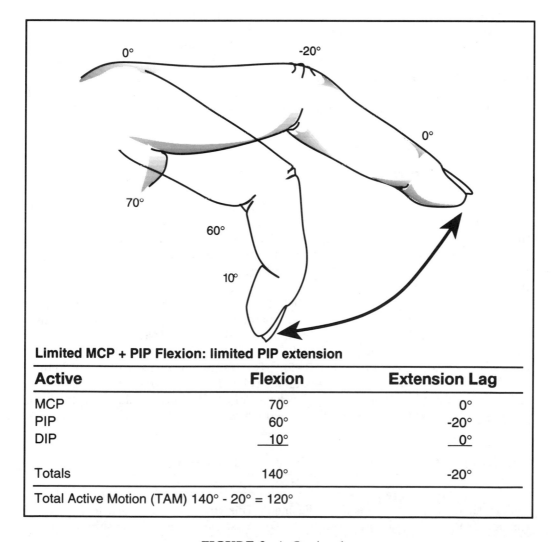

Limited MCP + PIP Flexion: limited PIP extension

Active	Flexion	Extension Lag
MCP	70°	0°
PIP	60°	-20°
DIP	10°	0°
Totals	140°	-20°

Total Active Motion (TAM) 140° - 20° = 120°

FIGURE 3–4. *Continued.*

of motion. In some cases greater passive than active motion may be noted in individual joint measurements with the adjacent joints in 0° extension. This finding suggests limited tendon glide due to adherence of the tendon to surrounding structures, relative lengthening of the tendon due to injury or surgical procedure, pathology, such as scarring within the muscle that limits muscle excursion, muscle weakness, or pain. Less obvious pathology not evident with individual joint measurements, where the proximal joints are supported in extension, may only be apparent with composite flexion or extension where greater muscle-tendon excursion and/or strength is required. In either case, flexor lag indicates the presence of greater passive than active flexion at a joint or joints, and extensor lag indicates the presence of greater passive than active extension. The presence, degree, and cause of flexor or extensor lag has a direct impact on treatment approach and technique.

DIFFERENTIAL DIAGNOSIS

The multitude of joints and multiarticular muscles that contribute to the positioning, precision, and power capabilities of the hand presents a complex puzzle of mobility. The hand's normally fluid motion may be affected by pathologic changes involving any number of soft tissue structures including the joint capsule, intrinsic muscles, oblique retinacular ligament, and extrinsic flexor or extensor muscles. Adherence, contracture, and painful conditions related to these inert and contractile tissue structures will result in dysfunction. Differentiation of the contributing factors will ultimately influence treatment decisions.

Intrinsic Tightness

As the interosseous and lumbrical muscles insert into the oblique fibers of the lateral bands and distally join the extensor mechanism, they cross the MP joint volar to the axis of rotation and the PIP joint dorsal to the axis of rotation. Both muscles are, therefore, maximally lengthened with the MP joint extended and the PIP joint simultaneously flexed. Conversely, they are in a slack position when the MP joint is flexed and the PIP joint extended.

To test for the presence of intrinsic tightness as described by Bunnell,[29] the MP joint is passively flexed and the PIP joint is simultaneously passively flexed. The MP joint is then passively extended and at the same time the PIP joint is passively flexed. If greater PIP flexion can be obtained with the MP joint flexed than with it extended, intrinsic contracture or adherence exists (Fig. 3–5).[30] The test is repeated with the MP joint in radial, then in ulnar, deviation to check for an isolated intrinsic contracture on either the radial or the ulnar aspect of the digit. The degree of PIP flexion with the MP extended is recorded as a measure of the degree of contracture.

Tightness of the Oblique Retinacular Ligament

Intrinsic contracture in the finger refers to contracture or adherence of the oblique retinacular ligament or Landsmeer's ligament. This structure runs volar to the axis of rotation of the PIP joint and dorsal to the DIP axis, making its relationship to the PIP

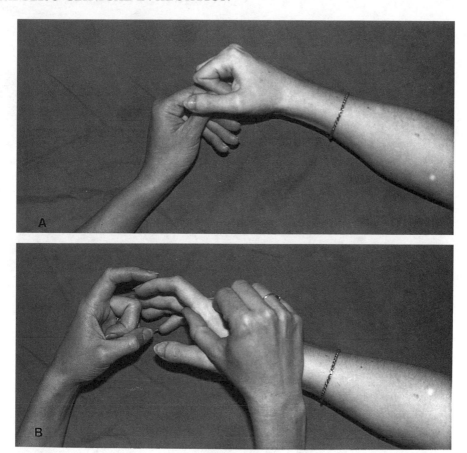

FIGURE 3–5. The result of the intrinsic tightness test is positive if greater passive PIP flexion is obtained with the MP passively flexed (*A*) than with the MP passively extended (*B*).

and DIP joints essentially the same as the intrinsics' relationship to the MP and PIP joints.[31] The test for contracture is therefore the same, only at the PIP and DIP joint level. The PIP and DIP joints are passively flexed. The PIP joint is then passively extended and the DIP joint passively flexed. Contracture of the oblique retinacular ligament is present if greater DIP flexion is obtained with the PIP joint flexed than with the PIP joint extended (Fig. 3–6A,B). The degree of DIP flexion with the PIP joint extended is measured and recorded.

Tightness of the Extrinsic Flexor and Extensor Tendons

Adherence or contracture of the extrinsic flexors is detected by passively maintaining the fingers and thumb in full extension while passively dorsiflexing the wrist. In the presence of flexor tightness, the increasing flexor tension that develops as the wrist is passively dorsiflexed will pull the fingers into flexion (Fig. 3–7,A). At the point when this tension is first detected by the evaluator, the position of the wrist is measured and recorded to indicate the degree of restriction.

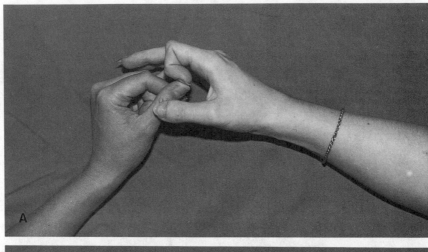

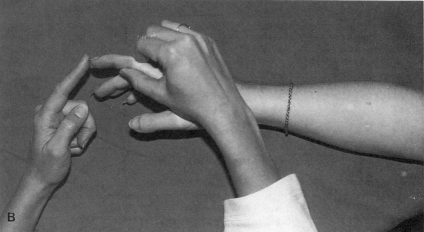

FIGURE 3–6. The result of the oblique retinacular ligament (Landsmeer's ligament) test is positive if greater passive DIP flexion is obtained with the PIP passively flexed (*A*) than with the PIP passively extended (*B*).

Flexor restrictions may also occur distal to the wrist, in which case the position of the wrist will not affect tendon tension. To test for suspected flexor restriction distal to the wrist, the MP joint is passively extended while the PIP and DIP joints are passively maintained in extension. The angle at the MP joint is measured when flexor tension is first detected.

Detection of extrinsic extensor tightness is simply a reverse process. The digits are passively maintained in full flexion while the wrist is passively flexed. If tension pulling the fingers into extension is detected by the examiner's hand as the wrist is brought into flexion, extrinsic extensor tightness exists. The position of the wrist when extensor tension is first detected is measured and recorded (Fig. 3–7,*B*).

As is true of the flexors, extensor restrictions can also occur distal to the wrist, producing a different pattern. To test for extensor tightness distal to the wrist, the PIP and DIP joints are maintained in passive flexion as the MP joint is passively flexed. The position of the MP joint is measured at the point extensor tension is first detected.

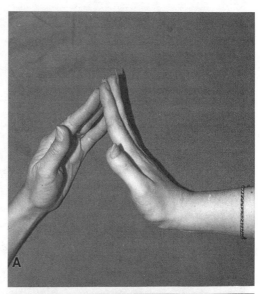

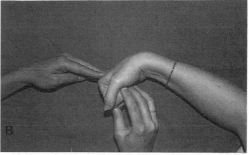

FIGURE 3–7. *A*, Extrinsic flexor tightness can be measured by passively extending the fingers, then dorsiflexing the wrist and noting the position of the wrist when tension is first detected in the flexors. *B*, Extrinsic extensor tightness can be measured by passively flexing the fingers, then passively flexing the wrist and noting the position of the wrist when tension is first detected in the extensors.

SELECTIVE TISSUE TENSION TESTING

Selective tissue tension testing helps to differentiate the source of dysfunction, particularly when pain is part of the primary complaint. Selective tissue tension testing involves the selective application of tension to specific inert and contractile structures through active, passive, and resistive movements.[32] Active movements, as mentioned earlier, demonstrate the degree of joint irritability (pain), the patient's willingness to move, and muscle-tendon action on the joint. Passive movements apply tension to inert structures (such as joint capsule and ligaments), which normally serve to allow, limit, and guide movement. Resistive movements (isometric contractions) test the contractile structures for irritability and ability to develop and sustain tension with minimal involvement of insert structures.

Inert Structure Assessment

"END FEEL"

The passive restraint or "end feel" perceived by the examiner at the passive end range of a normal joint has a slightly elastic quality. The "end feel" associated with an

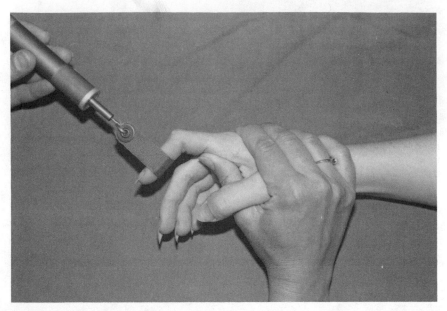

FIGURE 3–8. Torque angle can be measured using a thick string or loop attached to the distal end of a Haldex orthotic gauge and looped around a consistent point of the digit distal to the axis of the joint being measured. A specific force is applied toward extension at a right angle to the segment being moved. To measure flexion, a pencil eraser tip can be attached to the gauge and force applied toward flexion.

unyielding joint capsule contracture is more abrupt, having little or no elasticity. A bony block produces a very abrupt, hard "end feel." A very elastic "end feel" through a greater range may be related to swelling around the joint. Reported pain or muscle guarding perceived before reaching a definite joint "end feel" may indicate that joint capsule or other soft tissue irritability is limiting passive range prior to actual joint capsule contracture.

TORQUE RANGE OF MOTION

Brand[33] suggests a further step in quantifying the degree and type of passive tissue restraint by torque angle measurements. Torque angle measurements involve applying known forces at a constant distance from the joint with the proximal joints in a consistent position (Fig. 3–8). One torque angle refers to the resultant joint angle measurement at a specific force. Torque angle measurements refer to the resultant angles obtained with different levels of force. A torque angle curve is a line plot of the torque angle measurements of a joint and reveals the viscoelasticity of the joint's restraining tissue (Fig. 3–9).[33]

COLLATERAL LIGAMENTS

Radial and ulnar collateral ligament stress tests at the wrist, MP, and IP joints detect any joint instability due to ligamentous laxity or disruption. Stress tests are performed by stabilizing the proximal bone forming the joint and applying lateral stress to the distal bone forming the joint. Less significant ligamentous injury may result in localized

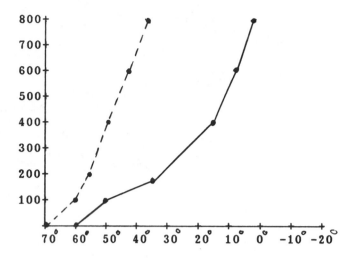

FIGURE 3–9. Torque angle curve. *Solid line* is the curve for a normal PIP joint; *dotted line* is the curve for a PIP joint with flexion contracture. The steeper curve of the dotted line shows that, for the joint with flexion contracture, increases in force produce less change in the joint angle.

pain and tenderness over the ligament with motion and stress testing, even though stability is not affected.

Contractile Structure Assessment

Passive movement may also be used to stress a contractile structure by applying force in a direction opposite to the muscle action to assess its irritability and extensibility. For example, Finklestein's test for tenosynovitis in the first dorsal wrist compartment involves full flexion of the thumb CMC, MP, and IP combined with ulnar deviation of the wrist to stress the abductor pollicis longus and extensor pollicis brevis tendons.[34,35] Reproduction of pain in this position indicates irritation of the stressed structures.

As previously mentioned, isometric contractions of isolated muscles or muscle groups test contractile structure for irritability and ability to develop and sustain tension with minimal involvement of inert structures. Reproduction of pain with isometric testing may indicate pathology such as tendonitis in the contractile unit.

The integration of all the information accumulated through these various tests should lead to identification of the restricting factors. Potential restrictions to hand mobility and the pattern each manifests is summarized in Table 3–4. Inconsistencies among test results should lead the examiner to look more closely at the patient's degree of effort. To clarify the results one may need to retest areas or pursue further testing.

STRENGTH

Testing of muscle group strength was included as part of the upper-quarter screening to identify gross weakness or imbalance for each upper extremity joint motion. Manual muscle testing of individual muscles is intended to identify more specifically the strength level of each muscle. Individual muscle testing is indicated when weakness or imbalance is found with gross testing; in the case of suspected neurologic involvement; in sequential evaluations to detect reinnervation following nerve injury, repair, or decompression; and for assessment before and after tendon transfers.

TABLE 3–4 Differential Diagnosis (Mobility)

Etiology	Manifested Pattern (Passive Motion)
Intrinsic tightness	Less PIP flexion with MP extended
Oblique retinacular ligament tightness	Less DIP flexion with PIP extended
Extrinsic extensor tightness	Proximal: Less MP/IP flexion with wrist flexed
	Distal: Less IP flexion with MP flexed
Extrinsic flexor tightness	Proximal: Less MP/IP extension with wrist extended
	Distal: Less IP extension with MP extended
Joint capsule	Adjacent joint position does not affect joint motion; elastic or hard "end feel"

Specific Muscle Testing

Muscles activating the wrist and hand include those innervated by the radial, median, and ulnar nerves. This section of the chapter focuses on clarifying techniques for palpation and testing of those muscles innervated by the radial nerve, the median nerve, and the ulnar nerve. Surface tendon relationships at the wrist have been emphasized because tendons of the muscles of the wrist and hand can often be more easily isolated for palpation than the muscle bellies.

Muscles innervated by the radial nerve include the extensor carpi radialis longus (ECRL), extensor carpi radialis brevis (ECRB), extensor carpi ulnaris (ECU), extensor digitorum communis (EDC), extensor digiti quinti (EDQ), extensor indicis proprius (EIP), extensor pollicis longus (EPL), extensor pollicis brevis (EPB), and abductor pollicis longus (APL). Because the EPL tendon crosses the ECRL tendon at the wrist, the palpating finger is placed ulnar to the EPL to slide the tendon radially. The ECRL tendon can then be palpated proximal to the second metacarpal as the patient dorsiflexes the wrist, as shown in Figure 3–10. Because of the lateral position of the ECU tendon as it inserts into the ulnar side of the fifth metacarpal, the ECU acts primarily as an ulnar deviator of the wrist with the forearm in pronation. The ECU tendon can best be palpated, as illustrated in Figure 3–11, just proximal and ulnar to the fifth metacarpal during ulnar deviation of the wrist. ECRL, ECRB, and ECU when all three are functioning are difficult to isolate and individually grade; however, dorsiflexion as a motion can be graded. Also, if one or more of these muscles is weak, some imbalance may be

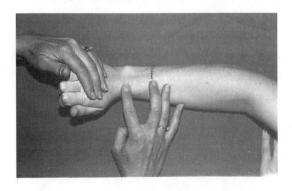

FIGURE 3–10. Palpation of the ECRL tendon.

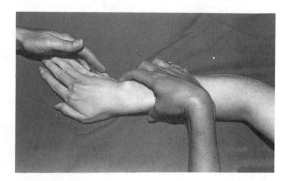

FIGURE 3–11. Palpation of the ECU tendon.

observed in a radial or ulnar direction during dorsiflexion and associated imbalance toward flexion during radial and ulnar deviation.

The EDC tendons to the index, long, and ring fingers can be palpated as they pass over their respective metacarpals, as shown in Figure 3–12. The EDC to the little finger is at times not present or exists as a slip from the ring finger EDC. The EDQ tendon can be palpated over the fifth metacarpal and the EIP tendon just ulnar to the index EDC tendon, as illustrated in Figure 3–13. Examination of each extensor tendon is important as ruptures or lacerations can be subtle. A laceration proximal to the juncturae tendinae involving the extensor of either the long or the little finger may not produce any evident loss of extension at the MP joint. Because of the tendinous connections of the juncturae tendinae, MP extension of the injured digits can still occur if the EDC tendon of the ring is intact. Because the little EDC tendon alone can fully extend the MP joint, disruptions of the EDQ tendon can also be overlooked unless the tendon is palpated. An EDQ tendon laceration can also be noted when extension of the little MP joint is weak against resistance. The same is true for interruption of the index EDC tendon or EIP tendon either of which could still extend the index MP joint independently.

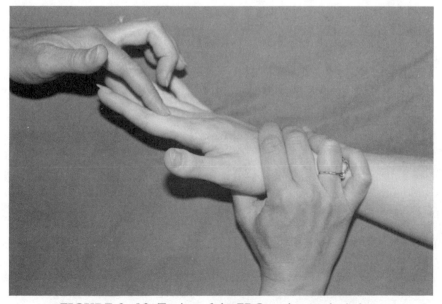

FIGURE 3–12. Testing of the EDC tendon to the index.

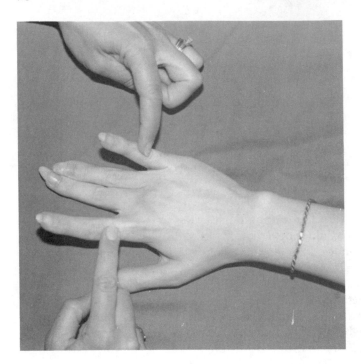

FIGURE 3–13. Testing of the EDQ and EIP tendons.

The EPL tendon can be palpated on the ulnar border of the anatomic snuffbox at the wrist and along its course to the distal phalanx of the thumb. The EPL is the only muscle capable of bringing the thumb CMC joint fully into the plane of the palm. Careful palpation and testing of the EPL tendon is particularly important because IP extension can also be accomplished by the intrinsic muscles to the thumb via their insertion into the extensor mechanism.

The APL tendon can be palpated at the base of the thumb metacarpal on the radial border of the wrist, as depicted in Figure 3–14. The EPB tendon can be palpated just dorsal to the APL as the thumb is brought into a position midway between radial and palmar abduction (Fig. 3–15).

Median innervated muscles include the flexor carpi radialis (FCR), palmaris longus (PL), flexor digitorum profundus (FDP), flexor digitorum superficialis (FDS), lumbricales

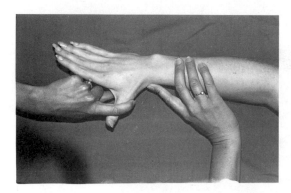

FIGURE 3–14. Palpation of the APL tendon.

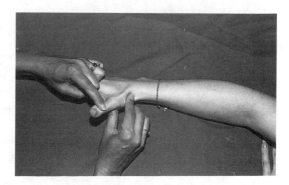

FIGURE 3–15. Palpation of the EPB tendon.

to the index and long, flexor pollicis longus (FPL), abductor pollicis brevis (APB), $\frac{1}{2}$ flexor pollicis brevis ($\frac{1}{2}$ FPB), and the opponens pollicis (OP).

The FCR with insertions into the second and third metacarpal bases is palpated volarly, radial to the midline of the wrist as the patient flexes the wrist. The PL tendon can be palpated just ulnar to the FCR tendon as the patient cups the palm and flexes the wrist simultaneously, as demonstrated in Figure 3–16.

Testing for the FDP is accomplished by stabilizing the wrist in neutral and the PIP joint in extension (Fig. 3–17). Substitution can occur with the wrist in extension and a tenodesis action. When testing the FDS the wrist is stabilized in neutral and the fingers not being tested are held in extension, as shown in Figure 3–18. Careful stabilization of the fingers in extension is important so as to prevent flexion of the DIP joints and substitution by the FDP. As with the FDP substitution can also occur with the tenodesis action. The FPL is tested by stabilizing the wrist in neutral and the MP joint in extension

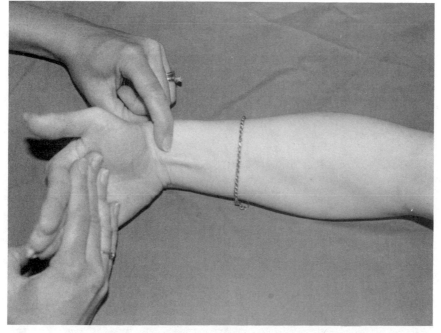

FIGURE 3–16. Palpation of the PL tendon.

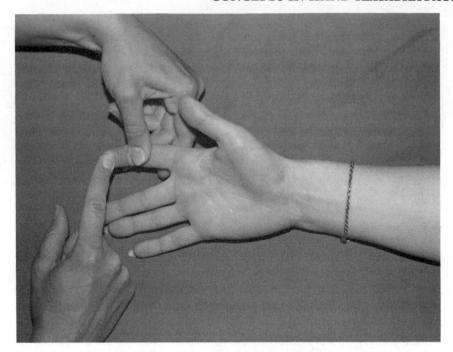

FIGURE 3–17. Testing for the FDP.

(Fig. 3–19). The median innervated lumbricales are discussed with the ulnar innervated lumbricales.

The APB muscle can best be palpated over the thenar eminence medial to the thumb metacarpal during palmar abduction of the thumb (Fig. 3–20). The OP muscle belly is palpated just radial to the APB next to the thumb metacarpal as the thumb is

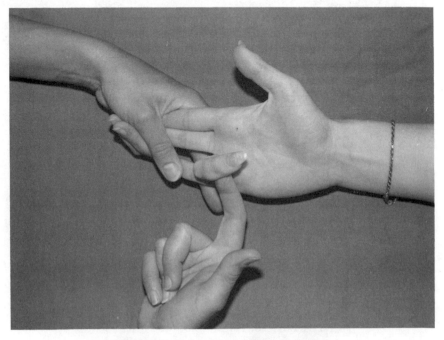

FIGURE 3–18. Testing for the FDS.

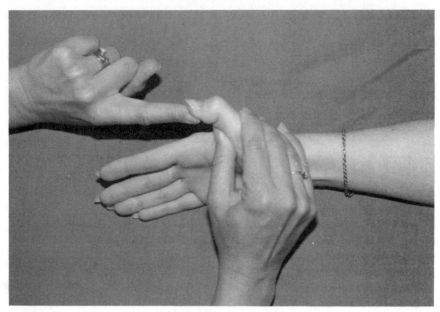

FIGURE 3–19. Testing for the FPL.

pronated for opposition, as shown in Figure 3–21. The FPB is palpated just distal to the APB. The function of FPB is difficult to isolate due to FPL substitution and dual median and ulnar nerves innervation.

Muscles innervated by the ulnar nerve include the flexor carpis ulnaris (FCU), flexor digitorum profundus (FDP) to the ring and little, the lumbricales to the ring and little, the four dorsal and three palmar interossei, the flexor digiti minimi (FDM),

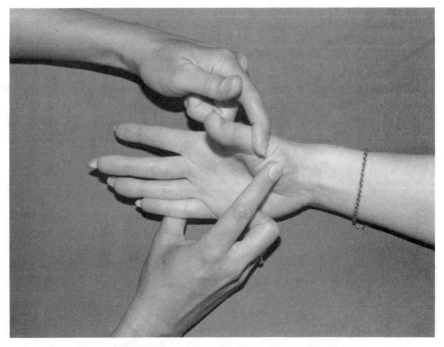

FIGURE 3–20. Palpation of the APB.

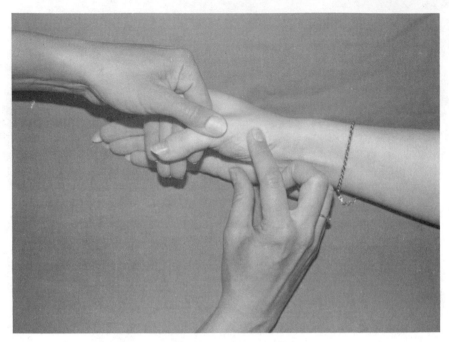

FIGURE 3–21. Palpation of the OP.

abductor digiti minimi (ADM), opponens digiti minimi (ODM), adductor pollicis, and $\frac{1}{2}$ flexor pollicis brevis ($\frac{1}{2}$ FPB).

The FCU is the strongest wrist flexor. The FCU tendon can be palpated just proximal to the pisiform on the volar aspect of the wrist as the wrist is actively flexed. Testing for the FDP to the ring and little fingers is the same as testing for the index and middle fingers, as described earlier.

The lumbricales, both median and ulnar nerves innervated, are difficult to test because they cannot be palpated easily. In addition, because the lumbricales function as MP flexors and IP extensors they cannot be isolated in the presence of the long flexor, extensor, and interossei function.

Intrinsic extension of the IP joint, by the combined action of the interossei and lumbricales, can be evaluated by supporting the wrist in dorsiflexion and the MP joint in hyperextension and asking the patient to extend the IP joint as demonstrated in Figure 3–22. Hyperextension of the MP joint reduces the mechanical advantage of the long extensors distally so that IP extension is primarily accomplished by the intrinsics. Although this position does not isolate individual muscles, it can help detect weakness or absence of intrinsic function as indicated by the presence of extensor lag or strength variation among fingers.

The palmar and dorsal interossei are tested for adduction and abduction, respectively (Figs. 3–23, 3–24). The fingers are placed on a flat surface to minimize flexor substitution for adduction and extensor substitution for abduction. The first dorsal interosseous can be isolated and palpated by having the patient abduct the index finger with the MP joint slightly flexed to avoid extensor substitution. The muscle belly of the first dorsal interosseous is palpated on the radial side of the index finger proximal to the metacarpal head, as depicted in Figure 3–25.

The hypothenar muscles consisting of the FDM, ADM, and ODM are tested as a

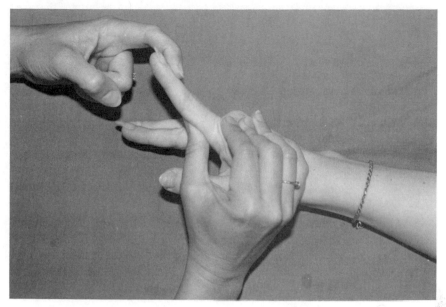

FIGURE 3–22. Evaluation of intrinsic extension of the IP joint.

unit because they are difficult to palpate individually. The hypothenar muscles are all active during flexion, abduction, and opposition of the fifth metacarpal and MP joint flexion and abduction. The muscle bellies are palpated along the midulnar border of the hand while the patient abducts the little finger with the MP joint slightly flexed (Fig. 3–26). This position avoids extensor substitution.

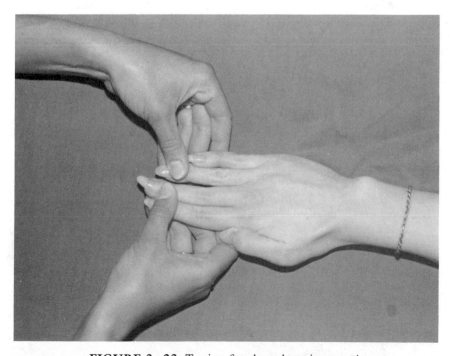

FIGURE 3–23. Testing for the palmar interossei.

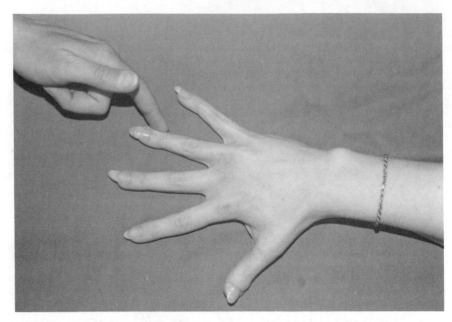

FIGURE 3–24. Testing for the dorsal interossei.

The adductor pollicis (ADD.P) can be most directly palpated dorsally, proximal to the first dorsal interosseous between the first and second metacarpals as the thumb is actively adducted (Fig. 3–27).

Substitution by the EPL or FPL can be eliminated or at least detected by holding the thumb IP joint in the direction opposite that of the substituting muscle while palpating the adductor muscle.

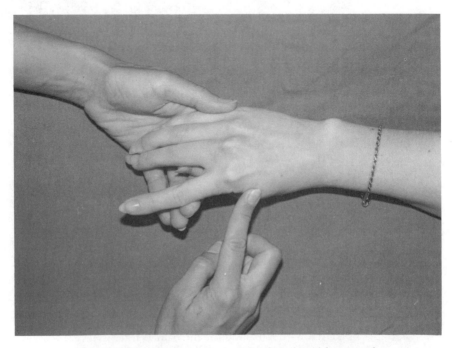

FIGURE 3–25. Palpation of the first dorsal interossei.

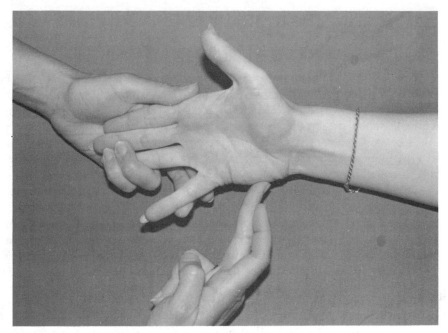

FIGURE 3–26. Palpation of the hypothenar muscles.

This section has provided an overview of muscle palpation and testing techniques for the muscles influencing the wrist and hand. For more specific information, the reader is encouraged to review the bibliography for additional resources on palpation and manual muscle testing.

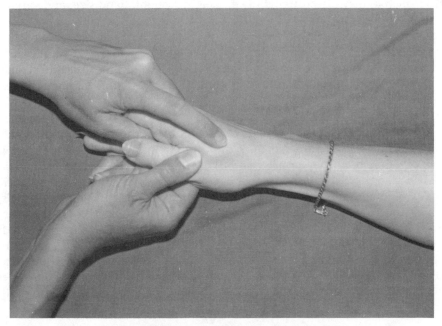

FIGURE 3–27. Palpation of the ADD.P.

Functional Strength

Grip and pinch strength represents the interaction and combined strength of the intrinsic and extrinsic muscles of the wrist and hand.

Recent studies by Mathiowetz and associates[36,37] demonstrated that the Jamar Dynamometer (± 3 percent callibration accuracy) by Asimow Engineering and the B&L Pinch Gauge (± 1 percent callibration accuracy) are the most accurate instruments available when callibration is maintained for measurement of grip and pinch strength. Using these instruments and standardized testing procedures, inter-rater reliability tests resulted in a correlation coefficient of .97. Test-retest reliability revealed the highest correlation coefficients were achieved with the mean of three trials (.80 or above). Lowest correlations were found with one trial. Subsequently, norms were established using these instruments and standardized testing procedures.[38,40] The Jamar Dynamometer measures grip strength in five different diameters; the first position is the smallest, the fifth position is the largest. Norms were developed for grip in the second position of the dynamometer, thumb pulp to index and long pulp pinch (palmar pinch), thumb pulp to lateral index pinch (lateral) and thumb tip to index tip pinch (tip pinch).

In all grip and pinch strength positions the mean right-hand score was greater overall than the mean left-hand score, regardless of hand dominance with the mean difference between the right and left hands being 11 percent for men and 14 percent for women. For these reasons and because of the low number of left hand–dominant subjects, norms were combined for right and left hand–dominant subjects. The contralateral hand is probably a closer standard for comparison than the norms unless both sides are involved. Differences between the right and left can be expressed as a percentage deficit. For example, 40 lb grip strength in the second position on the right hand compared with 100 lb on the left could be expressed as right-hand strength of approximately 40 percent compared with the left, or a 60 percent deficit.

Previous studies,[41-44] though not all using standardized testing procedures, indicated other factors may affect strength (e.g., height, weight, hand size, and variation in time of day).

In the normal hand, grip strength will vary with each of the five handle positions. The first position grip has been shown to be the weakest, followed by the fifth and fourth. Maximum grip strength usually occurs with the handle in the second position for women and the third position for men. Plotting all five positions on a graph creates a bell-shaped curve.

In the injured hand, grip testing in all five positions of the Dynamometer is indicated in situations when the average of three trials in the second position may not reveal the entire picture. In some cases this testing may validly result in a linear relationship rather than the normal bell curve. Absence of the bell curve should not necessarily be interpreted as lack of maximum effort. However, if three repeated trials in the same position reveal greater than 10 to 20 percent variation between trials, the patient may not be exhibiting maximum effort.[40] Results should be examined for consistency with other tests. For example, intrinsic weakness or limited finger flexion due to joint contracture may allow relatively normal strength in the larger handle positions but diminished strength in smaller diameter positions. The contralateral hand can again be used for comparison. Adequate norms are not available for all five positions. Testing positions, standard procedure, and available norms for grip and pinch strength are presented in Appendix C.

CIRCULATION

Circulatory impairment may contribute to cold intolerance, edema, and pain in the hand. Bluish, mottled, or pale discoloration of the hand may be present with vascular impairment due to peripheral causes or altered sympathetic response. Differences in skin temperature can be quickly assessed with the dorsum of the examiner's hand or with a temperature probe, and compared with the contralateral side. Clinically, circulation can be tested by palpation of the radial and ulnar pulses at the wrist and with the Allen test.[45]

The Allen test is performed by occluding the radial and ulnar arteries at the wrist using the evaluator's thumbs, while the patient quickly flexes and extends the fingers several times. The patient then relaxes the hand and one artery is released. The speed of refilling of the hand is noted. Refilling is indicated by return of color, and speed is quantified in terms of seconds or described as being quick, slow, or absent. The test is repeated, releasing the opposite artery.

The Allen test can also be performed on each digit.[46] The radial and ulnar digital arteries are milked proximally from the fingertips by the evaluator's thumbs, then released one at a time, while observing for filling of the finger. Lack of refilling when an artery is released is indicative of circulatory impairment involving that vessel.

NERVE COMPRESSION

Compression lesions distal to the arm may involve the radial, ulnar, or median nerve. Compression syndromes involving the median nerve include carpal tunnel, pronator syndrome, and anterior interosseous syndrome; radial nerve compression includes posterior interosseous syndrome and superficial radial nerve entrapment; and the ulnar nerve may be compressed in the canal of Guyon or in the cubital tunnel. In addition to specific muscle and sensibility testing, other provocative tests can help to identify various nerve compression syndromes.

Provocative tests for carpal tunnel syndrome include Phalen's[47] test and Tinel's sign.[48,49] Phalen's test is performed by passively flexing the wrist and holding it for 30 seconds. Reproduction of numbness or tingling in the median distribution is considered a positive test result. Reverse Phalen's testing is performed by passively dorsiflexing the wrist; results are positive if symptoms are reproduced.

Tinel's sign is produced by gentle percussion from distal to proximal along the nerve trunk. A true Tinel's sign is indicative of regenerating sensory axons and is positive at the most distal point that the patient perceives a tingling sensation that radiates distally in the distribution of the nerve. However, Tinel's sign may also be elicited at the site of a nerve compression.

Pronator syndrome may be characterized by pain in the forearm on resistance to pronation and flexion of the long and ring finger flexor digitorum superficialis. Tinel's sign may also be present at the site of compression.

There are usually no sensory abnormalities with anterior interosseous compression or posterior interosseous syndrome but muscle weakness or paralysis may be observed in the motor distribution of the nerve.

Superficial radial nerve compression is characterized by pain along the radial forearm with possibly Tinel's sign at the site of compression and hypesthesia in the distribution of the nerve.

Ulnar nerve compression at the canal of Guyon or cubital tunnel may be associated with a positive Tinel's sign at the site of compression and possibly also muscle weakness, depending on the severity of compression. Cubital tunnel compression pain and sensory symptoms may also be reproduced by full elbow flexion.

ASSESSMENT OF CLINICAL FINDINGS

The information obtained from the history and physical examination should fit together to form a picture of the nature and origin of the patient's dysfunction. A schematic example with significant findings highlighted is presented in Table 3–5. The history includes patient report and medical records indicating a crush injury to the right volar distal forearm with laceration and subsequent repair of the flexor digitorum profundus and flexor digitorum superficialis tendons to the long and ring fingers 5 weeks before the initial therapy visit.

Significant findings included the dense, adherent nature of the volar wrist scar, limited wrist dorsiflexion, the presence of long and ring finger flexor lag, the difference between the degree of active flexion with the proximal joints flexed versus extended, the presence of flexor tightness and minimal independent flexor digitorum superficialis function.

Assessment of information from the history and physical examination indicated that the limitations were primarily due to flexor adherence or tightness in the volar distal forearm in the area of injury and repair with possible secondary flexor weakness and volar capsule restrictions at the wrist joint. The existence of flexor weakness and volar wrist capsule restriction can be more accurately assessed once the flexor tightness and scar adherence begins to resolve.

Inconsistencies among components of the evaluation or between the history and physical examination should alert the therapist to possible errors or oversights and stimulate a closer look at psychosocial factors that may have influenced the patient's responses. Consultation with a counselor or psychologist can be helpful in identifying psychosocial or psychological issues that may interfere with successful rehabilitation.

IMPLICATIONS FOR TREATMENT

Assessment of the evaluation findings provides a basis for treatment. For example, a patient reported his problem to be swelling, stiffness, and soreness in the left-hand PIP joints during attempts to make a fist, following a distal radius fracture 2 months earlier. He further stated, and medical records confirmed, that he was casted for 6 weeks, during which time he reported swelling and inability to move his fingers fully. Objective examination revealed a swollen hand and wrist (555 ml on the right, 660 ml on the left by volumetric testing).

Measurement of joint mobility revealed capsular restrictions at the MP and PIP joints, limiting flexion to 50° at the MP joints and 90° at the PIP joints. Extrinsic flexor tightness was also demonstrated as the wrist was moved beyond 10° of dorsiflexion. Intrinsic tightness was present in the long and ring fingers such that, with the MP joints extended, the PIP joints could be flexed to only 45° as opposed to 90° with the MP joints flexed.

The patient's functional inability to make a fist and fully extend the digits and the PIP soreness appeared related to several factors that require specific variations in

TABLE 3–5 Assessment of Clinical Findings

Test	Findings
Upper-quarter screening	Within normal limits (WNL) at and proximal to the elbow
Forearm/wrist/hand observations	Well-healed incision with slightly elevated 4-in scar over volar wrist and forearm
Skin/scar	Scar was dense, adherent, and blanched with passive extension of wrist and digits
Volume	Injured right 650 ml; left 640 ml
Range of motion: Active and passive	
Wrist	20° dorsiflexion active and passive; otherwise WNL
Digits	
Thumb, Index, Little	WNL actively with wrist at 0°.
Long, Ring	MP joints
	WNL actively, passive PIP and DIP flexion WNL, PIP and DIP joint extension WNL, actively; PIP flexion 80° actively, DIP flexion 20° actively with proximal joints at 0; Composite flexion 40° PIP, 5° DIP; passive flexion WNL all joints
Intrinsic tightness	Negative
ORL tightness	Negative
Extensor tightness	Negative
Flexor tightness	Flexor tension all fingers beyond 5° wrist dorsiflexion
Strength	Deferred due to recent repairs; all muscles noted to be functioning with active testing; only 10° PIP flexion with independent FDS testing with "pulling" noted along length of scar
Sensibility	WNL
Circulation	WNL

treatment. The swelling must be initially controlled to allow other mobilization techniques to be most effective. Correction of the extrinsic flexor tightness and limited excursion is dependent on stretching the wrist and fingers simultaneously toward extension. Correction of the MP and PIP joint flexion limitations requires application of forces directed specifically to the capsular structures through exercise or splinting or both. Correction of the intrinsic tightness requires exercise and splinting in a position that combines MP extension and PIP flexion to lengthen the intrinsics maximally.

The general observation of the patient's inability to flex and extend the fingers fully in no way fully delineates the source of his dysfunction. By identifying specifics, treatment can be specific and more effective. More general treatment activities involving various patterns of hand use can still be integrated but must be modified to focus on improving structural limitations.

Evaluation and assessment are ongoing during treatment. In the words of Nancy Watts,[50] "As the patient's response is seen and felt, we adjust the pressure of our hands, the tone of our voice, or the speed of the movement in order to modify or maintain the patient's response and to shape it into the pattern we seek. At such moments, evaluation and treatment occur almost simultaneously in a circuit that links our performance to that of the patient. This is one of the skills we speak of as the 'art of clinical practice'."

Rigid treatment protocols destroy the art and science of clinical practice. Treatment guidelines should be specific enough to manage standard situations, broad enough to encompass the common exceptions and flexible enough to allow separate decisions for unusual cases.

SUMMARY

A systematic approach to the evaluation of the hand and upper extremity is presented in this chapter. General as well as specific components of a comprehensive hand evaluation must be considered. Differential diagnosis, selective tissue tension testing, evaluation of circulation, and provocative tests for nerve compression are also important. Clinical findings and the implications for treatment must be assessed.

Although the process may seem tedious initially, experience will allow the examiner quickly to screen uninvolved areas and efficiently to evaluate areas requiring greater attention. Information derived from the evaluation can then be integrated to achieve the best plan of care for each individual patient.

REFERENCES

1. Feinstein, A: Scientific methodology in clinical medicine: I. Introduction, principles and concepts. Ann Intern Med 61:564, 1984.
2. Feinstein, A: Scientific methodology in clinical medicine: IV. Acquisition of clinical data. Ann Intern Med 61:1162, 1964.
3. Feinstein, A: Clinical Epidemiology: The Architecture of Clinical Research. WB Saunders, Philadelphia, 1985.
4. Feinstein, A: An additional basic science for clinical medicine: IV. The development of clinimetrics. Ann Intern Med 99:843, 1983.
5. Rothstein, JM: On defining subjective and objective measurements. Phys Ther 69:577, 1989.
6. Peacock, EE: Biological principles in the healing of log tendons. Surg Clin North Am 45:2, 1965.
7. Panel Discussion 1: Tendon healing. In Hunter, JM, Schneider, LH, and Mackin, EJ (eds): Tendon Surgery in the Hand. CV Mosby, St Louis, 1987.
8. Banes, AJ, et al: Effects of trauma and partial devascularization on protein synthesis in the avian flexor profundus tendon. J Trauma 21(7):505, 1981.
9. Amadio, PC and Hunter, JM: Prognostic factors in flexor tendon surgery in zone 2. In Hunter, JM, Schneider, LH, and Mackin, EJ (eds): Tendon Surgery in the Hand. CV Mosby, St Louis, 1987.
10. Hoppenfeld, S: Physical Examination of the Spine and Extremities. Appleton-Century-Crofts, New York, 1976.
11. Waylett-Rendall, J and Seibly, D: A study of the accuracy of a commercially available volumeter. J Hand Ther 4:10, 1991.
12. Brand, P and Wood, H: Hand volumeter instruction sheet. US Public Health Service Hospital, Carville, LA.
13. American Academy of Orthopedic Surgeons: Joint motion: Method of measuring and recording. AAOS, Chicago, 1965.
14. Swanson, AB, Goran-Hagert, C, and Swanson, G: Evaluation of impairment of hand function. In Hunter, JM, et al (eds): Rehabilitation of the Hand. CV Mosby, St Louis, 1978.
15. Hillenbrandt, FA, Duvall, EN, and Moore, ML: The measurement of joint motion. III. Reliability of goniometry. Phys Ther Rev 29:302, 1949.
16. Low, LJ: The reliability of joint measurement. Physiotherapy 62:227, 1976.
17. Salter, N: Methods of measurements of muscle and joint functions. J Bone Joint Surg 37B:474, 1955.
18. Boone, DC: Reliability of goniometric measurements. Phys Ther 58:1355, 1978.
19. Amis, AA and Miller, JH: The elbow. Clin Rheum Dis 8:571, 1982.
20. Bird, HA and Stowe, J: The wrist. Clin Rheum Dis 8:559, 1982.
21. Wagner, C: Determination of the rotary flexibility of the elbow joint. Eur J Appl Physiol 37:47, 1977.
22. Hamilton, GF and Lachenbruch, PA: The reliability of goniometry in assessing finger joint angle. Phys Ther 49:465, 1969.
23. Hurt, SP: Considerations in muscle function and their application to disability evaluation and treatment. Am J Occup Ther 1:69, 1947.
24. Hurt, SP: Considerations in muscle function and their application to disability evaluation and treatment. Part I, Am J Occup Ther 1:209, 1947.

25. Hurt, SP: Considerations in muscle function and their application to disability evaluation and treatment: Joint measurement. Part II. Am J Occup Ther 1:281, 1947.
26. Colditz, J: Personal communication.
27. American Society for Surgery of the Hand: Clinical Assessment Committee Report. Presented March 10, 1976.
28. Strickland, JW: Results of flexor tendon surgery in zone II. Hand Clin 1 (1):1985.
29. Bunnell, S: Ischaemic contracture, local, in the hand. J Bone Joint Surg 35A:88, 1953.
30. Smith, R: Non-ischemic contractures of the intrinsic muscles of the hand. J Bone Joint Surg 53A:1313, 1971.
31. Zancolli, E: Structural and dynamic basis of hand surgery. JB Lippincott, Philadelphia, 1968, p 136.
32. Cyriax, J: Textbook of Orthopaedic Medicine. Vol I: Diagnosis of Soft Tissue Lesions. Williams & Wilkins, Baltimore, 1975.
33. Bell-Krotoski, BA, Berger, DE, and Beach, RB: Application of biomechanics for evaluation of the hand. In Hunter, JM, et al (eds): Rehabilitation of the Hand: Surgery and Therapy. CV Mosby, St Louis, 1990, p 139.
34. Cailliet, R: Hand Pain and Impairment. FA Davis, Philadelphia, 1982.
35. Kilgore, E and Graham, W: The hand-surgical and non-surgical management. Lea & Febiger, Philadelphia, 1977.
36. Mathiowetz, V, et al: Reliability and validity of grip and pinch strength evaluations. J Hand Surg 9A:222, 1984.
37. Mathiowetz, V, et al: Grip and pinch strength: Normative data for adults. Arch Phys Med Rehabil 66:72, 1985.
38. Fess, EE: The effects of Jamar Dynamometer handle position and test protocol on normal grip strength. Procedures of the American Society of Hand Therapists. J Hand Surg 7:308, 1982.
39. Smith, RO and Benge, MW: Pinch and grasp strength: Standardization of terminology and protocol. Am J Occup Ther 39(8):531, 1985.
40. Bechtol, CD: Grip test: Use of a dynamometer with adjustable handle spacing. J Bone Joint Surg 36A:820, 1954.
41. Mathiowetz, V, Rennells, C, and Donahoe, L: Effects of elbow position on grip and key pinch strength. J Hand Surg 10A:694, 1985.
42. Schmidt, RT and Toews, JV: Grip strength as measured by the Jamar dynamometer. Arch Phys Med Rehabil 51:321, 1970.
43. Pryce, JC: The wrist position between neutral and ulnar deviation that facilitates the maximum power grip strength. J Biomechanics 13:505, 1980.
44. Coulter, CL, Ferrin, VJ, and Smith, LK: Grip strength in normal children as measured by the Jamar dynamometer. Unpublished master's thesis, Texas Women's University.
45. Allen, E: Thromboangitis obliterans: Methods of diagnosis of chronic occlusive arterial lesions distal to the wrist with illustrative cases. Am J Med Sci 178:237, 1929.
46. Ashbell, T, Kutz, J, and Kleinert, H: The digital Allen test. Plast Reconstr Surg 39:311, 1967.
47. Phalen, G: The carpal tunnel syndrome: Seventeen years' experience in diagnosis and treatment of 654 hands. J Bone Joint Surg 48A:211, 1966.
48. Moldaver, J: Tinel's sign: Its characteristics and significance. J Bone Joint Surg 60A:412, 1978.
49. Kaplan, E: Translation of J. Tinel's "Four millement" paper. In Spinner, M: Injuries to the Major Branches of Peripheral Nerves of the Forearm, ed 2. WB Saunders, Philadelphia, 1978.
50. Watts, NT: Decision analysis: A tool for improving physical therapy practice and education. In Wolf, SL (ed): Clinical decision making in physical therapy. FA Davis, Philadelphia, 1985, p 7.

BIBLIOGRAPHY

Lehmukuhl, D and Smith, L: Brunstrom's Clinical Kinesiology, ed 4. FA Davis, Philadelphia, 1983.

Kendall, H, Kendall, F, and Wadsworth, G: Muscles, Testing and Function, ed 3. Williams & Wilkins, Baltimore, 1983.

Ranchos Los Amigos Hospital, Occupational Therapy Department, Guide for Muscle Testing of the Upper Extremity. Ranchos Los Amigos Hospital, Downey, California, 1978.

Daniels, L and Worthingham, C: Muscle Testing Techniques of Muscle Examination, ed 5. WB Saunders, Philadelphia, 1986.

Tubiana, R, Thromine, J and Mackin, E: Examination of the Hand and Upper Limb. WB Saunders, Philadelphia, 1984.

The Hand, Examination and Diagnosis. American Society for Surgery of the Hand, ed 2. Churchill Livingstone, New York 1983.

CHAPTER 4

Sensibility Testing

Anna Mae Tan, OTR

Sensibility testing is an important component of every hand evaluation because sensation is essential for hand function. Motor control alone does not ensure skillful use of the hand; rather, the synthesis of movement and sensibility endows the hand with its exquisite abilities. Through our fingertips, our sense of touch conveys sensory impressions that guide our hand to move a pen, catch a ball, or gently hold a child's hand.

The loss of sensibility has serious consequences for hand function. When sensibility is diminished, hand function is limited, precision movements are awkward, and objects cannot be manipulated with normal speed and skill. The greater the loss of sensibility, the more significantly hand function is impaired.

The objectives of this chapter are to (1) discuss the value of sensibility testing; (2) present basic concepts of sensory physiology; (3) present a neurophysiologic classification of sensory tests and discuss how to select the appropriate sensory tests based on this classification system; and (4) provide procedural guidelines for performing sensibility testing as well as recording, interpreting, and summarizing the results.

CONCEPTS OF SENSORY PHYSIOLOGY

Injuries to peripheral nerves may result in altered sensory perceptions that affect hand function. The ability accurately to assess sensibility helps the therapist and physician to diagnose and treat patients with nerve injuries. Test results can help determine whether an injury is a complete or incomplete nerve laceration or a compression neuropathy. Repeated sensibility testing provides a way to chart nerve regeneration after nerve repair or surgical decompression. Ultimately, the information obtained about a patient's sensibility helps to clarify functional impairment and identify therapy needs.

The sensory tests used clinically to assess sensibility are based on concepts of sensory physiology. Understanding the organization of the sensory system and a few basic concepts of sensory physiology provides a foundation for understanding sensory testing.

The sensory system is organized into serial chains of neurons that ascend from the

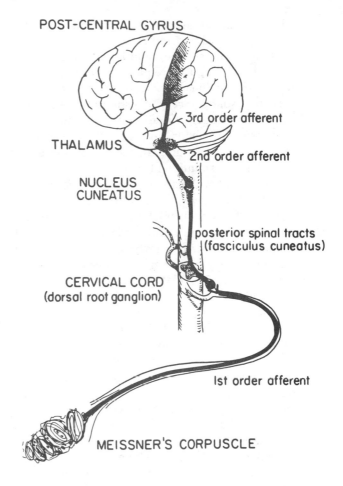

POST-CENTRAL GYRUS

3rd order afferent

THALAMUS

2nd order afferent

NUCLEUS
CUNEATUS

posterior spinal tracts
(fasciculus cuneatus)

CERVICAL CORD
(dorsal root ganglion)

1st order afferent

MEISSNER'S CORPUSCLE

FIGURE 4–1. The sensory system is organized into chains of neurons that transmit sensory information from sensory receptors in the skin to the brain. First-order neurons in the spinal cord or medulla convey impulses to third-order afferents in the thalamus that in turn convey impulses to the somatosensory cortex of the brain. (From Dellon,[2] p 29, with permission.)

hand to the brain (Fig. 4–1).[1–4] The receptor neurons are the first neurons in this sensory pathway. These neurons transduce sensory stimuli into electrical impulses and transmit these impulses along ascending axons to neurons in the spinal cord or medulla.[1,2] Neurons in the spinal cord conduct the sensory impulses to neurons in the thalamus, which in turn convey the impulses to the somatosensory cortex of the brain.[2,4] In the somatosensory cortex the impulses are decoded and the perceptions recognized.[4]

Receptor neurons respond only to stimuli within a defined area of the skin, called a *receptive field*.[1–3] Each neuron along that sensory pathway is also associated with this same receptive field.[1–3] If a stimulus is moved, a different receptive field and series of neurons is stimulated. We are able to perceive and differentiate one point from another because one series of neurons rather than another has been activated.[3]

The number of nerve fibers that innervate a receptive field is referred to as the *innervation density*.[2] The innervation density determines the amount of cortical representation of the area in the cerebral cortex.[4] The greater the innervation density, the greater the cortical representation of the area in the cerebral cortex.[4] Just as more sensory receptors innervate the palmar surface of the fingertips than the forearm, likewise a greater area of the cerebral cortex represents the palmar surface of the fingertips than the forearm.

All the cutaneous sensory receptors and their associated fibers adapt to an applied stimulus and may do so either slowly or rapidly.[3,4] Slowly adapting fiber-receptors respond to a stimulus throughout the application of the stimulus.[1-4] These fiber-receptors increase their impulse frequency as the stimulus intensity is increased, and function to convey information about constant touch and deep pressure.[2,4] Rapidly adapting fiber-receptors adapt quickly to a stimulus, responding briefly when the stimulus is first applied and then again briefly when the stimulus is removed. These fiber-receptors convey information about light transient movements.[2-4]

The sensory receptors are very specialized and respond uniquely to different stimuli.[1-4] Only a stimulus of the proper quality and intensity sufficient to reach the receptor threshold will activate a specific receptor.[1-4]

The *mechanoreceptors*[1-4] all respond to touch stimuli and transmit tactile perceptions needed for hand function. There are three different mechanoreceptors. The *Meissner's corpuscles* are rapidly adapting receptors that are responsive to brisk, light movements and low-frequency vibration (30 to 40 Hz).[1-4] *Pacinian corpuscles* are rapidly adapting receptors that are sensitive to deep moving pressure and high-frequency vibration (200 to 300 Hz).[1-4] The slowly adapting *Merkel's receptors* respond to constant touch stimuli.[1-4]

Neurophysiologists are just beginning to understand how sensory receptors respond to stimuli individually, and many mysteries remain about how the receptors interact to produce the complex perceptions we know as cutaneous sensibility. Further refining of this concept of receptor specificity and inter-receptor interactions will help us understand more fully how sensory features are encoded by the different fiber-receptors.

Sensory receptors transduce sensory stimuli into electrical impulses called *action potentials*.[5-8] Action potentials are generated by depolarization of the cell membrane.[5-8] Depolarization results from an increased flow of sodium ions across the openings in the receptor cell membrane. The cell membrane can be depolarized by an electrical impulse, mechanical deformation, or a chemical messenger.[5-8] In sensory testing we are depolarizing the cell membrane mechanically. The mechanical stretch from the stimulus activates the cell openings, allowing more ions to flow across the membrane.[6] The voltage of the membrane increases with the increased ion flow until the voltage is strong enough to reach the threshold of the axon and triggers the production of the action potential, which is self-propagated along the nerve.[5-8]

The *conduction velocity* of the action potential along a nerve is affected by the diameter of the nerve and whether the nerve is myelinated.[5-8] Fibers with larger diameters conduct impulses faster.[6,7] Myelination[6-8] also increases the conduction velocity by increasing the fiber diameter and providing a nodal arrangement that allows the propagation of the potential from node to node. The axons that convey information about touch are large myelinated fibers with high conduction velocities.[5,6,8]

After a nerve injury several factors may influence the fiber diameter or its myelination and affect the conduction velocity. Mechanical compression from nerve entrapments or scar tissue can decrease the fiber size and slow the conduction velocity of the impulse.[6-8] Damage to the myelin sheath will also cause slowing of nerve conduction and the conduction slowing will last until remyelination is complete.[6,8] After a nerve repair, the regenerating nerve fibers conduct impulses more slowly because their fibers are thin and do not regain their original diameter or full myelination for many years.[7,8]

CLASSIFICATION OF SENSORY TESTS

The sensory tests, currently found to be the most useful clinically, can be classified neurophysiologically into four types. They are innervation density tests, threshold tests, stress tests, and sensory nerve conduction studies.

Innervation Density Tests

Innervation density tests are a class of sensory tests that test the ability to discriminate between two identical stimuli placed close together on the skin. This ability is neurophysiologically based on the innervation density of the area being tested and a high level of cortical integrity.[1,2,13] The more richly innervated an area is, the sharper the contrast between the stimuli and the more easily the brain can distinguish the stimuli as distinct entities when the space between the two points is small. A high level of cortical integrity is needed for the brain to interpret the distinction correctly. The static and moving two-point discrimination tests are tests of innervation density.[2]

Clinical research[9-11] has demonstrated that innervation density tests are helpful in assessing sensibility after nerve repair and during nerve regeneration. Following nerve repair and during nerve regeneration, cortical integrity is impaired because the sensory pathway has been interrupted and the cerebral cortex becomes disorganized.[2,8] The regenerating fibers may not reestablish their continuity with the same sensory pathway (Fig. 4–2). As a result, a stimulus may activate a different set of neurons in the cerebral cortex then it did previously.[2,8] Innervation density test results are abnormal when there is cortical impairment and test results improve as more fibers reinnervate the receptive fields being tested and the brain reorganizes itself.

Experimental and clinical research[12-15] have demonstrated that innervation density testing is not as useful in assessing compression neuropathies because the cortical integration remains normal even if a few fibers are conducting to their correct cortical end points. The results of innervation density testing may be normal in patients with nerve compressions until all the nerve fibers are compressed at which time all sensory perceptions are lost.[13,14]

Threshold Tests

Threshold tests measure the intensity of the stimulus necessary to depolarize the cell membrane and produce an action potential. Vibratory testing and Semmes-Weinstein monofilaments are threshold tests.

Clinical research[13] has shown that threshold tests are useful in assessing diminished sensibility in nerve compressions and in monitoring nerve recovery after surgical decompression. Threshold test results are abnormal when a nerve is compressed and a greater stimulus force is required to activate a receptor. Conversely, the threshold test results return to normal as the nerve recovers from the compression.

During nerve regeneration, threshold tests reflect the progressive maturing of the reinnervated fiber-receptors. As they mature the threshold for stimulus perception gradually returns to normal.[7,8]

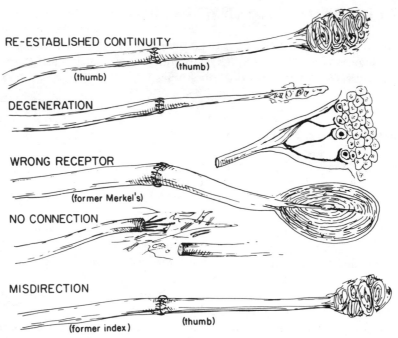

RE-ESTABLISHED CONTINUITY

(thumb)

(thumb)

DEGENERATION

WRONG RECEPTOR

(former Merkel's)

NO CONNECTION

MISDIRECTION

(former index)   (thumb)

FIGURE 4–2. After a nerve has been repaired and it is regenerating, the regenerating nerve fibers may follow different pathways. *A,* It is hoped that the majority of fibers will reestablish connections with the appropriate sensory receptors. *B,* Other fibers, however, will regenerate to damaged end organs. *C,* Some will regenerate to the appropriate receptive field but the wrong receptor. *D* and *E,* Still others may not connect at all or will be misdirected to the wrong fingers and reinnervate an incorrect receptive field. Reinnervation of nerve fibers into different receptive fields or receptors will generate different sensory impulses in response to stimuli than occurred prior to a nerve repair. (From Dellon,[2] p 211, with permission.)

Stress Tests

Stress tests are tests that combine the use of sensory tests with activities that provoke the symptoms of nerve compressions. The stress test consists of prestress baseline threshold testing, followed by provocative activities to stress the nerve, and then poststress threshold testing to assess any changes in nerve threshold. These tests are used in cases of mild nerve compression when patients report symptoms during activities but no abnormalities are detected by baseline sensory testing.

Sensory Nerve Conduction Studies

Sensory nerve conduction studies are electrophysiologic studies that assess the conduction of sensory action potentials along a nerve trunk. Sensory nerve conduction studies are electrophysiologic studies that assess the conduction of sensory action potentials along a nerve trunk.[7,8] The results can assist in assessing the type, degree, and location of sensory nerve injuries. Compression of the nerve or partial lacerations may be confirmed by slowing of conduction velocity or alteration in potential amplitudes.[7,8] Nerve injuries that result in loss of nerve continuity with wallerian degeneration of the distal nerve segment produce a conduction block at the site of the injury.[7,8] A conduction block can be identified electrodiagnostically 4 or 5 days after the acute interruption when the distal segment becomes inexcitable because of degeneration of nerve fibers.[5,7]

Nerve regeneration with reestablishment of nerve continuity is evident electrophysiologically by return of nerve conduction and a gradual increase in the conduction velocity as the nerve matures over time.[7,8]

SELECTING APPROPRIATE SENSORY TESTS

Before performing any sensory tests, the therapist needs to select the tests that are the most sensitive for the specific injuries. Table 4–1 shows different sensory tests that are useful for assessing nerve lacerations, nerve regeneration, nerve compressions, or performing general sensory screenings.

Assessing a suspected nerve laceration requires tests that can assess the continuity of the nerve. An innervation density test, threshold test, or a nerve conduction study will identify if there is loss of nerve continuity and absence of nerve conduction. Complete lacerations would result in loss of nerve conduction and absence of all sensory perceptions.[2,6-8] A partial laceration may be reflected by abnormal innervation density test scores,[9-11] abnormal values in threshold tests,[13-22] or abnormal nerve conduction studies.[2,6-8]

After a nerve has been surgically repaired and is regenerating, the therapist needs tests that assess the regeneration of the fibers and the cortical reorganization. Sensory tests are not helpful until the regenerating axons of the repaired nerve have reinnervated the area being tested.[8] The most useful procedure to monitor the advancement of the regenerating sensory nerve to the fingertips is the Tinel's sign.[8]

When the Tinel's sign has advanced to the area being tested, an innervation density test is helpful to assess the quality of the reinnervation and the cortical reorganization.[2,8-11] A threshold test is also helpful to follow the maturation of the nerve and the return to normal threshold.[7,8] Monthly reevaluations help the therapist to chart the recovery of the nerve and the progressive maturation.

Assessing nerve compression problems requires tests that are very sensitive to changes in receptor function and nerve conduction. Threshold tests,[11-19] stress tests, and electrophysiologic studies[7,8] are sensitive indicators of these changes. Vibrometry or Semmes-Weinstein monofilament testing results can show gradual changes in threshold

TABLE 4–1 Sensory Tests

Assessing Nerve Compression	Assessing Nerve Lacerations and Nerve Regeneration	Sensory Screening
Semmes-Weinstein monofilaments	Tinel's sign	Semmes-Weinstein monofilaments
Vibrometry	Semmes-Weinstein monofilaments	Static two-point discrimination test
Electrodiagnostic studies	Moving two-point discrimination test	
Stress tests	Static two-point discrimination test	
	Electrodiagnostic studies	

values as nerve compression progresses and similarly will demonstrate a return to normal values as a nerve recovers.[13-19] Vibrometry is slightly more sensitive than Semmes-Weinstein testing,[13-18] but more problems are associated with the current instrument used in vibrometry than with monofilaments. Stress testing is helpful in compressive neuropathies when the symptoms are transient or occur only when the hand is engaged in some provocative activity.[19] Nerve conduction studies will provide evidence of nerve compression and may help isolate the site of compression with test results that show slower nerve conduction velocity or conduction blocks.[7]

Innervation density tests are not as helpful when there is a nerve compression, until the nerve compression is so advanced that all perception is lost.[12-15] When the nerve compression is advanced, the therapist may also notice muscle atrophy indicating motor fiber involvement. For example, in advanced cases of carpal tunnel syndrome, patients frequently have atrophied thenar muscles when innervation density test results in the median nerve distribution of the hand are abnormal.

Assessing sensibility when no nerve injuries are reported or suspected can be performed easily through a sensory screening. This screening may confirm the presence of normal sensibility or identify overlooked or subtle signs of nerve injuries. A brief screening should be done on the fingertip pulps, including a threshold test and an innervation density test. This type of sensory screening will reflect the neurophysiologic status of the sensory system and the quality of the adaptive responses of the different fiber-receptor systems.

PERFORMING SPECIFIC SENSORY TESTS

General Guidelines

Sensory testing requires concentration by the patient and should be performed in a quiet distraction-free environment. The hand should be supported to avoid inadvertent movement of the hand by the testing instruments.

The sensory tests should be performed following accepted guidelines and should be scored and reported appropriately. There are no standardized methods for any of the current sensory tests used, but extensive clinical use by physicians and therapists has produced accepted guidelines. Consistency is best ensured when the same therapist sequentially evaluates the patient and the same test instruments are used.

The therapist needs to keep in mind the anatomic course of the nerves through the arm and the sensory distribution of the peripheral nerves in the hand. Sensibility may be tested anywhere along the course of any peripheral nerve. Knowing the anatomy and the course of the nerves through muscles and around vessels and bone, as well as the areas of sensory overlap, is essential for accurate diagnosis and treatment of nerve injuries. Having an anatomy textbook nearby during testing is helpful. Sensory deficits are frequently missed or overlooked when anatomy is forgotten, especially with digital nerve injuries. When a digital nerve injury is suspected, the therapist needs to remember that testing must be done along the side of the finger where the digital nerves course from the palm to the fingertip.

Tinel's Sign

The Tinel's sign is used to monitor the progression of nerve regeneration.[8] The Tinel's sign refers to the tingling sensation that radiates in the area of the cutaneous distribution of an injured nerve when the nerve segment is percussed. To elicit the sign, the nerve segment is percussed distally to proximally until a level is reached at which the abnormal tingling sensation is elicited.[8] This point marks the farthest point that the regenerating fibers have reached. The percussion should be performed gently using the fingertips, a blunt-tip pen, or a rubber pencil eraser. Care should be taken to ensure that the percussion is accurately applied along the course of the nerve.

The distance from the site of nerve injury or repair to the point where the Tinel's sign is elicited is measured and recorded in millimeters (Fig. 4–3). A rate of recovery can be calculated by dividing the millimeter distance by the days since the surgical repair[8] (millimeters per day). The rate of regeneration of the nerve fibers and the location where the Tinel's sign was elicited should both be reported.

Sunderland[8] provides the general rates for axonal regeneration that are the most widely accepted: 2 mm per day in the forearm, 1 to 2 mm per day at the wrist, and 1 to 1.5 mm per day in the hand. Sunderland points out that rate of regeneration can be affected by many factors and reports slower regeneration rates across suture lines, through scar tissue, or in older patients.

Tinel's sign located distal to the site of nerve repair indicates that some regenerating sensory nerve fibers have crossed the suture line or that the nerve fiber continuity has been restored with the nerve fiber below the lesion. This test does not provide any measure of the number of axons that are regenerating and cannot predict the outcome or quality of the sensory recovery.

Tinel's sign is not considered useful during the first month after nerve injury or repair.[8] During this time, the site of percussion is so close to the lesion that the force required to elicit the sign cannot be applied without the effects of the mechanical stimulation on the injured segment producing misleading distal tingling from stimulation of distal injured segments.

Static Two-Point Discrimination Testing

Static two-point discrimination testing assesses the ability to discriminate between two static points when simultaneously placed on the skin. This test can be performed with an adjustable caliper or a discrimination device (Fig. 4–4). Calipers have adjustable ends so the width between the ends can be varied in millimeter increments. The discrimination devices have several points preset at varying millimeter widths. To ensure instrument validity, all testing devices should be checked to make sure the millimeter calibrations are accurate. The ends should also be checked to be sure that they are smooth and blunt. Sharp edges will activate the nocioceptors rather than the mechanoreceptors.[1,3] During testing, the hand should be fully supported and vision occluded.

This test is not standardized and there are many clinical variations of the testing procedure. The author's preferred method is to test the fingertip pulp beginning with the two prongs spaced 2 mm apart. One or two points are randomly applied parallel to the longitudinal axis of the fingertip. This random sequencing of application is aimed at

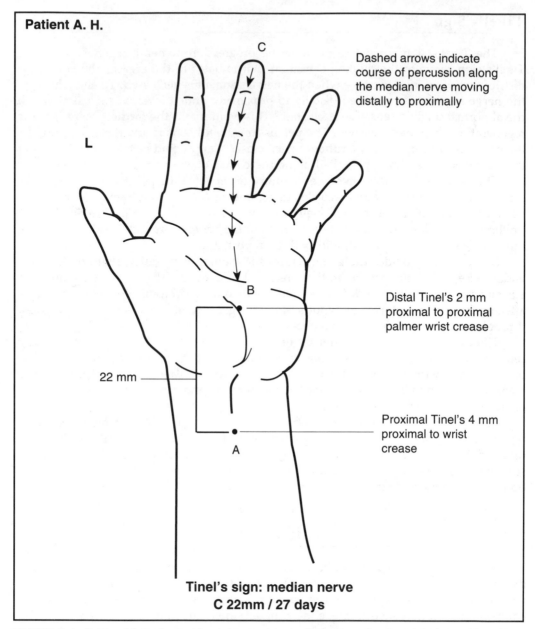

Patient A. H.

C

L

Dashed arrows indicate
course of percussion along
the median nerve moving
distally to proximally

B

Distal Tinel's 2 mm
proximal to proximal
palmer wrist crease

22 mm

Proximal Tinel's 4 mm
proximal to wrist
crease

A

**Tinel's sign: median nerve
C 22mm / 27 days**

FIGURE 4–3. For this patient with a regenerating median nerve, the site of the injury is marked as A. The distal Tinel's sign is marked as point B. The distance between A and B is measured and recorded as 22 mm per 27 days after surgical repair. This median nerve is recovering at a rate of approximately 1 mm per day and is following a normal rate of recovery.

reducing the patient's ability to guess the correct answer. Care should be taken to be sure that the two points are applied at the same time and with equal force. The pressure applied should be gentle and not enough to blanch the skin.

The patient is asked whether he or she feels one or two points in response to the stimulus application. If the patient cannot accurately detect two points 2 mm apart, the width between the two points is increased until the correct number of responses are

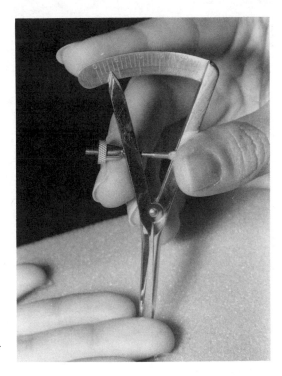

FIGURE 4-4. Static two-point discrimination testing.

obtained. Testing is concluded if the patient cannot detect two points at 20 mm apart. Test results are recorded as the millimeter width at which two points could accurately be perceived in several trials, as demonstrated in Figures 4-5 and 4-6. Guidelines for interpreting the functional significance of the scores are provided by the American Society for Surgery of the Hand.[20] Norms for static two-point discrimination by age and sex have also been delineated in a study by Louis and colleagues.[21] Accurate discrimination of two points between 2 and 5 mm apart is considered normal for adults at the fingertip pulps.[21]

Moving Two-Point Discrimination Testing

The moving two-point discrimination test, developed by Dellon,[2] is performed with the same instruments as those used for the static two-point test. Testing is done on the palmar surface of the fingertips proximally to distally with the patient's vision occluded and hand fully supported. Testing begins by orienting the patient to the test in an area of intact sensibility. The fingertips are tested beginning with the prongs spaced 5 mm apart. Testing progresses from higher values to lower values to orient patients to the test. The prongs are held perpendicular to the finger and moved parallel to the long axis of the finger. The testing stimulus is randomly alternated between one and two moving points. If the patient correctly perceives the stimulus, the spacing is then decreased until the patient can no longer accurately perceive the difference or is accurate at 2 mm distance. According to Dellon,[2] 7 of 10 trials must be correctly perceived to score this test.

Dellon[2] reports the normal value for moving two-point discrimination at 2 mm.

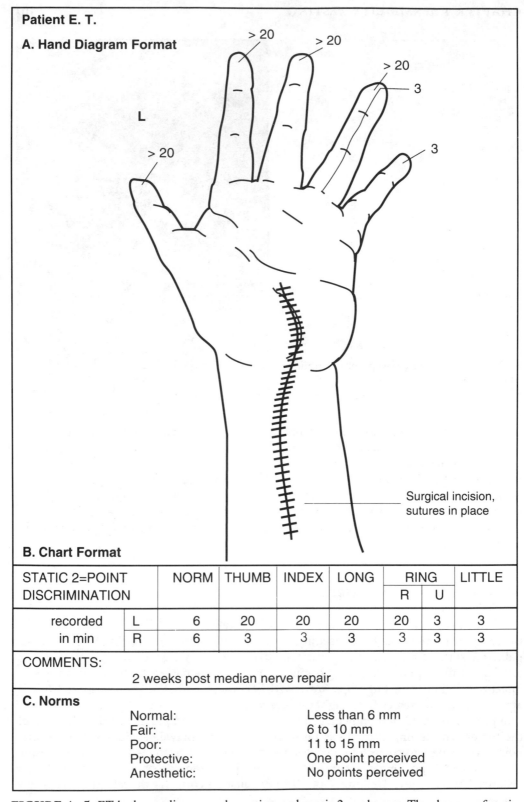

Patient E. T.

A. Hand Diagram Format

L

> 20
> 20
> 20
3
3
> 20

B. Chart Format

STATIC 2=POINT DISCRIMINATION		NORM	THUMB	INDEX	LONG	RING		LITTLE
						R	U	
recorded in min	L	6	20	20	20	20	3	3
	R	6	3	3	3	3	3	3

COMMENTS:

2 weeks post median nerve repair

C. Norms

Normal:	Less than 6 mm
Fair:	6 to 10 mm
Poor:	11 to 15 mm
Protective:	One point perceived
Anesthetic:	No points perceived

FIGURE 4–5. ET had a median nerve laceration and repair 2 weeks ago. The absence of static two-point discrimination documented in this sensory form would be expected. (Norms from the American Society for Surgery of the Hand, with permission.)

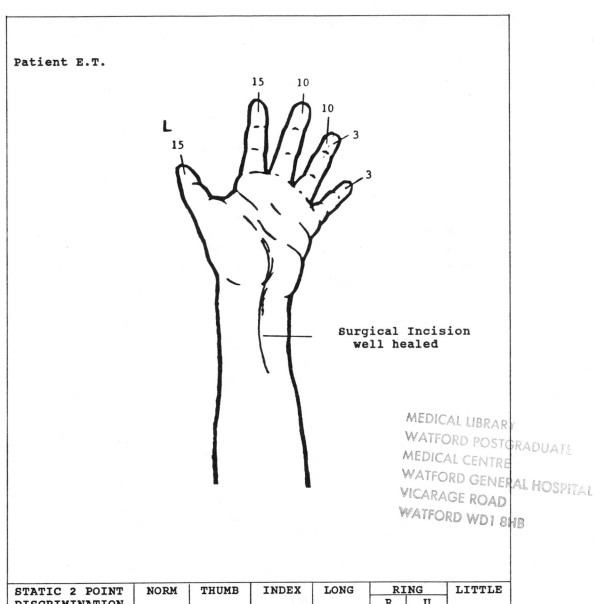

Patient E.T.

Surgical Incision
well healed

STATIC 2 POINT DISCRIMINATION		NORM	THUMB	INDEX	LONG	RING		LITTLE
						R	U	
recorded	L	≤ 6	15	15	10	10	3	3
in mm	R	≤ 6	3	3	3	3	3	3
COMMENTS: 10 months post median nerve repair								

FIGURE 4–6. Results of static two-point discrimination testing at 10 months after–median nerve repair show that the nerve fibers have regenerated to the fingertips and cortical reorganization is occurring. There is poor sensibility in the thumb and index and fair sensibility in the long finger.

Values for moving two-point discrimination by age and comparison of these values with static two-point discrimination have been compiled by Louis and associates.[21]

Semmes-Weinstein Monofilament Discrimination Testing

The Semmes-Weinstein monofilament discrimination test assesses the threshold of stimulus necessary for the perception of light touch to deep pressure. The Semmes-Weinstein monofilament discrimination test is performed using the Semmes-Weinstein Anesthesiometer monofilament testing set. These sets are available in sets of 20 monofilaments or five monofilaments. The larger monofilament set is recommended because it offers smaller intervals of testing stimuli. This larger range of filaments is valuable when testing early signs of nerve compression in which small changes in threshold are important to detect.

The monofilaments are hand-held probes consisting of nylon monofilaments inset at right angles to lucite rods. The probes are of equal length with increasing diameters. In the large 20-filament set the monofilaments are marked with a number ranging from 1.65 to 6.65.[19] This number represents the logarithm of 10 times the force in milligrams required to bow the monofilament (log 10 Fmg).[19]

A research study by Bell-Krotoski and Tomanak[22] assessed the force application repeatability of the monofilaments. The results of this research study demonstrate that if the monofilament lengths and diameters are accurate, then the filaments produce a stimulus force that is controlled, objective, and reproducible. This study highlights the importance of careful storage and replacement of altered filaments to ensure accuracy of the monofilaments.

The author's preferred testing procedure is the one credited to Bell-Krotoski.[20] The procedure is to test the fingertip pulps with the patient's hand fully supported and vision occluded. Testing should first be demonstrated on an area of intact sensibility. The patient is asked to give a verbal response when he or she feels the filament.

The monofilament is applied perpendicular to the palmar skin of the fingertip until it bows (Fig. 4–7). Filaments marked 2.44 through 4.08 are applied three times to the test area, whereas filaments 4.17 through 6.65 are applied only once per trial in a given area.[20] The lighter filaments should be applied three times to reach the required thresholds for these filaments.[21] The filaments should be applied slowly and accurately. Any filament application that moves across the finger should not be counted. Careless application techniques have been found to render the filaments less accurate in controlled measurements of the filament forces.[23]

Testing usually begins with filaments 2.44 or 2.83, which is considered the normal range of values. If the patient can accurately identify the touch of either of these filaments sensibility is normal in the area being tested, and testing can be discontinued. If the patient cannot identify the touch of these filaments, the therapist should progressively apply each next larger monofilament until touch pressure can be identified for all fingertips.

Test results can be recorded as the filament number of the monofilament perceived or the milligrams or grams of force at which the stimulus is perceived (Fig. 4–8). In reporting the results of testing one must remember that there is a range of normalcy. Filaments 1.36, 2.44, and 2.83 are all considered normal for constant touch perception and the most accurate value for each individual is the smallest filament perceived in a fingertip of intact sensibility on the injured hand or contralateral hand.[20] Because of the

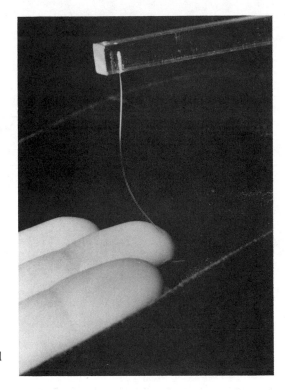

FIGURE 4–7. Semmes-Weinstein threshold testing.

range of normalcy, the author recommends testing fingers with filaments 2.44 and 2.83. This approach is particularly helpful if a patient has early signs of nerve compression. If the median innervated long finger of the noninvolved hand can accurately perceive filament 2.44, but the long finger of involved hand can only perceive filament 2.83, one must suspect median nerve compression in the carpal tunnel in the involved hand and additional stress testing should be performed. The touch thresholds can be equated with hand function based on research reported by Von Prince.[24]

Vibratory Testing

Vibratory testing assesses the threshold of stimulus needed to perceive vibration or brief touch stimuli and is assessed using a vibrometer.[2,15–18]

A vibrometer frequently used to assess vibratory perception today is the Bio-Thesiometer.[15,18] This vibrometer is an electrically controlled testing instrument that produces vibration at a fixed frequency (120 Hz) with a variable amplitude. A meter displays a readout in voltage.

Testing with the Bio-Thesiometer is performed by holding the vibrating head in contact with the fingertip being tested while slowly and gradually increasing the amplitude of the stimulus by turning the amplitude control knob (Fig. 4–9). Testing is done with the patient's hand supported and vision occluded. The patient is asked to report when vibration is detected.

The threshold is recorded as the voltage required to perceive the vibratory stimulus.

```
┌─────────────────────────────────────────────────────────────────────────────┐
│                                                                               │
│              Semmes-Weinstein Monofilament Test Results                       │
│                                                                               │
│   Patient A.T.                                                                │
│                                                                               │
└─────────────────────────────────────────────────────────────────────────────┘
```

Semmes-Weinstein Monofilaments		NORM	THUMB	INDEX	LONG	RING		LITTLE
						R	U	
filament	L	≤ 2.83	3.61	3.22	3.61	3.22	2.83	2.83
number	R	≤ 2.83	2.44	2.44	2.44	2.44	2.44	2.44

COMMENTS:

Nighttime paresthesias in left thumb and long fingers, and aching on ulnar side of hand.

Norms   Filament Numbers

Normal light touch	1.65 – 2.83
Diminished Light touch	3.22 – 3.61
Diminished protective sensation	3.84 – 4.31
Loss of protective sensation	4.56 – 6.65
Untestable	6.65

FIGURE 4–8. The results of Semmes-Weinstein monofilament testing for AT document diminished light touch in the median nerve distribution of the hand and confirm the diagnosis of carpal tunnel syndrome. Notice that the results of testing in the left ulnar nerve distribution are within the normal range but are higher than those for the right nonsymptomatic hand. This patient also had ulnar nerve compression. The signs were subtle and evident only by comparison with the test results of the right hand. (Data from Semmes, J and Weinstein, S: Somatosensory Changes after Brain Wounds in Man. Harvard University Press, Cambridge, 1980.)

Voltage can then be converted into microns of displacement (stimulus amplitude) from the calibration chart supplied by the manufacturer.

The mean normal baseline value of the vibratory threshold has been reported by Szabo and colleagues[15] as 0.015 μm. The opposite hand can provide the normal baseline value for each patient.

There are limitations with vibratory testing that result from problems inherent in the testing instrument, thus limiting its clinical usefulness. During testing, it is difficult to hold the vibrometer head steady, and patients may perceive pressure from the device placed on the hand before they perceive vibration. The vibrometer also does not allow any variability of the vibration frequency. The fixed frequency of 120 Hz may stimulate only some of the functioning sensory receptors and not others.[2,3]

Therapists who want to do research may find a vibrometer helpful. Clinically, I recommend using the information provided with Semmes-Weinstein monofilament testing rather than vibratory testing with the Bio-Thesiometer.

On the horizon are clinical vibrometers that provide variable amplitude with variable frequencies.[16] As the sophistication of these testing instruments improves, the usefulness of vibratory testing as a clinical test is likely to improve as well.

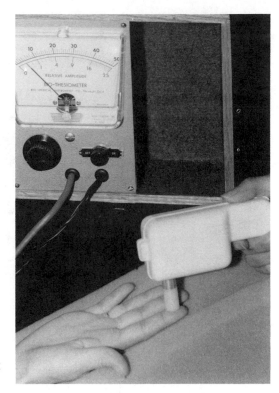

FIGURE 4–9. Vibratory threshold testing using a Bio-Thesiometer.

Sensory Nerve Conduction Studies

Sensory nerve conduction studies assess the conduction of sensory action potentials along a nerve trunk.[7] In nerve conduction studies, a stimulating current, applied through surface or needle electrodes, evokes a sensory action potential that is self-propagated by the nerve and is recorded at some distance in either direction along the nerve (Fig. 4–10).

The recorded sensory action potentials are passed through an amplifier that is connected to different monitoring devices. An oscilloscope displays the potential for visual monitoring, while an audioamplifier and speaker allow acoustic monitoring. The visual displays on the oscilloscope screen may be photographed or the signals fed through a fiberoptic system and permanently recorded on paper. Computers are often used to store, average, or manipulate the test data.

The nerve conduction velocity and sensory latency of the action potentials are studied the most extensively, though recently attention is being paid to the amplitude, duration, and configuration of the action potential.[7] The *sensory latency* (recorded in milliseconds) is the interval of time between the onset of the stimulus and the onset of a response. *Distal sensory latency* refers to latency recorded over the distal segment of the nerve. *Proximal sensory latency* is the time from the stimulus to the onset of the impulse when the recording electrode is placed proximal to the stimulating electrode. Recently, to increase the sensitivity of testing, researchers have compared the test times with those of another nerve or with those of a different segment of the same nerve.[7]

The amplitude, duration, shape, and configuration of the sensory response are studied manually or by computer. A change in configuration is believed to suggest lack

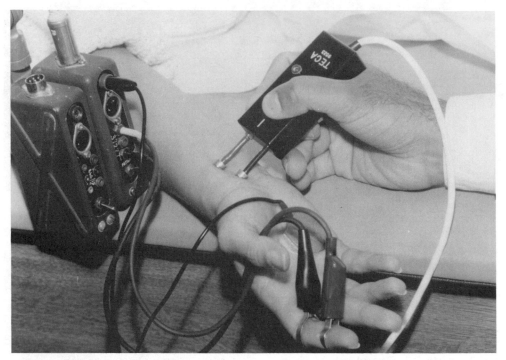

FIGURE 4–10. Nerve conduction testing for carpal tunnel syndrome.

of uniform conduction along the course of the nerve and may suggest focal demyelination without conduction block.[7,8]

Stress Testing

Stress tests combine the use of sensory tests with provocative activities to reproduce the symptoms of nerve compressions. The stress test consists of prestress baseline sensory testing, activities to stress the nerves and provoke the symptoms, and poststress sensory testing. The sensory tests chosen should be those most sensitive for evaluation of nerve compressions; namely, the threshold tests. Semmes-Weinstein monofilaments or vibrometry are the most useful because they have been shown to detect early signs of nerve compression.

The provocative activities the patients are asked to perform help most when they closely simulate the activities that produce the symptoms of the patient (Fig. 4–11). Skillful interviewing of the patient by the therapist is necessary to obtain a good picture of the potentially stressful activities, and careful attention to detail is often needed to reproduce the motions and forces of the provocative activities. Factors such as repetitiveness, force, mechanical stresses, posture, vibration, and temperature should be considered when simulating activities.

Many nerve compression problems are cumulative in nature, and many activities may work together to produce the symptoms. Work tasks, combined with recreational and self-care activities, may produce similar repetitive trauma that cumulatively leads to symptoms. In these cases baseline sensory testing is done initially; then repeat testing

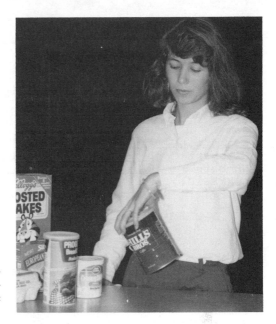

FIGURE 4–11. Stress testing is most informative when the tasks to be performed reproduce the movements or activities that cause the reported symptoms.

may be performed at the end of a workday, at the end of a workweek, or after an active weekend.

Reporting the results of stress testing should include the baseline sensory test results of both the involved and contralateral hands and the results of repeat sensory testing after the provocative activity was performed (Fig. 4–12). A description of the activity used to provoke the symptoms should also be provided. This description should include all the parameters such as the force, repetitions, resistance, motions, posture, and time to elicit symptoms. This report is especially important to document if repeat testing is needed to assess job modifications or splinting.

CORRELATING SENSIBILITY WITH HAND FUNCTIONS

Sensibility evaluations can provide information about the acuity of the sensory system and cortical integrity. The most accurate way to correlate this information with hand function is to include dexterity tests and activity of daily living assessments as part of the overall evaluation. This combination will allow the therapist to assess how sensibility is influencing hand function and will identify the need for sensory reeducation, patient education on sensory precautions, desensitization, splinting, or activity modifications.

WRITING A SENSIBILITY TESTING SUMMARY

The therapist testing sensibility is responsible for synthesizing all the test results and bringing some meaning to those results for the referral source. To do this task, the therapist must review constantly the clinical research on sensibility testing and communicate with other therapists in the field. Often the most important information in the

Stress Test Results

Patient K.M.

A.   Baseline Test

Semmes Weinstein		NORM	THUMB	INDEX	LONG	RING		LITTLE
						R	U	
Filament	L	≤ 2.83	2.83	2.83	2.83	2.83	2.83	2.83
Numbers	R	≤ 2.83	2.83	2.83	2.83	2.83	2.83	2.83

COMMENTS:
           Nocturnal paresthesias in left thumb, index, and long
           fingers.

B.   Post Stress Test

Semmes Weinstein		NORM	THUMB	INDEX	LONG	RING		LITTLE
						R	U	
Filament	L	≤ 2.83	3.22	3.61	3.61	3.22	2.83	2.83
Numbers	R	≤ 2.83	2.83	2.83	2.83	2.83	2.83	2.83

FIGURE 4–12. KM complained of symptoms of numbness and tingling in the median nerve distribution of her hand when she worked as a supermarket checker. *A*, Sensibility testing in the clinic with her hand at rest did not document any sensory abnormalities. *B*, Stress testing was done with simulation of the movements involved in scanning groceries at a supermarket check out. After 30 minutes of simulated grocery scanning KM complained of paresthesias and the Semmes-Weinstein monofilament testing documented the sensory abnormalities in the median nerve distribution of her hand.

entire sensibility test battery is the summary paragraph the therapist includes at the end of the report. Summaries must be interpretive, accurate, and concisely written. This skill improves with experience and practice, as well as with knowing what information is most valuable to the referring physician.

A sample summary paragraph for a patient who was tested for possible carpal tunnel syndrome might be written as follows:

Sensibility test results for Mr. Handy confirm your tentative diagnosis of carpal tunnel syndrome. Elevated threshold numbers for Semmes-Weinstein monofilament tests in the median nerve distribution reflect loss of protective touch. Impaired static two-point discrimination in the median nerve distribution, as well as flattening of the thenar eminence indicative of thenar atrophy, reflects significant nerve compression. Mr. Handy's slower times on dexterity testing and the difficulty he has in keeping pace at work may be due to loss of sensory feedback when he works with vision occluded.

When the patient reports symptoms of nerve compression but test results are not abnormal, this information may suggest the need for additional stress testing or confirm a more subtle compression that helps confirm a quicker recovery. A sample of a summary paragraph for a patient with these test results might be written like this:

Sensibility test results for Ms. Fingering reflect normal values for all of her fingers and her thumb. No abnormal test results were found in the ulnar nerve distribution where Ms. Fingering reports symptoms of numbness and tingling. Discussion of her symptoms revealed that they are typically transient in nature and occur most frequently after heavy word processing. Ms. Fingering demonstrated that she leans on her elbow while keying in the data, and this positioning may be contributing to her symptoms. Suggestions for better positioning to eliminate pressure on the ulnar nerve in the cubital tunnel were provided. Ms. Fingering will monitor her symptoms and if they increase stress testing and work site assessment may be helpful.

A patient who had a surgical repair of the median nerve in the forearm 2 months earlier may just be beginning to show signs of an advancing Tinel's sign, and a follow-up summary paragraph on sensory status could be written as follows:

Mr. Sawblade is now 2 mo postsurgical repair of the median nerve in his forearm. His Tinel's sign has advanced 58 mm from the site of repair in the 62 days since his surgery. His recovery rate is just under 1 mm per day. Further nerve regeneration will need to progress through an area of extensive soft tissue injury in his forearm and will be carefully monitored. Mr. Sawblade has been instructed in sensory precautions, has been taught how to care for the anesthetic areas of his hand and arm, and is following these instructions appropriately.

SUMMARY

This chapter reviewed concepts in sensory physiology and presented a classification system for sensory tests. The selection of appropriate sensory tests, followed by discussion of Tinel's sign, static and moving two-point discrimination, monofilament discrimination, vibratory testing, sensory nerve conduction studies, and stress testing were discussed. Information on correlating sensibility with hand function and suggestions for writing sensibility testing summary were also included.

Therapists testing sensibility do not need to feel overwhelmed by the number of sensory tests available, or confused by the test results. Clinical research has demonstrated the usefulness of the sensory tests currently available to assess the different types of nerve injuries. Careful selection of tests that are sensitive for the type and level of peripheral nerve injury the patient has will provide the therapist with helpful information about the patient's condition and therapy needs. An interpretative, concise, and accurate summary of sensory findings and recommendations is critical in communicating findings with the referral source and devising a treatment plan.

REFERENCES

1. Martin, JH: Receptor physiology and submodality coding in the somatic sensory system. In Kandel, ER and Schwartz, JH (eds): Principles of Neural Science, ed 2. Elsevier, New York, 1985, pp 287–300.
2. Dellon, AL: Evaluation of Sensibility and Re-education of Sensation in the Hand. Williams & Wilkins, Baltimore, 1981, p 29.
3. McIntyre, AK: Cutaneous receptors. In Sumner, AJ (ed): The Physiology of Peripheral Nerve Disease. WB Saunders, Philadelphia, 1980.
4. Kandel, ER: Central representation of touch. In Kandel, ER and Schwartz, JH (eds): Principles of Neural Science, ed 2 Elsevier, New York, 1985, pp 323–325.

 5. Baichi, RL: Excitation and conduction in nerve. In Sumner, AJ (ed): The Physiology of Peripheral Nerve Disease. WB Saunders, Philadelphia, pp 1–40.
 6. Koester, J: Resting membrane potential and action potential. In Kandel, ER and Schwartz, JH (eds): Principles of Neural Science, ed 2. Elsevier, New York, 1985, pp 50–57.
 7. Kimura, J: Electrodiagnosis in Diseases of Nerve and Muscle: Principles and Practice. FA Davis, Philadelphia, 1989, p 64.
 8. Sunderland, S: Nerves and Injuries, ed 2. Churchill Livingstone, New York, 1978.
 9. Gelberman, RH, et al: Digital sensibility following replantation. J Hand Surg 3(4):313, 1978.
10. Moberg, E: Objective methods for determining the functional value of sensibility in the hand. J Bone Joint Surg 40B(3):454, 1958.
11. Werner, JL and Omer, GE, Jr: Evaluating cutaneous pressure sensation of the hand. Am J Occup Ther 24:347, 1970.
12. Lundborg, G, et al: Median nerve compression in the carpal tunnel—functional response to experimentally induced controlled pressure. J Hand Surg 7(3):252, 1982.
13. Gelberman, RH, et al: Sensibility testing in peripheral nerve compression syndromes. J Bone Joint Surg 65A:632, 1983.
14. Szabo, RM, Gelberman, RH, and Dimick, MP: Sensibility testing in patients with carpal tunnel syndrome. J Bone Joint Surg 66A(1):60, 1984.
15. Szabo, RM, et al: Vibratory testing in acute peripheral nerve compression. J Bone Joint Surg 9A(1):104, 1984.
16. Lundborg, G, et al: Digital vibrogram: A new diagnostic tool for sensory testing in compression neuropathy. Plast Reconstr Surg 65(4):466, 1980.
17. Dellon, AL: Clinical use of vibratory stimuli to evaluate peripheral nerve injury and compression neuropathy. Plast Reconstr Surg 65(4):466, 1980.
18. Dellon, AL: The Vibrometer. Plast Reconstr Surg 71(3):427, 1983.
19. Bell, JA: Light touch–deep pressure testing using Semmes-Weinstein monofilaments. In Hunter, et al (eds): Rehabilitation of the Hand, ed 3. CV Mosby, Philadelphia, 1990, pp 585–593.
20. American Society for Surgery of the Hand: The Hand, Examination and Diagnosis, ed 2. Churchill Livingstone, New York, 1983, p 106.
21. Louis, et al: Evaluation of normal values for stationary and moving two point discrimination in the hand. J Hand Surg 9A(4):552, 1984.
22. Bell-Krotoski, J and Tomanak, L: The Repeatability of Testing with Semmes-Weinstein monofilaments. J Hand Surg 12A(11):155, 1987.
23. Levin, SL, Pearsall, G, and Ruderman, RJ: Von Frey's method of measuring pressure sensibility in the hand: An engineering analysis of the Weinstein-Semmes Pressure Anesthesiometer. J Hand Surg 3(3):211, 1978.
24. Von Prince, K and Butler, B: Measuring sensory function of the hand in peripheral nerve injuries. Am J Occup Ther 6:385, 1967.

CHAPTER 5

Functional Evaluation of the Hand

Patricia A. Totten, OTR, CHT
Sharon Flinn-Wagner, MEd, OTRL, CVE

Returning the patient to a former level of productive living is the ultimate goal of the hand therapist. Even if the patient has a devastating injury or disease that has impaired hand function, the therapist must strive to help the patient achieve satisfactory function. Standard evaluation tools are used to assess range of motion, strength, and sensibility to quantify and qualify dysfunction and pathology. Unfortunately, interpretations from these measurements are limited in scope, allowing the therapist to make only general conclusions about the patient's functional status. A clear example is seen in the case of a woman with rheumatoid arthritis who, despite joint deformities and documented limited motion, is functionally independent due to the substitution patterns she has developed to perform self-care and cooking tasks. To better understand a patient's functional ability, the therapist should systematically draw from all appropriate means of assessment available. Data gathered from standard evaluation techniques, interviews, questionnaires, observations, and functional tests shed light on deficient areas in need of treatment.

The objectives of this chapter are to (1) review the history of functional testing; (2) present information regarding factors that influence clinical reasoning; (3) review terminology associated with functional patterns of movement; (4) discuss methods of functional evaluations including questionnaires, interviews, observations, and functional tests; (5) discuss the qualities of standardized functional tests; (6) describe some commonly used standardized functional tests; and (7) describe documentation of patient performance on functional tests.

HISTORY OF FUNCTIONAL TESTING

The concept of returning a patient to productive function has its roots in occupational therapy. One of the earlier documentations outlining treatment intervention dates back to 1915 when goals were set to help patients overcome disabilities and progress toward reestablishing a "capacity for industrial and social usefulness."[1] World War I gave impetus to the field of therapy; the development of antisepsis and anesthesia allowed many soldiers to survive their wounds, thereby increasing the demand for rehabilitation. In *The Army Manual on Occupational Therapy*, Bird T. Baldwin made valuable contributions in the form of records which "enable the examiner to determine which mode of treatment leads to the greatest and most consistent gains in a particular case . . ."[2]

Following World War I, therapists became more interested in upper extremity function as new developments evolved in the medical field: tendons were being repaired, new antibiotics were discovered, and surgeons were able to save limbs which, in previous years, would have been amputated.[3] Dr. Wynn Parry of the Royal Air Force in England published a text on hand rehabilitation in 1958, proposing the team approach to treating hand patients in which the physician, physiotherapist, occupational therapist, and patient collectively work toward a common goal.[4] This ideal collection became a model for American therapy centers and occupational therapists began specializing in the treatment of upper extremity peripheral nerve injuries and amputations.[5] Therapists became skilled in developing techniques to assist patients in the following areas: activities of daily living (ADLs), work simplification, rehabilitation for the disabled homemaker, and training in the use of upper extremity prosthesis.[6] As medical advances were made in the treatment of poliomyelitis during the 1950s, therapists expanded their remedial efforts to include the treatment of the more chronic conditions such as arthritis, congenital defects, stroke, and deficits resulting from traumatic injury.[6] Interest in the treatment of these chronic conditions spurred therapists to explore functional assessments. During the 1960s, a greater understanding of rheumatoid arthritis hand deformities and function occurred, thus contributing to the development of functional evaluations. Data assimilated from these evaluations led therapists to develop joint protection techniques[7] and to report valuable information to surgeons regarding a patient's preoperative baseline versus postoperative performance.[8]

In the early stages of hand therapy, upper extremity function was tested by observing patients picking up and manipulating coins and common household objects. These common practices were replaced with more standardized methods of testing. In the evolution of functional testing, specificity was practiced. Tests were structured to be administered to each patient in the same manner: (1) parameters listed the physical setup of the test; (2) testing material became standardized; and (3) requirements were made to ensure uniform delivery of the test (such as specific instructions read to each patient and postures that each patient must assume during the testing procedure). In 1969, the Jebsen test of hand function,[9] incorporated seven subtests designed to measure hand performance in various activities, such as handwriting, and the manipulation of small common objects and 1-lb cans.

Throughout the 1970s more objective tests, such as the physical capacities evaluation (PCE) of hand skill introduced by Bell and associates,[10] established norms for three disability groups: paraplegia, left hemiplegia, and right hemiplegia. Functional evaluations tested "the status of hand skill regardless of vocational potential . . . determining the need for occupational therapy services. Functional evaluations were chosen to measure progress toward fulfilling treatment goals, thereby determining the effectiveness of the treatment, and the need for further, or cessation of treatment . . ."[10]

As new technology emerged in the late 1970s and 1980s, many upper extremity clinics began to experiment with innovative apparati such as the Baltimore Therapeutic Equipment (BTE) Work Simulator. This computerized rehabilitation device allows the patient to work with various tool handles so that specific muscle groups can be exercised or home and job tasks can be simulated with a graded resistance. Although normative data have not yet been compiled for all of the tool handles,[11] a therapist may make some decisions through the course of treatment regarding the patient's isometric or isotonic efforts.

CLINICAL REASONING AND THE FUNCTIONAL EVALUATION PROCESS

A familiarity with normative upper extremity anatomy, function, and impairment will enable the clinician to make some assumptions regarding the patient's functional status. Expectations regarding a patient's functional outcome can be made from the following sources: the referring physician; pertinent case studies in textbooks; rehabilitation nurses; information about the patient's functional role in society; and the patient's anticipated goals. The model of assessment of occupational performance developed by Rogers and Masagatani[12] in 1985 (Fig. 5–1) outlines pertinent factors that the therapist should consider while assessing and treating the patient. The clinical reasoning process presented in this model will enhance the therapist's ability to use the aforementioned information and systematically assimilate a series of evaluations and treatment priorities. Treatment processes are influenced by the therapist's past experiences, resourcefulness, and preferences. Clinical judgment may be clouded when the therapist has preconceived biases and limited access to tests or resources; however, the opposite can also be problematic. Entrepreneurs, therapists, and manufacturers have flooded the present market with evaluation tools and testing equipment. This wealth of resources can be overwhelming to the inexperienced therapist. Preference should be given to tests that have been standardized, field tested, and accompanied by reports explaining how the measurements can be used to make judgments regarding patient function.[13] The therapist drawing from a comprehensive knowledge base "using valid and reliable assessment tools will increase the mathematical probabilities of making the correct clinical decisions."[13]

TERMINOLOGY ASSOCIATED WITH FUNCTIONAL PATTERNS OF MOVEMENT

Functional Patterns of Movement of the Shoulder and Elbow

The term "function" is frequently used without regard to a specific anatomic pattern of movement. Although the focus of this text is the hand, hand function is dependent on the action of the proximal joints that enable the hand to reach most efficiently. Rather than define shoulder movement solely in terms of goniometric measurements, the therapist should refer to the standards set by the American Shoulder and Elbow Surgeons.[14] External and internal rotation are measured not only from the classic

ASSESSMENT OF OCCUPATIONAL PERFORMANCE
Developed by Joan Rogers, 1945

ASSESSMENT LEVEL	ASSESSMENT CONTENT	PRIMARY METHOD
1. What **does** the patient do routinely?	TEMPORAL ADAPTATION (Lifestyle) Coordination of daily habits in self-care, work, and leisure occupations	History-taking: Patient Collateral
2. What **can** the patient do?	OCCUPATIONAL PERFORMANCE (Skill) Self-care: Feeding Dressing Hygiene and grooming Bathing Work: Paid employment Volunteer Home management Meal planning/preparation Shopping Housekeeping (dusting, bed-making and the like) Money management Gardening Home repair Time management:	Performance testing in actual or simulated situations
3. What factors facilitate or hinder occupational performance?	OCCUPATIONAL PERFORMANCE COMPONENTS (Skill Abilities and Specifics) Biologic: Functional vision/hearing Postural balance/functional mobility Endurance Psychologic: Cognitive Orientation Attention Concentration Memory Problem-solving Judgment Emotional Motivation for occupation Personal causation Social: Functional communication written Verbal Social support Presence Attitude Environment Architectural barriers Products	Standardized and unstandardized tests
4. What are the patient's self-perceptions of occupational performance?	PERCEPTIONS OR COMPETENCE	Interview

FIGURE 5–1. Occupational performance assessment developed by Joan Rogers.[12]

starting position of shoulder abduction to 90° with the elbow in 90° of flexion, but also in the plane of the scapula. For example, active internal rotation can be documented as the highest vertebral level a patient can reach while positioning the dorsum of the hand against the back and striving to reach upward with a hitchhiking thumb. Hoppenfeld,[15] in his classic text, *Physical Examination of the Spine and Extremities*, reviews the proximal positions of upper extremity function, referred to as the Apley "scratch test." Abduction and external rotation are assessed when the patient reaches behind the head to touch the superior medial angle of the opposite scapula. Internal rotation and adduction are assessed when the patient reaches across the midline to touch the opposite acromion. Internal rotation is tested when the patient reaches behind the back to touch the inferior angle of the opposite scapula, as seen in Figure 5–2.

The Examination Data Form outlined by the American Shoulder and Elbow Surgeons also includes a functional checklist in which the evaluator addresses proximal upper functions such as using the back pocket, performing rectal hygiene, washing the opposite underarm, using the hand overhead, combing the hair, using the hand and arm at shoulder level, carrying 10 to 15 lb with the arm at the side, as well as throwing and lifting.[14] Although these are important functions that should be recognized, they are measured rather subjectively, with responses falling in the categories of normal, mild compromise, and other descriptions of performance.

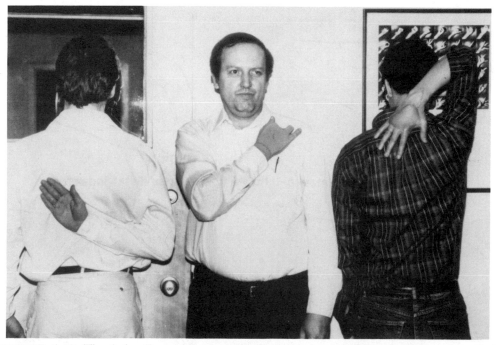

FIGURE 5–2. The Apley "scratch" test evaluating a patient's active range of motion. *Left*, Internal rotation and adduction; patient reaches behind back to touch inferior angle of the opposite scapula. *Middle*, Internal rotation and adduction (less demanding); patient reaches across midline to touch opposite acromion. *Right*, External rotation and abduction; patient reaches behind head to touch superior medial angle of opposite scapula.

Functional Patterns of Movement of the Hand

Adult hand prehension patterns are dependent on (1) a sensate and mobile hand that can assume various postures, (2) adequate finger length, and (3) sufficient width and depth of the palm.[16] In a comprehensive review of relevant literature, Cassanova and Grunert[16] report that a multitude of distinct terms, 334 in all, were used to describe the forms of prehension. They propose a readily identifiable system for static and dynamic prehension pattern nomenclature based on numbering the digits with roman numerals I through V. These patterns are then classified using the digital landmarks or contact surfaces such as metacarpophalangeal (MP), proximal interphalangeal (PIP), or distal interphalangeal (DIP) joint; proximal, middle, or distal phalanx; radial or ulnar aspect of the digit; or tip or pad aspect of the digit. Excellent examples of these patterns are demonstrated in Figures 5–3 through 5–7.

Hand function has also been described by Melvin,[17] who divides hand usage patterns into four categories:

1. Finger-thumb prehension
   a. Objects are held between the thumb and fingers of a single hand.
   b. Finger-thumb patterns include tip, lateral, and three-point pinch patterns.
2. Full hand prehension
   a. Palm of the hand forms one of the gripping surfaces (gross power and cylindrical grasp).

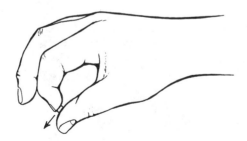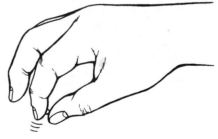

A, B.   I pad distal-to-II tip ↔ I tip-to-II pad distal (index roll).

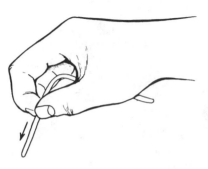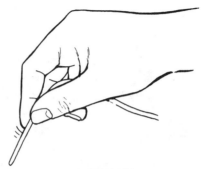

C, D.   I tip-to-II tip ↔ I pad distal-to-II pad distal (pinch).

FIGURE 5–3. Prehensile patterns: Dynamic thumb–index finger pad pinches. (From Casanova and Grunert,[16] p 240, with permission.)

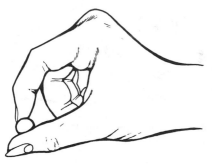 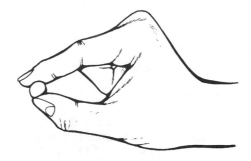

A. **I pad distal–to–II tip** (tip-to-tip opposition, tip prehension).

B. **I tip-to-II pad distal** (round pinch).

FIGURE 5–4. Prehensile patterns: Static thumb–index finger "other" pinches. (From Casanova and Grunert,[16] p 240, with permission.)

3. Nonprehension
   a. The hand is used as an extension of upper extremity (hook grip, hand used to push objects).
   b. The fingertips (usually the index or long finger) are used to apply pressure (smoothing sheets while making a bed or pressing pie dough into a pie pan).
   c. A fingertip (usually the index or long finger) is used for precision or sorting (pushing buttons, turning pages, dialing a telephone).
   d. The heel or the ulnar side of the hand is used to apply pressure (kneading bread dough).
4. Bilateral prehension
   a. Bilateral prehension requires the palmar surfaces of both hands to hold an object which is too large, cumbersome, or heavy to be held with a single hand.

Swanson[8] reports that the average hand "utilizes only an estimated 10 percent of its skill potential" and defines three categories of movement patterns: fixed posture, integrated motions, and percussive movements. With fixed postures, much like Melvin's classification of nonprehension hand patterns,[17] the hand acts as a terminus for the proximal arm. Functional upper extremity movements in which the hand assumes a fixed posture include "scooping, receiving, pushing, pointing, hooking, resting the palm or knuckles."[8] Integrated motions occur when the digits work together to manipulate small objects in the basic grasp, release, and pinch patterns. Pulp, lateral, and tip pinch

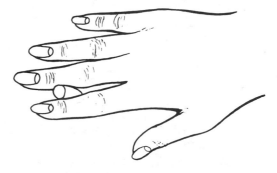

FIGURE 5–5. Prehensile patterns: Static index finger–middle finger pinch. (From Casanova and Grunert,[16] p 240, with permission.)

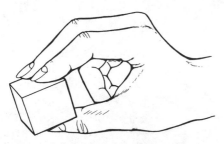

A. I pad distal–to–II & III pads distal (chuck or three-fingered pinch, palmar prehension, three-jawed chuck grasp, three-point fixation, finger thumb prehension, precision grip, chuck, three-jaw chuck, chuck grip, three-chuck pinch, three-digit or chuck pinch).

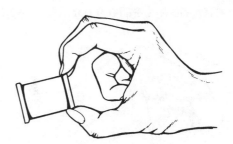

B. I tip–to–II & III tip (precision translation).

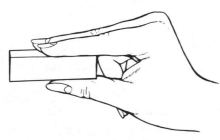

C. I pad distal–to–II & III pads distal and middle (multilateral thumb finger pinch, three-point prehension, three-point palmar pinch, three-jaw or three-jaw chuck, three-point, palmar, radial digital, cylindrical radial palmar, palmar tripod, terminoterminal tridigital pinch, terminoterminal tridigital pinch).

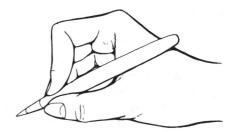

D. I pad distal–to–web–to II pad distal and II radial distal (web-of-thumb).

FIGURE 5–6. Prehensile patterns: Static three-finger pinches—pads and tips. (From Casanova and Grunert,[16] p 241, with permission.)

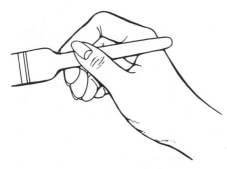

A. I pad distal–to–II pad distal and radial proximal and III radial distal (unnamed).

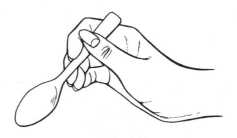

B. I pad distal–to–II pad distal and radial proximal and III dorsal distal (teaspoon finger grip).

FIGURE 5–7. Prehensile patterns: Static three-finger pinches—radial index finger. (From Casanova and Grunert,[16] p 241, with permission.)

are examples of integrated motions. Pulp pinch is performed between the flat surfaces of the thumb and an opposing digit; lateral pinch is performed between the lateral surface of the thumb and the side of another digit, and tip pinch is done between the tips of the thumb and an opposing digit. Percussive movements rely on a proximal joint to move a distal joint, and are usually accomplished with the PIP, MP, wrist, elbow, and shoulder joints, or even with the whole body.[8] During percussive movements the hand acts as an instrument for the more proximal joints. Typing and playing an instrument are examples of percussive movements. Swanson recommends that hand function be documented using (1) range-of-motion measurements of the joints of the hand, (2) flexion of the DIP crease to the palmar crease in terms of centimeters, and (3) the patient's ability to grasp cylinders ranging from 2.5 to 10 cm and spheres measuring from 5 to 12.5 cm.[8]

Strength

A patient's ability to function is also related to muscle strength. When presented with a patient with a lower motor neuron (LMN) dysfunction, muscle disease, or orthopedic dysfunction, a manual muscle test should be done. Hand grip has been an indicator for determining strength since 1880.[18] Grip strength has been correlated to function in the areas of hand dominance and overall physical fitness.[18] Bechtol,[19] in 1954, produced a grip dynamometer with adjustable hand spacings which measured hand grip force in pounds. Bechtol's article suggests that adult grip strength is altered according to the size of the object being grasped. Figure 5–8 illustrates a sample of the

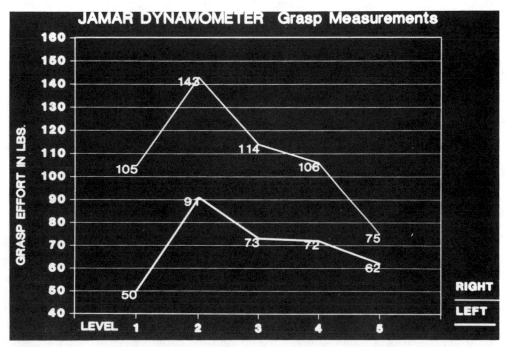

FIGURE 5–8. Plotted right-handed (*top line*) and left-handed (*bottom line*) efforts on the Jamar Dynamometer. Vertical axis represents grasp effort in pounds. Horizontal axis represents each handle level on the Jamar Dynamometer.

bell-shaped curve that should be created when a patient puts forth maximum effort on all five levels of the dynamometer. Pryce's research[20] revealed that maximal grip strength occurred when the wrist was positioned in 0 to 15° of extension. In testing hand strength, the American Society for Surgery of the Hand[21] recommends that the second handle position be used in determining grip strength and that three trials should be averaged.

An adapted sphygmomonometer may be used to measure grip when the patient is unable to use the Jamar Dynamometer because of arthritis, a sensitive palm, or a weakened grasp. According to Melvin,[17] the cuff of a sphygmomanometer is rolled up and secured, so that when inflated to a specific mmHg reading, it maintains a constant circumference. The reported recommended standards are for circumference sizes of 6, 7, and 8 in with mmHg readings of 20, 30, and 40, respectively. The patient is instructed to grip the inflated cuff firmly. The average of three trials is recorded. Normative data for this method have been compiled on a cuff measuring 8 in starting at 40 mmHg.[22]

Pinch strength may be measured by the pinchmeter. Usually, three types of pinch are assessed: key or lateral pinch; three-point pinch or three-jaw chuck, or tip-to-tip pinch (thumb to each opposing finger). According to the American Society for Surgery of the Hand,[21] the average of three trials is recorded. The author suggests that the pinchmeter should be positioned with the gauge facing down to prevent the patient from receiving visual feedback while exerting maximum effort.

Function may also be affected by the patient's ability to control movements. Cerebellar dysfunction and lesions of the basal ganglia may affect voluntary movement and maintenance of upright posture.[23] Endurance is an important component of function and should be noted by the length of time or number of repetitions that a patient is able to perform an activity prior to experiencing fatigue. Endurance deficits were first recognized in association with lower motor neuron problems,[24] but patients with upper extremity dysfunction experience decreased endurance secondary to prolonged immobilization and injury.

METHODS OF FUNCTIONAL EVALUATION

The functional evaluation process is analogous to a research study. Gay[24] describes descriptive research as "collecting data to test hypotheses using questionnaires, interview, or structured observations." In addition to these three assessment tools, functional evaluations incorporate standardized functional tests to allow objective measurement of patient performance.

Questionnaires

Well-constructed questionnaires serve as screening tools and gather information independent of the therapist, saving time and expense. Assuming that the patient is a reliable reporter, responses on a functional questionnaire provide clues to areas that should be targeted in the subsequent evaluation process. A questionnaire (Fig. 5–9) may be brief and uncomplicated so that a patient, family member, or clinical secretary may complete it as the patient awaits the initial therapy visit. If the patient completes the form independently, the therapist will learn about the patient's ability to follow directions. A questionnaire might be used for a patient who has suffered a left cerebral

Therapy Department

Name: _____   Activity Analysis:
Date: _____   Brief

The answers to this questionnaire will help your therapist learn about any difficulties that you may encounter while performing your usual daily activities.

Please place a check in the appropriate column as you read through the list.

Can you manage the following activities?	Easy	Difficult	Unable to do	Not applicable
1. PERSONAL HYGIENE				
a. bathing				
b. toileting				
2. DRESSING				
a. upper				
b. lower body				
3. FOOD PREPARATION				
a. snack				
b. meal				
4. DINING				
a. feed self				
b. drink from cup/glass				
5. FORMER HOBBIES				
6. FORMER WORK TASKS				

FIGURE 5–9. ADL assessment. Example of a brief activity analysis questionnaire.

vascular accident (CVA), and complains of experiencing increased flexor tone and pain in his right-dominant upper extremity. A questionnaire completed by a family member may reveal that the patient is particularly concerned about writing, getting his right hand open for hygiene purposes, and dressing the upper body independently.

When a patient complains of difficulties performing certain activities, the therapist may choose to follow up with an actual activity analysis or issue a more detailed questionnaire (Fig. 5–10), breaking down activities into their component parts. The

Therapy Department

Name: _____   Activity Analysis
Date: _____   Food Preparation

    The answers to this questionnaire will help your therapist learn about specific problems that you may encounter while performing activities that relate to food preparation.

    Please place a check in the appropriate column. Add any comments if you wish to explain your situation.

Can you manage the following activities?	Easy	Difficult	Unable to do	Not applicable	Comment/ solution
1. OPENING					
a. cans					
b. jars					
c. packaged goods					
2. COOKING/BAKING					
a. pick up pan/kettle					
b. fill pan /kettle					
c. carry pan/kettle to stove					
d. turn stove/oven on/off					
e. measure ingredients					
f. stir ingredients					
g. break an egg					
h. drain vegetables pour from kettle					
i. remove hot dish from oven					

FIGURE 5–10. ADL assessment. Example of a detailed activity analysis questionnaire.

questionnaire should also include space for the patient to list his or her expectations of therapy. This will provide the patient with an opportunity to elaborate on concerns not addressed on the form or to express matters that he or she may feel are too personal to discuss outright with the therapist. Upon reviewing the questionnaire, the therapist will be able to recognize and appreciate the patient's problems and standard of acceptable performance.

Interview

Interviews are probably the most common means of assessment when evaluating a new patient. Interviews serve to probe responses received in the questionnaire and to clarify a pattern of dysfunction. An example of a right hand–dominant woman with the diagnosis of rheumatoid arthritis may be posed. The patient comes to the clinic 4 weeks after right thumb MP joint fusion and carpal tunnel decompression. A thumb spica splint is fabricated that encompasses the radial hand, forearm, and wrist yet allows thumb interphalangeal (IP) joint motion. The patient is instructed to wear the splint at all times, except when performing active range-of-motion exercises for the right wrist, thumb IP joint, and fingers. The therapist, upon review of the questionnaire, notes that the patient has particular difficulty and heightened pain during cooking tasks. Upon questioning the patient, the therapist learns that the patient removes her splint to prepare meals and whenever her hand contacts water.

The interview may also assist the therapist in determining how the patient is coping with disability-related circumstances (i.e., employer-employee relations or law suits) and what is important to the patient's sense of well-being. Pain scales may also be included in the interview process. The interview serves as a bridge between the knowledge a therapist has about the presenting diagnosis, the unique pattern of dysfunction that has affected the patient, and the objective tasks that should be selected to quantify the pattern of dysfunction.

Observation

Observation is the most critical component of the therapist's assessment in that it allows the therapist to synthesize a profile of a patient's condition. Observations are helpful in teaching the therapist how a patient may function outside of the clinical setting. Although informal observations can be made, formal observations that can be measured and reproduced allow the therapist to summarize a patient's status and make predictions regarding the patient's response to treatment.

Observations of the patient fall into two categories: spectator observations or staged observations. Spectator observations occur when the therapist assumes the role of a spectator and discretely observes the patient's function in the clinic. Staged observations are designed by the therapist to evaluate a specific aspect of the patient's function, with the patient being a passive or active participant in the test.

SPECTATOR OBSERVATION

Spectator observation may include surveillance of the patient's postoperative dressing, the level of assistance that a patient accepts from a family member, the manner in which the extremity is held in relation to the body, or the method the patient uses to take off a coat upon entering the clinic. While reviewing a questionnaire with a truck driver 6 weeks after distal phalanx amputation of the small finger, the therapist may note that the patient denies difficulties with hand function as he simultaneously gestures with the affected finger positioned in extension and abduction.

STAGED OBSERVATION

Patient Unaware

Opportunities to learn more about a patient may be staged when the therapist appears to drop a pen or goniometer in the general direction of the patient or when the therapist presents an appointment card to the patient at his midline. Notations are made regarding the patient's response: does the patient choose to interact with the affected extremity; does the affected extremity move spontaneously or with difficulty; are any compensatory techniques used? These observations are documented during the initial evaluation and are reassessed routinely until the grasping pattern is integrated into the body scheme spontaneously.

Patient Actively Involved

Staged observations that depend on active participation of the patient quantify a patient's dysfunctional level. Staged observations are nonstandardized but should be set up in the same manner whenever presented to the patient in subsequent trials. Consistent use of the same test format allows the therapist to make comparisons against baseline data as the patient progresses through treatment. Examples of staged observations are outlined in an article by Carthum, Clawson, and Decker.[25]

---

1. *One-Handed Activities*

A. Safety pin test   Timed test. A 1-in safety pin is held in the uninvolved hand while the involved hand opens and closes the safety pin.

B. Button test   Timed tests requiring the subject to unbutton and button several buttons. This test uses two button boards.
     1) Board 1: Composed of three buttons, sizes ½ in, 1 in, and 1⅝ in, with similar-sized buttonholes
     2) Board 2: Composed of six buttons, all ⅞ in in diameter with similar-sized buttonholes

2. *Two-Handed Activities*

A. Knife and fork test   Timed test. Patient uses standard eating utensils to cut through a piece of plasticized clay.

B. Shoelace test   Timed test. Using three sets of holes, patient unties the bow, removes the entire lace, replaces the lace, then ties the bow.

Staged observations can be developed to quantify and qualify any functional deficit. An example of a staged observation may be presented using the case of Mrs. X, who suffers from rheumatoid arthritis and reports that her joint deformities and decreased range of motion interfere with kitchen tasks, specifically cutting vegetables and picking up heavy pots and pans. Through an activity analysis, the therapist may evaluate the patient's ability to cut vegetables by posing specific tasks for the patient to perform.

1. Method
   a. Trial of grasping knives with different-sized handles
   b. Trial of different cutting techniques (i.e., using a dagger type of hold, using the traditional approach, or using a rocking method)
   c. Trial of cutting mediums (i.e., various grades of putty or actual fruits or vegetables)

    d. Trial of various cutting surfaces (i.e., a traditional cuttingboard or an adaptive cuttingboard with a stabilizing nail to secure the object being cut)

2. Procedure (for test-retest situations)
    a. Testing should always employ the same knife, cutting technique, cutting medium, and cutting surface.
    b. The setup should always be placed a specific number of inches or centimeters from the table's edge.
    c. The cutting medium should be of the same size as that introduced during the initial evaluation.

3. Measuring Performance
    a. The patient is instructed to cut approximately ¼-in slices from a putty roll. The therapist counts the number of slices completed in a 1-minute period.

4. Variations/Treatment Implications
    a. Upon noting difficulty, the therapist may decide to downgrade the resistance of putty, offer the patient a rocker knife or builtup handle, or plan a splint to better align and stabilize the metacarpophalangeal joints. The patient should be taught joint protection techniques and isometric exercises to improve upper extremity strength.
    b. Upon noting ease when performing the task, the therapist may opt to upgrade the resistance of the putty and teach the patient the importance of balancing work activities with rest.

When testing the patient's ability to lift heavy pans, the therapist may initially have the patient lift an empty pan and evaluate the grasp pattern. Measured water may be added and the distance carried could be noted. Adaptations may include using two hands to carry the pan or instructing the patient to slide it across the countertop in order to reach the stove.

Functional Tests

Functional tests are formal observations that require specific guidelines for administration and measurement so that the test results can be used to qualify patient performance when compared with normative data. Once the data-gathering process is complete in regard to (1) the patient's available range of motion, (2) method of using the hand, and (3) an understanding of the patient's goals in relation to returning to the home or work environment, the therapist determines which functional tests may be used as indicators of baseline function. Functional tests assess a broad spectrum of hand and upper extremity function including ADLs, gross and fine motor ability, tool usage, manipulation, dexterity, grasp and release of objects, unilateral and bilateral hand use, and sensibility.[26] A patient's performance may be scored according to one or more of the following methods: (1) time limit (quantity completed in a specified time period), (2) qualitative scoring (the way an object is grasped), (3) work limit (timed to completion), and (4) subjective data (pain, complaints).[26]

STANDARDIZED VERSUS NONSTANDARDIZED FUNCTIONAL TESTS

In 1987, Mcphee[27] reviewed and analyzed 41 known hand function tests. He concluded that no single hand function test was appropriate for all patients. How is the therapist to know which functional test is appropriate for which patient? To develop baseline information about the patient and then follow up with testing at regular intervals to determine patient progress, a standardized test of function is preferred. A standardized test is defined as an instrument that must satisfy all of the following conditions[28]:

1. A statement that defines the purpose or intent of the test
2. Correlation statistics or another appropriate measure of instrument validity
3. Correlation statistics or another appropriate measure of instrument reliability
4. Detailed descriptions of the equipment used in the test
5. Normative data, drawn from a large population sample, that are divided into categories according to appropriate variables such as hand dominance, age, sex, or occupation
6. Specific instructions for administering, scoring and interpreting the test

In choosing a test, the therapist notes whether the tests have been proven statistically valid and reliable; that is, do "they appropriately measure what they purport to measure and do they measure consistently with their measurement unit, between examiners and from trial to trial."[28] In this day of accountability, the therapist should select tests that are consistently reproducible and provide objective information about patient performance and progress. If the functional test is used to quantify performance by using normative data, the guidelines and instructions that accompany the test must be closely followed. Normative data cannot be correlated to makeshift versions of the test or to a test that has been used in the interim as part of the treatment process.[28]

DESCRIPTIONS OF COMMONLY USED STANDARDIZED FUNCTIONAL TESTS

Standardized functional tests serve as a means to measure objectively patient performance. The chapter appendix summarizes standardized functional tests with regard to the length of time needed to administer, the validity and reliability, and the approximate cost. The more common tests are further described as follows:

Bennett Hand Tool Test

The Bennett hand tool test is composed of a wooden rectangular base and two upright boards. The upright board, placed at the patient's left, contains screws and two sizes of bolts with accompanying washers. A screwdriver and various-sized wrenches are provided. The examiner reads the directions and times the patient as he or she disassembles the left wooden upright using hands and tools then replaces the screws and bolts on the opposite upright. Normative data are based on the time to complete the task and are compared to those of other workers or applicants in various lines of work (Fig. 5–11).[29]

Box and Block Test

The box and block test comprises a wooden box with two side-by-side compartments separated by a raised partition. The partition is placed at the patient's midline. The test includes a rectangular box that houses several 1-in wooden cubes. The examiner pours the blocks into a compartment and then reads the directions to the patient while demonstrating that the patient must pick up one block at a time and transfer it

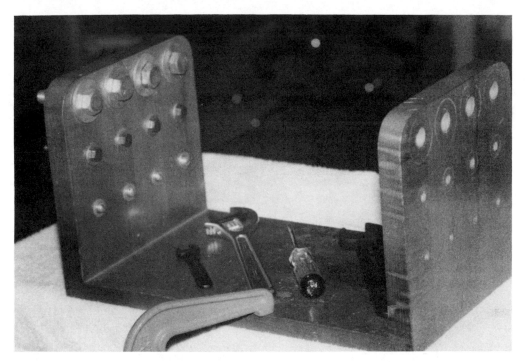

FIGURE 5–11. Bennett hand tool function test: Consists of two wooden uprights with bolts and screws that are removed from the left upright and mounted on the right upright using tools and fingers.

over the partition so that it lands in the other compartment. A 15-second practice test is included for each hand. The actual test for each hand lasts 1 minute. Scoring is dependent on the number of blocks transferred. Normative data are listed by gender and age group (Fig. 5–12).[30]

Crawford Small Parts Dexterity Test

The Crawford small parts dexterity test consists of a wooden board with separate wells for metal pins, collars, and screws. A metal plate containing holes for pins and threaded holes for screws fits over a portion of the board. Tweezers and a small screwdriver are provided. The test is divided into two parts, each with its own set of normative data. Part I, "Pins and Collars," measures dexterity as the patient uses tweezers to insert small pins upright into close-fitting holes and then to fit small collars over the protruding pins. Part II, "Screws," measures dexterity in starting screws into threaded holes and screwing them down with a screwdriver (Fig. 5–13).[31]

Jebsen-Taylor Hand Function Test

The Jebsen-Taylor hand function test is composed of seven subtests that represent various hand activities. The test must be fabricated according to the specifications of the Jebsen and Taylor article.[53] The seven subtests include (1) writing, (2) turning over 3 by 5–in cards (which simulates page turning), (3) picking up small common objects, (4) simulated feeding, (5) stacking checkers, (6) picking up and placing large empty cans, and (7) picking up and placing 1-lb cans. The examiner reads the directions to the

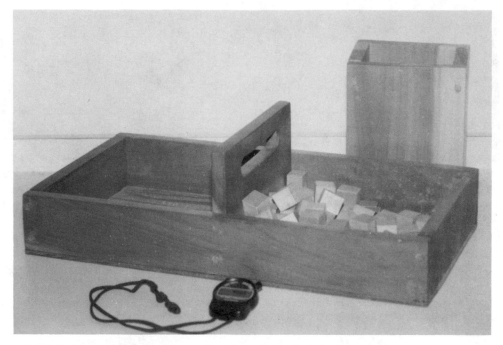

FIGURE 5–12. Box and block test: Consists of wooden blocks and a two-compartment box with a partition. To ensure a random distribution the blocks are poured from the wooden box shown in the back right of the picture.

patient and records the time that the patient requires to complete each subtest with the nondominant and then the dominant hand. The results are compared with normative data available relative to gender and age (Fig. 5–14).[9]

Minnesota Rate of Manipulation Test (MRMT)

The Minnesota rate of manipulation test is composed of a rectangular base having several holes. Large checkerlike disks painted black on one side and red on the other are provided. The patient is seated at a table. The board is placed on the table in front of the patient and the examiner reads the instructions to the patient. Five tests may be performed: (1) placing, (2) turning, (3) displacing, (4) one-hand turning and placing, and (5) two-hand turning and placing. The test is timed, and the performance is compared with normative data.[32]

Nine-Hole Peg Test

The nine-hole peg test is composed of a base having nine holes, and nine pegs that are contained in an area separate from the base. The object of the test is for the patient to place the nine pegs in the holes in any order. Instructions are read to the patient, and the patient practices the test with each hand. The test is timed and the patient's performance is compared with normative data for gender and age group (Fig. 5–15).[33]

Purdue Pegboard Test

The Purdue pegboard test includes a testing board with two columns of holes aligned vertically down the center of the board. At the top of the board, four recessed cups may be found. These cups contain small metal pegs, washers, and collars. There

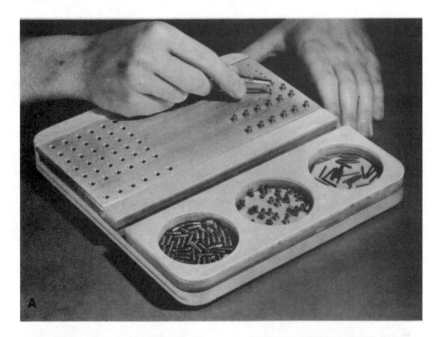

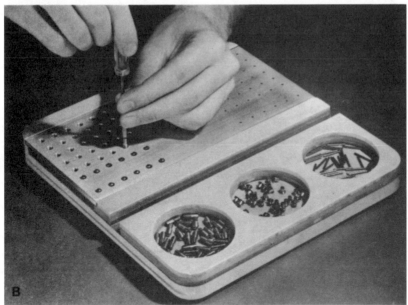

FIGURE 5–13. Crawford small parts dexterity test measures fine eye-hand coordination. *A*, Part 1 (Pins and Collars) requires the use of tweezers to inset metal pins into holes and place collars over the pins. *B*, Part 2 (Screws) requires the use of a screwdriver to fasten small screws into a metal plate. (From Crawford, JE and Crawford, DM: Crawford Small Parts Dexterity Test Manual. The Psychological Corporation, Harcourt Brace Jovanovich, San Antonio, TX, 1981, with permission.)

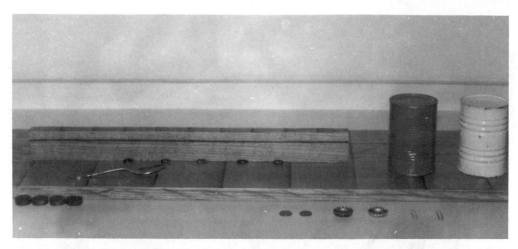

FIGURE 5–14. Jebsen-Taylor Hand Function Test. Constructed of wooden board and common household objects, the test is composed of seven subtests. Components of these tests are depicted above: stacking checkers, simulated feeding, manipulation of small objects, and lifting and placing empty and 1 lb cans.

are five subtests from which to choose: (1) right hand; (2) left hand; (3) both hands; (4) right, left, and both hands; and (5) assembly. The examiner reads the instructions to the patient, times the patient, and scores the patient's performance against normative data based on gender and job types (such as applicants for factory work or applicants for assembly jobs).[34]

Valpar Work Samples

The Valpar Corporation[35] has developed 19 work samples that are useful to the therapist and vocational rehabilitation specialist. San Diego worker norms are most frequently used by those evaluating upper extremity function.[35] Four work samples frequently used in hand clinics are described as follows:

Valpar Small Tools Mechanical Work Sample No 1. This test requires the patient to work the small hand tools such as screwdrivers, pliers, and wrenches. The patient must reach into a square hole in the front of a five-sided hinged box and work within the confines of the box. Each panel on the box requires a different set of tools to

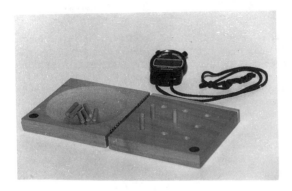

FIGURE 5–15. Nine-hole peg test: Patients are timed as they place and remove the nine pegs in the wooden grid.

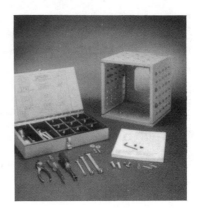

FIGURE 5–16. Valpar Corporation Work Sample (VCWS) 1—Small Tools (Mechanical). The patient assembles panels of the work sample using tools such as screwdrivers, wrenches, a nut driver, and a pair of pliers. (Note: Illustration is to demonstrate components of work sample, not how the actual test is administered.) (From Valpar International Corporation, PO Box 5767, Tucson, AZ 85703-5767, with permission.)

accomplish tasks such as inserting fasteners, screws, bolts, and hitch pin clamps, as seen in Figure 5–16. The examiner may elect to have the patient assemble one or all of the panels and even disassemble the entire work sample as well. Instructions are read to the patient and the patient is timed. Patient performance is compared with normative data compiled on specific populations.

Valpar Upper Extremity Range-of-Motion Work Sample No. 4. This test consists of a five-sided box lined with two sizes of machine bolts and a container of corresponding hex nuts. The patient must reach through a square opening in the front of the box and fasten the nuts on the appropriate pegs. The patient must use shoulder, upper arms, elbows, wrists, hands, and fingers to complete the test. The patient must rely on finger dexterity and the sense of touch to perform the test. The right and left hands are tested separately, the test is timed, and the patient's performance is compared with normative data (Fig. 5–17).[35]

Valpar Simulated Assembly No. 8. The Valpar simulated assembly is administered while standing. The testing equipment is composed of a machine with a rotating horizontal well and two bins—one containing metal pins and one containing a black spacer and a white cap. Using the components listed previously, the patient must perform a three-step assembly onto the revolving well. An automatic counter built into

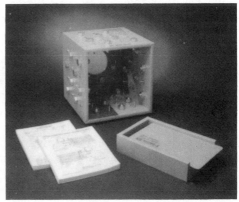

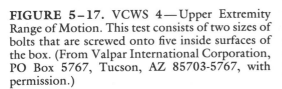

FIGURE 5–17. VCWS 4—Upper Extremity Range of Motion. This test consists of two sizes of bolts that are screwed onto five inside surfaces of the box. (From Valpar International Corporation, PO Box 5767, Tucson, AZ 85703-5767, with permission.)

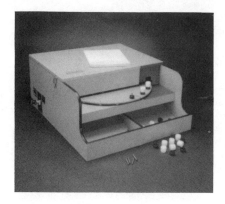

FIGURE 5–18. VCWS 8 — Simulated Assembly. This unit consists of an assembly wheel and assembly parts that are fitted into the wheel. The number of completed assemblies is tallied by the unit. (From Valpar International Corporation, PO Box 5767, Tucson, AZ 85703-5767, with permission.)

the machine records the number of assemblies completed in a 20-minute period of time. The patient's performance is compared with normative data (Fig. 5–18).[35]

Valpar Whole Body Range-of-Motion Work Sample No. 9. This test is administered while standing or crouching/kneeling. This work sample consists of a two-part adjustable frame that must be adjusted according to the patient's height. The frame contains four attached panels with permanently attached bolts placed in the pattern of a triangle, square, and kidney. Three Plexiglas forms in the shapes of a triangle, square, and kidney as well as Plexiglas nuts are provided. The bottom panel is obscured by a fifth panel that juts out from the frame at an angle.

The examiner reads the directions to the patient, who transfers the objects onto the appropriate bolts and tightens the designated number of nuts into place. The test requires reaching at shoulder level, over the head, and at knee level while performing the manipulation tasks. The bottom panel requires the patient to rely upon sense of touch as vision is occluded by the jutting panel. The transfers are timed, and the performance is compared with normative data (Fig. 5–19).[35]

TIMELY INTRODUCTION OF STANDARDIZED TESTS

When using standardized tests as part of the evaluation battery, the clinician must be aware of the diagnosis and the healing status of the involved structure(s). A functional test may not be indicated upon the patient's initial therapy visit when wound care, edema reduction, and splinting are the primary concerns. The therapist should be informed of precautions and the timing involved in the progression of treatment.

METHODS OF DOCUMENTATION

When documenting the patient's performance on a standardized test, the therapist must strive for objectivity but may consider using descriptive phrases to inform the reader of the prehensile pattern used, the patient's chosen method of approach, or any difficulties that the patient encountered when performing the test. The following case studies illustrate documentation of objective and subjective performance on standardized tests.

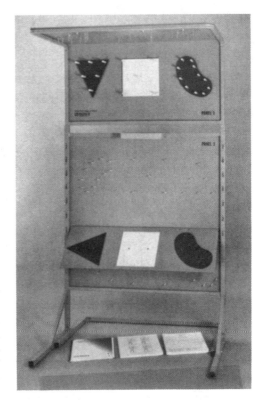

FIGURE 5–19. VCWS 9—Whole Body Range of Motion. Three shapes are mounted on this adjustable frame that accommodates a patient's height. The shapes are moved from panel 1 to panel 4 and are fastened into place with booted nuts. (From Valpar International Corporation, PO Box 5767, Tucson, AZ 85703-5767, with permission.)

CASE STUDY NO. 1. INFORMATION REGARDING ADL FUNCTION

Mrs. X is a right hand–dominant woman with a 10-year history of rheumatoid arthritis. Her primary problem is of MCP joint subluxation and ulnar deviation in her right hand. Mrs. X and her physician are considering MP joint arthroplasties of the index through small fingers. A functional evaluation has been requested to define Mrs. X's limitations, and if surgery is decided upon, to provide a baseline with which to compare post-operative results.

A questionnaire identified the client's concerns in her role as a homemaker, and the Jebsen-Taylor hand function test was selected as one component of the total functional evaluation. Performance on the test revealed that with the left nondominant hand, Mrs. X was able to score within normal limits (WNL) on four of seven subtests. She scored below normal limits (BNL) on the subtests for writing, picking up small objects, and card turning. She relied on three-point pinch when stacking checkers and picking up small objects such as bottlecaps, but slid small flat objects (3 by 5–in cards, a penny, and a paperclip) to the table's edge before securing the objects in her hand. With the right dominant hand, she scored WNL on two of seven subtests. Mrs. X scored BNL on card turning, manipulation of small objects, and stacking small objects. She could not complete the task requiring lifting and placing lightweight and 1-lb cans. Mrs. X relied on thumb-tip pinch to the radial aspect of her index finger and lateral pinch patterns. She also slid flat objects to the table's edge before grasping them. The contractures of the MP joints appeared to interfere with her ability to open her hand to accommodate the cans. After the subtest was presented, Mrs. X reported that she relies on a two-handed method to grasp large items at home.

CASE STUDY NO. 2. INFORMATION REGARDING INTERIM PERFORMANCE

Mr. Y is a 48-year-old, right hand–dominant automobile mechanic who sustained amputations of the right dominant long, ring, and small fingers at the middle phalanx level. An interview identified the patient's concerns in his worker role as a mechanic and several tests were selected. The Bennett hand tool test and the Valpar Small Tools Mechanical Work Sample requiring the use of a screwdriver and pliers were administered. The patient was tested at 6 and 8 weeks after the injury.

6 WEEKS AFTER INJURY

As compared with normative data compiled on airline mechanics, Mr. Y performed in the 15th percentile, with a time of 6 minutes and 45 seconds on the Bennett hand tool test. He manipulated bolts with the thumb and index finger rather than use a normal three-point pinch. Contact with finger stumps was avoided by grasping tools with the thumb and index or with a dagger type of grasp. On both panels of the Valpar Work Sample, Mr. Y demonstrated performance in the BNL range as compared to San Diego employed worker norms. On the panels requiring screwdriver and pliers usage, Mr. Y scored in the 40th and 30th percentiles, respectively. When grasping tools, he relied upon the thumb, index, palm, and proximal phalanx of the small finger. Rather than relying upon his digits to manipulate the tools, Mr. Y used a great deal of wrist flexion to complete the tasks.

8 WEEKS AFTER INJURY

Mr. Y scored in the 85th percentile, with a time of 4 minutes and 52 seconds on the Bennett hand tool test. While manipulating bolts, he used the thumb and index finger as well as a three-point pinch pattern. During the Valpar section of the evaluation requiring tool usage, Mr. Y grasped tools in the usual power-grip hand posture and maintained contact on the tools with his finger stumps. However, when tightening the bolts, he resorted to the dagger type of grasp, avoiding contact with the finger stumps. As compared with normative data for the Valpar Small Tools Mechanical Work Sample, Mr. Y scored in the 100th percentile and the 90th percentile on the panel requiring screwdriver and plier use, respectively. The score for the screwdriver panel is within normal limits; however, the score for plier use is BNL, as scores range from 0 to 150 percent. Mr. Y was noted to use a normal grasp pattern on all tools without excessive wrist flexion.

CASE STUDY NO. 3. CLINICAL DECISION MAKING

Mr. Z, a 43-year-old, right hand dominant man sustained a crush-amputation injury to his right dominant hand at work. This injury resulted in the loss of the index finger, long finger, and the middle and distal phalanges of the ring finger. He also suffered a laceration to the proximal palm. Mr. Z attended therapy for 4 weeks for wound care, edema control splinting, and active range-of-motion exercises. The referring physician has recommended that Mr. Z undergo a functional assessment and be followed up with appropriate treatment, resistive exercises, and a work-hardening program.

A questionnaire and subsequent interview reveal that Mr. Z is married and employed at a factory that fabricates metal shelving units. Mr. Z states that he caught his right dominant hand in a machine press and then tried to free his hand by jerking and twisting his arm. Mr. Z's only hobby was bowling with his wife and friends. Although he initially related that he had no problems with ADLs, he did state that he experienced difficulty with tasks that required fine motor manipulation such as buttoning, zippering, and shoe-tying. He went on to relate that he had difficulty writing, opening locks with keys, and picking up objects. His goals are to return to work and resume bowling.

Mr. Z reported that he was in good health and was concerned about the extent of his injury. His primary complaint was of hypersensitivity along the palmar laceration and at the tip of his amputated ring finger. The physical examination, results of functional tests, and subsequent treatment and intervention are outlined in Table 5–1.

In order to assist the patient in returning to his hobby of bowling, the therapist and patient jointly decided that the right hand prehension pattern and the size of the right ring finger would interfere with the patient's ability to hold the ball. Transfer of dominance training was initiated so that the patient could learn to bowl with the nondominant left side. This was done by outlining a series of exercises that first focused on proximal strengthening and gross motor control. Dominance retraining proceeded with activities requiring a combination of proximal stabilization with distal control, coordination, and strengthening. Activities included (1) having the patient pinch weighted bean bags with the left hand and then throw the bean bags onto designated targets; (2) directing the patient to use a pulley with the left upper extremity to simulate the bowling motion; (3) instructing the patient to use a weight during his home program to simulate the bowling motion; (4) instructing the patient to use the pliers handle on the BTE Work Simulator in a three-point pinch pattern for sustained pinch; and (5) instructing the patient to move weights with his left hand (via three-point pinch pattern) ranging from 5 to 12 pounds using shoulder forward flexion.

Mr. Z progressed through his treatment program, which required him to work in the clinic for approximately 2 hours, three times a week, for 2 months. During his course of treatment, his clinical program and home program of exercises and activities were upgraded 1 to 2 times per week. He spent an additional month performing an intensified exercise and work hardening program requiring him to be engaged in activities for 4 to 6 hours per session. He was also instructed in safe biomechanical maneuvers. As treatment progressed, decreased hypersensitivity was noted in the area of the palmar laceration and the right ring finger. Mr. Z was able to actively flex the right ring finger MP joint to 95°. Right shoulder strength

TABLE 5–1 Case Study: Functional Evaluation Findings and Treatment Implications

Evaluation	Findings	Treatment Plan
1. Wound	Well healed, some areas with thick scarring	Decrease scarring 1. Massage 2. Pressure garment, stents
2. Posture/Range of Motion	Forward shoulders	Improve posture 1. Education re: posture 2. Strengthen scapular retractors 3. Pectoralis minor stretch
	Range of motion (ROM) WNL except: (R) ring MP extension/flexion −10/75° (AROM) 0/85° (PROM)	Increase MP joint flexion 1. A/PROM exercises
3. Strength	Manual muscle test (general) Right upper extremity Shoulder forward flex 4/5 Elbow ext/flex 4/5 Wrist ext/flex 4/4 Thumb ext/flex 4/4 Ring finger ext/flex 3+/3+ Small finger ext/flex 4/4 Left upper extremity WNL Jamar Dynamometer/pinch meter—testing deferred until 6 weeks after injury 2° to healing and hypersensitive ring finger and palmar scar (sphygmomonometer effort = 50 mm Hg)	Increase BUE strength 1. Theraband, pulleys, and BTE Work Simulator for BUE 2. PREs for wrist, including isotonic/isometric program; adapt weights with builtup handles 3. Putty exercises for thumb and small finger pinch 4. 6 weeks after injury, begin isometric gripping with padded dowel, progress to isotonics
4. Sensibility	Hypersensitivity on tip of ring finger and palm Semmes-Weinstein monofilament test results: diminished light touch in areas of (R) ring tip and of palmar scar Phalen's test Right (+) Left (−)	Desensitization program Issue an adapted bike glove to protect areas of decreased sensation and hypersensitive areas; insert piece foam in tip of glove designated for ring finger 1. Educate patient to avoid flexed wrist posture 2. Consider right wrist cock-up splint for night
5. Functional tests: tests given at 4 weeks postoperatively		
a. Nine-Hole peg test	(R) 42 sec (mean 17.7 sec) (L) 26 sec (mean 18.9 sec)	Instruct patient in bilateral and unilateral fine motor tasks (i.e., buttoning, turning key, tying laces)

TABLE 5–1 (*continued*)

Evaluation	Findings	Treatment Plan
b. Box and Block test	(R) 35 blocks (mean 83 blocks) (L) 75 blocks (mean 80 blocks)	Instruct patient in tasks requiring prehension of items ranging from 1–2 in, including stacking blocks picking up objects, and placing large pegs into a grid
c. Jebson-Taylor hand function test	(R) hand 6/6 subtests BNL (L) hand 6/6 subtests WNL (test for lifting and placing 1-lb cans postponed until 6 weeks)	Issue a builtup handle for writing and eating utensils; practice turning pages in a book, playing cards; practice picking up small objects (other than those used in test), and wide objects for gross grasp
d. Valpar whole body range-of-motion test work sample No. 9	Test completed within 1600 sec, which corresponds to BNL performance in the 5th percentile; patient required 11 rest breaks secondary to ring finger hypersensitivity and BUE fatigue	Instruct patient in tasks which require reaching, lifting, and carrying in overhead, crouching, and kneeling positions; instruct patient to use hands to assemble and dissemble nuts and bolts
e. Valpar upper extremity range-of-motion work sample	(R) 468 sec = 10% = BNL (L) 410 sec = 45% = BNL Observations: Patient relied on (R) thumb to small finger prehension; required 12 breaks, complaining of hypersensitivity; (L) hand prehension used three-point tip, and lateral pinch	Instruct patient to fasten loose nuts on bolts, alternating hands; also initiate twisting and pinching putty
f. Endurance testing: BTE II Work Simulator	Used large tools to simulate gross grasp and proximal unilateral arm movement: steering tool, ladder, long arm tool, short arm tool with forearm stabilized; baseline data for 2-minute trial tests; (R) and (L) power readings were within 15% of one another, which may indicate similar strength; frequent complaints of upper extremity fatigue; patient seen lifting ring finger off handle, relying on thumb and index grasp	Instruct patient in ADL tasks requiring similar motions (i.e., sweeping, raking); initiate endurance training using pulleys or 2-minute periods with the BTE Work Simulator, adjusting the resistance as needed.

(*continued*)

TABLE 5-1 (*continued*)

Evaluation	Findings	Treatment Plan
6. Functional Tests: Tests given 6 weeks postoperatively		
a. Valpar small tools mechanical work sample No. 1	Panels selected to test hand use with screwdrivers (panel 1), pliers (panel 2), and wrenches (panel 4) Patient Performance Panel No. 1: 910 sec = 45% = BNL Panel No. 2: 315 sec = 10% = BNL Panel No. 3: 1435 sec = 40% = BNL	Instruct patient in wrist weight program, wrist weight well, use of similar tools on assembly boards in clinic Monitor right wrist excursion and complaints of pain secondary to the (+) right Phalen's test
b. Endurance testing: BTE Work Simulator	Used tools simulating pliers, screwdriver, and key turning to test repetitive pinch and grip with and without wrist motion; patient demonstrated 80–90% more power with left hand performing 2-minute baseline studies	Upgraded wrist and digital strengthening program

was WNL (grade 5), whereas right pinch and grip strength was 75 percent of that of the left nondominant hand. Mr. Z's performance on the nine-hole peg and the box and block tests slightly improved but was still BNL. His performance was WNL on seven out of seven of the Jebsen-Taylor subtests and the Valpar tests (Nos. 1 and 9), using both upper extremities. Mr. Z reported no discomfort in the entire right upper extremity and stated that bowling with his left hand was steadily improving.

Three months postoperatively Mr. Z returned to his former job in a medium-duty work capacity (lifting and carrying a maximum weight of 50 pounds). Six months postoperatively he returned to his physician for a follow-up visit and to be evaluated for a cosmetic prothesis. Although Mr. Z reported that he was doing well with his job tasks, he complained of shooting nocturnal pains in his right volar wrist and occasional pain in the thumb and index finger. The diagnosis of carpal tunnel syndrome was confirmed by electromyographic (EMG) findings and sensory testing. The patient was instructed to wear a wrist extension at night and periodically during the day. An appointment was made with the physician to reevaluate the status of the carpal tunnel syndrome in 1 month's time.

SUMMARY

Functional assessments complete the physical evaluation process by providing information about the patient's ability to function despite possible limitations in motion, strength, and sensibility. Using the evaluation methods of interview, questionnaire, observation, and functional tests, the therapist attempts to qualify and quantify the patient's functional goals and status. Functional evaluations are used to identify a patient's limitations so that appropriate treatment may be implemented. When accurately administered on an interim basis, functional evaluations provide feedback regarding the patient's response to treatment. The resultant findings inform the patient and rehabilitation team about the patient's abilities and limitations, thus assisting the decision-making process regarding therapy, surgical intervention, or return to a functional status in the community.

REFERENCES

1. Dunton, WR: Principles of Occupational Therapy. AOTA Bulletin No. 4, 1923, as quoted in Hopkins, HL and Smith, HD: Willard and Spackman's Occupational Therapy, ed 5. JB Lippincott, Philadelphia, 1978, p 13.
2. Baldwin, BT: Occupational therapy applied to restoration of function of disabled joints. Walter Reed Monography, Washington, DC, April 1919, p 5.
3. Bunnel, S: Surgery in World War II—Hand Surgery. Office of the Surgeon General, Department of the Army, Washington, DC, 1955.
4. Wynn-Parry, CB, et al: Rehabilitation of the Hand. Butterworth & Co. London, 1973 (first edition 1958).
5. Spackman, CS: A history of the practice of occupational therapy for restoration of physical function. Am J Occup Ther 22(68):1917–1967, 1968.
6. Hopkins, HL: An historical perspective on occupation therapy. In Hopkins, HL and Smith, HD: Willard and Spackman's Occupational Therapy, ed 5. JB Lippincott, Philadelphia, 1978, pp 15–16.
7. Cordery, JC: Joint protection—a responsibility of the occupational therapist. Am J Occup Ther 19(5):285, 1965.
8. Swanson, AB: Evaluation of disabilities and record keeping. In Swanson, AB: Flexible Implant Resection Arthroplasty in the Hand and Extremities. CV Mosby, St Louis, 1973.
9. Jebsen, RW, et al: An objective and standardized test of hand function. Arch Phys Med 6:311, 1969.
10. Bell, E, Jurek, K, and Wilson, T: Hand skill measurement. Am J Occup Ther 30(2):80, 1976.
11. Berlin, S and Vermette, J: An exploratory study of work simulator norms for grip and wrist flexion. Vocational Evaluation and Work Adjustment Bulletin, 61, Summer 1985.
12. Rogers, J and Masagatani, G: Clinical reasoning of occupational therapists during the initial assessment of physically disabled patients. In Focus; Skills for Assessment and Treatment. AOTA, Rockville, MD, 1988, p 67.
13. Bear-Lehman, J and Abreu, BC: Evaluating the hand: Issues in reliability and validity. Phys Ther 1025–33, 1989.
14. Norris, TR: History and physical examination of the shoulder. In Nicholas, JA and Hershman, EB: The Upper Extremity in Sports Medicine. CV Mosby, Philadelphia, 1990, pp 41–90.
15. Hoppenfeld, S: Physical Examination of the Spine and Extremities. Appleton-Century-Crofts, New York, 1976.
16. Cassanova, JS and Grunert, BK: Adult prehension: Patterns and nomenclature for pinches. J Hand Ther 2:231, 1989.
17. Melvin, J: Rheumatic Disease: Occupational Therapy and Rehabilitation, ed 2. FA Davis, Philadelphia, 1982.
18. Schmidt, RT and Toews, JV: Grip strength as measured by the Jamar Dynamometer. Arch Phys Med Rehab 52:321, 1970.
19. Bechtol, CO: Grip test; use of a dynamometer with adjustable hand spacing. J Bone Joint Surg (Am) 36A:820, 1954.
20. Pryce, JC: Wrist position between neutral and ulnar deviation that facilitates maximum power strength. J Biomechanics 13:505, 1980.
21. American Society for Surgery of the Hand: The Hand: Examination and Diagnosis. Churchill Livingstone, New York, 1988.
22. Daniels, L and Worthington, C: Muscle Testing: Techniques and Manual Examination. WB Saunders, Philadelphia, 1972.
23. Trombly, CA and Scott, AD: Evaluation of motor control. In Trombly, CA and Scott, AD (eds): Occupational Therapy for Physical Dysfunction. Williams & Wilkins, Baltimore, 1977.
24. Gay, LR: Educational research: Competencies for analysis and application. Charles E Merril, Columbus, 1981, p 153.
25. Carthum CJ, Clawson, DK, and Decker, JL: Functional assessment of the rheumatoid hand. Am J Occup Ther 23:122, 1969.

26. Apfel, E: Preliminary development of a standardized hand function test. J Hand Ther 3(4):191, 1990.
27. Mcphee, SD: Functional hand evaluations. Am J Occup Ther 41(3):158, 1987.
28. Fess, EE: Documentation: Essential Elements of an Upper Extremity Assessment Battery. In Hunter, JM, et al (eds): Rehabilitation of the Hand. CV Mosby, Philadelphia, 1990.
29. Bennett, GK: Hand Tool Dexterity Test Manual. The Psychological Corporation, Harcourt Brace Jovanovich, San Antonio, 1981.
30. Mathiowetz, V, et al: Adult Norms for the Box and Block Test of Manual Dexterity. Am J Occup Ther 39:386, 1989.
31. Crawford, JD and Crawford DM: Small Parts Dexterity Test Manual, Revised. The Psychological Corporation. Harcourt Brace Jovanovich, San Antonio, 1981.
32. Minnesota Rate of Manipulation Tests, Examiners Manual. American Guidance Services, Circle Plains, MN, 1969.
33. Mathiowetz, V, et al: Adult norms for the nine hole peg test of finger dexterity. Occup Ther J Res 5(1):24, 1985.
34. Instructions and Normative Data for Model 32030 Purdue Pegboard, Lafayette Instrument Co, Lafayette, IN, 1969.
35. Valpar International Corporation, PO Box 5767, Tucson, AZ, 85703-5767.
36. Instructions for 32021 O'Connor Finger Dexterity Test. Lafayette Instrument Co, Lafayette, IN.
37. Pennsylvania Bi-manual Work Sample, Examiner's Manual. American Guidance Services, Circle Plains, MN, 1945.
38. Potvin, AR, et al: Simulated activities of daily living examination. Arch Phys Med Rehab 53:476, 1972.
39. Smith, H: Smith hand function test. Am J Occup Ther 27:244, 1973.

APPENDIX: SUMMARY OF STANDARDIZED TESTS OF HAND FUNCTION

Test	Purpose									Methodology	Reliability	Validity	Standardization	Approximate Time to Setup, Administer, and Score	Approximate Cost	Source	Comments
	ADL	Dexterity	Grasp/Release	Gross Motor	Manipulation	Physical Demands	Tool Use	Strength	Dx								
Apfel's Pickup Test[26]	✓	U	✓		✓					Transfer of 19 standardized common objects requiring varying prehension patterns. Transfer is made from specified positions on a felt board to a box.	Inter-rater reliability demonstrated by having two testers time subjects simultaneously. Scores: Pearson $r = .997, p > .001$	Correlated with the box and block test. Validity for dominant hand was very good (Pearson $r = -.861$, $p < .001$) Validity for nondominant hand was less adequate (Pearson $r = -.586, p < .1$)	56 male and female normal volunteers from 20–79 y.o., mean age 41.2 yr Average scores (times) for dominant and nondominant hands	Less than 10 min	$	Constructed from items procured from household, local hardware and department stores Apfel article	Although norms available, author reports test is in preliminary development stage
Bennett Hand Tool Dexterity Test (HTDT)[29]		B	✓		✓		✓	✓		Remove nuts/bolts from left upright with tools/fingers. Replace nuts/bolts on right upright with tools/fingers.	Test retest (.81–.88)	Correlation with forced choice supervisory ratings and standardized tests including Crawford Small Parts, MRMT, Pennsylvania Bi-manual Work Sample, Purdue Pegboard	Raw scores male and female workers, applicants, injured workers, mentally retarded individuals, and various occupations	Less than 30 min	$$	Available from The Psychological Corporation FRED SAMMONS	
Box and Block Test of Manual Dexterity[30]		U	✓		✓					Grasp as many as 150 blocks which are randomized in a compartment of a partitioned box	Inter-rater Reliability Right hand = .976 Left hand = .937	Correlated with MRMT and General Aptitude Test Battery	628 male and female volunteers from 20–94 y.o. Average scores (times) by age, sex, dominance	Less than 10 min	$	Constructed from items procured from lumberyard Mathiowetz article	

(continued)

143

Test	Purpose									Methodology	Reliability	Validity	Standardization	Approximate Time to Setup, Administer, and Score	Approximate Cost	Source	Comments
	ADL	Dexterity	Grasp/Release	Gross Motor	Manipulation	Physical Demands	Tool Use	Strength	Dx								
Crawford Small Parts Dexterity Test (CSPDT)[31]	✓	HP B			✓		✓			Part I: Use of tweezers to place small metal pins into a metal grid. Tweezers are then used to place metal collars over pins. Part II: Twist screws into metal grid and tighten with a screwdriver. May be performed on a time-limit or work-limit basis	Reliability coefficients for work-limit scores ranged from: Part I (.80–.91) Part II (.90–.95) Reliability coefficients for time-limit scores were as follows: Part I (.90) Part II (.89)	Correlated with the HTDT, MRMT, Pennsylvania Bi-manual Work Sample, Purdue Pegboard Also correlations drawn between Parts I and II or CSPDT Correlations ranged from high to moderate to low (refer to test manual for details)	Population sizes range from: Large groups (100+) Small groups (50–99) Very small groups (under 50) Norms are listed in terms of race, sex, injured workers, mentally handicapped, and various occupations	Less than 30 min	$	Available from The Psychological Corporation	
Jebsen-Taylor Hand Function Test Original Version[9]		U	✓		✓			1 lb.	H RA TQ	Made up of 7 subtests including: 1. Writing 2. Turning 3 × 5″ cards 3. Picking up small objects 4. Simulated feeding 5. Stacking checkers 6. Pick-up/ place empty cans 7. Pick-up/ place 1-lb. cans	Normal subjects: Difference between means of age groups by subtests/ hand was statistically significant to $p < .05$ except in subtest #4 for women	Not reported in article	Normal subjects were categorized in terms of sex and age. Age groups, range from 1. (20–29) 2. (30–39) 3. (40–49) 4. (50–59) 5. (60–99)	Less than 30 min	$	Constructed from items procured from a lumberyard, grocery store, hardware store Jebsen-Taylor article	

Test			Description	RH/LH	Not reported in article	Not reported in article	Not reported in article	Normative sample	Time	Cost	Construction	Comments
Jebsen Test of Hand Function (Australian Version)[9]	✓	U ✓ ✓	✓	Tests grip strength and incorporates use of original 7 Jebsen subtest items		Not reported in article	Not reported in article	Male and female volunteers 16–90 y.o.; percentile scores available for age, sex, hand dominance	Less than 30 min	$$	Jamar Dynamometer Items constructed in the Jebsen-Taylor hand function test	Cost is higher because Jamar Dynamometer is included
Jebsen Test of Hand Function (Specific for R/L Hemiplegia)[9]	✓	U ✓ ✓	✓	RH LH	Use of 7 Jebsen subtest items	Not reported in article	Not reported in article	49 male and female volunteers s/p CVA. Mean age 66 y.o. Population consisted of: (RH) = 22 (LH) = 27 Norms available for: 1. Females: RH using L non-dominant side R dominant side 2. Females: LH using R dominant side L non-dominant side 3. Males: RH using L non-dominant side R dominant side 4. Males: LH using R dominant side L non-dominant side	Less than 30 min	$	Items constructed in the Jebsen-Taylor hand function test	

(continued)

Test	ADL	Dexterity	Grasp/Release	Gross Motor	Manipulation	Physical Demands	Tool Use	Strength	Dx	Methodology	Reliability	Validity	Standardization	Approximate Time to Setup, Administer, and Score	Approximate Cost	Source	Comments
Minnesota Rate of Manipulation Test (MRMT)[32]		U B	✓		✓					Large checkerlike disks are moved in relation to a rectangular base. Includes 5 subtests: 1. Placing 2. Turning 3. Displacing 4. One-hand turning and placing 5. Two-hand turning and placing	Reliability tests: 2 Trial (.87–.95) 4 Trial (.93–.97)	Correlated with Pennsylvania Bi-manual test, and 4 other tests. T-scores (.75) of papermill machine operators, validity coefficients	Millworkers— individuals in the young, old, or blind category	Time is dependent on which test(s) is (are) administered	$$$	Available from: Lafayette Instrument Co. J.S. Preston	
Nine-Hole Peg Test[33]		U	✓		✓					Pick up, place, and remove 9 pegs in relation to starting position and holes in a square base	Not reported in article	Not reported in article	246 male and female volunteers from 18–60 y.o. Average scores listed by age and sex	Less than 10 min	$	Available from: 1. Susquehanna Rehab 2. Rolyan 3. North Coast Medical	
O'Connor Finger Dexterity Test[36]		U	✓		✓					Place 3 metal pins in each of the 100 board holes	Not reported in article	Not reported in article	Standard norms for sex	Less than 30 min	$$	North Coast Medical San Jose, CA 95125 J.A. Preston	
Pennsylvania Bi-manual Work Sample[37]		B	✓	✓	✓					Assembly and disassembly of 20 nuts and bolts	Split halves method (.89)	Correlated with MRMT and O'Connor finger dexterity test	Raw scores for 16–50+ y.o., sex, education, and industry	10 min assembly 5 min disassembly	$$	J.A. Preston	
Purdue Pegboard[34]		U B	✓	✓	✓					Pick up and place metal pins in board holes. Metal collars and washers may be placed over pins.	Test-retest correlations for three trials (.84–.91)	Normative data for male and female job applicants, workers Intercorrelation studies	Average scores listed by age, sex,	Time is dependent on which test(s) is (are) administered	$$	North Coast Medical San Jose, CA 95125 J.A. Preston	

Purpose

Test	D B			P MS	Description / Subtests	Reliability	Norms	Time	Cost	Comments
Simulated Activities of Daily Living Examination (SADLE)[38]	✓	✓ ✓ ✓	✓	✓	education, and occupation 5 subtests may be utilized: 1. Right hand 2. Left hand 3. Both hands 4. Right and left and both hands (R + L + B) 5. Assembly Test battery includes standing, walking, and various ADL subtests: 1. Putting on a shirt 2. Managing 3 visible buttons 3. Zipping a garment 4. Putting on gloves 5. Dialing a telephone 6. Tying a bow 7. Manipulating safety pins 8. Picking up coins 9. Threading a needle 10. Unwrapping a Bandaid 11. Squeezing toothpaste 12. Cutting with a knife 13. Using a fork	Test-retest on young adult normal subjects with a 1-month interval between the 1st and 2nd examination. Excluding standing tests, "zipping a garment," and "using a fork," reliability coefficients are significantly greater than zero at the .05 level (r ≥ .47)	Discussion regarding comparison to quantitative examination of neurological function (QENF) Mean performance ratings are listed for each subtest with regard to age, ranging from 18–74 y.o. 1. Young adults 2. Older adults 3. Oldest adults Also, information available on performance of P and MS patients.	Less than 60 min	$	Test is constructed from items procured from a department and drug store and therapy equipment Parts of test do not reflect present-day ADL or therapy equipment, i.e., 1. Dialing a phone 2. Using putty-like material for simulated dining tasks

(continued)

Test	Purpose: ADL	Dexterity	Grasp/Release	Gross Motor	Manipulation	Physical Demands & Worker Traits	Tool Use	Strength	Dx	Methodology	Reliability	Validity	Standardization	Approximate Time to Setup, Administer, and Score	Approximate Cost	Source	Comments
Smith Hand Function Evaluation[39]	✓	U B	✓		✓			✓		Tests grasp/release, ADL, writing, and hand strength	Information not available to author	Information not available to author	Information gathered on 91 non-handicapped individuals. Norms given for age groups	?	$$	Jamar Dynamometer Items procured from department and hardware stores	
Valpar Small Tools Mechanical Work Sample No. 1[45]		✓	✓	✓	✓	✓	✓	✓		Test requires use of small hand tools such as screwdrivers, pliers, and wrenches. The evaluee must reach through a hole in front of a 5-sided box in order to assemble hardware on one panel at a time. Disassembly of the entire unit may also be tested. Panel 1: Screwdrivers Panel 2: Hitchpins/pliers Panel 3: Nutdriver/Allen wrench Panel 4: Wrenches Panel 5: Small screwdriver wrenches	Panel 1 (.84) Panel 2 (.90) Panel 3 (.82) Panel 4 (.83) Panel 5 (.89) Total assembly (.83) Total disassembly (.80)	Valpar recommends test-retest with local norms	Methods, time, motion (MTM) standards developed for each panel. Normative data available for disassembly section also. Percentiles range from 5–150%, with average performance listed at 100% Populations for Valpar tests listed in key.	Dependent on number of panels selected. Panel No. Time to Complete 1 Up to 20 min 2 Up to 5 min 3 Up to 20 min 4 Up to 29 min 5 Up to 35 min	$$$$	Valpar International Corporation PO Box 5767 Tucson, AZ 85703-5767	

148

Test	Type	Description	Reliability	Norms recommendation	Norms data	Time	Cost	Source
Valpar Upper Extremity Range-of-Motion Work Sample No. 4[35]	U	Test requires evaluee to reach through a hole in front on a 5-sided box in order to fasten two sizes of bolts onto the panels.	Dominant (.97) Other (.99) Disassembly (.91)	Valpar recommends test-retest with local norms	Normative data supplied for dominant and non-dominant hands	Less than 30 min for subjects other than mentally retarded	$$$$	Valpar International Corporation PO Box 5767 Tucson, AZ 85703-5767
Valpar Simulated Assembly Work Sample No. 8[35]	B	The evaluee must perform a 3-step assembly (using metal pins, spacers, and caps) into a revolving horizontal wheel	Reliability (.99)	Valpar recommends test-retest with local norms	Normative data supplied using methods, time, motion (MTM)	20 min	$$$$	Valpar International Corporation PO Box 5767 Tucson, AZ 85703-5767
Valpar Whole Body Range-of-Motion Work Sample No. 9[35]	B	Test is administered while standing, kneeling, or crouching. The evaluee must transfer and fasten 3 plastic forms on 4 panels placed at various heights	Reliability (.95)	Valpar recommends test-retest with local norms	Normative data supplied using San Diego employed worker norms	Less than 30 min	$$$$	Valpar International Corporation PO Box 5767 Tucson, AZ 85703-5767

U = Unilateral
B = Bilateral
HP = Hand preference
I lb = 1 pound
H = Hemiparetic
RA = Rheumatoid arthritis
TQ = Traumatic quadriplegia (C6–C7)
RH = Right hemiplegia
LH = Left hemiplegia
L = Left
R = Right
P = Parkinson
MS = Multiple sclerosis
D = Dominance
CVA = Cerebral vascular accident

$ = Under $50
$$ = $50 – $250
$$$ = $250 – $1000
$$$$ = $1000 – $2500

Concepts in Clinical Treatment

CHAPTER 6

Wound Management

Mark Walsh, PT, MS, CHT
Elaine Muntzer, PT, CHT

The importance of wound management cannot be understated. The role of the therapist in managing wounds grows each day with the advent of hand therapy as a specialty, the early discharge of patients, and a greater reliance by the physician on the professional health community to provide more services than traditionally expected. This higher level of care requires an increased knowledge and places a greater responsibility on the hand therapist. The hand therapist now must be able to recognize the characteristics of a wound to provide early intervention and to formulate a goal-oriented, logical treatment plan for hand-injured patients.

There are various ways to characterize wounds, as well as different—at times diametrical—methods of treatment. The information in this chapter is not presented as absolute and unyielding, but as a basis for knowledge needed to evaluate and treat the wounded hand. The objectives of this chapter are to (1) develop an approach to wound management based on the concepts of wound healing; (2) provide a basis for evaluation of wound characteristics; (3) develop a rational, problem-solving approach to treatment based on currently available methods; (4) discuss the characteristics and methods of treatment of edema; and (5) examine the characteristics of and therapeutic intervention during the late maturation phase of wound healing.

EVALUATION

Evaluation is the requisite groundwork on which assessment of status, formulation of goals, and establishment of treatment are based. The components of wound evaluation are outlined in Table 6–1. If approached in a logical sequence, the difficulty of evaluation is diminished. A thorough evaluation includes history, subjective information, and objective evaluation.

TABLE 6–1 Components of Wound Evaluation

A. History
    1. Injury—etiology, date of onset, injury components
    2. Social/Occupational—age, dominance, vocational/avocational, alcohol, nicotine, caffeine, family support
    3. Medical—system review, previous injury, medications, allergies
B. Subjective report
    1. Pain, sensory changes
    2. Functional problems
C. Objective evaluation
    1. General observation
        a. Wound, surrounding tissue, extremity
        b. Location
    2. Wound
        a. Size, shape, depth measurement
        b. Classification
            (1) Primary/delayed primary
            (2) Secondary
        c. Exudate characteristics
        d. Wound bed
            (1) Necrotic, granulative, epithelial budding
            (2) Vital structure involvement
        e. Wound margins
            (1) Extent
            (2) Change
        f. Grafts/flaps
            (1) Adherence
            (2) Drainage
            (3) Vascularity

History

Relevant social history encompasses the patient's age, hand dominance, occupation, and avocational interests. The therapist must be aware of the patient's living and transportation arrangements and family support. The preceding are necessary in determining if outside assistance is required or if the patient will be self-sufficient with the program. Alcohol, tobacco, and caffeine use is important to note, as these factors affect wound healing.[1] Abstinence from nicotine and caffeine is requisite for the patient with circulatory compromise, arterial repair, and digital replantation. Excessive use of alcohol may affect compliance with the home program.

MECHANISM OF INJURY

Obtaining a history that includes date of wounding, etiology, thermal, mechanical, or traction components and the injury environment will begin to provide answers about the wound itself and the surrounding tissues. The mechanism of injury is important, especially if caused by thermal or compressive forces, which damage tissues outside the actual wound margins. In these injuries, one should note margins of demarcation because of the increased potential for infection. A traction component may cause a local or peripheral nerve injury. Environmental factors may delay wound healing and increase the risk of infection.

MEDICAL HISTORY

The patient's medical history may have a profound effect on wound healing. Systemic diseases such as diabetes mellitus, peripheral vascular disease, hepatic disease, hematolytic disorders, and malnutrition may affect wound healing and increase the potential for infection. Certain medications such as anti-inflammatories, steroids, and anticoagulants may retard wound healing by suppressing clotting time or initial wound inflammatory response.[2] A patient may be allergic to certain medications, topical agents, or cleansing additives. The open wound provides a direct systemic access to topical agents or medication such as iodine derivatives. A patient who has had an adverse reaction to iodine or shellfish may experience adverse systemic or local effects. The patient taking prophylactic or therapeutic antibiotics should be reminded to complete the course of medication as prescribed.

Subjective Information

The patient's subjective complaints and concerns are important in evaluation of a wound. The location and description of pain or its absence will lend clues about the extent of tissue involvement. Throbbing discomfort may be related to dependency of the upper extremity and not to the wound itself, while intractable pain unrelieved by elevation may indicate arterial involvement or infection. Reported burning discomfort may be related to a possible neurologic component or the presence of a chemical irritant. The presence of hypersensitivity in the wound or surrounding tissues may imply ischemia, cutaneous nerve exposure, or local nerve irritation. For example, the median palmar cutaneous nerve may be involved with a carpal tunnel release or a radial cutaneous nerve injury with laceration of the first dorsal compartment tendons. A nerve injury would be accompanied by subjective complaints of sensory alteration. The therapist needs to ascertain whether the sensory component is in a dermatomal or peripheral distribution or is related to the actual wound. The absence or presence of sensation within the wound can assist in determining the depth of tissue damage. In the case of thermal injury, the less sensation present the greater the depth of tissue destruction. The depth of involvement can also be obtained by the patient's report of hand function. Loss of motion or sensation or the presence of a joint contracture may indicate underlying tendon, neurologic, or periarticular involvement.

Objective Evaluation

LOCATION

A common mistake is confining evaluation and treatment to the wound itself. The wound, surrounding tissues, and entire extremity should be inspected for edema, color changes, or excessive warmth to determine the extent of tissue involvement or presence of infection. The location of the wound is noted, using anatomic landmarks to describe boundaries. Intimate knowledge of hand anatomy is required, as there may be underlying vital tissues not visible in the wound such as tendon, bone, periarticular, or neurovascular structures. A wound located over vital structures requires caution with debridement to avoid exposure of or damage to the underlying structures. Any exposed vital structures should be noted, as demonstrated in Figure 6–1. Treatment should proceed only after notifying and consulting with the attending physician.

The location has implications for wound healing and infection also. The volar circulatory supply of the hand is more perpendicular to the dermis and the dorsal supply is more longitudinal.[3] A dorsal avulsion injury would have better viability than a similar volar injury because of less extensive capillary damage. A dorsal injury may, however, have delayed wound healing due to venous congestion, as the principal venous return occurs dorsally.[4]

CONFIGURATION

The shape and size of the wound can be measured with a ruler or traced onto transparent paper. Depth can be determined using a sterile applicator to mark surface level or by aspirating sterile water that has been placed in the wound and noting the volume. Assessment of the wound margins will help determine the extent of tissue involvement. Dusky areas of decreased temperatures may indicate arterial compromise and decreased tissue viability. Venous and arterial status is assessed by observing the color and noting blanching and refill. In general the greater the refill time, the greater the circulatory compromise.

INFLAMMATORY RESPONSE

The therapist must learn to differentiate between the normal inflammatory response and the prolongation of the response, which may herald infection with its cardinal signs of edema, erythema, elevated temperature, and pain. The presence of erythema may be the normal inflammatory response lasting 5 to 7 days. Erythema lasting longer than 5 days, especially when accompanied by swelling and warmth, may indicate a more significant problem such as vascular compromise or infection (Fig. 6–2). An extended area of erythema may indicate cellulitis, a spreading infection in the tissue planes, and streaking redness may indicate lymphangitis. Areas of suspect color changes and edema should be outlined with surgical skin marker to allow sequential assessment of changes (Fig. 6–3).

EXUDATE

The presence of drainage and description of its color, odor, and consistency, are extremely important to note in assessing a wound's status and progress. Characteristics of the various types of exudate are described in Table 6–2. If there is any concern about exudates being purulent, a wound culture should be taken to identify the potential source of infection and allow specificity of antibiotic treatment. Eschar present in the wound implies avascularity, as in the case of a thermal or severe crushing injury. Eschar, usually white or white-yellow, adheres to the wound bed, and requires enzymatic or surgical debridement. This eschar should not be confused with fibrinous or proteinaceous exudate, which is easily debrided, revealing the wound bed. The color and extent of granulation tissue in comparison to the amount of necrotic tissue should be noted. The presence of epithelial buds, small pink islets forming within the wound, implies a partial-thickness wound with improving circulation and evidence of healing by secondary intention.

The therapist should determine if there is any undermining occurring beneath apparently healthy dermal and subcutaneous tissue. A fissure, a tunnel that could connect with a fascial compartment or synovial sheath system, may also be present; if so, its depth should be measured.

TABLE 6-2 Wound Exudate Characteristics

	Serous	Serosanguineous	Fibrous/ Proteinaceous	Purulent
Color	Yellow	Yellow-red to red	White to white-yellow	Green/brown/ white-yellow
Odor	No	No	No	Yes
Adherency	No	No	Yes	No
Consistency (viscosity)	Thin, transparent to wound base	Thin-thick, transparent?	Gel-like, nontransparent	Viscous, nontransparent
Wound type	Primary Secondary	Primary Secondary	Secondary	Primary Secondary

WOUND CLASSIFICATION

Wounds may be classified according to type of closure (Fig. 6-4), including primary intention, delayed primary intention, healing by secondary intention, grafts, and flaps (Chapter 2). Wound healing by secondary intention may be classified and treated according to a color scheme of black, yellow, or red (Fig. 6-5).[5] A black wound is covered with dark, thick eschar that impedes epithelialization and wound contraction. The yellow wound, ranging from ivory to green-yellow, is present with superficial injury or after removal of eschar. These wounds are covered with adherent fibrinous exudate and debris or purulent drainage. As necrotic tissue and debris are removed, red granulation tissue may appear in the wound bed and margins.

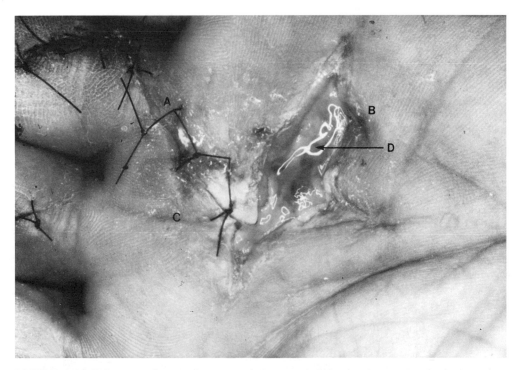

FIGURE 6-4. Primary and secondary wound closure. *A*, Primary closure; *B*, secondary wound closure; *C*, wound maceration; *D*, nonpurulent serous and proteinaceous wound exudate.

Many wounds present as a combination of colors, and management is by treating the most serious color initially. A black wound is treated by debridement of the eschar, leaving a yellow wound. The yellow wound is managed by cleansing and dressing techniques to assist in removal of debris. When the desired red wound bed has been obtained, care is directed toward providing a protective environment and atraumatic dressing changes.

GRAFTS AND FLAPS

Evaluation of grafts and flaps requires some special considerations. A graft is an avascular tissue transfer that requires nourishment from the wound bed, whereas a flap retains its viability with an intact circulatory supply. Table 6–3 reviews the characteris-

TABLE 6–3 Graft and Flap Characteristics

	Tissue Layers	Vascularity/ Take	Common Drainage	Donor Site Closure
Split thickness	Epidermis/ superficial dermis	3 days	Serous Sanguineous	Secondary Intention
Full thickness	All skin appendages Nerve ending except a) some sweat glands b) some pacinian capsules	5–7 days	Serous Sanguineous	Primary
Pedicle flap dermis and axial/random subcutaneous fat		Approximately 3 weeks	Serosanguineous	Primary or Skin Graft
Musculocutaneous	Dermis and muscle			
Fasciocutaneous	Dermis and fascia			
FREE FLAP		Immediate	Serosanguineous	Primary or skin graft
Cutaneous	Dermis and subcutaneous fat			
Myocutaneous	Dermis and subcutaneous fat, muscle			
Myo	Muscle only			
Osteo	Bone alone or in combination			
Joint	Joint and bone			

tics of grafts and flaps.[6-8] In general the thicker the graft, the longer the time required for capillary infiltration. The graft must adhere to the granular bed for capillary infiltration to occur.

A split-thickness graft (STG) should be viable in 3 to 5 days and a thick split-thickness (TSTG) or a full-thickness graft (FTG) in 7 to 10 days, displaying pink color, blanching, and adherence to the wound bed. Blanching is monitored by compressing the graft with a sterile applicator to determine refill of the capillaries. Adherence is determined by gently applying pressure and sliding the applicator in a longitudinal direction and observing for motion at the graft. In the case of the TSTG or FTG, motion may be detected as the epidermis separates from the dermis; this superficial motion does not necessarily indicate nonadherence of the graft. With care of any graft, initial postoperative dressing change is not performed without consulting the attending physician. Flap viability is determined similarly by noting pink color and refill time. It generally takes approximately 3 weeks for recipient capillary infiltration of the flap to occur.

CLINICAL WOUND MANAGEMENT

Clinical wound management requires a knowledge base of wound cleansing techniques, modalities, and agents. A thorough understanding of wound anatomy is necessary for proper debridement. The combined effects of cleansing and debridement lay the foundation for wound healing enhancement. The proper application of a wound dressing is of paramount importance. The dressing provides the proper environment for healing and plays an important role in the prevention of infection.

Cleansing

Clinical management of the open wound includes cleansing to (1) assist in removal of exudate and necrotic tissue; (2) decrease surface contamination, and (3) control wound pathogens. The various agents and methods available for cleansing are often employed without rationale for their use or recognition of their effects on the wound bed and surrounding tissues. Studies exist that both support and decry the use of certain wound cleansing preparations.

TOPICAL CLEANSING AGENTS

Commercially available surgical scrub solutions containing iodophors with surfactant or hexachlorophene are not safe for cleansing open wounds. They contain toxic anionic detergents that damage tissue defenses and may potentiate development of infection. An in vitro study by Rodenheaver and colleagues[9] found that povidone-iodine antiseptic solution (Betadine) offered no therapeutic benefit to contaminated wounds when compared with 9 percent saline solution. Peacock and Van Winkle[10] state that utilizing povidone-iodine preparation to cleanse or dress wounds is unsupported by any meaningful data. An in vitro study by Linneaweaver and associates[11] compared the toxicity of four commonly used antimicrobial cleansers — 1 percent povidone-iodine (Betadine), 0.5 percent sodium hypochlorite (Dakins), 0.25 percent acetic acid, and 3 percent hydrogen peroxide — to assess their effect on human fibroblasts and on bacteria (*Staphylococcus aureus*). The study concluded that at 100 percent strength, all four solutions were 100 percent fibroblast toxic. At any dilution, the hydrogen peroxide and acetic acid were more injurious to fibroblasts than to bacteria. The povidone-iodine at a dilution of 1:1000 and sodium hypochlorite at a dilution of 1:100 were bacteriocidal without being cytotoxic. When using wound cleansing agents, the therapist must weigh the bactericidal effects against the potentially cytotoxic effects.

WHIRLPOOL

Cleansing of either delayed primary or secondary wounds occurring during the inflammatory or fibroplastic phase of wound healing can be accomplished by several methods. The whirlpool is an effective modality for cleansing and debriding superficial necrotic material, and in assisting with antibacterial treatment of the open wound. The mechanical effect of whirlpool helps to stimulate granulation tissue, softens tissues, and increases circulation to the affected areas. This increase in circulation in turn raises the level of oxygen, antibodies, leukocytes, vital cellular nutritional components, and systemic medications such as antibiotics, and enhances metabolite removal. The whirlpool also creates sedation and an analgesic effect that may aid in reducing pain.[12]

Additives

The first consideration for the use of whirlpool is to determine the additive to be used. Additives that have been found to be bactericidally effective are povidone-iodine solution,[13] sodium hypochlorite 5.25, household chlorine bleach,[14] and chloramine T.[15] The proper dilutions for these 3 compounds in the average hand tank of 22 to 36 gal are listed in Table 6–4. The choice of whirlpool additive may also be determined by the physician or may be based on patient allergy to an additive. Finally, the therapist must be aware that whirlpool additives will create an aerosol that may potentially cause lightheadedness, dizziness, or syncope if the area is not adequately ventilated.

Temperature, Duration, and Aeration

The temperature of the whirlpool is recommended to be 98°F or less, and preferably 94°F. Studies have shown that temperatures greater than 98°F increase volume of the affected upper extremity regardless of position or the performance of exercise during treatment.[16,17] The duration and level of agitation depend on the viability of the surrounding tissues and on the wound itself.

Skin grafts, prior to 3 to 5 days for a STG and 7 to 10 days for an FTG, may not tolerate the high shearing forces and turbulence created by the whirlpool because they are not adherent to the granular bed and do not have sufficient ingrowth of capillaries. Whirlpool use prior to these times is contraindicated. The aeration of the whirlpool should be minimal and the duration, during the initial phase, is 5 minutes. As the graft ages and its stability improves, duration and aeration may be increased.

TABLE 6–4

Whirlpool	Additive	Dilutions
22–36 gal	Betadine	4 oz
	chlorine bleach	26 oz
	chloramine T;	20–38 g
	chlorazene	

These same principles apply for tissue flaps. If the whirlpool temperature is too low or the patient gets chilled, vasoconstriction of the supporting or infiltrating vessels could result, causing flap ischemia and possibly partial or total loss of the flap. In general the younger the flap in postoperative days the more minimal the agitation, shorter the duration, and the closer the water temperature should be to normal body temperature.

The painful open lesion also deserves special considerations to avoid stimulating neural tissue, thereby increasing pain. Whirlpool temperatures close to or at body temperature (98.6°F) with minimal agitation, directed away from the wound, may assist debridement while minimizing pain. Whirlpool duration is usually determined by patient comfort and may last as long as 20 minutes.

Special Considerations

The therapist should also consider the extremity's circulatory condition—venous and arterial—which must be able to tolerate the temperature and turbulence created by the whirlpool. Sensibility must not be compromised to a level that would prevent the patient's ability to protect himself or herself from further injury. Traumatized tissues that require immobilization may not be able to tolerate whirlpool because of underlying fractures, joint injuries, or soft tissue damage such as an early tendon repair. Therefore, whirlpool would be contraindicated.

Finally, the therapist must consider the position of the extremity in the whirlpool. The dependent position may encourage the development of or increase in edema.[17,18] This increase in edema may compromise venous and arterial circulation, increase pain, and restrict desired motion. A towel roll or pad should be placed over the edge of the tub to minimize the pressure placed on the axilla. The extremity can be supported with either a towel sling or an extremity rest available from the whirlpool manufacturer.

Contraindications for the use of the whirlpool are the same as those for superficial heat, with consideration given to objectives of the treatment, condition and type of wound, and the condition of the surrounding tissues and extremities.

IRRIGATION

Although not commonly used, a second method available for cleansing a wound is irrigation, which is the flushing of sterile water or antiseptic solution into the wound using a Water Pik or syringe. The objectives of this method are the same as for whirlpool; however, the therapeutic effect is confined to the local area surrounding the wound and eliminates the unwanted systemic effects of the whirlpool. The special considerations discussed for whirlpool also apply to irrigation. The Water Pik, which mechanically pumps water at a particular volume, velocity, and force while being an effective wound cleanser and debrider, may cause damage to delicate tissues. The syringe allows manual control of the velocity and force, which, although inconsistent, enables the therapist to direct a gentler, less damaging flow. Use of irrigation may not have the antimicrobial effect of whirlpool because of the insufficient duration of exposure of the tissues to the cleansing solution. Irrigation—either mechanical or manual—is performed with the extremity held over a basin to contain the runoff. Duration is determined by therapist and patient tolerance. Treatment may be terminated once the loose superficial and exudative material has been removed and the objectives of cleansing have been achieved.

Debridement

Debridement of the open wound removes exudates, devitalized tissue, and tissue contaminated by bacteria and foreign substances. Devitalized tissue provides a culture medium for bacteria, inhibits leukocyte phagocytosis and subsequent destruction of bacteria, and impedes epithelialization.[19] Debridement may be accomplished by either mechanical or enzymatic means.

MECHANICAL DEBRIDEMENT

Mechanical debridement may employ whirlpool, sterile instruments, or wet-to-dry dressings. To prevent damage to vital structures when manually debriding one must know their precise location in relationship to the wound. Caution should be used with mechanical debridement in patients receiving anticoagulant therapy, as clotting time is reduced. Manual debridement of contaminants and devitalized tissue may be preceded by whirlpool or irrigation. When debriding, fragile neovascularization and migrating epithelium at the wound margins must not be disrupted. Wet-to-dry dressings are sometimes used for debriding. This method of nonselective debriding tends to damage vascularized and epithelialized tissues.

ENZYMATIC DEBRIDEMENT

Enzymatic debridement may be indicated in a wound bed containing copious amounts of coagulum (fibrinous protein-rich exudate) or eschar. This technique may also be useful for the patient who does not tolerate manual debridement or in areas where the safety of manual debridement is questionable, such as over the neurovascular bundle on the volar aspect of the thumb. The hydrolysis of coagulum by enzymatic debridement has been found to prolong the effective period of antibiotic action.[20] Clinically useful enzymatic agents must (1) cause rapid lysis of eschar, (2) be inactive on normal tissue, (3) be nontoxic and nonirritating; and (4) be readily applicable.[21] Enzymatic debridement uses fibrinolytic enzyme preparations such as Travase, Elase, and Collagenase. Their use is confined to exudate and necrotic tissue to avoid damage to wound defenses and to new epithelium and granulation tissue. Use on large areas for prolonged periods may promote sepsis and should be avoided.[21] The softened debris resulting from enzymatic debridement should be removed by daily cleansing to avoid providing a medium for bacterial growth.

Wound Dressing and Topical Agents

The purpose of wound dressings is to provide a clean or sterile environment, prevent surface contamination and mechanical stress, and aid in positioning. Dressings should be applied so as not to unnecessarily restrict motion, inhibit sensory input, cause shearing forces, or compromise circulation. Dressings are applied with a contact, intermediate, and outer layer (Fig. 6–6). Types of contact layers are adherent, dry gauze, or nonadherent such as Adaptic. The intermediate and outer layers are compressive or noncompressive. The clinical decision as to specific topical ointment and dressings used depend on wound type and the state of wound healing and surrounding tissues.

There is some controversy as to whether the use of topical ointments is indicated

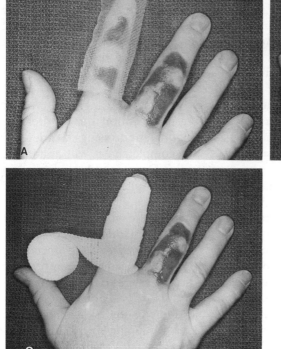
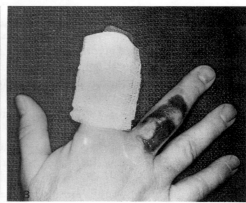

FIGURE 6–6. Three layers of dressings for granulating wound. A, Nonadherent layer, B, sterile gauze intermediate layer; and C, outer layer of Kling.

and if any bactericidal effects are evidenced.[22] Topical ointments may aid in nonadherence of dressings, encourage epithelialization, and promote tissue pliability, therefore allowing increased range of motion. Clinical decision as to use may be based on the hydrophilic or the hydrophobic properties of the preparation. Hydrophobic ointments such as Bacitracin or Neosporin provide a moist environment for dry wounds, whereas hydrophilic agents such as Betadine encourage drying and are helpful with macerated wounds or those with serous, sanguineous, or fibrinous drainage. Ointment may be applied directly to the wound with a sterile applicator or applied to the contact layer of dressing for the patient with a painful wound or marginal tissues.

PRIMARY CLOSURE

The primarily closed wound with well-approximated margins re-epithelializes rapidly. By the fourth or fifth day, the wound has developed resistance to surface contamination and needs dressing only to avoid environmental stress or aid in positioning soft tissues and joints. The dry, primarily closed wound may be dressed with dry sterile dressing or with a hydrophobic ointment and nonadherent contact dressing such as Xeroform to provide surface hydration, to encourage healing, and to decrease skin dryness and tightness. The wound should be monitored for maceration as indicated by white, wrinkled, wet wound margins. The primarily closed wound with small amounts of drainage may be dressed with a hydrophilic ointment and nonadherent dressing such as Adaptic, which permits wound drainage to the intermediate layer to encourage drying.

SECONDARY CLOSURE

Dressing of the open wound depends on the state of the wound bed and presence of exudate. A contact layer of dry sterile dressings is adherent to an open wound and absorbs exudate. This adherence may result in the disruption of neovascularization and re-epithelialization during dressing changes; therefore, caution must be used when applying this dressing type. Dry or wet-to-dry dressings nonselectively debride the wound and their use is not encouraged in the clean epithelializing wound bed. In the case of unwanted adherence, the dressing may be loosened with sterile water or normal saline. Nonadherent contact layers provide moisture, decrease shearing forces, avoid disruption of wound surface and margins, and decrease discomfort during dressing changes. Adaptic and Xeroform are commonly used nonadherent dressings. Scarlet Red is a nonadherent dressing, although, if allowed to dry completely, it will adhere. A biologic contact dressing such as porcine xenograft or E-Z Derm may be indicated in partial-thickness wounds with clean wound beds, to promote rapid epithelialization and protect against dehydration.

Some wounds have exposed vital tissue such as tendon; these wounds must be kept moist at all times with the use of a hydrophobic agent to prevent dehydration.

An intermediate or outer layer of compressive dressings may be used for edema reduction or for securing a graft to the wound bed. Precautions used with compressive dressings are to avoid vascular compromise, allow indicated range of motion, monitor for infection and areas of decreased sensation, and ascertain the level of patient reliability. Compression may be provided by fluffing multiple layers of sterile gauze for bulk, while using Kerlix, Ace, or Coban wrap as an outer layer. Wrapping should be noncircumferential and applied distal to proximal without undue tension. Vascular status must be closely monitored. A slowed blanch/refill time, along with blue or white tissues of fingertips, indicates arterial compromise as depicted in Figure 6–7, whereas purple discoloration indicates venous congestion. Sensory changes or intractable throbbing pain unrelieved with elevation are indicative of circulatory compromise. Compressive dressings are contraindicated in the presence of vascular repair or replantation usually for 21 days[24] to allow for adequate circulatory status.

An intermediate layer of noncompressive dressings, usually gauze pads, provides a sterile or clean environment, absorbs exudate, provides protection from trauma, and aids in positioning the digits and in maintaining the palmar arches and web spaces. Application of both the intermediate layer and outer layer consisting of Kling, Kerlix, and/or elastic bandage secures the inner layers and should allow for the desired range of motion and sensory input. Shearing forces across the wound or over fragile skin and bony prominences should be avoided. Monitoring of and precautions for noncompressive dressings are the same as for compressive dressings because increase in edema or shifting of dressings may create compression.

GRAFTS AND FLAPS

A wound not primarily closed or allowed to heal by secondary intention may be covered with a graft or a flap. The graft first survives by plasmatic diffusion; nourishment is then provided by transudate from the wound bed. Ultimate survival requires vascularization of the graft. Infection or anything that acts as a barrier to capillary infiltration may result in its loss. These barriers may be blood, hematoma formation, or wound exudate that separates the graft from the wound bed.

Grafts

Postoperative goals are to avoid fluid accumulation, prevent shearing forces, and inhibit contraction. These goals are accomplished with elevation, immobilization, and pressure. Time until initial postoperative dressing change ranges from 24 hours to 5 days after application. The advantage of early dressing change is that if seroma or hematoma is present, it can be evacuated from beneath the graft. Evacuation is accomplished by incising with a sterile blade, aspirating with sterile syringe, or rolling gently toward the margins with a sterile cotton-tip applicator. The disadvantage of early dressing change is its potential to disrupt the graft. To minimize stress to the graft, the dressing is removed while placing counterpressure to the graft at the dressing graft interface with gloved hand or sterile applicator. Redressing is with a nonadherent contact layer, bulky fluff to fill any concavity providing an even pressure distribution, and a gentle noncircumferential pressure layer with Coban or elastic wrap if there is no circulatory compromise.

Immobilization allows for protection from external trauma, especially shearing forces, and prevents loss of motion by maintaining tissues in their lengthened position. A dorsal hand graft requires immobilization in the protected position. A fingertip graft may be protected with a thermoplastic gutter splint or a cast, which also provides even circumferential compression. Unrestricted active range of motion is initiated after graft "take" and consultation with the referring physician. The usual time table is 5 days for an STG and 7 to 10 days for an FTG.[24] The graft should be protected from shearing forces for 7 to 14 days; compression garments may usually be worn at 14 days. When the graft is fully healed, it may be lubricated with moisturizing cream to decrease dryness and tightness.

The donor site for an FTG is primarily closed and is treated as indicated for a primarily closed wound. A split-thickness donor site is an abraded area similar to a second-degree burn, and postoperative care will be according to the preference of the attending surgeon.

Flaps

Flaps are indicated when the wound bed is not suitable for the rapid vascularization necessary for graft survival or when subcutaneous tissue is needed, such as with a partial fingertip amputation.[6] Flap care includes elevation and positioning for edema control, active and passive range of motion to uninvolved digits or joints, and wound care. A flap is dressed to provide optimal wound environment and to maintain homeostasis. Special care is exercised to avoid crimping of or traction on a pedicle flap or compression of the arterial supply of a free flap. Clean technique is used, with topical ointment if necessary and a contact layer of nonadherent dressing applied around the pedicle or flap. Care must be taken to avoid maceration, and often the area between the pedicle and other tissues must be padded with dry sterile dressing. For example, a thenar flap dressing uses sterile gauze that is rolled and positioned to support the digit from beneath and maintain the relationship of recipient to donor site. The digit is then protectively positioned with Kling, avoiding pressure over the PIP joint. Elastic wrap provides the outer layer, used to immobilize the thumb and affected digit protectively to avoid crimping of or traction on the pedicle. If there is significant drainage or accumulation of wound byproducts and necrotic tissue, whirlpool for 5 to 10 minutes with minimal agitation may be undertaken after consultation with the attending physician. Compression wrapping for edema control and for flap shaping may be initiated as a general rule 3 weeks postoperatively and after the vacularization of the flap is confirmed.

INFECTION CONTROL

Infection control techniques are designed to protect the patient, who is vulnerable to further infection because of compromised immune response; the public; the therapist; and other patients. These techniques encompass care of the wound and disposal of wound care byproducts, dressings, debrided material, and items used in wound care. As clinicians, our approach to sterile technique used for the prevention of infection requires the use of sterile field, gloves, instruments, and dressings in an undisturbed environment. Clean technique or reverse isolation uses clean field and gloves, sterile instruments, and clean and/or sterile dressings. Disposal of any items used in treatment of a draining wound or from a patient with infectious disease must be disposed of according to specific institutional guidelines. The importance of thorough handwashing before and after each patient contact cannot be overstated.

HIV Precautions

Recent concern over the increasing numbers of patients with acquired immune deficiency syndrome (AIDS) has resulted in a greater focus on wound care and infection control. The primary human immune deficiency virus, HIV, targets macrophages and T lymphocytes. Impedance of macrophages and T lymphocytes contributes to the clinically observed delay or nonhealing of the wound and to the severity and duration of the infection. Because an HIV-infected patient may not be diagnosed at time of treatment, the clinician should be watchful for common hand infections that recur or do not readily respond to treatment and may be accompanied by delayed or nonhealing wounds.[25,26] In addition one must be alert for signs of HIV-associated secondary infections, such as herpes zoster, tuberculosis, and salmonellosis. Observations from the medical history may reveal more obvious opportunistic diseases such as Kaposi's sarcoma, *Pneumocystis carinii* pneumonia, *Mycobacterium avium* intracellular, and cytomegalovirus.[27]

Wound management includes use of a disposable, waterproof, sterile underliner, and sterile gloves and instruments. Masks, goggles, and gowns are recommended when there is the possibility of contact with blood, blood products, or body fluids. One should be cautious when handling scissors, forceps, and scalpels to avoid puncturing of gloves or skin. Clinical precautions include following institutional guidelines for infection control and the Centers for Disease Control (CDC) recommendations found in the *Morbidity and Mortality Weekly Report* (MMWR).[28] HIV-infected patients should be scheduled at the end of the treatment day, if possible, to minimize exposure of themselves and others and to allow thorough disinfecting after treatment. By drying or using a dilution of 1:10 household bleach or 70 percent alcohol the HIV virus is readily inactivated.[26,29]

CLINICAL MANAGEMENT OF HIV PATIENT

Hand therapy management of the HIV-infected patient presents a challenge because of delayed wound healing and complicating medical factors. The need for immobilization and elevation for infection control may be prolonged. Prolonged infection and poor wound healing alters the normal time sequence for inflammation, fibroplasia, and maturation, resulting in the potential for joint restrictions, soft tissue tightness, and tendon adherence. During active infection, early preventive intervention is through the use of protective position splinting and constant elevation. Frequent monitoring of wound and edema status, check of splint fit, and avoidance of constrictive dressings are essential.

When infection has been controlled and the patient's general condition and specific wound status permit, gentle active range of motion is initiated. Active motion may need to be isolated joint by joint to avoid shearing stress. As wound granulation progresses, light, functional activities are added. As a result of the precarious condition of the immune system in these patients, the wound may never reach the maturation phase. Ongoing therapy management may fluctuate constantly to address the changing wound and infection status.

EDEMA

One of the most important problems a therapist will face is controlling and eliminating edema in the hand-injured patient. The presence of edema can inhibit wound healing by decreasing arterial, venous, and lymphatic flow. Edema increases the risk of infection and decreases motion, which could lead to remodeling of collagen in the shortened position causing a permanent loss of motion.[10,30] Fibrosis may be increased by compromised vascular flow creating tissue hypoxia, increased cell permeability and stagnating interstitial fluids containing increased quantities of protein.[31] The different types of edema and their characteristics and methods of treatment are outlined in Table 6-5. The control of edema is important even when not apparently visible, as interstitial fluid volume will increase 30 to 50 percent above normal before detection.[32,33] Therefore, edema control must be initiated as soon as possible after injury and should include the entire upper extremity.

Edema can be monitored by recording skin temperature,[34] which will increase or decrease according to the amount of edema present. Edema can also be evaluated by measuring the disappearance of RTSA and Na [^{131}I] by lymphatic reabsorption.[35] A more practical and accurate way to measure and monitor edema would be the use of circumferential measurements or volumetrics[36] (Chapter 3). When using circumferential measurements it is vitally important to standardize the location of each measurement so it is reproducible. Circumferential measure is probably most useful when only one or two digits are involved or a Volumeter is unavailable. The Volumeter uses water displacement for the measurement of edema and has been found to be accurate within 10 ml.[36] The proper use of the volume, described by Brand and Wood,[37] accompanies each Volumeter.

Elevation

One of the simplest and most effective ways to control edema is through elevation of the extremity and hand above the level of the heart. In theory, elevation decreases arterial hydrostatic pressure and assists in lymphatic and venous drainage, thereby decreasing interstitial volume.[38,39] The patient should be comfortably positioned with the extremity in the optimal position: the hand and wrist above the elbow with the wrist in neutral or slight extension, and the elbow above the level of the heart.[40] The therapist should exercise caution with the extreme of positioning for replants and revascularization to avoid compromising arterial flow and venous drainage. When using slings the therapist must pay close attention to hand-wrist position and closely monitor motion of the more proximal joints and cervical spine to prevent iatrogenic stiffness. Caution must also be exercised to avoid patient dependence on the sling as the only means of edema

TABLE 6–5 Edema Types, Causes, Characteristics, and Treatment Methods

Type	Cause	Characteristic	Treatment Methods
Acute	Inflammatory response (trauma, infection)	Elevated protein content; immediately reducible; displacable (temporarily); redistributable; soft to palpation; uniformly distributed	1. Elevation 2. Active exercise/ range of motion (ROM) 3. Intermittent compression (vasopneumatic devices, string wrap) 4. Retrograde massage 5. Conductive cooling 6. Electromodalities (High Voltage Galvanic Stimulation)
Dependent	Increased arterial pressure; decreased venous pressure	Unaltered protein content(?); uniformly distributed; pitting	1. Elevation 2. Active exercise/ROM 3. Massage 4. Compression (intermittent or continuous)
Fibrotic	Prolonged inflammatory response	Elevated protein content; not easily reducible; "brawny" —hard to palpation; compartmental— articular facial, dorsal hand, local wound	1. Continuous pressure (pressure garments, Coban, Ace, Tubagrip) 2. Elevation 3. Active exercise/ROM 4. Continuous Passive Motion 5. Massage 6. Electromodalities (HVGS, AC muscle stim) 7. Thermal modalities of heat (moist heat, paraffin, Fluidotherapy)
Factitious (self-inflicted)	Venous/lymphatic statis	Uniformly distributed; elevated protein content(?); glovelike demarcation (circumferential); pitting to fibrotic (depends on duration present)	1. Resistant to all methods 2. Casting 3. Continuous observation 4. Continuous compression 5. Active exercise/ ROM (functional activities) 6. Professional counseling

FIGURE 6-1

FIGURE 6-2

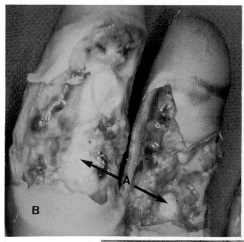

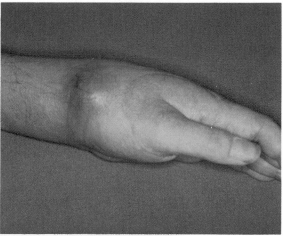

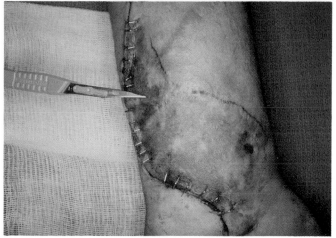

FIGURE 6-3

FIGURE 6–1. Open wound of fingers demonstrating exposure of flexor tendons (*A*) and skin maceration of the wound margins (*B*).

FIGURE 6–2. Infected puncture wound characterized by erythema, edema, and elevated temperature.

FIGURE 6–3. Proximal flap circulatory compromise. Note use of skin marker to delineate level of compromise.

FIGURE 6-5

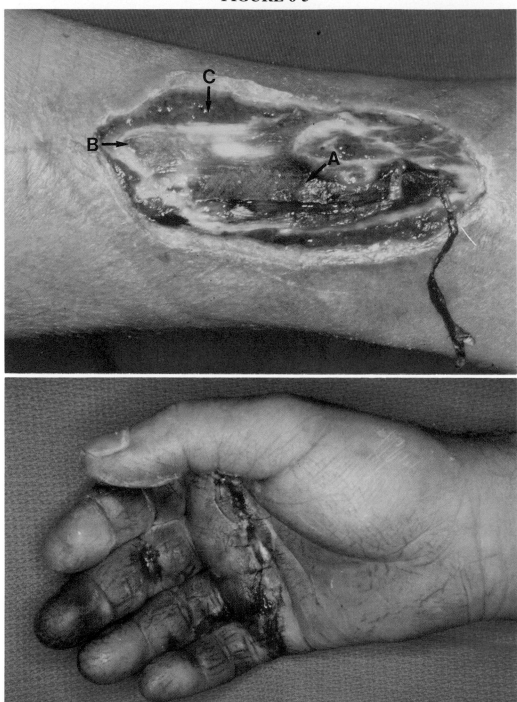

FIGURE 6-7

FIGURE 6–5. Wound demonstrating combination of black (*A*), yellow (*B*), and red (*C*).

FIGURE 6–7. Crush injury with volar degloving. Note the significant arterial compromise and questionable viability of the middle finger.

reduction. We prefer to avoid the use of slings because of this concern. Keeping the extremity elevated without a sling elicits active involvement in the treatment from the patient.

Active Exercise

Active exercise in conjunction with elevation is another effective means of edema control.[40] Exercise creates muscle pumping, soft tissue movement, and compression— all of which play a role in maintaining equilibrium between extravascular and intravascular fluid volumes. The primary effect of exercise is to increase lymphatic flow and venous return to the heart by lowering capillary hydrostatic pressure, thereby decreasing intersitital volume.[33] All the joints of the extremity should be moved actively and passively through their full available ranges, except those joints unsafe to move secondary to injury. Active motion may also be augmented by isometric contraction. An example of active exercises is differential tendon gliding and intrinsic pumping. Although beneficial in assisting with venous and lymphatic flow and in maintaining motion, passive range of motion and the use of continuous passive motion devices should be used as an adjunct to, and not as a replacement, for active exercise.

Intermittent Compression

External compression is also an effective tool for edema control and is used in a variety of methods including massage, intermittent compression, and continuous compression. Massage is a form of intermittent compression and augments venous and lymphatic flow, as well as interstitial tissue compression.[41] Retrograde massage may be limited to a single digit or may include the entire extremity. A duration of 5 to 10 minutes or to patient tolerance is recommended.

VASOPNEUMATIC DEVICES

Vasopneumatic devices are another form of intermittent compression. The duration of treatment depends on the type of edema. Edema that is acute or dependent in nature may require only 2 hours of compression per treatment.[42] Fibrotic chronic lymphatic or prolonged factitious edema may require 8 to 72 hours of continuous intermittent compression to reduce edema.[43] During these prolonged periods the appliance should be removed every 2 to 4 hours to allow for active exercises. The compression-to-release ratio is usually 3:1 or 4:1, with compression lasting at least 60 to 90 seconds. Compression should be at least 25 mmHg and never greater than diastolic pressure. For the upper extremity, compression usually is 60 mmHg if tolerated by the patient.[43] Intermittent compression can also be used to assist in augmenting joint motion by positioning the fingers in the restricted position to obtain stretch. The compression provides the passive stretch and may assist in increasing motion by applying a low-load, long-duration stress. Precautions should be taken because of the poor control over the amount of force being applied. The therapist should also use caution in treating patients who have locally infected wounds, fractures, and a history of cardiac disease, as the increase in intravascular fluid volume and external pressure may place an increased demand on the heart. Vasopneumatic devices are contraindicated in the presence of acute wound infection, infections beyond the local boundaries of the wound, compartmentalized or systemic infection such as lymphangitis or cellulitis, and unstable fractures or external fixation devices.

Vasopneumatic compression should not be performed until 3 weeks after the revascularization procedure and after consultation with the attending physician. An open wound is not necessarily a contraindication for vasopneumatic intermittent compression use. The wound should be covered with a noncircumferential dressing of adequate amount to absorb the increased exudate and avoid the contamination of the appliance. The individual should be supplied, if possible, with a separate appliance and the sleeve disinfected after each use. In the presence of soft tissue reconstruction procedures, vasopneumatic compression is contraindicated until 5 days after STG, 7 to 10 days after FTG, and 3 weeks after flap separation, so as not to compromise capillary infiltration and venous drainage.

STRING WRAPPING

Another method of intermittent compression would be string wrapping (Fig. 6–8). This approach could include one or more digits or the entire hand to the level of the wrist. Wrapping occurs distal to proximal for 5 minutes with the extremity elevated. During this time retrograde massage can be performed. Flowers[44] has found that combined string wrapping and retrograde massage are more effective than either technique alone. Following the removal of the string, active exercises are initiated. The entire procedure may be repeated three to four times per day.[45]

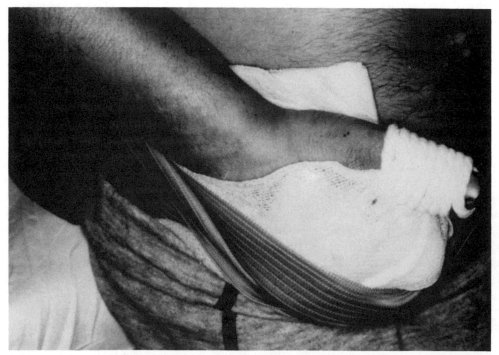

FIGURE 6–8. String wrapping of a single digit while the groin pedicle flap is still attached to the donor site.

Continuous Compression

Continuous compression can be achieved with Coban, Ace wraps, compressive garments, or air cast splint. When using Coban or Ace wrap for continuous or intermittent compression, hands are always wrapped distal to proximal in a "figure 8" fashion to avoid a tourniquet effect. The Coban or Ace should be left on for at least 1 hour and preferably at night, thus allowing free use of the fingers during the day for function and exercise (Fig. 6–9). Compressive garments or materials such as Isotoner gloves, Jobst compression garments, and Tubagrip are effective in controlling edema and should be applied in conjunction with the other methods of edema control previously discussed. Consideration must be given to the arterial, venous, and lymphatic status with the gradient of pressure adjusted by using the millimeters of mercury specified by Jobst or the manufacturer for Tubagrip.

COMPRESSIVE MATERIALS

Using compressive material or garments deserves special consideration with open wounds. The therapist should be aware of the shearing forces on the new epithelium created by donning garments or wrapping with compressive materials. Frictional and shearing forces may also be created under the garment by active range-of-motion exercises or functional activities. This approach may cause a problem, especially when the garment overlays recent skin grafts, flaps, or newly epithelialized tissue, as in a burn or donor site. Compressive garments may also compromise a delicate circulatory status

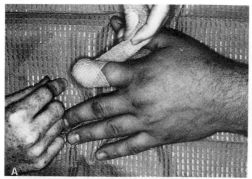
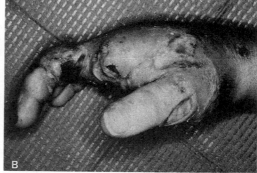
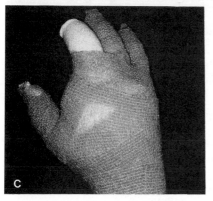

FIGURE 6–9. *A*, Coban wrap for edema control and stump shaping. Note that the wrap is applied in a figure-eight manner, starting distally and working proximally. *B*, Edematous hand with open wound. *C*, Same hand with dressing and Coban wrap.

resulting in hypoxia and necrosis. In general, avoiding external compressive materials until at least 5 days after STG, 10 days after FTG, and 3 weeks after flap reconstruction is best.

Care should be taken when compressive garments are placed over dressings to avoid creating excessive pressure per square inch over the wound. Maceration of the wound should be avoided by frequent dressing changes, at least twice per day or more often if wound exudate is excessive. Compressive materials may impede soft tissue mobility and interfere with the patient's ability to perform essential active exercises necessitating the removal of the garment or wrap for exercise. Static and dynamic splinting may be used in conjunction with these compressive garments, keeping in mind the precautions previously discussed.

Thermal Agents

Thermal agents have a limited and adjunctive role only for the control of edema. Superficial heating increases tissue extensibility[46] and is a potent vasodilator.[47] The increased capillary pressure causes a diffusion of fluid out of the capillaries into the interstitial tissues. The net effect of superficial heat alone may increase edema, vascular compromise, and local tissue ischemia, resulting in decreased metabolic byproduct removal and delayed wound healing. Superficial heat is appropriate after the inflammatory phase and when applied with limb elevation.

Cryotherapy, on the other hand, causes vasoconstriction and a decrease in capillary infiltration, metabolic rate, and pain. During the initial inflammatory phase, cryotherapy effectively reduces acute edema. Avoid overcooling which may delay wound healing as a result of vasospasm and tissue ischemia.[48] Cryotherapy is contraindicated in the presence of arterial repair. Other physical agents such as electrical stimulation may be of assistance in edema reduction (see Chapter 8 for information on physical agents and electrical stimulation).

SCAR MANAGEMENT

Optimal management of scar tissue during the late maturation phase begins with proper care of the injured tissues from time of injury through the inflammatory and fibroplastic phases. Scar tissue management focuses on the control of stresses placed on the healing tissues. Prolonged inflammatory response is avoided by proper early wound management, infection prevention, minimizing stress to the wound, protection of the uninjured tissues, and edema control. Early active and passive motion provides controlled stress encouraging optimal remodeling of scar tissue. Edema reduction allows increased motion, adequate arterial support for tissue nutrition, and the removal of traumatized biologic material and wound-healing byproducts. Early initiation of protective position splinting will reduce the development of shortened remodeled scar.

The late maturation phase is characterized by scar that is predominantly extracellular in nature, with high collagen content and rapid turnover. Morphologically the scar remains active for years, changing slowly in size, shape, texture, and strength.[30] Scar formation is influenced by chemical mechanisms, patient's age and race, condition of adjacent tissue condition, and the size and extent of the wound. The greater the amount of scar, the more difficult it is to alter physiologically. During the final phase of wound healing scar management is achieved via external mechanisms of control and applying the concept of low-load, long-duration stress.

Thermal Agents

The application of thermal agents for tissue heating has been found effective in temporarily increasing tissue extensibility. Lehman and associates[46] found that tendon elongation or extensibility could be increased by heating tissues to temperatures greater than 45°C. This extensibility was enhanced with the application of constant stretch during and immediately after the heat application.[46] The effectiveness of heat, however, was questioned by Hamilton,[49] who found no significant improvement in PIP motion in patients receiving heat and exercise or exercise alone. The use of heat modalities may be initiated after the acute inflammatory phase. Precautions must be observed in areas of impaired sensation or compromised circulation. To provide increased tissue extensibility the heating modality of choice must elevate tissue temperature to greater than 40°C and be applied in conjunction with stretch. In the hand, effective superficial heating agents are paraffin, hot packs, and Fluidotherapy.[39,47,50,51] Prolonged stretch may be applied by using Coban or Ace wrap to position the digit or hand in the desired position. Whirlpool should not be used as a superficial heating modality because of possible increase in edema[16,17] and should be limited to open wound care only.

Selective deep-tissue heating for improved extensibility may be provided with the use of ultrasound. At present, ultrasound has not been demonstrated structurally to alter scar tissue, although it does provide selective deep-tissue heating. Stress applied during or immediately after, ultrasound has been shown to be effective in increasing tissue extensibility and improving residual length.[53] To obtain the thermal effect, ultrasound application must be of sufficient duration and intensity. For the hand and wrist, ultrasound is applied in the continuous mode with an intensity of 1.0 watt per cm² or less directly to the area with contact medium or with underwater technique using a water temperature 36.7 to 38.8°C to avoid tissue cooling. Duration of application in general is 5 minutes per 25 cm² of surface area.[52]

Massage

Although a paucity of research and literature on the effects of massage on scar tissue exists, massage is widely used for scar tissue management and is noted to be clinically efficacious prior to exercise. Massage may alter scar through a combination of mechanical stress and thermal effects.[53] The movement, occurring between the therapist's contact with the patient's tissue, and between the scar and the surrounding tissue may create a local thermal effect resulting in increased tissue extensibility. Mechanical stress may also be created by the physical movement of the scar and surrounding tissues, assisting with improved collagen organization. Massage possibly provides a continuous compression, which may decrease local interstitial fluid content, resulting in a temporary increase in tissue extensibility.

Clinically massage is the manual application of combined pressure and low friction movements. Massage is applied perpendicular to the scar or in small circular motions, with firm pressure to facilitate movement of the scar and surrounding tissues away from structures to which it may be adhered. Duration of massage depends on patient tolerance and the size of the affected area. A general guideline is a 5- to 10-minute application, avoiding erythema or discomfort. A lubricant should be used to protect against injurious friction and superficial tissue damage in the newly forming scar. Gentle massage may be initiated during the early phases of wound healing to closed wounds which demonstrate a small amount of tensile strength. In areas of flaps, skin grafts, and wounds healed by secondary intention, and in patients with prolonged wound healing, massage should be used with caution, as previously discussed. Massage should not be instituted over an infected or acutely inflamed area.

Mechanical Vibration

Mechanical vibration as a procedure to provide mechanical stress to scar tissue has been advocated for clinical use, although not supported in the literature. Considerations, precautions, and time frame for using vibration are the same as those for massage. The use of vibration may, through accommodation, also assist in desensitization of hypersensitive scar and surrounding tissues.

Compressive Techniques

The techniques with which to apply compression for scar management include compressive garments and materials, dressings, or inserts to improve pressure distribution. Various theories have been postulated regarding the effects of compression on scar. The application of pressure of 25 mm Hg decreases the blood flow, causing local hypoxia and decreasing fibroblast synthesis of collagen.[54] Pressure may mechanically force fluid out of the tissue, resulting in closer approximation of cross-links. Increased tissue extensibility may result from disruption of the anchoring contractile fibrils and the acceleration of degradation of ground substance components.[55] Using compression materials and garments for scar management remains unsupported by strong scientific research in the literature.

The more mature the scar the less effect any mechanical stress will have on the organization of collagen. As a result, clinical management should not be delayed until after wound closure. Wound dressings may be applied for compression, with the precaution of avoiding wound ischemia. In areas of skin bridging such as the axilla, antecubital fossa, and digital web spaces, early application of pressure dressings is important to avoid soft tissue contraction. Materials such as Coban, Ace wrap, and Tubigrip stockinette for temporary use and custom-made garments such as Jobst for prolonged use provide uniform circumferential compression. Adjunctive compression inserts to increase local compression or improve conformance of pressure over concave areas may be fabricated from silastic Elastomer (Fig. 6–10), or from Otoform, dermal pads, or felt. As fibroblastic activity is without interruption, application of pressure is most efficacious when continuous, at least 23 hours a day, and when initiated as soon as wound status permits. The same precautions for initiation and use apply as discussed in the use of compression for edema control. The therapist should closely monitor vascularity of the wound and surrounding tissues to avoid ischemia. The wrap-on garment should not interfere with joint motion or inhibit sensory input. Attention to scar fragility is important, as garments do create friction and shearing forces and maceration, which can result in superficial breakdown and blister formation. Patient reliability is a final consideration, especially with application of compression wrap. Inappropriate applica-

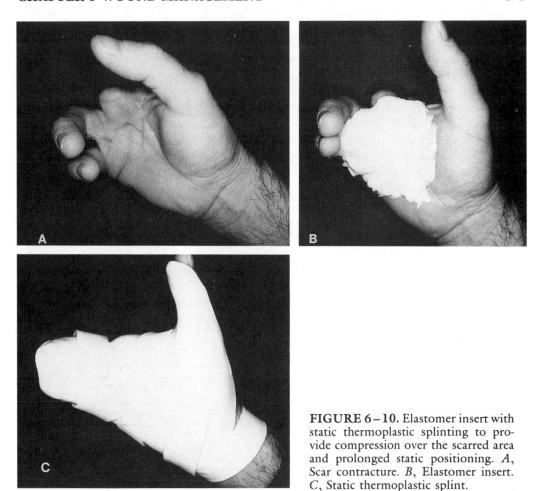

FIGURE 6–10. Elastomer insert with static thermoplastic splinting to provide compression over the scarred area and prolonged static positioning. *A*, Scar contracture. *B*, Elastomer insert. *C*, Static thermoplastic splint.

tion alters the amount and distribution of pressure, possibly resulting in further tissue damage.

Splinting

Scar tissue remodeling can be assisted with the use of splinting. Although splinting is addressed in depth in Chapter 9, some specifics deserve attention. Early initiation of splinting as a preventive measure may result in less need for corrective management during maturation. Preventive short-term immobilization during the inflammatory phase for up to 5 days in a resting or functional position may help avoid a prolonged inflammatory response. Protective position splinting may be necessary during the inflammatory and fibroplasia phases to assist in preventing contractures of injured and uninjured structures. Protective positioning may be necessary only for those digits, or part of a digit or the hand, that are injured and affected by lack of mobility. During the maturation phase, splinting is used for scar management through application of low-load, long-duration stress.[56] The primary considerations in stress application are the direction and amount of the force and its duration (see Chapter 9 to determine the appropriate use of static and dynamic splinting design, force, and duration).

SUMMARY

The role of the hand therapist in patient wound management has been progressively expanding. An increased knowledge base of the biology of wound healing and improvement in evaluative skills and clinical wound management expertise are essential for optimal patient care. Proper initial management is requisite in prevention of a prolonged inflammatory response resulting in edema, soft tissue and periarticular tightness, decreased motion, and the potential for permanent loss of function. Preventive management through the inflammatory and fibroplasia phases causes optimal scar tissue formation and less need for prolonged management in the maturation phase. A thorough initial evaluation and constant reevaluation are necessary to assess the patient's needs and to establish and revise the plan of care. Management in the overlapping inflammatory and fibroplasia phases incorporates wound care and dressings to provide an optimal environment for healing, edema control measures, active and passive motion, and splinting. Intervention during the maturation phase focuses on scar tissue management with modalities, massage, compression, and low-load, long-duration splinting. As research in the laboratory and in the clinical setting is expanding the knowledge of wound biology and management, we would encourage the reader to pursue updated literature and continuing education courses on this topic.

REFERENCES

1. Goldner, RD: Postoperative management. Hand Clin 1(2):206, 1985.
2. Weiss, HG: Platelet physiology and abnormalities of platelet function. N Engl J Med 293:536, 1975.
3. Beasley, RW: Hand Injuries. WB Saunders, Philadelphia, 1981, p 23.
4. Gray, H: Anatomy Descriptive and Surgical, ed 15. Bounty Book, New York, 1927, p 593.
5. Cazzell, JZ: Wound care forum—the new RYB color code. Am J Nurs 1342, 1988.
6. Grad, JB and Beasley, RW: Fingertip reconstruction. Hand Clin 1(4):667, 1985.
7. Browne, EZ: Skin grafts. In Greene, DP (ed): Operative Hand Surgery. Churchill Livingstone, New York, 1982, p 1283.
8. Winspur, I: Distant flaps. Hand Clin 1(4):729, 1985.
9. Rodenheaver, G, et al: Bacterial activity and toxicity of iodine-containing solutions in wounds. Arch Surg 117:181, 1982.
10. Peacock, EE and Van Winkle, W: Surgery and Biology of Wound Repair. WB Saunders, Philadelphia, 1970.
11. Linneaweaver, W, et al: Cellular and bacterial toxicities of topical antimicrobials. Plast Reconstr Surg 75:394, 1985.
12. Walsh, MT: Hydrotherapy: The use of water as a therapeutic agent. In Michlovitz, SL (ed): Thermal Agents in Rehabilitation. FA Davis, Philadelphia, 1986, p 119.
13. Ziegenfus, RW: Povodine-iodine as bactericide in hydrotherapy equipment. Phys Ther 49:582, 1969.
14. Aston, S: Burns in children. Ciba Clin Symp 28:14, 1976.
15. Steve, L, Goodhart, P, and Alexander, J: Hydrotherapy burn treatment: Use of chloramine-T against resistant microorganisms. Arch Phys Med Rehabil 60:301, 1979.
16. Schultz, K: The effect of active exercise during whirlpool on the hand. Unpublished thesis, San Jose State University, San Jose, CA, 1982.
17. Walsh, MT: Relationship of hand edema to upper extremity position and water temperature during whirlpool treatments in normals. Unpublished thesis, Temple University, Philadelphia, 1983.
18. Magness, J, Garret, T, and Erickson, D: Swelling of the upper extremity during whirlpool baths. Arch Phys Med Rehabil 51:297, 1970.
19. Edlich, RF, et al: Fundamentals of wound management in surgery. In Smith Kline & French (Dist): Technical Factors in Wound Management. Chirurgecom, South Plainfield, NJ, 1977.
20. Rodenheaver, GT, et al: Proteolytic enzymes as adjuncts to antibiotic prophylaxis of surgical wounds. Am J Surg 127:564, 1974.
21. Hummel, RP, et al: The continuing problem of sepsis following enzymatic debridement of burns. J Trauma 14(7):572, 1974.
22. Geronemus, RG, Mertz, PM, and Eaglstein, WH: Wound healing: The effects of topical antimicrobial agents. Arch Dermatol 115:1311, 1979.

23. Rao, VK, Nightingale, G, and O'Brien, BM: Scanning electron microscope study of microvenous grafts to artery. Plast Reconstr Surg 71(1):98, 1983.
24. Salisbury, RE, Reeves, S, and Wright, P: Acute care and rehabilitation of the burned hand. In Hunter, JM, et al (eds): Rehabilitation of the Hand, ed 2. CV Mosby, St Louis, 1984, p 585.
25. Kelen, GD, et al: Unrecognized human immunodeficiency virus infection in emergency department patients. N Engl J Med 318(25):1645, 1988.
26. Johnson, CD and Glickel, SZ: AIDS and the hand therapist. J Hand Ther 2(3):157, 1989.
27. Glatt, AE, Chirqwin, K, and Landesman, SH: Current concepts in treatment of infections associated with human immunodeficiency virus. N Engl J Med 313(22):1439, 1988.
28. Centers for Disease Control: Update: Universal precautions for prevention of transmission of human immunodeficiency virus, hepatitis B virus, and other blood bourne pathogens in health-care settings. MMWR 37(24):377, 1988.
29. Centers for Disease Control: Recommendations for prevention of HIV transmission in health care settings. MMWR (Suppl) 36:2S, 1987.
30. Kelly, M and Madden, JW: Hand surgery and wound healing. In Wolfert (ed): Acute Hand Injuries; A Multispecialty Approach. Little Brown, Boston, 1980, p 49.
31. Saferin, E and Posch, J: Secretans disease: Post traumatic hand edema of the dorsum of the hand. Plast Reconstr Surg 58:703, 1976.
32. Guyton, A: Textbook of Medical Physiology, ed 6. WB Saunders, Philadelphia, 1981.
33. Guyton, A: Basis Human Physiology: Normal Function and Mechanism of Disease, ed 2. WB Saunders, Philadelphia, 1977.
34. Hambury, H, Watson, K, and Toth, A: The Use of Differential Skin Temperature Measurements in the Evaluation of Post-traumatic Edema Control. Med Biol Eng Comput 13:202, 1975.
35. Lotveit, T and Lotveit, A: Absorption of edema following ankle fractures. Scand J Clin Lab Invest 31:155.
36. Fess, E and Moran, C: Clinical Assessment Recommendations. Publication of American Society of Hand Therapists, Garner, NC, 1981.
37. Brand, P and Wood, H: Hand Volumeter Instruction Sheet. United States Public Health Service Hospital, Carville, LA.
38. Vasudevan, S and Melvin, J: Upper extremity edema control: Rationale of treatment techniques. Am J Occup Ther 33:520, 1979.
39. Abramson, D: Physiologic basis for the use of physical agents in peripheral vascular disorders. Arch Phys Med Rehabil 49:216, 1965.
40. Whitson, T and Allen, B: Management of the burned hand. J Trauma 7:895, 1971.
41. Wood, EC: Beard's Massage Principles and Techniques. WB Saunders, Philadelphia, 1974, p 48.
42. Sanderson, RG and Fletcher, WS: Conservative management of primary lymphedema. Northwest Med 64:584, 1965.
43. The Jobst Extremity Pump: Clinical application of an overview of the pathophysiology of edema. Jobst Institute, Toledo, 1985.
44. Flowers, KR: String wrapping versus massage for reduction digital volume. Phys Ther 68(1):57, 1988.
45. Hunter, JM and Mackin, ED: Edema and bandaging. In Hunter, JM, et al (ed): Rehabilitation of the Hand. CV Mosby, St Louis, 1984, p 146.
46. Lehman, J, et al: Effect of therapeutic temperatures on tendon extensibility. Arch Phys Med Rehabil 51:81, 1970.
47. Abramson, D, et al: Changes in blood flow, oxygen uptake, and tissue temperature produced by a topical application of wet heat. Arch Phys Med Rehabil 42:305, 1961.
48. Michlovitz, SL: Cryotherapy: The use of cold as a therapeutic agent. In Michlovitz, SL (ed): Thermal Agents in Rehabilitation. FA Davis, Philadelphia, 1986, p 73.
49. Hamilton, G: Mobilization of the proximal interphalangeal joint: The influence of heat, cold and exercise. Phys Ther 47:111, 1967.
50. Abramson, D, et al: The effect of altering limb position on blood flow, O_2 uptake and skin temperature. J Appl Physiol 17:191, 1962.
51. Borrel, R, et al: Comparison of in vivo temperatures produced by hydrotherapy, paraffin wax treatment, and Fluidotherapy. Phys Ther 60:1273, 1980.
52. Ziskin, MC and Michlovitz, SL: Therapeutic ultrasound. In Michlovitz, SL (ed): Thermal Agents in Rehabilitation. FA Davis, Philadelphia, 1986, p 141.
53. Chamberlain GJ: Cyriax's friction massage: A review. J Ortho Sports Phys Therapy 4:16, 1982–1983.
54. Kischer, CW and Sheltar, MR: Alteration of hypertrophic scars induced by mechanical pressure. Arch Dermatol 111:60, 1975.
55. Baur, PS, et al: Wound contractions, scar contractures and myofibroblasts: A classical case study. J Trauma 18:8, 1978.
56. Arem, AJ and Madden, JW: Effects of stress on healing wounds: Intermittent noncyclical tension. J Surg Res 20(2):93, 1976.

CHAPTER 7

Therapeutic Exercise: Maintaining and Restoring Mobility in the Hand

Barbara Stanley, PT

The hand is a mobile structure, capable of performing tasks as complex as playing a piano or as simple as grasping a hammer. This great freedom of movement results from the unique anatomy of the hand and from the ability of the structural components (joints, tendons, skin, and so on) to glide with relation to each other. The tendency for the hand to become stiff is one of the most debilitating complications associated with hand rehabilitation. The development of joint contractures and tendon adhesions resulting from injury and immobilization can significantly impair hand function long after the original injury has healed. Therapeutic exercise is a valuable tool for maintaining and restoring mobility in the hand. The use of "early, controlled motion" to influence scar formation and maintain gliding plains of motion is an integral component of any hand rehabilitation program.

The objectives of this chapter are (1) to outline the rationale for use of therapeutic motion to maintain and restore mobility in the hand; (2) to present guidelines for the selection and application of exercise to maintain and restore joint mobility and tendon glide; (3) to outline how exercise programs can be adapted to allow early motion when structures in the hand are injured; and (4) to identify treatment modalities that compliment an exercise program, including thermal agents, splinting, continuous passive motion, and neuromuscular electrical stimulation.

THE ROLE OF THERAPEUTIC MOTION IN MAINTAINING AND RESTORING MOBILITY: TREATMENT RATIONALE

Movement is the activity necessary to maintain joint mobility and gliding tendon function. Immobilization, or even restricted movement, is the primary reason joint stiffness and restricted tendon glide occur. Even a normal hand, when immobilized for a prolonged period of time, will develop secondary shortening of periarticular structures, as well as adhesion formation within joints and between tendons and surrounding structures.[1,2] The deleterious effects of immobilization become more pronounced when combined with trauma and edema. Trauma, from injury or surgery, produces scar. The inflammatory edema associated with trauma envelops the tissues of the hand, producing scar wherever the edema is found. Scar tissue that is allowed to form without the benefits of controlled movement becomes dense and restrictive, potentially binding together normally gliding plains of motion.

Therapeutic motion can help maintain connective tissue mobility and favorably affect scar tissue formation by influencing the physiologic process of collagen formation. Collagen is the primary component of scar and connective tissue (tendon, ligaments, joint capsules). The physical stress that results with movement affects collagen formation in several ways. Movement enhances the normal orientation of collagen fibrils and prevents increased cross-link formation in newly synthesized collagen.[2,3] Motion-induced stress also increases collagenous strength and hypertrophy in ligament and tendon.[2]

The key to successful treatment of the stiff hand is prevention: Joint motion that is not lost to contracture is joint motion that does not have to be regained. Following injury, the use of "early, controlled motion" influences collagen formation so as to maintain and restore gliding planes of motion. When contractures and tendon adhesions do develop, therapeutic exercise is one of many treatment methods used to restore motion through collagen remodeling.

EVALUATION: GENERAL CONSIDERATIONS

The evaluation process begins with the therapist determining which structures need to be immobilized, which structures can be moved without restriction, and which structures can be moved only under certain conditions. The effects of exercise on skin, bones, joints, tendons, nerves, and vessels should be systematically considered, with each structure classified in one of the aforementioned categories. When movement is allowed, but only under certain restrictions, these restrictions should be clearly defined. For example, following a proximal phalanx fracture, active motion may be permitted only if the fracture site is manually supported

Objective measurements of active, passive, and torque-angle range of motion, as well as grip and pinch, should be recorded. These measurements are used to identify limitations and provide a baseline against which to compare subsequent measurements to assess the effectiveness of the exercise program. Documentation of skin color, skin temperature, and edema measurements provides guidelines regarding the tissue response to the exercise stress. When exercise is used to maintain mobility, the evaluation findings, as well as a knowledge of the rehabilitative process, should be used to anticipate what limitations in motion will most likely occur. For example, the presence of excessive edema on the dorsum of the hand frequently results in metaphalangeal (MP) joint extension contractures and intrinsic tightness. By anticipating these problems, intrinsic stretching and isolated metacarpophalangeal (MCP) flexion exercises can be used to prevent the development of fixed contractures.

When the purpose of the exercise program is to restore motion, the hand should be evaluated to determine if limitations in motion are a result of secondary changes in joints and soft tissues, rather than a result of pain, edema, muscle atrophy, or muscle deinnervation. If decreased motion is a result of joint and soft tissue tightness, the therapist should determine the specific structure(s) that is (are) limiting movement, including the joint, skin, ligament, muscle, or tendon (see Chapter 3). Based on this information, an exercise program can be developed specifically to stress those structures that are limiting motion.

DEVELOPING AN EXERCISE PROGRAM

When developing an exercise program to maintain and restore motion in the hand, the following factors should be considered: the mode of exercise (passive versus active versus resisted), the amount of stress that is to be applied to the hand, and the ability of the stress to be selectively directed toward the structure that is limiting the motion.

Exercise Mode: Passive Versus Active Versus Resistance

Therapeutic exercise can be performed passively, actively, or against resistance. Passive exercise is produced entirely by an external force. The external force may be applied by gravity, a machine, another individual, or the patient.[4] Active exercise is performed by an active contraction of the muscle crossing the joint.[4] Muscles contracting against resistance perform resistive exercise. The decision to use passive, active, or resisted exercise depends on the purpose of the exercise as well as an understanding of the advantages and disadvantages of each exercise form. All three forms of exercise are contraindicated when the stress produced would be disruptive to the healing process of a repaired or injured structure.

PASSIVE EXERCISE

Passive exercise is used to maintain joint and soft tissue mobility, as well as the mechanical elasticity of muscle. In addition, passive exercise decreases edema, assists circulation, enhances synovial diffusion, and decreases pain.[4] Passive motion is indicated when pain, paralysis, spasticity, and weakness prevent a patient from actively maintaining full joint range of motion (ROM). Passive range of motion (PROM) is also used when joint mobilization and stretching techniques are required to improve joint and soft tissue mobility. During the early phase of wound healing, gentle, controlled passive exercise may be preferred over active exercise to influence collagen formation without inflicting pain. In the case of rheumatoid patients with acute synovitis, Melvin[5] feels that active exercise may actually increase muscle tension and joint compression, and she therefore recommends the use of passive motion within the patient's pain-free, available range.

ACTIVE EXERCISE

Like PROM exercise, active range-of-motion (AROM) exercise maintains mobility, enhances synovial diffusion, and decreases pain. In addition, AROM exercise provides several advantages over PROM exercise, the most important of which is the ability of active exercise to produce tendon glide. Because it can apply stress to joints, soft tissue, and tendons, active exercise is the preferred method of exercise when the integrity of repaired structures is not a consideration. Active exercise also maintains the physiologic elasticity and contractility of muscles, as well as providing a stimulus for bone integrity. When compared with passive exercise, active exercise is more effective in reducing edema because of the active muscle contraction required. Active-assistive exercise is a type of AROM exercise in which assistance is provided by an outside force, either manually or mechanically, because the muscles that move the joint need help to complete the motion.[4]

RESISTANCE EXERCISE

By increasing muscular strength, resistance exercises increase the amount of stress the patient can actively exert on stiff joints and restricted tendons. Muscular strength plays a particularly important role in restoring tendon glide, which will be discussed later.

Exercise Dosage: Controlling the Amount of Stress Applied

Whether the exercise is performed passively, actively, or against resistance, the therapist must determine the amount of stress that the exercise is to impart on the tissues of the hand. The total amount of stress is a product of the intensity, duration, and frequency.[6,7] This concept is more commonly referred to as the "exercise dosage," and describes how hard the patient should actively contract a muscle or passively stretch a joint (force/intensity), how long the force is to be sustained (duration), the number of exercise repetitions performed at each exercise session, as well as the number of exercise sessions per day (frequency).

The total amount of stress, and the manner in which the stress is applied (force/intensity, duration, frequency) depend on the purpose of the exercise and the phase of wound healing occurring in the hand. For example, when the purpose of the exercise program is to maintain the ROM of normal joints, active exercise through the full ROM performed one time a day is sufficient to maintain the integrity of connective tissue structures. Such an exercise program might be prescribed to maintain shoulder mobility for a patient who is being immobilized for a wrist fracture.

A totally different exercise dosage would be needed after a flexor tenolysis. Although the tenolysis involves surgical removal of scar tissue to restore tendon glide and active motion, the procedure itself is a source of trauma to the tissues, resulting in edema and further scar formation. The exercise program used after tenolysis requires frequent exercise sessions (every hour), performed for short periods of time (5 to 10 minutes). Frequent exercise sessions are chosen to keep the tendon gliding in the newly forming bed of scar. Short duration exercise sessions are used to prevent the patient from overexercising, which may actually contribute to the postsurgical inflammatory process.

After surgery or injury, determining the appropriate amount of stress is an ongoing process that should reflect the current stage of wound healing. The stress that is applied should favorably influence the biologic process of collagen synthesis and formation. Unfortunately there are no specific guidelines for how to determine the "ideal" stress.[3,8,9] Therapy becomes a balancing act, with the therapist constantly modifying the amount of stress, and the way in which that stress is applied. If too much stress is applied, tissue damage and inflammation result. When the stress is insufficient to influence collagen formation, motion-limiting scar forms, resulting in joint contractures and tendon adhesions. A general look at the wound healing process as it relates to therapeutic exercise will offer some insight as to how the exercise stress should be modified with each stage of wound healing.

WOUND HEALING STAGES

Inflammatory Phase

During the inflammatory phase, immobilization is indicated to rest tissues traumatized by either surgery or injury. Therapeutic motion started too early will only aggravate the trauma, perpetuating the inflammatory response.

Fibroplasia Phase

The inflammatory phase subsides as the wound enters the fibroplasia phase, accompanied by an increase in both the collagen content and the tensile strength of the wound. During the fibroplasia phase, the newly formed collagen is immature but gaining in strength, and is favorably influenced by exercise induced stress. Arem and Madden[10] have shown that scar elongation is not possible after 14 weeks of scar maturation, but a 3-week-old scar can be significantly lengthened when subjected to tension. When exercise is used, the amount of stress applied is dictated by the condition of injured or repaired structures. Initially, AROM exercises and joint mobilization may be introduced to maintain gliding surfaces. The total stress applied should be very low, consisting of a gentle force applied only a few repetitions per day. The exercises should always be performed in the pain-free range. Any signs of increased edema, pain, or warmth are indications that the applied stress is excessive and should be reduced. As the patient progresses through the fibroplasia phase, increasing resistance to movement will be felt as the tensile strength of the collagen increases. As a result, the total stress applied is also increased with exercise sessions occurring more frequently, for longer periods of time, and with increasing intensity.

Scar Maturation Phase

During the scar maturation phase, collagen synthesis plateaus and the strength of the wound increases. Ideally, whatever joint stiffness and loss of tendon excursion developed during the inflammatory and fibroplasia stages have resulted from immature scar that can still be favorably altered by therapeutic exercise. This possibility does not always occur, as evidenced by the presence of fixed joint contractures and unyielding tendon adhesions. High-intensity forces are not biologically effective in remodeling scar. According to Peacock, "most individuals who place reliance on brute force to activate incarcerated tendons are still thinking of rupturing adhesions, rather than applying stimuli to encourage secondary remodeling of scar tissue."[11] The ability to influence collagen formation and restore motion relies on the prolonged metabolic turnover of scar collagen and is best achieved with a low-load, long-duration stress.[10,12-14] The stress must be of a mild, prolonged nature and applied at the end range of joint motion. Flowers and Michlovitz[7] use the term total end range time (TERT) to describe the total amount of time the joint or tendon spends at the end of its available range.

The ability of therapeutic exercise to produce permanent lengthening changes in fixed contractures is limited because therapeutic exercise cannot maintain long-duration forces at the end range of motion. In treating joint contractures, exercise techniques such as passive stretching and joint mobilization should be used to stretch or "prime" the tissues temporarily whereas methods that maximize TERT (such as splinting or serial casts) provide the force necessary to produce permanent lengthening changes. Once the ideal tissue length has been achieved, active, passive, and resisted exercise are used to maintain the increased motion.

Exercise Selection: Directing the Stress to the Appropriate Structure

The corrective stress must be applied to the structure that is limiting motion, whether that structure is scar tissue limiting tendon glide or skin tightness limiting joint motion. When the corrective stress is applied to the wrong tissue, the exercise will not only be ineffective in restoring motion, but also may result in tissue damage. For example, limited finger flexion can result from flexor tendon adhesions, extrinsic extensor tightness, intrinsic tightness, or joint contractures. If the corrective force is applied to the joint (i.e., passive isolated joint stretching), when the limitation is due to extrinsic extensor tightness, the exercise will not restore finger flexion. Exercise-induced tissue damage can occur following flexor tendon repair, when ROM exercises must be performed to prevent proximal interphalangeal (PIP) flexion contractures. The challenge here is to direct the corrective force to the PIP joint, and not to the surgically repaired flexor tendon. By passively flexing the surrounding distal interphalangeal (DIP), MP, and wrist joints, the flexor tendon system is put on slack, allowing the extension force to be directed to the PIP joint. If these precautions are not taken, the extension force would be applied to the tendon, as well as the joint, possibly resulting in tendon rupture.

GENERAL EXERCISE CONSIDERATIONS

Before initiating any exercise program, the therapist must first address the general problems of muscle co-contraction and muscle imbalance.

Minimize Muscle Co-contraction

Therapeutic exercise will be of limited benefit in restoring motion if the patient is tense and co-contracting. *Muscular co-contraction* is simultaneous contraction of the agonist and antagonist muscles for a particular motion. A patient may subconsciously co-contract the muscles if it is anticipated that the exercise will produce pain. Co-contraction also occurs when the patient "strains" or tries too hard to perform active exercise. Frequently, co-contraction can be eliminated by dispelling the patient's fear that therapy is synonymous with pain. Relaxation can be encouraged by verbal cuing, general stretching exercises, and deep breathing techniques. Biofeedback can be used to monitor and reduce muscle tension in the contracting antagonist muscle.

Re-establish Normal Muscular Balance

The synergistic relationship of the wrist extensors and finger flexors is essential for normal hand function. The role of the wrist extensors is to stabilize the wrist, usually in a position of slight extension to facilitate finger function. After injury or periods of immobilization, there is a tendency for patients to assume a flexed wrist posture due to inhibition and wasting of the wrist extensor musculature (Fig. 7–1). The process of selective extensor weakness has been documented in the quadriceps and triceps muscle as well.[15-17] When this normal, synergistic relationship is disrupted, any attempts at active finger flexion are accompanied by wrist flexion rather than wrist extension. Positioning of the wrist in flexion not only limits full finger flexion by placing tension on the extrinsic extensor system, but also diminishes the length tension relationship of the flexor musculature, resulting in decreased flexor strength. In some cases, the wrist extensors will be so inactivated, the patient will use the finger extensors rather than the wrist extensors to extend the wrist, thereby further diminishing function.

Frequently, muscular balance can be easily restored by instructing the patient to hold the wrist in slight extension when performing active finger exercise. For other patients, muscle reeducation techniques will be needed. Active wrist extension exercises with the fingers held lightly in a fist will reeducate the wrist extensors without competition from the long finger extensors. Early strengthening exercises of the wrist extensors will help restore them to their important role of wrist stabilizers. When exercise alone does not remedy the problem, splinting can be used to position the wrist in extension, while biofeedback and electrical stimulation can be used to retrain the extensor musculature.

EXERCISES TO MAINTAIN AND RESTORE JOINT MOBILITY

Limitations in joint motion can result from contracture of the periarticular structures of the joint; changes in the muscle tendon systems, skin or retinacular ligaments that

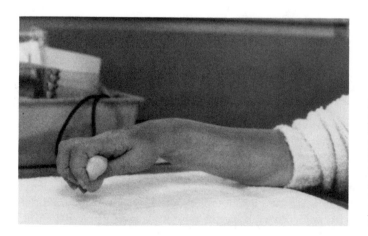

FIGURE 7–1. Following injury or immobilization, inhibition of the wrist extensors produces a flexed wrist posture. Note that the extrinsic finger extensors must now contract to support the wrist, which prevents the MCP joints from flexing to grasp the putty.

cross the joint; or both. The therapist must carefully consider which structure(s) is (are) limiting motion and selectively stress that structure. The following section will discuss the selection and application of passive, active, and resisted exercises to maintain and restore joint mobility.

Passive Stretching Exercises

GENERAL CONSIDERATIONS

Passive exercise can be done through the available range of motion (PROM) to maintain joint and soft tissue mobility, or a passive stretch can be applied at the end range of motion to lengthen pathologically shortened soft tissue structures, thereby increasing motion.[4] The potential abuses of passive stretching are numerous, including mobilization of unprotected joints, stretching of the wrong joint or soft tissue structure, and the infliction of additional tissue trauma.[8,9,18] The hand is particularly vulnerable to damage because excessive external forces can easily overpower and disrupt the supporting structures of the small joints of the fingers and thumb.

When performed properly, passive stretching can be an integral part of any therapy program designed to increase motion. The corrective force should be applied in a gentle, slow, sustained manner. When more than one structure is responsible for limitations in joint motion, separate exercises should be incorporated. For example, PIP joint flexion may be limited by joint tightness and intrinsic tightness. In this situation, passive PIP flexion should be performed with the MCP joint in extension to stretch the intrinsic system and passive PIP flexion should be performed with the MCP flexed, putting the intrinsic system on slack and allowing the joint structures to be stretched.

Stretching exercise should be used with caution when osteoporosis is suspected. Vigorous stretching of joints following prolonged immobilization is discouraged, as immobilization tends to decrease the tensile strength of connective tissue (tendons and ligaments).[4] Precaution should be used when stretching edematous tissue, which is more susceptible to injury than normal tissue. When possible, the ROM of the contralateral extremity should be used as a guideline so that stretching does not occur beyond the normal range. Newly united fractures should be stabilized either manually or with splints.

PASSIVE STRETCHING — JOINT CONTRACTURES

When joint contractures are present, passive stretching should be preceded by joint mobilization. Joint mobilization refers to passive traction and/or gliding movements to joint surfaces that maintain or restore the joint play normally allowed by the capsule. The ability to use joint mobilization requires a high level of knowledge and skill that is beyond the scope of this text. For further information the reader is referred to work of Kaltenborn[19] and Maitland.[20]

When stretching a joint, the hand or digit should be positioned to eliminate resistive force from surrounding muscle-tendon systems. The segment proximal to the joint being mobilized should be stabilized while the corrective force should be applied to the segment distal to the joint being mobilized. For example, if a PIP joint flexion contracture is stretched by applying the corrective force through the distal phalanx without stabilizing the proximal phalanx, the exercise will serve only to hyperextend the normal

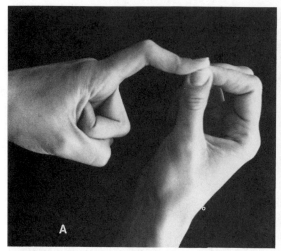 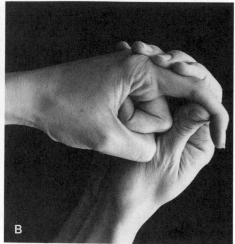

FIGURE 7–2. Passive stretching of a PIP flexion contracture. *A*, Inadequate stabilization of the adjacent joints produces hyperextension of the normal MCP and DIP joints. *B*, With proper stabilization, the corrective force is directed to the stiff PIP joint.

MCP and DIP joint (Fig. 7–2). As a general rule, the corrective force should be applied to the distalmost portion of the segment distal to the joint being mobilized. This approach will provide a longer lever arm and increase the amount of force that can be transmitted to the joint structures. In keeping with the principles of joint mobilization, the use of a joint distraction will avoid joint compression during the stretching procedure.

Finger Joints

Each joint should be stretched individually. To avoid tension from the extrinsic muscle-tendon systems, the wrist should be kept in neutral and the adjacent MCP, PIP, or DIP joints should be allowed to flex and extend passively.

Contractures of the MCP joints in extension, particularly of the little finger, are more difficult to reverse than MCP flexion contractures. Stretching the fingers into abduction is important when MCP extension contractures develop to assist in the stretching of tight collateral ligaments. The patient can be instructed to stretch the fingers independently into abduction by intertwining the fingers of both hands into a praying position. MCP hyperextension is frequently overlooked because it is nonessential for performing activities of daily living. The fact that MCP hyperextension is one of the first motions lost following injury, particularly with arthritis, indicates the importance of this movement in maintaining normal baseline function.[5]

Thumb Joints

The MP and interphalangeal (IP) joints of the thumb should be treated the same as IP of the fingers and ranged into flexion and extension. The carpometacarpal (CMC) joint of the thumb offers a unique combination of movements, including flexion/extension, abduction/adduction, and axial rotation. When stretching the CMC joint, the force should always be applied proximal to the MCP joint to prevent injury to the collateral ligaments of the MCP joint.

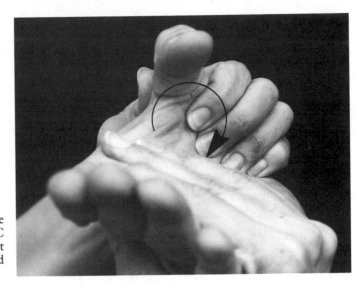

FIGURE 7–3. Passive stretching of the thumb CMC joint into rotation. Note that the corrective force is applied proximal to the MP joint.

The CMC joint of the thumb also demonstrates a small degree of axial rotation, which, when combined with CMC abduction and flexion, produces thumb opposition. This small degree of axial rotation should be maintained with passive stretching because this rotation is essential for pulp-to-pulp opposition and is very difficult to restore once a contracture starts to develop. Passive stretching of the thumb into axial rotation is seen in Figure 7–3.

Maintenance of the thumb web space, essential for a functional hand, is dependent not only on the mobility of the CMC joint motion but also on supple skin and soft tissue in the web space. To keep the web space soft tissue as flexible as possible, passive stretching should also occur in the midposition between thumb palmar abduction and extension. This position puts the web space soft tissue on maximal stretch (Fig. 7–4).

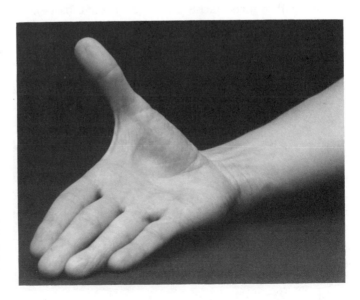

FIGURE 7–4. The skin and soft tissue of the thenar web space is on maximal stretch when the thumb CMC joint is positioned between palmar abduction and extension.

Carpometacarpal and Intermetacarpal Joints

The articulations between the distal carpal row and the bases of the second through fifth metacarpals form the CMC joints. These plane synovial joints allow 1° of freedom —flexion and extension. Due to strong ligamentous support the second and third CMC joints are relatively immobile while the fifth joint demonstrates 10 to 20° of flexion. Together these joints form the palmar arches, which in combination with the intermeta-carpal joints, allow the hand and digits to conform optimally to the shape of the object being held.

One recommended procedure for stretching these joints is for the therapist to face the patient's hand, placing his or her thumb in the patient's palm and fingers on the dorsal surface of the patient's hand. Using his or her fingers, the therapist then rolls the patient's metacarpals over the therapist's palmarly placed thumbs, thereby increasing the palmar arch (Fig. 7–5).[4]

Wrist Joint

The wrist is capable of flexion, extension, and radial and ulnar deviation. The extrinsic muscles of the fingers cross the wrist joint, potentially influencing wrist ROM. To eliminate their effect, the corrective force should be applied proximal to the MCP joints, allowing the fingers to flex naturally with wrist extension and to extend with wrist flexion.

Distal Radioulnar Joint

When stretching the distal radioulnar joint into pronation and supination, the humerus should be stabilized to prevent substitution through internal-external rotation of the shoulder. The corrective force should be applied to the distal forearm, not to the hand. Stretching should be performed with the elbow in flexion and extension, as pronation in the extended position may be caused by tightness of the biceps brachii.[21]

PASSIVE STRETCHING: MUSCLES

Muscle is composed of innervated contractile tissue (muscle fibers) that are inter-woven with noncontractile tissue (connective tissue). Limitations in joint motion may result from changes in the contractile and noncontractile components of muscle. While

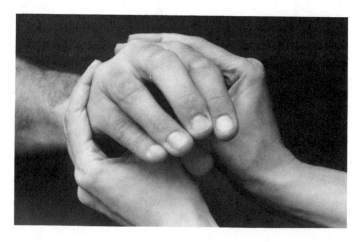

FIGURE 7–5. Range of motion of the CMC and interme-tacarpal joints of the hand.

passive stretching procedures are capable of elongating both components, active inhibition techniques facilitate stretching of the contractile element of muscle. Active inhibition techniques reflexively relax the muscle fibers to be elongated prior to the stretching maneuver.[4,22,23] The contract-relax exercise is an example of an active inhibition technique. In this exercise the patient performs an isometric contraction of the tight muscle before passive lengthening is engaged. Active inhibition stretching is particularly effective in restoring supination, as motion may be limited due to pronator hyperactivity.[24]

When stretching muscle-tendon systems that cross multiple joints, the muscle must be stretched over one joint at a time, and then all joints simultaneously, until optimum length of soft tissues is achieved. To minimize compressive forces in the small joints, stretching should start with the small, distal joints and proceed proximally.[4]

Intrinsics (Interossei and Lumbrical Muscles)

With the PIP and DIP joints held in flexion, the MCP joint is gently stretched into extension (Fig. 7–6).

Extrinsic Extensors (Extensor Digitorum Muscle)

First the DIP, the PIP joints, and finally the MCP joints are flexed. With these joints stabilized in flexion, the wrist is slowly flexed until the patient perceives a stretch on the dorsum of the forearm (Fig. 7–7).

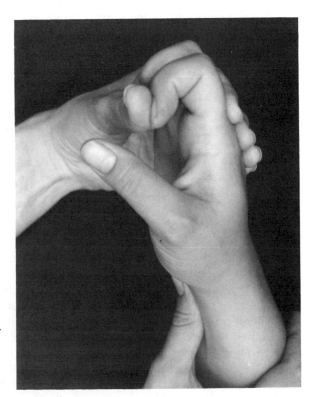

FIGURE 7–6. Passive stretching of the intrinsic musculature. With the PIP and DIP joints held in flexion, the MCP joint is gently stretched into extension.

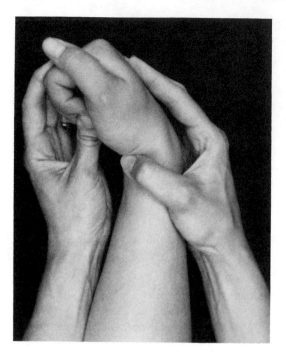

FIGURE 7–7. Passive stretching of the extrinsic extensor system. With the DIP, PIP, and MCP joints stabilized in flexion, the wrist is slowly flexed until the patient perceives a stretch in the dorsum of the forearm.

Extrinsic Flexors (Flexor Digitorum Profundus/Superficialis Muscles)

First the DIP, the PIP, and finally the MCP joints are extended. With these joints maintained in extension, the wrist is slowly extended until the patient feels a stretch in the volar forearm (Fig. 7–8).

PASSIVE STRETCHING: LIGAMENTS

Oblique Retinacular Ligament

The oblique retinacular ligament passes volar to the PIP joint and dorsal to the DIP joint, acting to extend the DIP joint when the PIP joint is extended. Tightness of the oblique retinacular ligament will limit DIP flexion, particularly when the PIP joint is extended. To stretch this structure, the PIP joint should be stabilized in extension while a passive stretch is applied to the DIP joint into flexion.

Active Exercise

When used to maintain mobility, active exercise should be performed through the full available joint ROM. Depending on the nature of the injury, the therapist should anticipate what structures may become tight and incorporate active exercises to prevent limitations in motion. Composite motions, such as fisting and thumb opposition to each digit, should be encouraged, as they reproduce normal functional activities. Exercise is not limited to the hand and wrist but should include the elbow, shoulder, and cervical area to prevent secondary limitations in motion from disuse.

When active exercise is used to restore mobility in the presence of increasing tissue resistance, fast, ballistic movements are discouraged by instructing the patient to main-

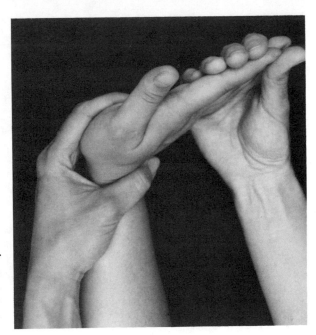

FIGURE 7–8. Passive stretching of the extrinsic flexor system. With the DIP, PIP, and MCP joints stabilized in extension, the wrist is slowly extended until the patient feels a stretch in the volar forearm.

tain the end range position so that a gentle stretch can be applied. Just as with passive exercises, active exercises should be selected that apply stress to the specific structure that is limiting joint motion. When active exercise is used to restore motion in stiff joints, care must be taken to ensure that the corrective force is directed toward the stiff joint and not dissipated in the adjacent normal joints. The following exercises are useful for isolating the corrective force to the appropriate joint.

Blocking Exercises

When the DIP joint is stiff moving into flexion, generalized fisting exercises will result in increased flexion of the normal MCP and PIP joints, which offer less resistance to motion. Blocking exercises developed by Bunnel[47] eliminate this problem by having the patient manually stabilize the middle phalanx (Fig. 7–9A). This action immobilizes the MP and PIP joints, thus directing the active force toward the stiff DIP joint. When the PIP joint is stiff, the patient or therapist stabilizes the proximal phalanx, encouraging isolated flexion of the PIP joint. When multiple fingers are involved, the use of a Bunnel block allows for proper stabilization without manual assistance (Fig. 7–9B). Although these exercises were designed to restore finger flexion, the principle is applicable to all joints, in flexion or extension.

Isolated MP Joint Flexion (Tabletop Exercise)

When MP flexion is limited, active MP flexion should be performed with the IP joints in extension (Fig. 7–10). Active positioning of the MP joints in flexion and IP joint extension (intrinsic plus position) isolates the intrinsic muscles which are the primary flexors of the MP joint. Care should be taken to position the thumb in extension while performing the tabletop exercise. The natural tendency of the thumb to adduct during finger flexion limits full MP flexion of the index and middle fingers.

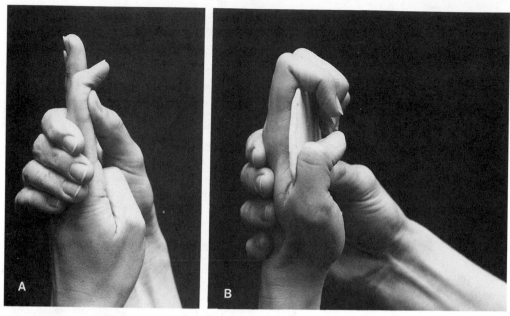

FIGURE 7–9. Blocking exercises. *A*, By stabilizing the PIP and MCP joints in extension, the active flexor force is directed to the stiff DIP joint. *B*, The use of a Bunnel block is helpful when stabilizing more than one finger. Here the block is stabilizing the MCP joints to encourage PIP joint flexion.

Resistance Exercise

Immobilization produces muscle atrophy, with complete inactivity resulting in decreased strength at a rate of 5 percent per day.[25,26] With the stiff hand, muscles that are significantly weaker than normal must work against joints that are resistant to motion. Resistance exercise not only increases muscle strength and endurance, but also improves the ability of the patient actively to mobilize stiff joints.

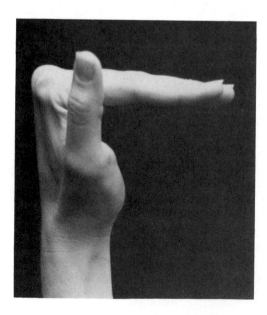

FIGURE 7–10. Tabletop exercise isolates the MCP joints. Care should be taken when performing this exercise to keep the thumb in extension to allow for full flexion of the index MCP joint.

Resistance exercise can be classified as either static (isometric) or dynamic (isotonic or isokinetic). Isometric exercise, used early in the rehabilitative process, allows for strengthening without the stress to joints and soft tissue produced by dynamic exercise. Strength gains made with isometric exercise occur only at the joint angle at which the exercise is performed. As a result, the patient should exercise at several different joint angles throughout the range of motion. Isotonic exercise occurs when a muscle is subjected to a constant or variable resistance throughout the available range of motion.[4] Constant resistance exercise uses free weights, weight pulley systems, elastic material, and putty whereas variable resistance exercise uses equipment such as the Baltimore Therapeutic Equipment (BTE) work simulator. With isokinetic exercise, the velocity of muscle shortening and lengthening is controlled, while the resistance is varied. The advantage of isokinetic over isotonic exercise is that near-maximal tension is produced by the muscle throughout the entire range of motion.[4] The disadvantage of isokinetic exercise is that the use of specialized equipment, such as the Cybex or Orthotron, is required.

Resistance exercises that strengthen functional muscle groups rather than individual muscles should be selected. The tools available for increasing strength are limited only by the therapist's imagination. Graded putty exercises are useful for strengthening the intrinsic muscles. The putty can resist finger abduction/adduction to strengthen the interossei, it can be pinched into a cone to strengthen the lumbricals and the thenar musculature (Fig. 7–11) or it can resist finger flexion and extension to strengthen the extrinsic musculature. The patient should be cautioned to exercise only as directed because excessive putty use is associated with inflammatory problems in some patient populations.[27] Strengthening the synergistic motions of finger flexion and wrist extension is important for increasing grip strength. Numerous devises claiming to be superior in increasing grip strength are available. The most therapeutically appropriate devises are those that (1) allow isotonic rather than isometric contraction of the finger flexors, (2) conform to the shape of the patient's hand (unlike a tennis ball where the patient's hand must conform to the shape of the ball), (3) do not put excessive force into the palm of the hand, and (4) allow easy adjustment of the resistance level. Resistance exercises should be performed in wrist flexion, extension, and radial and ulnar deviation to increase forearm strength using free weights or a weight well.

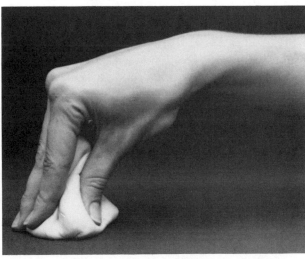

FIGURE 7–11. Correct technique is important when performing resistance exercises. To strengthen the intrinsic musculature, the putty is pinched into a cone with the PIP and DIP joints held in extension. If the PIP and DIP joints flex during the exercise, the patient is substituting with the extrinsic flexors.

One area that should not be overlooked is the use of resisted exercise to counteract disuse atrophy. Muller found that a single daily contraction at 50 percent of maximal effort is sufficient to maintain muscle strength when normal muscle innervation is present.[25] Resistance exercises performed on the uninjured extremity have been shown to maintain and increase strength in the opposite extremity due to the cross-over effect of training.[28,29] This cross-over phenomenon was not observed when the injured extremity was immobilized, possibly because of central changes associated with motor learning.[30]

EXERCISES TO MAINTAIN AND RESTORE TENDON GLIDE

Active flexion and extension of the fingers and thumb depends on the ability of the extrinsic tendon system to glide in relation to surrounding structures. Adhesion formation can occur at any point along the course of the tendon, limiting tendon excursion in proximal and distal directions. Favorable remodeling of the scar around a tendon is best accomplished by applying stress to the tendon, which in turn transmits the stress to the adjacent scar.[31] The most efficient way to restore tendon glide is to lengthen the adhesion in both distal and proximal directions so that every gain in motion made in one direction can be used to improve motion in the other direction.[13] For example, if the extensor tendon is scarred to surrounding structures, active finger extension exercises stretch the adhesion proximally while active and passive finger flexion exercises stretch the adhesion distally. Frequently, restoring proximal glide to a scarred tendon is more difficult because the only way a proximal force can be applied is through contraction of the muscle either actively or by electrical stimulation. As a result, restoration of proximal tendon glide is limited by the strength, endurance, and tolerance of the patient, whereas distal stretching of the adhesion can be accomplished more easily through passive stretching or progressive splinting.

Passive Versus Active Exercise

The ability of active motion to produce substantially more tendon excursion than passive exercise makes it the exercise of choice when the goal of therapy is restoring tendon glide. Although not comparable to active exercise, passive motion does produce tendon excursion.[32] When active motion is contraindicated, such as following tendon repair, the tendon excursion produced by passive motion may be used to minimize the formation of dense, restrictive adhesions. This is the rationale behind the use of early mobilization programs following flexor and extensor tendon repair.[33-35]

The following section will discuss exercise selection for maintaining and restoring tendon glide when the integrity of repaired structures is not a consideration. Because of their unique anatomic and functional requirements, exercises for the flexor and extensor systems will be considered separately.

Flexor Tendons

The dextrous movement of the fingers in flexion is dependent not only on gliding of the flexor tendons with respect to surrounding structures, but also on isolated gliding of the profundus tendon with respect to the superficialis tendon within each finger and the gliding of one superficialis tendon with respect to another. Adhesions can form at any point in the system limiting motion in one or more of the gliding planes described earlier. For the exercise program to be successful, the therapist must first identify which planes of motion have become adherent and then select specific exercises to stress the restrictive scar.

BLOCKING EXERCISES

In addition to mobilizing stiff finger joint, blocking exercises also produce gliding of the flexor tendons with respect to surrounding structures, and gliding of the profundus with respect to the superficialis. DIP joint flexion, with the PIP joint stabilization in extension, inactivates the flexor digitorum superficialis (FDS) tendon, producing glide of the flexor digitorum profundus (FDP) with respect to the FDS and surrounding tissue. PIP joint flexion with stabilization of the MCP joint in extension encourages gliding of the FDS with respect to the surrounding tissue. This exercise does not selectively move the FDS with respect to the FDP unless the patient is encouraged not to bend the DIP joint. If the therapist can passively extend the distal phalanx without encountering resistance, the superficialis is being exclusively used to flex the finger.

A slight variation on this exercise is important to mention. Frequently patients with flexor tendon adhesions will present with substantial FDP pull-through when the finger is blocked in extension, but limited to no pull-through as the finger moves into a fist. When this occurs, continued blocking with the finger extended will no longer exert force on the tendon adhesion. Instead, blocking exercises should be performed with the MCP and PIP joints flexed to the point where the patient starts to lose DIP motion (Fig. 7–12). This simple modification will ensure that the flexor force is being directed to remodeling the adherent scar.

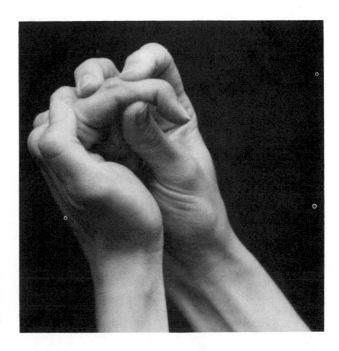

FIGURE 7–12. To increase the difficulty and effectiveness of the blocking exercise, the exercise is performed with the PIP and MCP joints stabilized in increasing amounts of flexion.

TENDON GLIDING EXERCISES

Many authors have studied and reported on the excursion of flexor tendons.[36-40] Wehbé and Hunter[41,42] examined tendon glide through in vivo, cadaver, and electromyographic studies. In the in vivo studies, flexor tendons were tagged intraoperatively with a buried suture at the wrist level. Radiographs taken postoperatively showed the amount of gliding of each flexor tendon with the digits and wrist in various positions. Based on their results, a simple exercise program was developed using the three positions which provided maximum differential gliding for both flexor tendons, as illustrated in Figure 7–13.[41-43] With the hook position, maximum gliding is achieved

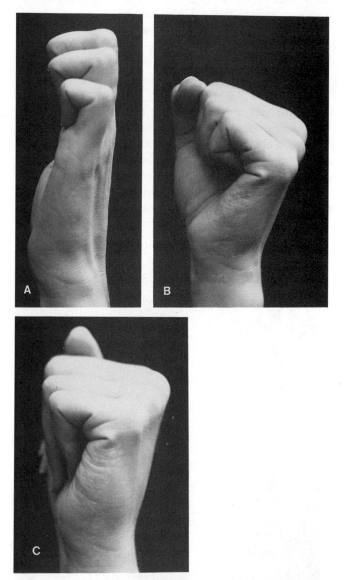

FIGURE 7–13. Tendon gliding exercises. All three positions should be preceded by full finger extension to achieve maximal gliding of the flexor tendons. A, Hook position. B, Fist position. C, Straight fist position.

between the two flexor tendons. With the fist position, the profundus tendon achieves maximum gliding with respect to sheath and bone as well as a substantial amount of gliding over the superficialis tendon. Finally, the straight-fist position produces maximum gliding of the superficialis tendon with respect to the flexor sheath and the bone. Maximum flexor pollicis longus gliding is obtained by flexing the IP and MCP joints of the thumb fully. Keeping in mind that adhesions need to be stretched distally as well as proximally, each of the three positions should be preceded by full finger extension. The study also indicated that wrist motion and effort greatly amplify tendon excursion in the fingers and in the thumb.[41,43] Once a patient is able to perform the exercises with the wrist in neutral he should be instructed to perform the same exercises with the wrist in extension and flexion. Wrist and finger extension followed by wrist and finger flexion produces the maximum total excursion of the flexor tendons with respect to surrounding structures. Increased patient effort produced an increase in the amplitude of the flexor tendons by up to 44 percent.[42]

ISOLATED SUPERFICIALIS EXERCISES

Unlike the profundus tendons to the third, fourth, and fifth digits, which are interdependent because they share a common muscle belly, the muscle bellies of the superficialis tendons are independent, allowing independent PIP flexion of each digit. The formation of adhesions between the superficialis tendons can prevent independent FDS movement. Isolated superficialis exercises, as seen in Figure 7–14, are done by flexing one finger at a time at the PIP joint, with the uninvolved hand keeping the other fingers in extension. This exercise produces gliding of the superficialis tendons not only

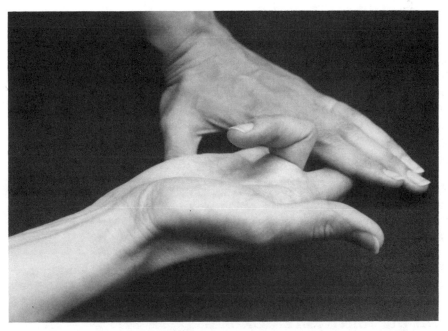

FIGURE 7–14. Isolated superficialis exercises are performed by flexing one finger at a time while stabilizing the uninvolved fingers in full extension.

with respect to other superficialis tendons, but also with respect to the profundus tendon which is rendered inactive when the other three profundus tendons are held in extension.

EXTRINSIC FLEXOR STRETCHING

Distal stretching of the tendon must not be overlooked and can be accomplished with extrinsic flexor stretching. Full distal tendon excursion is present when simultaneous wrist and finger extension is equal to the uninvolved extremity. When active exercise is not sufficient to produce full extension, passive manual stretching and splinting can be incorporated.

Extensor Tendons

Restoration of normal glide in the digital extensor tendons presents a unique challenge. The extensor tendons over the dorsum of the hand are thin, broad structures that are very susceptible to the formation of scar. At the finger level, the EDC, interossei, and lumbrical tendons form a complex extensor mechanism. Adhesions can form at any point along the system, limiting active and passive finger flexion as well as active finger extension. The loss of active extension in the presence of full passive extension is referred to as an extensor lag. Overcoming an extensor lag is not an easy task, considering that the extrinsic extensors are substantially weaker than the extrinsic flexors, making the proximal stretching of adhesions more difficult to achieve. For example, the extrinsic finger extensors can generate only 38% of the tension of all the extrinsic finger flexors.[14] In addition, simultaneous flexion of all finger joints requires extensive mobilization of the extensor mechanism. As a result extensor tendon adhesions may prove more disabling by limiting finger flexion than finger extension.[11]

The specific exercise selected to facilitate extensor tendon glide depends on the location of the adhesion. Lack of full active extension at the MCP joint indicates an adhesion of the EDC, which is the sole extensor of the MCP joint. Metacarpal fractures or extensor tendon lacerations over the dorsum of the hand frequently result in EDC adhesions. An extensor lag present at the PIP and DIP joints indicates an adhesion of the complex extensor expansion, which is composed of the EDC, lumbricals, and interossei. Adhesions in this area are very difficult to treat.

MCP JOINT EXTENSOR LAGS

Movement of the fingers from a fist to a hook position eliminates the intrinsic muscles, allowing for isolated gliding of the extrinsic finger extensors (Fig. 7–15).[44-48] When patients have a hard time actively maintaining the PIP and DIP joints in flexion, they can be instructed to hold a pencil in their flexed fingers or the PIP and DIP joints can be taped or strapped into flexion. Once the patient is able to perform the exercise with the wrist in neutral, the exercise should be repeated with the wrist in flexion and extension to produce maximal EDC excursion.

PIP AND DIP JOINT EXTENSOR LAGS

Unlike the flexor system, extension of the PIP and DIP joints depends on the combined action of the extrinsic extensor and intrinsic muscles. The intricate relation-

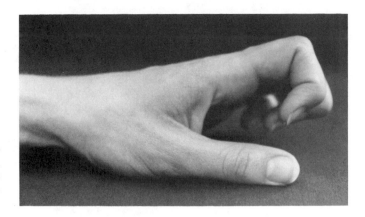

FIGURE 7-15. The extrinsic extensors can be isolated by extending the MCP joints with the PIP and DIP joints maintained in flexion.

ship of the EDC, lumbrical, and interossei have been analyzed through EMG and cadaver studies.[44-50] The lumbrical is the major extensor of the IP joints and contracts strongest with the MCP in flexion and the IP in extension.[45,48] As a result, active PIP and DIP extension should be performed with the MCP joint held in flexion, as seen in Figure 7-16. This position not only encourages intrinsic extension but also directs the force of the extrinsic extensor tendon more distally.[51] As extension improves, the patient can be progressed to a more difficult exercise. With the palm flat on a table, the patient is asked to lift the middle and distal phalanx of his or her finger off the table, as illustrated in Figure 7-17. The proximal phalanx should remain on the table during this exercise to ensure that the extensor force is directed toward the distal phalanx, and not MCP hyperextension. When the hand is flat on the table, and the patient cannot actively lift the middle and distal phalanx off the table, the exercise can be made easier by placing a pencil or dowel under the proximal phalanx.

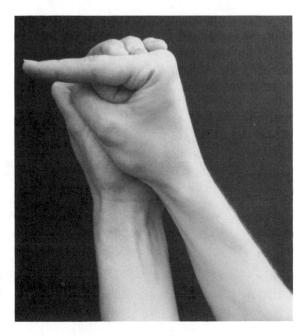

FIGURE 7-16. Active extension of the PIP and DIP joints with the MCP joint stabilized in flexion encourages intrinsic extension.

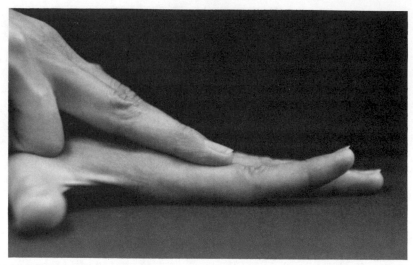

FIGURE 7–17. Terminal extension exercises are performed by stabilizing the MCP joint in extension while lifting the middle and distal phalanges off the table.

DIFFERENTIAL EXTENSOR TENDON GLIDE

Adhesions between the EDC tendons are frequently a problem with injury over the dorsum of the wrist. Figure 7–18 suggests that differential tendon glide can be restored by alternately moving each digit into graded flexion, while the adjacent digits are held in extension.[35] Combinations of dynamic flexion and extension splinting can be used to create a shear between these tendons, thus improving differential excursion.

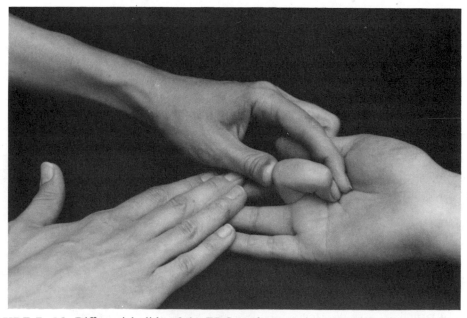

FIGURE 7–18. Differential glide of the EDC tendons can be restored by alternately moving each digit into graded flexion while the adjacent digits are held in extension.

EXTRINSIC EXTENSOR STRETCHING

The manner in which extensor tendon adhesions are stretched distally depends on the location of the adhesion. Adhesions distal to the MCP joint are not affected by the position of the wrist. When the adhesion is proximal to the MCP joint, maximal stretch occurs with simultaneous wrist and finger flexion.

A note of caution is needed when stretching is used to restore full finger flexion. When an extensor tendon adhesion limits both active extension and passive flexion, aggressive efforts at restoring finger flexion may result in an increasing extensor lag. In such cases elongation of the extensor unit by dehiscence or gap formation should be suspected. This possibility is particularly true after extensor tendon repairs and finger fractures.[11] When the restoration of passive flexion occurs at the expense of active extension, the therapy program should focus on increasing proximal extensor pull-through via active exercise and strengthening, while minimizing aggressive stretching into flexion.

Resistive Exercise

Maximizing muscle strength is an important component of any program to manage tendon adhesions because active contraction of the muscle is the only way (with the exception of electric stimulation) an increased proximal pull can be exerted on tendon adhesions. Whenever possible, resistance exercises should promote a sustained contraction of the muscle, which will not only increase strength but also provide the most favorable force for scar remodeling. Sustained contractions provide the low-load, long-duration force at the end range of motion that encourages lengthening changes of the scar collagen. Activities such as raking and sanding require sustained contraction of the FDS and FDP. These activities are effective only if each fingertip comes in direct contact with the tool handle, to ensure that the flexor muscle is actively contracting and exerting tension on the motion limiting adhesion. As a result, the tool handle should be built up with adhesive-backed foam that is progressively cut back as the patient's active flexion improves (Fig. 7–19). Adaptations to the sander, such as incorporating a Hand Helper, can facilitate FDP versus FDS pull-through. For the intrinsic and extrinsic extensor musculature, activities such as ceramics or sanding with an extension block and Theraband will promote finger extension (Fig. 7–19).

With an understanding of the anatomy of the flexor, extensor, and intrinsic musculature, countless other exercises can be developed that will increase muscle strength and promote tendon glide. To strengthen the FDS muscle, isolated superficialis exercises can be performed into putty. The patient can also flex the PIP joints against a clothespin held in the palm. The FDP muscle can be strengthened by having patients grasp a dowel with their hand and either push the dowel into progressively resistive putty or prevent the dowel from being pulled out by their other hand. As finger flexion improves, the patient is required to grasp progressively smaller dowels. The BTE Work Simulator can also be used to increase flexor strength (Fig. 7–20).

When an extensor lag is present, use of a Velcro roll (Fig. 7–21) provides an inexpensive means of applying graded resistance to the finger extensors. A 12 by 6 in board is lined with two strips of hook Velcro, approximately 2 in apart, while a metal can is wrapped with two strips of pile Velcro approximately 2 in apart. To strengthen the intrinsic extensors, the patient is asked to roll the can along the board by moving the PIP and DIP joints from flexion into extension, while keeping the MP joints straight. To

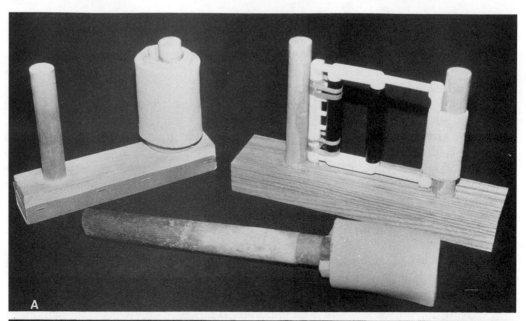

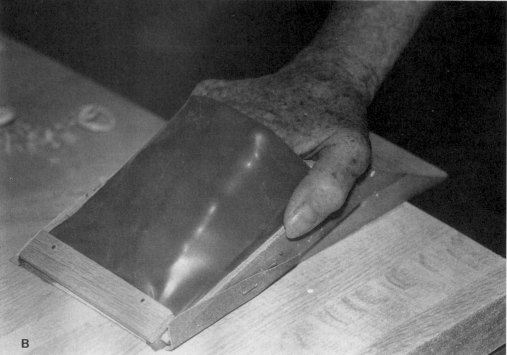

FIGURE 7–19. Sanding not only increases strength but encourages proximal tendon excursion. *A,* Adapted sanders for improving finger flexion. Adhesive-backed foam is used to build up the handle so that each fingertip comes in direct contact with the sander. *B,* A triangular-shaped sander with an elastic band stretched over the dorsum of the fingers encourages resisted intrinsic extension.

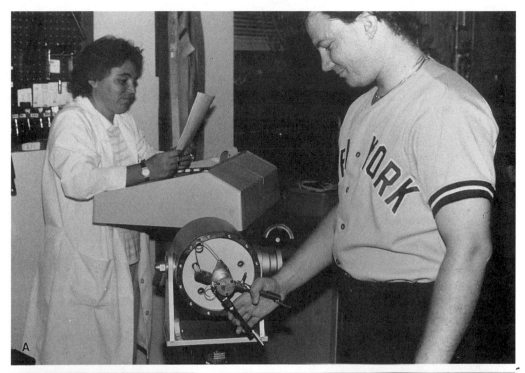

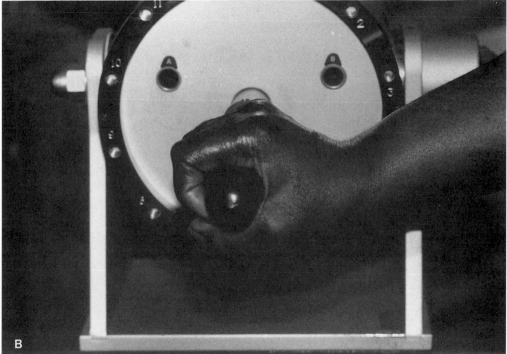

FIGURE 7–20. BTE work-simulator tools 162 (pliers) (*A*) and 167 (screwdriver) (*B*) can be used to increase flexor strength.

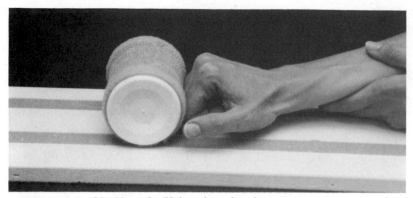

FIGURE 7–21. Use of a Velcro board to increase extensor strength.

strengthen the extrinsic extensors, the patient is asked to roll the can by moving the MCP joints from flexion to extension, while keeping the IP joints flexed. The amount of resistance is graded by adding or subtracting strips of Velcro. These same exercises can be performed into putty or against Theraband. The BTE tool number 701 with a block used for MCP extension is another method for strengthening the intrinsic musculature (Fig. 7–22).

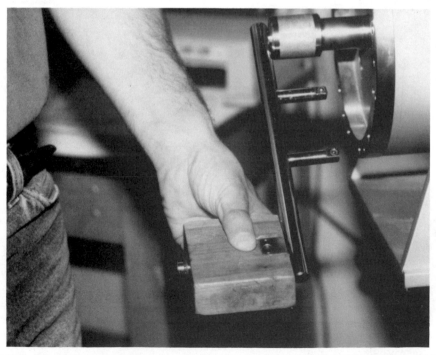

FIGURE 7–22. BTE work-simulator tool 701 places the hand in an intrinsic-plus position for strengthening the intrinsic extensors.

MODIFYING AN EXERCISE PROGRAM WHEN STRUCTURES IN THE HAND ARE INJURED

Developing an exercise program to maintain and restore range of motion is a challenging task when the therapist must consider the status of repaired structures in the hand. The repaired structure, whether tendon, skin, nerve, or bone, becomes the weak link in the hand, frequently requiring immobilization and, in the best of circumstances, limiting the amount of stress that can be applied to surrounding joints and tissues. One of the fundamental goals of any rehabilitation program is to provide controlled motion, as early as possible, to influence the healing process. The following exercise adaptations allow the therapist to use therapeutic movement to maintain joint mobility and tendon glide while protecting repaired structures.

Protected Range-of-Motion Exercises

Protected ROM exercises selectively mobilize joints and tendons while minimizing stress on repaired structures. Protected ROM exercises can be performed passively or actively and are accomplished by placing the repaired structure in a protected position while adjacent tissues are carefully mobilized. An example of protective exercise can be seen following radial nerve injuries, where tendon transfers of the pronator teres, flexor carpi ulnaris, and flexor digitorum superficialis may be performed to restore wrist, thumb, and finger extension. After surgery the hand must be immobilized with the wrist, MCP joints, and thumb in extension to allow the transfers to heal in a shortened position without tension. Approximately 4 weeks after surgery, protected active motion may be performed to restore joint mobility while minimizing the stress placed on the tendon junctures. With the wrist, PIP, and DIP joints positioned in extreme extension, placing the tendon transfers on slack, the MCP joints can be actively flexed.[52] In this situation, protected motion allows early MCP flexion, preventing the formation of difficult MCP extension contractures that could result from prolonged immobilization. With the wrist positioned in extension, the exercise is repeated, this time allowing the PIP and DIP joints to flex while the MCP joint is maintained in extension. Protected ROM exercises are most frequently used following tendon repairs, tendon transfers, crush injuries, and replantations.

Active Exercise: Controlling the Intensity of the Applied Force

An important consideration when using early active exercise to restore motion is the amount of force the exercise exerts on the tissue in the hand. This is particularly important following tendon repair or tenolysis, when early active motion is needed to prevent adhesions formation, but excessive active stress may result in tendon rupture. Currently, there is no specific formula or technique for calculating and controlling the amount of force that is exerted with active motion, but the following general conclusions can be made based on clinical experience. Passive-hold, also known as place-hold, is the form of active exercise that applies the least amount of force on the tendon while producing the same tendon excursion as would occur with active motion.[53,54] In the passive-hold exercise, the joint is passively placed in the desired position and the patient is asked to actively maintain that position while the passive support is removed. Gentle active motion produces less stress to tendons than gentle blocking exercises, as blocking exercises produce more shear by selectively moving one tendon against adjacent structures.

THERAPEUTIC METHODS THAT ENHANCE THE EFFECTIVENESS OF EXERCISE

Thermal Agents

The use of thermal modalities can enhance the effectiveness of exercise to increasing motion. The use of heat prior to exercise facilitates stretching of connective tissue with less risk of tissue damage.[55,56] Thermal agents such as hot packs, Fluidotherapy, paraffin, and continuous-wave ultrasound at 3 MHz are all capable of heating soft tissue structures in the hand (see Chapter 8). Although "heat-and-stretch" techniques are a routine clinical practice, well-controlled clinical studies have failed to demonstrate the benefits of heat-and-stretch over stretch alone. Allowing the tissue to cool in a lengthened position encourages permanent lengthening changes.[56]

Splinting

Creative splinting can provide a useful adjunct to exercise. Passive and active assisted ROM can be accomplished through the use of a Velcro trapper. By strapping the involved finger to an adjacent uninvolved finger, this simple splint provides ROM when joint stiffness or tendon adhesions limit PIP and DIP joint motion.

Splinting is especially useful for stabilizing mobile joints so that the corrective exercise force can be directed to the stiff joint or adherent tendon. For example, exaggerated flexion of the MCP joint is often seen when tendon adhesions located in the finger prevent gliding and motion of the PIP and DIP joint. As the patient strains to flex the digit, the flexion force goes toward additional MCP flexion rather than PIP and DIP flexion. Fabrication of a simple ring splint, as seen in Figure 7–23, supports the MCP in extension, preventing hyperflexion of the joint as well as positioning the flexor tendon at a mechanical advantage for stretching of the motion-limiting adhesion. The splint can be fabricated in reverse to prevent hyperextension of the normal MP joint, when flexion contractures or tendon adhesions prevent full extension of the DIP and PIP joints. Small cylinder casts or splints can also be used to isolate the FDS and FDP with respect to each other. For example, when FDP pull-through is restricted in the presence of a gliding FDS tendon, attempts at active finger flexion result in increasing amounts of PIP flexion rather than DIP flexion. Removable cylinder casts or splints can be fabricated that immobilize the PIP joint, allowing for DIP flexion and isolated pull-through of the profundus tendon. Likewise, when FDS pull-through is restricted in the presence of a gliding FDP tendon, casts can be fabricated immobilizing the DIP joint in extension, while allowing PIP joint motion. These splints can be worn during exercise or active use of the hand.

Dynamic splinting is used to provide resistance to increase muscle strength, as well as to apply a corrective passive stretch to tendon adhesions and joint contractures (see Chapter 9). A forearm-based dynamic extension splint provides an extension force that

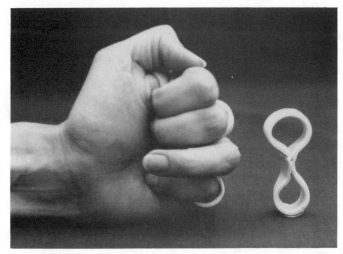

FIGURE 7–23. This ring splint is worn on the middle and little fingers to prevent excessive flexion of the ring finger MCP joint when PIP joint motion is restricted by stiffness or tendon adhesions.

not only stretches flexor tendon adhesions distally but also strengthens the flexor musculature when finger flexion is performed against the rubberbands. By immobilizing the PIP joint with a Velcro strap and extending the dorsal outrigger of the splint so that the finger cuff rests on the distal phalanx rather than the proximal phalanx, the splint can be used to isolate the profundus tendon. For patients with an extensor lag at the DIP and PIP joints, a simple exercise splint can be fabricated that stabilizes the MCP joint in flexion while resisting PIP and DIP joint extension, as seen in Figure 7–24.[57] Static adjustable and serial static provide an effective method of stretching tendon adhesions and joint contractures when passive and active stretching techniques fail (see Chapter 6).

Continuous Passive Motion

Continuous passive motion (CPM) is the application of continual, reciprocal passive joint motion by a mechanical device, such as the one shown in Figure 7–25, that controls the range, rate, and force of movement. Introduced in 1970 through the work

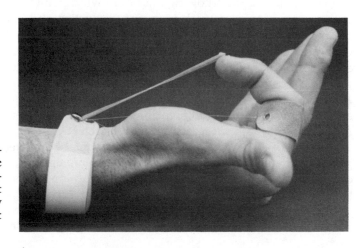

FIGURE 7–24. This exercise splint strengthens the intrinsic musculature by resisting PIP and DIP joint extension while statically maintaining MCP joint flexion.

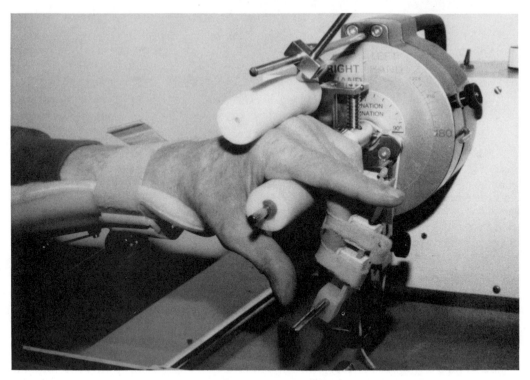

FIGURE 7–25. The Kinetec Hand and Wrist CPM machine.

of Salter and colleagues,[58] CPM is now believed to play a role in stimulating the healing and regeneration of cartilage, ligaments, and tendons, preventing joint stiffness and influencing adhesion formation.[58,59]

CPM is more effective in preventing than in correcting passive limitations in motion.[59] Most useful during the early phases of wound healing, CPM helps maintain the potential for motion by influencing the orientation of the collagen fibrils. Once the contracture becomes fixed, other methods of treatment such as splinting prove more effective in altering collagen formation. As a result, CPM is used clinically to prevent contracture formation following injuries in which tendon strength and skeletal stability are not a consideration, such as in open reduction and internal fixation of fractures,[60] crush injuries, and burns.[61] CPM can also be used to maintain the motion achieved during surgical procedures to release scar,[59] such as capsulectomies,[58,62,63] surgical elbow contracture release,[63,64] and Dupuytren's surgery.[63] With Dupuytren's surgery, CPM has proved effective in maintaining motion following PIP joint releases but has not proved advantageous in comparison to other forms of exercise for MCP joint releases.[63] CPM may have a select role in influencing adhesion formation after tenolysis, although this notion has not been substantiated by research.[54]

When used postoperatively, CPM should be initiated immediately. As for the wearing schedule, CPM should be used a minimum of 8 hours per day,[59] with some clinical studies reporting the best results in those patients who wore the machine the longest.[65] In a study by Prosser,[65] CPM was most effective in 22 patients when used during the first 3 weeks after surgery or injury, with a plateau in measurements noted at 7 days following injury. This result is not surprising considering that the first 3 weeks of wound healing are associated with accelerated collagen production, rather than increased tensile strength of the wound.

CPM can play a *limited* role in correcting passive limitations in motion. Clinical study suggests CPM is more effective when the limitation in passive motion is due to specific capsular restrictions rather than to muscle tendon unit tightness.[65] CPM should only be used for contractures with a soft "end feel," when the collagen is still responsive to mild stress. When soft "end feel" contractures are present, CPM has the advantage over splinting, of being able to work multiple joint contractures in opposite directions of motion. To maximize TERT and enhance the effectiveness of CPM on collagen formation, the unit should be programmed to pause at the end range of motion to provide a prolonged stretch on shortened tissues. TERT can also be increased if the unit is programmed to return only a small percentage of the available opposite range of motion. For example, if CPM is being used to stress mild PIP extension contractures, the unit can be set to maintain the end range of extension for 6 seconds and then to move only 15° into PIP flexion before returning into extension. CPM may be the therapists only alternative in managing stiffness and contractures for patients unable to tolerate exercise or splinting because of pain and anxiety.[61,63]

To use CPM effectively, the therapist must understand its limitations. CPM cannot replace active motion. Despite numerous adaptations in the device, CPM is still limited in achieving the extremes of joint motion, particularly of full digital flexion. Other factors such as cost, achieving proper fit, the lack of specificity regarding treatment parameter, and the tendency for patients to become overly reliant on the CPM device should all be considered by the therapist.[66]

Neuromuscular Electrical Stimulation

Neuromuscular electrical stimulation (NMES) provides a useful adjunct to exercise programs aimed at maintaining and restoring range of motion. NMES can be used as a tool for muscle reeducation when muscle imbalance is a problem. When the patient is unable to demonstrate a strong active contraction of the muscles responsible for moving a stiff joint or adherent tendon, NMES can augment AROM exercises. This fact is particularly important when tendon adhesions are limiting active motion, as NMES is the only way an increased stress can be exerted on tendon adhesions in a proximal direction. NMES can also be used to increase muscle strength following prolonged immobilization. Considerations for clinical use of NMES in each of the aforementioned situations are presented in Chapter 9.

HOME EXERCISE PROGRAM

The success of any therapeutic exercise program depends on patient cooperation. An exercise program that is conscientiously performed by the patient three to four times a day, 7 days a week, will prove far more effective than one that is performed only under therapist supervision while the patient is in the clinic. Patient cooperation is encouraged by providing a written home exercise program, preferably with illustrations, that specifies all applicable exercise parameters. A portion of each therapy session should be set aside for patients to demonstrate their exercise program to the therapist, to ensure that the exercises are being done correctly and in the proper sequence. One of the most difficult tasks for the therapist is to convince the patient that pain should not be a part of the exercise program. Patients should be instructed to monitor the response of their hand to the exercise program and adjust the exercise dosage if pain and increased edema occur after an exercise session. According to Brand, "patients are most compliant when they believe that they hold the key to successful rehabilitation."[14]

CLINICAL DECISION MAKING: CASE STUDY HISTORY

TS is a 50-year-old, right hand–dominant man, who sustained a laceration to the dorsum of his right hand when he punched someone in the mouth. The patient did not seek immediate medical treatment. A severe infection resulted from the human bite wound and the patient was hospitalized for a course of intravenous antibiotics and debridement. During the debridement the surgeon noted a partial tear of the EDC to the index finger, just proximal to the MCP joint. The tendon laceration was repaired secondarily once the infection was under control. A splint was fabricated to immobilize the wrist in 45° of extension, the index MP joint in 20° of flexion, and the index IP joints in extension. The patient was referred to therapy 2 weeks after the injury.

Therapeutic Management

2 WEEKS POST INJURY/3 DAYS POST TENDON REPAIR

Evaluation

Even though the infection had subsided, a significant amount of dorsal edema was present. Because of the quantity and dorsal location of the edema, the finger joints had assumed the position of least resistance, with the MP joints in extension and the IP joints in flexion. The incision was healing well. Passive and active range of motion measurements were taken of the unimmobilized fingers (Table 7–1). Range of motion of the shoulder and elbow was within normal limits. Two-point discrimination testing results were normal.

Treatment

What were the current and anticipated problems? This patient's primary problems were continued edema, and the presence of MP extension and IP flexion contractures. Anticipated problems included the formation of dense internal scar (secondary to the edema and immobilization) that could limit flexor and extensor tendon glide. TS's case was complicated by the tendon laceration, which required continued immobilization of the wrist and index finger.

What were the treatment goals? How were they accomplished?

1. Reduce edema — With the protective splint in place, edema reduction was accomplished through retrograde massage, elevation, active exercise, and compression wrapping of the fingers and palm.
2. Position the MP and IP joints in a functional position — A removable splint insert

TABLE 7–1 Range of Motion Measurements

		2 Weeks After Injury		3½ Weeks After Injury		10 Weeks After Injury	
		AROM	PROM	AROM	PROM	AROM	PROM
Index finger	MP			10/40		5/80	0/95
	PIP	NT*		0/40	NT	0/100	0/90
	DIP			0/85		0/85	0/90
Middle finger	MP	0/30	0/40	0/85	0/90	0/90	0/100
	PIP	30/50	20/65	5/60	0/90	0/95	0/00
	DIP	20/30	10/60	0/30	0/75	0/80	0/85
Ring finger	MP	0/25	0/40	0/80	0/90	0/95	0/100
	PIP	30/60	25/95	10/70	5/95	0/95	0/105
	DIP	30/40	20/60	0/45	0/80	0/80	0/90
Little finger	MP	0/10	0/35	0/70	0/80	0/100	0/105
	PIP	40/50	35/60	30/55	30/90	10/85	10/95
	DIP	20/30	10/40	5/40	5/70	5/75	0/90

*NT = Not tested.
Measurements are recorded as extension/flexion.

was fabricated for the long, ring, and little fingers to position the MP joints in flexion and IP joints in extension. The insert was attached to TS's forearm-based splint when he was not exercising. The insert was progressively remolded to accommodate improved MP flexion and IP extension.

3. Improve joint mobility and tendon glide — A home therapeutic exercise program was established. The patient was instructed to perform five repetitions of each exercise and to repeat the program six to seven times each day. All exercises were performed with the protective splint in place.

A. Passive stretching — Gentle stretching exercises were performed to the unimmobilized fingers and thumb, emphasizing MP joint flexion, IP joint extension, and thumb abduction and rotation. Because of the dorsal location of the edema and the prolonged positioning of the wrist and MP joints in extension, extrinsic extensor tightness was anticipated and the patient was instructed to begin composite MP, PIP, and DIP joint stretching into flexion.

B. Active exercise — Tendon gliding exercises were initiated to produce differential glide of the flexor tendons. Tabletop exercises were initiated to encourage isolated MP joint flexion. Blocking exercises of the thumb MP and IP joints and thumb abduction and opposition exercises were performed. AROM of elbow and shoulder joints was performed once a day.

3½ WEEKS AFTER INJURY; 2 WEEKS AFTER TENDON REPAIR

Two weeks after the tendon repair, TS was allowed to remove the splint to begin cautious mobilization of the repaired tendon. The surgeon opted for early mobilization for two reasons: (1) the tendon had been only partially lacerated and (2) the surgeon was concerned about the ability of the extensor tendon to glide through the postinfection scar. When the patient was not exercising, continued immobilization of the repaired tendon was required for an additional week.

Evaluation

By 3½ weeks after infection, the edema had become very brawny. Active flexion of the index finger MP joint was limited. Passive flexion of the long, ring, and little fingers was significantly better than the active flexion, indicating the presence of flexor tendon adhesions. A 30° flexion contracture of the little finger PIP joint was noted.

Treatment

What were the current problems? The presence of brawny edema indicated that the internal scar was maturing and would be more difficult to mobilize. Although aggressive blocking exercises and the initiation of resistance exercise were needed to mobilize the adherent flexor tendons, the exercises could not jeopardize the integrity of the repaired extensor tendon. Protected ROM exercises were needed to produce gliding of the index extensor tendon and the index MP joint flexion. The flexion contracture of the little finger PIP joint was not responding to passive stretching, indicating the need for splinting to provide a low-load, long-duration stress.

What were the treatment goals? How were they accomplished?

1. Scar control — This was accomplished by deep pressure and retrograde massage, superficial heat, and the use of Elastomer and Coban over the dorsal scar.
2. Improve joint mobility and tendon glide — The following exercises were added to the program:
   A. Protected active motion — A protected active exercise was designed to allow flexion of the index MP joint while minimizing the stress applied to the repaired extensor tendon. The patient was instructed to position his wrist in full extension and then actively flex the index MCP joint to 40° or until he felt slight tension along the dorsum of his hand, whichever occurred first. Overstretching of the extensor repair was prevented by positioning the wrist in extension and by limiting the amount of MP joint flexion. With the index MP joint in flexion, the patient actively extended the MP joint to initiate proximal gliding of the extensor tendon. The patient was encouraged to keep the index PIP and DIP joints in slight flexion to isolate the EDC muscle and tendons. Five repetitions of the protected active exercises were performed every other hour.

      The patient was instructed to increase the amount of MP flexion gradually. To avoid the formation of an extensor lag at the MP joint, the patient was only allowed to increase MP flexion if he was able to maintain full MP extension. By the fourth week, gentle passive stretching into flexion was initiated to regain the last degrees of MP flexion.
   B. Active exercise — Isolated superficialis exercises and blocking exercises with the fingers positioned in increasing amounts of flexion were initiated to encourage differential tendon glide for the long, ring and little fingers. Blocking exercises were started for the index finger IP joints with the index MP joint positioned in extension.
   C. Resistance exercise — Putty exercises for gross grip, isolated superficialis glide and thumb and finger pinch were initiated to promote flexor tendon pull-through. The active and resisted exercises were performed four times a day, 10 repetitions each exercise. These exercises were performed while the splint was worn.
   D. Passive stretch — A finger-based, volar splint was fabricated to stretch the little finger PIP joint into extension. The patient was instructed to wear the splint at

night so that the finger could be free during the day to work on increasing flexor tendon pull-through.

6½ WEEKS AFTER INJURY; 5 WEEKS AFTER TENDON REPAIR

Evaluation

Dense, internal scaring was present in the dorsal hand. TS presented with full passive and active joint motion except for a 25° extensor lag at the index MP joint. Despite the full passive joint motion, extrinsic extensor tightness was present in the extremes of wrist flexion. Grip measurements on the right were 50% of the left non-dominant hand.

Treatment

What were the primary problems? The remaining problems included decreased pull-through of the extensor tendon, extrinsic extensor tightness, and decreased strength.

1. Passive stretching—The patient was instructed to perform passive extrinsic extensor stretching.
2. Resistance exercise—Exercises were selected to strengthen the EDC muscle, including, isolated EDC extension against a Velcro roll and full finger extension into putty. Sanding with a finger extension block was initiated to provide a sustained proximal pull to the extensor tendon. Strengthening exercises were initiated with a Hand Helper to increase grip, and Progressive Resistive Exercises using free weights and the BTE Work Simulator to increase forearm and upper extremity strength.

10 WEEKS AFTER INJURY; 8½ WEEKS AFTER TENDON REPAIR

By 11 weeks after injury, grip measurements on the injured hand were 90% of the noninjured hand. The extensor tendon lag had resolved and the patient was able to return to work as a stuntman.

SUMMARY

Whether the diagnosis is a carpal tunnel release, rheumatoid arthritis, or replantation of a finger, therapeutic exercise provides the stress necessary to maintain and restore joint mobility and tendon glide. The development of an exercise program is based on knowledge of the anatomy of the hand, the diagnosis or surgery performed, and the phase of wound healing. An initial evaluation should be performed to identify limitations and establish baseline measurements. The therapist chooses passive, active, or resistance exercises to mobilize restricted tendons and joints or to strengthen muscle. Each exercise must be carefully selected to ensure that the corrective force does not jeopardize the integrity of injured or newly repaired structures. An exercise dosage is established and modified according to the wound healing process occurring in the hand. Therapeutic methods, such as thermal modalities, splinting, CPM, and NMES are used when needed to enhance the effectiveness of the exercise program. The patient is responsible for following through with a written home exercise program. Therapeutic exercise is most effective when used early in the rehabilitative process, before joint contractures and motion-limiting tendon adhesions occur.

REFERENCES

1. Akeson, WH, and Amiel, D, and Woo, S: Immobility effects of synovial joints: The pathomechanics of joint contracture. Biorheology 17:95, 1980.
2. Akeson, WH, et al: Collagen cross-linking alterations in joint contractures: Changes in the reducible cross-links in periarticular connective tissue collagen after nine weeks of immobilization. Connect Tissue Res 5:15, 1977.
3. Donatelli, R and Owens-Burkhart, H: Effects of immobilization on the extensibility of periarticular connective tissue. J Sports Phys Therapy 3:2, 1981.
4. Kisner, C and Colby, LA: Therapeutic Exercise; Foundations and Techniques, ed 2. FA Davis, Philadelphia, 1990.
5. Melvin, JL: Rheumatic Disease in the Adult and Child, ed 3. FA Davis, Philadelphia, 1989, p 457.
6. Bell-Krotoski, JA, Berger, DE, and Beach, RB: Application of biomechanics for evaluation of the hand. In Hunter, JM, et al (eds): Rehabilitation of the Hand, ed 3. CV Mosby, St Louis, 1990, p 141.
7. Flowers, KR, and Michlovitz, SL: Assessment and management of loss of motion in orthopaedic dysfunction. Postgrad Adv Phys Ther 5, 1988.
8. Grauer, D, et al: The effects of intermittent passive exercise on joint stiffness following periarticular fracture in rabbits. Clin Orthop 220:259, 1987.
9. Frank, C: Physiology and therapeutic value of passive joint motion. Clin Orthop 185:113, 1984.
10. Arem, AJ and Madden, JW: Effects of stress on healing wounds. J Surg Res 29:93, 1976.
11. Peacock, EE: Wound Repair, ed 3. WB Saunders, Philadelphia, 1984, p 119.
12. Kottke, FJ, Pauley, DL, and Ptak, RA: The rationale for prolonged stretching for correction of shortening of connective tissue. Arch Phys Med 47:345, 1966.
13. Sapega, AA, et al: Biophysical factors in range of motion exercises. Phys Sports Med 9:57, 1981.
14. Brand, PW: Clinical Mechanics of the Hand. CV Mosby, St Louis, 1985, p 68.
15. Young, A, et al: Effects of joint pathology on muscle. Clin Orthop 219:21, 1987.
16. Mac Dougall, JD, et al: Biochemical adaptation of human skeletal muscle to heavy resistance training and immobilization. J Appl Physiol 43:700, 1977.
17. Shakespeare, DT, et al: The effect of knee flexion on quadriceps inhibition after meniscectomy. Clin Sci 65:64P, 1983.
18. Michelsson, JE, and Riska, EN: The effect of temporary exercising of a joint during an immobilization period. An experimental study on rabbits. Clin Orthop 144:321, 1979.
19. Kaltenborn, FM: Mobilization of the Extremity Joints: Examination and Basic Treatment Techniques. Olaf Norlis Bokhandel, Universitetsgaten, Oslo, 1980.
20. Maitland, GD: Peripheral Manipulation, ed 2. Butterworth, Boston, 1977.
21. Norkin, C and Levangie, P: Joint Structure and Function: A Comprehensive Analysis. FA Davis, Philadelphia, 1983, p 206.
22. Tanigawa, MC: Comparison of the hold-relax procedure and passive mobilization on increasing muscle length. Phys Ther 52:725, 1972.
23. Sady, SP, Wortman, MA, and Blanke, D: Flexibility training: Ballistic, static or proprioceptive neuromuscular facilitation? Arch Phys Med Rehabil 63:261, 1987.
24. Kapandji, IA: The Physiology of the Joints. ed 5. Churchill Livingstone, New York, 1982, p 124.
25. Muller, EA: Influence of training and of inactivity on muscle strength. Arch Phys Med 51:449, 1970.
26. Booth, F: Physiologic and biochemical effects of immobilization on muscle. Clin Orthop 219:15, 1987.
27. Evans, RB, Hunter, JM, and Burkhalter, WE: Conservative management of the trigger finger: A new approach. J Hand Ther 1:59, 1988.
28. Stromberg, BV: Contralateral therapy in upper extremity rehabilitation. Am J Phys Med 65:135, 1986.
29. Hellebrandt, FA, Houtz, SJ, and Kirkosian, AM: Influence of bimanual exercise on unilateral work capacity. J Appl Physiol 2:446, 1950.
30. Rose, DL, Radzyminski, SF, and Beatty, RR: Effect of brief maximal exercise on the strength of the quadriceps femoris. Arch Phys Med Rehabil 157, 1957.
31. Strickland, JW: Biologic rationale, clinical application, and results of early motion following flexor tendon repair. J Hand Ther 2:71, 1989.
32. McGrouther, DA and Ahmed, MR: Flexor tendon excursions in "no-man's land." Hand 13:129, 1981.
33. Duran, RJ, et al: Management of flexor tendon lacerations in Zone 2 using controlled passive motion postoperatively. In Hunter, JM, et al (eds): Rehabilitation of the Hand. CV Mosby, St Louis, 1990, p 410.
34. Kleinert, HE, Klutz, JE, and Cohen, MJ: Primary repair of Zone 2 flexor tendon lacerations. AAOS Symposium on Flexor Tendon Surgery in the Hand. CV Mosby, St Louis, 1975, p 91.
35. Evans, RB: Therapeutic management of extensor tendon injuries. In Hunter, JM, et al (eds): Rehabilitation of the Hand. CV Mosby, St Louis, 1990, p 492.

36. Bunnell, S: Surgery of the Hand, ed 3. JB Lippincott, Philadelphia, 1986, p 48.
37. Kaplan, EB: Functional and Surgical Anatomy of the Hand, ed 2. JB Lippincott, Philadelphia, 1965, p 12.
38. McGrouther, DA and Ahmed, MR: Flexor tendon excursions in "no-man's land." Hand 13:129, 1981.
39. Simmons, BP, and de la Caffiniere, JY: Physiology of finger flexion. In Tubiana, R (ed): The Hand. Vol 1. WB Saunders, Philadelphia, 1981, p 383.
40. Silverman, PM, Willette-Green, V, and Petrilli, J: Early protective motion in digital revascularization and replantation. J Hand Ther 2:91, 1989.
41. Wehbé, MA and Hunter, JM: Flexor tendon gliding in the hand. Part I. In vivo excursions. J Hand Surg 10A:570, 1985.
42. Wehbé, MA, Hunter, JM: Flexor tendon gliding in the hand. Part II. Differential gliding. J Hand Surg 10A:575, 1985.
43. Wehbé, MA: Tendon gliding exercises. Am J Occup Ther 41:164, 1987.
44. Stack, HG: A study of muscle function in fingers. Ann R Coll Surg Eng 33:307, 1963.
45. Long, C and Brown, MA: Electromyographic kinesiology of the hand: Muscle moving the long finger. J Bone Joint Surg (Am) 46:1683, 1964.
46. Landsmeer, JMF and Long, C: The mechanism of finger control, based on electromyograms and location analysis. Acta Anat (Basel) 60:330, 1965.
47. Long, C: Intrinsic-extrinsic muscle control of the fingers: Electromyographic studies. J Bone Joint Surg (Am) 50:973, 1968.
48. Long, C: Muscle and tendon kinesiology. In Lamb, DW and Kuczynski, K (eds): The Practice of Hand Surgery. Blackwell Scientific Publications, Great Britain, 1981.
49. Bunnel, S: Surgery of the Hand, ed 2. JB Lippincott, Philadelphia, 1948, p 469.
50. Blackhouse, KM and Catton, WT: An experimental study of the functions of the lumbrical muscles in the human hand. J Anat 88:133, 1954.
51. Valentin, P: The interossei and the lumbricals. In Tubiana, R (ed): The Hand. WB Saunders, Philadelphia, 1981, p 244.
52. Reynolds, C: Preoperative and postoperative management of tendon transfers after radial nerve injury. In Hunter, JM, et al (eds): Rehabilitation of the Hand. CV Mosby, St Louis, 1990, p 696.
53. Hunter, JM, Singer, DI, and Mackin, EJ: Staged flexor tendon reconstruction using passive and active tendon implants. In Hunter, JM, et al (eds): Rehabilitation of the Hand. CV Mosby, St Louis, 1990, p 427.
54. Cannon, NM: Enhancing flexor tendon glide through tenolysis . . . and hand therapy. J Hand Ther 2:122, 1989.
55. Warren, CG and Lehmann, JF: Heat and stretch procedures: An evaluation using rat tail tendon. Arch Phys Med Rehabil 57:122, 1976.
56. Lehmann, JF, et al: Effect of therapeutic temperatures on tendon extensibility. Arch Phys Med Rehabil 51:481, 1970.
57. Wehbé, MA: Personal communication, 1984.
58. Salter, RB, et al: Clinical application of basic research on continuous passive motion for disorders and injuries of synovial joints: A preliminary report of a feasibility study. J Orthop Res 1:325, 1984.
59. Coutts, RD, et al: Symposium: The use of continuous passive motion in the rehabilitation of orthopedic problems. Contemp Orthop 16:75, 1988.
60. Gastings, H and Carroll, C, IV: Treatment of closed articular fractures of the metacarpophalangeal and proximal interphalangeal joints. Hand Clin 4:4, 1988.
61. Covey, MH, et al: Efficacy of continuous passive motion devices with hand burns. J Burn Care Rehabil 9:397, 1988.
62. Frykman, GK, et al: CPM improves range of motion after PIP and MP capsulectomies: A controlled prospective study. 44th Annual Meeting of American Society for Surgery of the Hand, San Antonio, TX, 1989.
63. Skirven, T, Bora, FW, and Osterman, AL: The use of continuous passive motion in hand rehabilitation. 42nd Annual Meeting of the American Society for Surgery of the Hand, Seattle, WA, 1987.
64. Peart, RE, Bora, FW, and Osterman, AL: Treatment of chronic elbow contractures with surgical release and CPM. 44th Annual Meeting of the American Society for Surgery of the Hand, Seattle, WA, 1989.
65. Prosser, R: The value of continuous passive motion in hand therapy. 10th World Congress of Physical Therapists, Sydney, Australia, 1987.
66. Dimick, MP: Continuous passive motion for the upper extremity. In Hunter, JM, et al (eds): Rehabilitation of the Hand, ed 3. CV Mosby, St Louis, 1990, p 1140.

CHAPTER **8**

Physical Agents and Electrotherapy Techniques in Hand Rehabilitation

Susan Michlovitz, MS, PT
Laura R. Segal, PT

Physical agents and electrotherapy devices can serve as important adjuncts in hand rehabilitation when appropriately selected and incorporated into an overall treatment plan. These devices can be used in programs aimed at reducing pain and guarding muscle spasm, controlling edema and inflammation, restoring range of motion, and facilitating tissue healing. The hand therapist must be aware not only of the biophysical effects of each agent, but also of the contraindications and precautions when considering use of these techniques. In this chapter, techniques and rationales for selected procedures with physical agents are described. Clinical decision making with these techniques are illustrated through case studies.

The objectives of this chapter are to (1) describe selected techniques with physical agents and electrotherapy devices; (2) discuss indications, contraindications, and precautions for use; (3) discuss options for home programming; and (4) illustrate the clinical decision-making process when using these devices.

As the extent of this chapter permits only an overview, the interested reader is referred to additional current references.[1,2]

CRYOTHERAPY

Application of cold is an age-old remedy for managing acute inflammation, edema, and pain. The physiologic effects produced by cold serve as the underlying rationale for its therapeutic use. Various cooling agents are available for clinical use and home treatment.

The standard regimen for controlling potential edema from acute trauma is ice, compression, and elevation. In addition, electrical stimulation and pulsed ultrasound have been included in these treatment programs. Their applications will be discussed later in this chapter. The basic reasons for using cold for edema management are to lessen interstitial fluid infiltration by reducing capillary permeability[3] and to reduce secondary hypoxic injury by slowing tissue metabolism.[4] In addition, the analgesic effects of cooling can enhance patient cooperation with exercise and encourage muscle pumping action for edema control.

Cold is thought by most clinicians to control edema. Interestingly, though, if one reviews the research literature, mixed results following cold application are reported. It should be noted, however, that most studies included animal models. Controversial results from animal studies with cryotherapy for controlling swelling are probable due to variations in application such as (1) prolonged duration (1 hour or longer) of cold application, at low temperatures, and (2) lack of compression and elevation following cold. More commonly, in the clinic, cold is applied for 10 to 20 minutes with at least 1 hour between applications, followed by a compression wrap and elevation. Shorter-duration cold applications than those found in animal studies will most likely not have adverse effects. The concept of cold followed by compression or cold and simultaneous intermittent compression versus cold alone has been supported in clinical studies.[5,6] Evidence found in an animal model study of ligamentous injury suggested that cold can decrease the inflammatory response, as measured by reduction cells such as polymorphonuclear leukocytes and lymphocytes.[7] A few testimonials have been reported in the literature regarding use of contrast baths for edema control, but to our knowledge no documented clinical research supports this notion.

Cold can reduce pain by elevating the pain threshold[8] and providing a counterirritation.[9] Judicious application of cold in selected patients may enhance their ability to exercise. Persons with painful disorders such as reflex sympathetic dystrophy (RSD) may benefit from cryotherapy. On occasions when the therapist or patient or both have been overzealous with exercise, cold can be applied after exercise. If this application needs to be done on a routine basis, though, we believe the exercise program may be too vigorous for its intended use.

Conductive cooling agents such as commercial gel packs, wet ice packs, ice massage, and cool whirlpools (65°F to 70°F) are all common methods of lowering tissue temperature. Wet ice packs (chipped ice wrapped in a terrycloth towel) can produce a greater skin temperature reduction than can commercial gel packs.[10] Gel or ice packs may have a moist towel interface to be used against the skin surface to enhance conductivity. Ice massage applied for approximately 5 minutes is most efficacious for application over a localized area (e.g., for tendinitis). Cool whirlpools may be incorporated in desensitization programs when having the limb in a dependent position is not a concern. Commercial gel packs are probably the most practical cooling agent for home use, as they can be easily stored in the freezer between applications.

Certain precautions should be considered prior to determining cryotherapy use in persons with underlying joint stiffness (i.e., rheumatoid arthritis) because lowering tissue temperature of joint capsular structures increases stiffness.[11] Cold intolerance can occur following a crush injury or replant of one or more digits or a hand. In addition, cold is a potent vasoconstrictor of smooth muscle[12] and can reduce circulation, which should be a precaution in its use in patients with peripheral vascular insufficiency (e.g., replanted digits). As cold can impair wound tensile strength,[13] it should be used judiciously directly over a healing wound during the first 2 to 3 weeks following insult. Cryotherapy for 1 to 2 hours around the knee has resulted in neuropraxia and axonotmesis of the peroneal nerve.[14,15] Certainly the data could also be applied to the upper extremity; for example, where the ulnar nerve is superficial at the medial aspect of the elbow.

SUPERFICIAL HEATING AGENTS

Elevation of tissue temperature can reduce pain and lessen the viscoelastic properties of connective tissue, making manual techniques and active exercise easier to perform. The pain-relieving properties of heat may be due to its counterirritation effects,[9] ability to elevate pain threshold,[8] and enhancement of local blood flow via vasodilation.[16] Heat can alter viscoelastic properties of connective tissue by reducing viscosity and elastic stiffness. Animal laboratory studies by Warren and colleagues,[17] Gersten,[18] and Lehmann and associates[19] suggest that connective tissue will tolerate a stretch with less risk of tissue damage if tissue temperature is elevated prior to stretch. Unfortunately, this notion has not yet been tested through well-controlled clinical trials.

Several heating agents are available to elevate tissue temperature. In the hand, the affected tissues are within 1 to 2 cm of the skin surface; therefore, paraffin, warm whirlpool, and Fluidotherapy can all be used for generalized heating of the hand and wrist including muscle and joint structures.[20] Moist hot packs are too cumbersome to be conveniently wrapped around the hand. When well-focused heating (i.e., over a specific tendon or joint) is desired, continuous-wave ultrasound at 3 MHz is suggested.[21]

Paraffin

Paraffin baths contain a mixture of paraffin wax and mineral oil. This mixture has a lower specific heat than water, allowing for tolerance of higher temperatures. Paraffin is used at temperatures ranging from 118°F to 130°F. The lower temperature range of 118°F to 120°F is suggested when the skin is freshly healed.[22] The "dip-and-wrap" technique for 15 to 20 minutes is the most frequently chosen option. A hot pack in towels may be wrapped around the paraffin glove to enhance heating. The hand should be elevated to reduce the likelihood of an increase in interstitial fluid. Paraffin baths can be inexpensively purchased for home use (Fig. 8–1) and are safer and more practical than warming paraffin in a stovetop double boiler.

Whirlpool

Warm whirlpools at 98°F to 104°F are sometimes chosen for heating and desensitization. Patients recovering from Colles' fractures were treated using whirlpool at 96°F to 110°F, followed by exercise, for 12 treatment sessions. This approach was compared with the same patient population treated with exercise alone for 12 treatment sessions. There were no significant long-term differences between the two methods of treatment in pain, edema, range of motion, or strength.[23]

In another study, pain, range of motion, and hand volume in four groups of patient's post-traumatic injury were compared, including whirlpool (109.5°F); whirlpool and exercise; paraffin (125.6°F) in elevation and paraffin followed by exercise.[24] There was a significant decrease in pain and increase in range of motion in all groups. Whereas

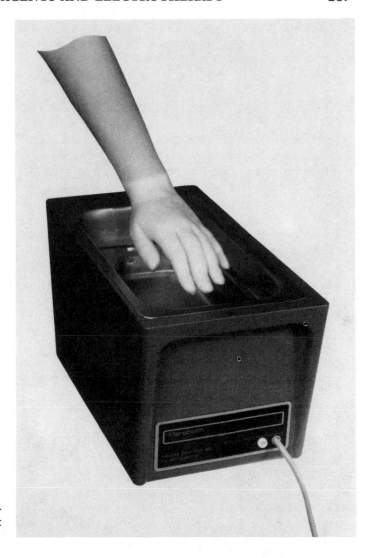

FIGURE 8–1. Home paraffin unit. (Courtesy Talcott Laboratories, Houston, PA.)

daily increases in hand volume were higher following whirlpool, there was no significant increase in hand volume over a 3-week period. Therefore, the decision between paraffin and whirlpool prior to exercise may be one of practicality and of patient and therapist preferences.

Fluidotherapy

Fluidotherapy is the trade name of an air-fluidized heating cabinet (Henley International, Sugar Land, Texas). The hand and wrist are immersed in medium of Cellex (cellulose) particles (Fig. 8–2). Warm air is forced from the bottom through the particles, forming an air-fluidized bed. Both the temperature of the bed and the amount of agitation can be controlled. Temperatures of 114°F to 116°F are used for heating, whereas lower temperatures are suggested for desensitization, if edema is of concern. We are not aware of any clinical studies (using patient populations) supporting the

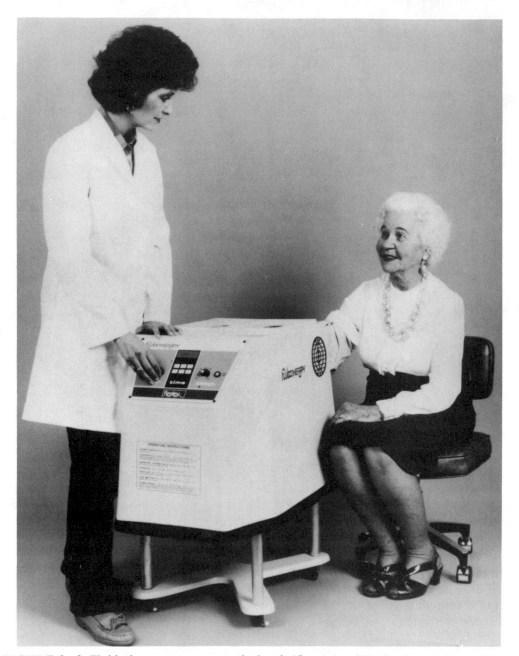

FIGURE 8–2. Fluidotherapy treatment to the hand. (Courtesy of Henley International, Sugar Land, TX.)

efficacy of Fluidotherapy compared with that of other heating agents. With Fluidotherapy and with whirlpool, however, exercise can be performed during immersion. It is necessary to cover the wound with an occlusive dressing prior to entry into the cellulose medium.

A home model Fluidotherapy unit is available. This unit may be appropriate, with carefully selected patients, where daily desensitization or vigorous heat application, or both, are warranted.

Precautions with Heating Agents

Precautions should be taken when using heating modalities on patients with vascular insufficiency,[25] uncontrolled edema, over areas of malignancy, infection, and diminished or absent sensation for pain and temperature. In addition, during the acute stages after injury and when bleeding may not be under control, heat should be avoided. Caution should also be exercised when using heat with infants and geriatric patients, as their thermoregulatory mechanisms are not fully developed or are depressed, respectively. (NOTE: These precautions also apply to continuous wave ultrasound).

ULTRASOUND

Ultrasound is used in medicine for diagnosis, therapeutic rehabilitation and destructive surgery. Low intensities—(under 1 mW per cm^2)—are used for diagnostic procedures; range of 0.25 W per cm^2 to 2.0 W per cm^2 for therapy; and greater than 10 W per cm^2 for destructive surgery. In therapy, ultrasound is used in low intensities to control inflammation and edema and to enhance healing. At higher intensities ultrasound becomes a heating agent to improve tissue extensibility and reduce pain and stiffness.

Sound waves at a frequency of greater than 20,000 Hz or cycles per second (cps) are inaudible to the human ear and are defined as ultrasound. As the frequency of sound increases, so does the ability to focus the energy and produce a collimated beam. At frequencies commonly used for therapy (1 MHz and 3 MHz), the beam is collimated for specific applications to well-delineated areas (i.e., for treating tendons and ligaments).

As the ultrasound beam (pressure wave) passes into tissue, some of the energy is scattered (reflected) and most is absorbed, particularly at tissue interfaces. Ultrasound at 1 MHz can be absorbed at depths of up to 5 cm. As frequency increases, the depth at which ultrasound energy is available for absorption decreases. This attenuation is primarily due to increased tissue frictional resistances at higher frequencies. Ultrasound at 3 MHz is mostly absorbed within the first 2 cm depth of tissue. Therefore, a frequency of 3 MHz may be more appropriate for use in hand rehabilitation. Certainly, the physical rationale for using 3 MHz ultrasound is apparent; now clinical studies of comparison between 1 and 3 MHz are needed.

Ultrasound energy is emitted in pressure waves from a piezoelectric crystal (located in the applicator) as a result of an applied electrical voltage across the crystal. The energy can be emitted in a continuous mode (uninterrupted) or in a pulsed mode (interrupted) (Fig. 8–3.) Power output of therapeutic ultrasound is measured in watts. The intensity is described as the power (watts) per unit area of the effective radiating area (ERA) of the crystal (in cm^2). Crystals are available with ERA for most hand therapy applications ranging between 0.5 cm^2 and 5.0 cm^2. Generally, the smaller the ERA, the easier is direct coupling between a small or irregular surface and the ultrasound applicator.

Intensities for therapeutic ultrasound range from 0.25 W per cm^2 to 2.0 W per cm^2. There has been a trend in the past decade to use lower intensities of ultrasound than in the past.[26,27] Recent work done by Dyson[26] supports the use of low-intensity ultrasound for tissue healing.

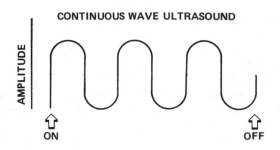

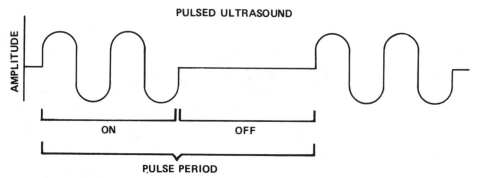

FIGURE 8–3. Continuous wave and pulsed wave ultrasound. (From Michlovitz, SL: Thermal Agents in Rehabilitation, ed 2. FA Davis, Philadelphia, 1990, p 139, with permission.)

Biophysical Effects of Ultrasound

The use of continuous-mode ultrasound to selectively heat tissues of high collagen content and at tissue interfaces is well known.[28,29] The pain-relieving effects of ultrasound are most likely due to thermal mechanisms.[30] Nonthermal (mechanical) effects of (pulsed) ultrasound include acoustical streaming and stable cavitation.[26] *Acoustical streaming* refers to the movement of fluids along the boundaries of cell membranes as a result of the mechanical pressure wave. This streaming has been implicated in the changes in ion fluxes and subsequent changes in cellular activity found with ultrasound applicator.[26] *Cavitation* is the vibrational effect on gas bubbles by an ultrasound beam. If the bubbles pulse (but do not implode, or collapse) then *stable cavitation* occurs. Stable cavitation can result in diffusional changes along cell membranes. These claims are based on animal studies for the reported increases in capillary density,[31] increases in fibroblastic activity (in vitro),[32] and increases in wound closure[33] after pulsed ultrasound application. Such studies serve as a solid scientific framework on which to build more information on the bioeffects of ultrasound.

Clinical Applications of Ultrasound

REDUCING JOINT STIFFNESS AND PAIN

Continuous-wave ultrasound has been used primarily for pain control[30,34] and as a heating agent to reduce stiffness and enhance viscoelasticity of connective tissue, such as joint capsules.

For more vigorous heating of the hand and wrist, intensities of about 1.0 W per cm^2 are suggested for heat-and-stretch applications. Time of application is 3 to 5 minutes per field (one-and-a-half to two times the ERA).[35] When ultrasound is used to provide heat, all precautions that apply to heat application are relevant.

For pain control (e.g., in patients with RSD[34] and in those with neuromas), ultrasound at intensities of 0.75 W per cm^2 or lower, applied over the involved peripheral nerve, are suggested.

EDEMA/INFLAMMATION CONTROL

Preliminary results of laboratory[36] and clinical[37] studies suggest that pulsed ultrasound application during the acute stages following trauma may assist in edema control. Certainly this is an interesting area for further clinical investigation. Pulsed ultrasound has also been reported to be effective in controlling symptoms occurring secondary to tendonitis.[38] In another study on tendonitis, continuous-mode ultrasound was no more effective than placebo.[39]

PHONOPHORESIS

Phonophoresis is the technique of driving medication across the skin into tissue via ultrasound. This technique is used to manage inflammatory conditions such as tendonitis and neuritis. Anti-inflammatory medications, such as 10% or 1% hydrocortisone[40], dexamethasone, and 0.25% triamcinolone acetonide, are added to an aqueous coupling solution and applied to the skin. This step is followed by continuous-mode ultrasound using intensities sufficient for mild heating. Perhaps the combined effects of heating and the mechanical driving force of the acoustic pressure wave may support this rationale. To our knowledge, the use of pulsed ultrasound has not been studied for phonophoresis. Recent clinical studies suggest that phonophoresis may be no more effective for reducing pain secondary to inflammation than is ice[41] or ultrasound alone.[42]

WOUND HEALING

Dyson and Suckling[43] and Roche and West[44] have reported healing of varicose and stasis ulcers with pulsed ultrasound at 3 MHz. This technique involves use of a sterile coupling medium and moving the ultrasound applicator around the perimeter of the wound. Intensities of less than 0.75 W per cm^2 pulsed at 20% duty cycle, 3 MHz are given.

USE OVER SURGICALLY REPAIRED TENDONS

There has been controversy in hand rehabilitation regarding the use of ultrasound over repaired tendons. Most of the available published data are preliminary and not definitively conclusive. Different animal models using different protocols were reviewed. Ultrasound at 1.1 MHz, 0.8 W per cm^2 pulsed for 5 minutes and applied 5 days a week for 6 weeks over freshly repaired rabbit Achilles' tendons resulted in a reduced breaking strength as compared with control subjects.[45] Ultrasound at 1 MHz, 1 W per cm^2, applied for 5 minutes while moving applicator over tenotomized rabbit Achilles' tendons resulted in greater tensile strength than in control subjects. Ultrasound in this study was administered on 9 consecutive days following tenotomy.[46]

Turner, Powell, and Ng[47] reported no beneficial effects or adverse changes in mechanical strength of repaired cockeral tendons in an ultrasound-treated group versus a control group. In this study, ultrasound was applied from weeks 3 to 8, three times per week, using 3 MHz, 1 W per cm^2 pulsed 20% duty cycle at 4 minutes. When ultrasound was instituted 4 weeks after surgical repair of flexor tendons in the hen, there were no adverse responses reported in tensile strength. In fact, functional return (as measured by grasp of the hen foot around a perch) was enhanced in the group treated with ultrasound. Ultrasound at 3 MHz, 0.75 W per cm^2, was applied for 5 minutes over a total of 20 days.[48] The results produced in this group could be frequency dependent, intensity dependent, and animal model dependent.

Certainly, this is an area for more research prior to making definitive conclusions. Evidence is inconclusive if ultrasound can be used to enhance tendon repair. Based on a review of the literature, we recommend that continuous-wave ultrasound not greater than 0.5 W/cm^2 be used over tendon repairs until the late fibroplasia phase. If ultrasound is used earlier, consider using low-intensity (0.75 W per cm^2 or less) pulsed mode with a moving applicator technique.

Other Ultrasound Treatment Considerations

A coupling medium is required between the ultrasound applicator and the skin surface to optimize ultrasound transmission. A commercially available aqueous-based gel is the most practical. Water coupling has been used in the past, but the availability of smaller applicators may preclude the need for this. If the ultrasound applicator heats up during treatment, coupling may be poor or the crystal may be damaged.

In addition, with continuous-wave and pulsed ultrasound, the applicator should be kept moving about 4 cm per sec[35] to prevent potential adverse responses. The center of the ultrasound beam has a higher intensity and may cause hot spots. Temporary cessation of blood flow[49] and platelet aggregation and endothelial damage[50] have been reported with the use of a stationary sound head. These phenomena may result from the standing wave formation (the interaction of the longitudinal wave and the reflected wave at tissue interfaces).

Ultrasound can be used over metal implants, but caution should be used when applying ultrasound over areas of methyl methacrylate cement.[51] One should avoid undue ultrasound exposure over epiphyseal plates in children, but low intensities with a moving application can be used if necessary.[51]

Ultrasound should not be used over areas of malignancy. Again one must remember that, when using ultrasound to elevate tissue temperature, the same contraindications and precautions apply as with the other heating agents discussed. By carefully selecting intensities, patients, and techniques (i.e., moving sound applicator and complete coupling), ultrasound can be a beneficial adjunct in hand rehabilitation.

ELECTRICAL STIMULATION

Electrical stimulation can be indicated in programs to reduce pain, to increase muscle contraction secondary to atrophy or neuromuscular dysfunction, and to enhance tissue healing. Electrical stimulation uses, categorized according to function, are listed in Table 8–1.[52] The clinician needs a clear understanding of the various currents produced by the electrical modalities. Describing currents for electrical stimulation has been a source of great confusion. In recent years, an effort has been made to standardize the nomenclature used in discussing these currents (Table 8–2).

TABLE 8–1 Electrical Stimulation Techniques[52]

TENS: Transcutaneous electrical nerve stimulation, used for pain control
NMES: Neuromuscular electrical stimulation, describes muscular stimulation through stimulation of an intact peripheral nerve
FES: Functional electrical stimulation, describes use of NMES for orthotic substitution
EMS: Electrical muscular stimulation, describes direct stimulation of denervated muscle
ESTR: Electrical stimulation for tissue repair, describes electrical stimulation for decreasing inflammation, enhancing tissue healing, controlling edema, administering iontophoretic agents, and improving vascular status

TABLE 8–2 Currents for Electrical Stimulation

DC: Direct current is the continuous unidirectional flow[1] of charged particles; this current never changes direction or is interrupted.
AC: Alternate current is an uninterrupted bidirectional flow of charged particles taking on a symmetric or asymmetric appearance.[2]
Pulsed current: Formerly described as interrupted AC or DC, this is the unidirectional or bidirectional flow of charged particles that periodically ceases for a finite period of time. Monophasic waveform is a "pulse that deviates in one direction from the zero current baseline and returns to the baseline" after a finite time.[3] Biphasic waveforms are pulses that deviate in both directions from the zero current baseline. A biphasic waveform can be symmetric or asymmetric.[4]

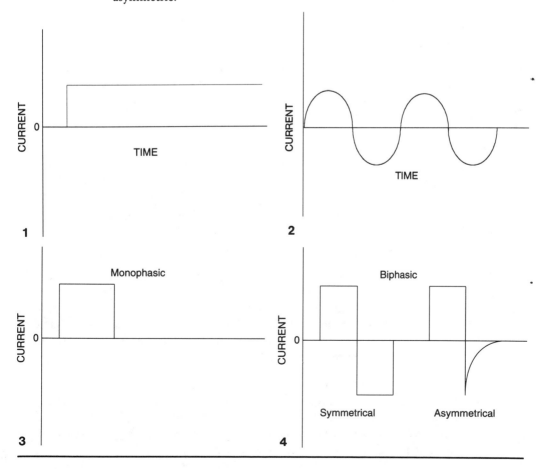

Transcutaneous Electrical Nerve Stimulation for Pain Control

The hand therapist is frequently faced with the difficult task of alleviating pain. Transcutaneous electrical nerve stimulation (TENS) is a treatment modality that has proven effective in controlling both acute and chronic pain syndromes. Reports of successful results with TENS are quite diverse. Many different electrical stimulation units (i.e., portable TENS and clinical models such as high-voltage pulsed-current and interferential stimulation) are available. These units have several stimulus characteristics (pulse rate, pulse duration, amplitude) that can be set manually and used for pain control.

Many theories have been postulated regarding the physiologic basis of pain modulation owing to TENS. The two most recognized theories used to date to explain TENS and its effect on pain are (1) the gate control theory proposed by Melzack and Wall in 1965[53]; and (2) the reported release of endogenous opiates during application of acupuncturelike TENS to chronic pain patients.[54]

Both theories have been under much scrutiny over the past decade. Freeman, Campbell, and Long[55] challenge the theory that endogenous opiates are released in response to TENS application. They state that chronic pain patients treated with TENS at 10 to 100 Hz did not show a decrease in pain relief after receiving an injection of naloxone (an endogenous opiate antagonist), which suggests that chronic pain relief is not mediated by increased release of endogenous opiates.[55]

STIMULUS MODES

Stimulus modes, which are the combination of parameters chosen to influence pain relief, are set by adjusting the stimulus parameters of the TENS unit, including the frequency (pulse rate), pulse duration, pulse width, and intensity (amplitude). Also available are units that allow for alteration in frequency modulation. The most commonly used stimulus modes are detailed here.

Conventional Mode

This mode of TENS is the most frequently used stimulation mode. Settings for the conventional mode consists of frequencies of 50 to 150 pulses per second (pps) and pulse durations of 20 to 100 microseconds (μsec). Intensity is just below muscle contraction. The patient experiences a tingling sensation. This mode supposedly activates large myelinated proprioceptive alpha and beta nerve fibers.[56]

Acupuncturelike Mode

This mode consists of low frequencies of 1 to 4 pps and pulse duration of 150 to 250 μsec. Intensity is set to patient's tolerance, producing a muscle contraction in myotomes that are segmentally related to the pain producing structure.[56]

The differences between acupuncturelike and conventional TENS are interesting to note. With chronic pain patients analgesia is reported to be effected with acupuncturelike TENS if conventional TENS has not been successful.[57]

Burst Mode (Pulse-Train)

Burst or pulse-train TENS is similar to acupuncturelike TENS. This mode combines low-frequency pulse rates (1 to 4 Hz) with a high internal frequency (70 to 100 Hz). The high pulse rates are emitted in fixed trains or bursts of 5 to 7 Hz per pulse between a carrier low-frequency wave. Pulse width is 250 μsec and intensity is high.[56] This mode may decrease accommodation to stimulation more effectively than with conventional TENS.

Brief-Intense Mode

This stimulation mode has the lowest patient tolerance level of the four modes discussed. Settings for the brief-intense mode consist of about 100 pps, pulsed width of 150 to 250 μsec, and intensity to patient tolerance. A tetanic muscle contraction is produced or muscle fasciculation occurs, depending on electrode placement.

According to Melzack,[58] brief-intense mode stimulation may disrupt the memory-like process for pain. He also suggests that this stimulation mode is most successful at decreasing pain for prolonged periods of time.[58]

CHOOSING STIMULUS PARAMETERS

Many studies have reported relative analgesic effects of TENS when stimulus modes were compared. One such report indicates analgesic effects lasting 20 to 30 minutes with acupuncturelike TENS, as compared with the relatively short analgesia following conventional stimulation. On the other hand, conventional TENS has also been reported to have analgesic effects lasting up to several hours.[59]

In a clinical setting, the therapist usually first tries conventional TENS because of the greater patient tolerance to this mode; then, depending on success in reducing painful syndromes, one of the previously outlined modes is chosen for the various explanations given. The analgesic effects of conventional TENS primarily occur when the current is on, but there may be some carry-over effect.

Acupuncturelike TENS can be appropriate for chronic pain conditions when conventional TENS has not been successful. Brief-intense TENS may be useful when performing certain exercise (i.e., mobilizations or wound care techniques) but may not be tolerated by some patients.

ELECTRODE PLACEMENT

In the cases in which pain transmission can be specifically attributed to a particular nerve, a high degree of pain relief can be achieved with stimulation of these peripheral nerves. This fact strongly supports the idea that maximal pain relief can be achieved if stimulation can be directed to the particular nerves involved.[60] There is agreement that persistent attempts at finding proper electrode placement as well as treatment parameters will influence one's relative success in attaining analgesia with TENS.

One method of identification and stimulation of specific nerves has been described by Berlant.[60] The therapist holds one electrode in the palm of the hand while the patient holds the second corresponding electrode. The stimulus is regulated to the therapist's tolerance; then, using one finger, the therapist touches the patient in an attempt to elicit a radiating sensation indicating localization of the peripheral nerve involved in the painful response. For example, if the volar aspect of the finger is painful, the therapist moves along the distribution of the median nerve to determine at which site the radiating sensation of the electrical stimulation is greatest. An electrode is then placed over that site.

A study performed by Waisbrod and associates[61] on chronic peripheral neuropathies found TENS treatment beneficial, as long as the stimulation was placed proximal to the lesion. Careful diagnosis of peripheral neuropathy appears essential for achieving advantageous results.

Mannheimer[62] outlines several methods of electrode placement that may be tried when treating various painful syndromes including (1) acupuncture, motor or trigger points; (2) stimulating the site of greatest tenderness or pain; (3) stimulating distant or contralateral sites; (4) specific dermatome or spinal segmental levels; (5) superficial points along peripheral nerves; (6) linear pathways; and (7) multiple electrodes applied to diffuse areas along anatomic sites using parallel or crossed techniques.

TENS FOR ACUTE AND CHRONIC CASES

Several studies have substantiated the usefulness of TENS on acute pain as compared with analgesics.[63,64] Quinton, Sloan, and Theakstone[65] measured pain and mobility following the use of TENS and placebo TENS for the first 3 days following emergency treatment of acute hand infections. Although specific TENS parameters were not mentioned, their findings indicate a statistically significant decrease in the use of mild analgesics and opiates as compared with the placebo TENS group. In addition, range-of-motion measurements for the TENS group were increased within the first 3 days.

Several studies have been done trying to minimize pain experienced with arthritis in the acute, as well as the chronic, stages. A study on induced acute arthritis of rabbit joints suggests conventional TENS may be useful for treating acute inflammatory arthritis by decreasing synovial fluid pressure volume and leukocyte count.[66]

Chronic joint pain can be treated with TENS when considering joints consisting of periosteum, synovium, and a capsule all supplied by the nonmyelinated sensory fibers (C fibers).[67] Both acupuncturelike and conventional TENS used peripherally can be a valuable tool in treating chronic pain conditions.[57]

Application of TENS for postoperative pain control can be quite successful. A reduction in narcotic intake has been reported when TENS is used postoperatively. Patients are generally seen preoperatively to establish stimulus parameters and to familiarize the patient with the treatment program. Sterile electrodes are placed adjacent to the incision, and TENS treatment begins in the recovery room and is used continuously for the first 48 to 72 hours.[64]

Electrical Stimulation for Muscle Dysfunction

Neuromuscular electrical stimulation (NMES) is often used clinically in programs for muscle reeducation, orthotic substitute (functional electrical stimulation, or FES), muscle strengthening, and range-of-motion exercises. When using NMES, especially for the upper extremities, the electrodes should be custom trimmed to ensure specific muscular stimulation, due to the small muscle groups. (Caution: The smaller the electrode, the higher the current density.) Electrodes should not be placed over bony prominences because of possible discomfort, and care must be taken to keep enough separation between electrodes to permit sufficient depth of penetration of the current.

ORTHOTIC SUBSTITUTION

FES is the use of NMES in place of orthosis. FES has been used for muscle reeducation in patients suffering from gait dysfunction and shoulder subluxation after cerebral vascular accident (CVA) or head trauma and to stabilize a proximal joint for use of a more distal joint (i.e., as a wrist extension orthosis during grasp and release activities).

When used correctly for shoulder subluxation, FES may not only prevent further joint separation, but also provide normal glenohumeral alignment when sitting or standing.[68] The advantage of such stimulation in lieu of using a sling includes normal joint alignment and a decrease in capsular stretch caused by gravity.[68] This result is accomplished by gradually increasing wearing time to reduce fatigue while increasing tolerance. The therapists at Ranchos Los Amigos use a time on–time off schedule of 24 seconds on and 2 seconds off in the reeducation of a subluxating shoulder. This approach is used to reposition the shoulder into normal alignment throughout the day if possible.[68] Stimulus parameters include tetanizing frequencies (30 to 50 pps), variable on-off time (in seconds) to reduce fatigue, and a ramp-up (surge on) to enhance patient comfort and reduce muscle guarding.

MUSCLE STRENGTHENING FOR DISUSE ATROPHY

There was an emergence of great interest in the use of electrical stimulation to increase muscle strength in 1978. At that time, the Russian stimulation technique was introduced at a Canadian symposium by Dr. Kots, a Russian physician. Kots claimed muscle strength increases of as high as 30 to 50%. He reported using 50 Hz bursted alternating current −10 seconds on; 50 seconds off. Since that time, many unsuccessful attempts have been made to duplicate these reported results.

Several studies have compared muscle strengthening with and without the use of electrical stimulation using the quadriceps muscle as a model.[69] For the most part, these studies conclude that electrical stimulation alone and electrical stimulation superimposed on voluntary effort can provide strength gains equivalent to but no greater than voluntary exercise alone. Therefore, cutaneous electrical stimulation may be a useful technique when attempting to strengthen poorly motivated patients or those who have difficulty producing a maximal volitional contraction.[70,71]

The use of electrical stimulation for muscle strengthening is probably accomplished by a combination of factors, the first of which is the short-term reeducation of muscle (increase in voluntary control, neural factors) followed by the longer-term stimulation result of actual muscle hypertrophy.[72] The use of electrical stimulation for both short-term and long-term muscle atrophy will be discussed in subsequent sections.

Electrical stimulation can also be used quite effectively on the patient with short-term muscle atrophy, (e.g., following immobilization or surgery). In these instances, muscle reeducation is beneficial because of the decreased sensory input or physical inhibition secondary to joint pain or postsurgical pain.[73]

Myofibrillar ATPase has been shown to decrease with immobilization. This fact may be responsible for the resultant decrease in muscle function. After using electrical stimulation on the immobilized part, there was no decrease in myofibrillar ATPase. Therefore, the use of NMES during immobilization may help prevent muscular atrophy due to immobilization.[74] When using electrical stimulation to decrease muscle atrophy, the strongest muscle contraction should occur for 30 to 60 minutes per day. Total stimulation time depends on on and off times (in seconds). A window placed in a cast or splint is often used for electrode placement and monitoring skin reactions.

NMES has also shown beneficial results when treating long-term atrophy. A study at Rancho Los Amigos on long-term atrophy changes with muscular stimulation concluded that actual changes in the quality of the muscle occurs with prolonged use (11 weeks) of electrical stimulation. These changes include hypertrophy of both fast- and slow-twitch fiber types, increased force output, and increased resistance to fatigue. In this study, stimulation was performed to produce 1½ hours of on-time per day, 7 days per week for 10 to 11 weeks. A maximum contraction was not tolerated by these patients; therefore, a 3 to 3+/5 level of muscular contraction was generated.[73]

RANGE OF MOTION

NMES can play an important role in improving range of motion.[75] NMES can be successfully used with patients who cannot tolerate traditional range-of-motion (ROM) regimens. The analgesic effects as well as the decrease in muscle guarding often associated with traditional ROM programs may contribute to the success.[68]

One example of use is maintaining ROM following a tenolysis procedure. The most important aspect of the postoperative management is ensuring that the patient actively pulls the tendon through the lysed region. NMES can be used as part of an early rehabilitation program by stimulating and assisting in active range of motion (AROM), thereby improving tendon gliding. In addition, NMES may decrease postoperative pain and edema as a result of increased muscle pump activity it produces. Short periods of stimulation (5 to 10 minutes) and frequent sessions (three to four per day) are recommended. The choice to use NMES after tenolysis depends on the quality of the tendon and the extent of the lysis. Certainly, NMES is not appropriate if the integrity of the tendon is in question.

ELECTRICAL MUSCLE STIMULATION FOR DENERVATED MUSCLE

Electrical muscular stimulation (EMS) has been used following peripheral nerve injury to prevent muscle wasting and atrophy. The number of studies that say electrical stimulation is effective for denervated muscle equals those that suggest it is ineffective. A study done by Herbison, Teng, and Gordon[76] concluded that no difference in mean muscle fiber diameter or muscle weights was found between treated and untreated rats. Many of the studies demonstrating positive effects with electrically stimulated animal models using periods of stimulation and intensities that would neither be practical nor comfortable for our patients. To stimulate denervated muscle, pulsed current at 3 msec or longer duration is required.

Electrical Stimulation for Tissue Repair

Although not extensively studied, the available laboratory and clinical evidence strongly suggests that electrical stimulation for tissue repair (ESTR) can be used by therapists to increase the rate of healing of open wounds. ESTR has been shown to influence wound healing by increasing blood flow,[79,81] decreasing microorganisms,[82] and influencing tissue growth.[77,82,83] The increase in blood flow may be due, in part, to the inhibition of sympathetic induced vasoconstriction, attributed to the use of the negative electrode.[77]

A decrease in microorganisms has been found in vitro, with the use of low-amperage direct current; however, high-volt pulsed current (HVPC) was not found to have a bactericidal effect. The authors suggested that an increase in treatment time, greater than 30 minutes, and an in vivo application may yield better results.[81]

The influence of tissue growth has been attributed to the anodal (positive-current) stimulation. The anode may activate a mechanism for tissue growth and repair.[82] Early epithelial cell migration has been detected under the anode in the early stages of wound healing.

Clinicians and researchers alike have chosen a variety of stimulus parameters to influence wound healing. In addition, electrode polarity must be considered when setting up a treatment program. Although not thoroughly studied, alternating electrode polarity during treatment to achieve an optimal rate of healing may be beneficial, particularly if plateaus in healing occur. A recent study using polarity in alternation to effect skin flap survival in pigs has provided further evidence to support this idea.[84]

HVPS is currently being used clinically for assistance with wound care. Kloth and Feedar[85] reported excellent results of accelerated wound healing with the use of HVPS on dermal ulcers. They used 105 pps at a voltage just below muscle contraction, 45 minutes a day, 5 days per week. A sterile electrode was placed in the wound, with the other electrode on the skin.[85]

PRECAUTIONS WITH ELECTRICAL STIMULATION

Electrical stimulation should not be used on patients with demand cardiac pacemakers. The effects of pregnancy have not yet been determined. Stimulation at intensities sufficient to cause muscle contraction are not advisable over areas where motion may cause tissue damage. Stimulation over the anterior surface of the neck may cause laryngeal muscle spasm, impairing breathing.

CLINICAL DECISION MAKING

Choice of a therapeutic technique should be based on the goals of treatment and special patient circumstances such as stage of healing and associated medical problems. These goals are determined after a thorough evaluation of the patient including history of present problems and objective measures.

A plan of care, which can include a physical agent or electrotherapy treatment, is then developed. The minimum number of treatment modalities should be selected to achieve a therapeutic goal. If too many modalities are used in one treatment session, it is difficult to tell which (if any) are effective. For example, if one chooses to control pain, then heat, cold, ultrasound, and electrical stimulation can all be selected. But if Fluidotherapy, cold packs, TENS, and ultrasound were applied to reduce hypersensitivity of a painful neuroma, treatment time would be prolonged and the clinician would be unable to determine which modality was responsible for the results of intervention. Contraindications and precautions should also be kept in mind. The clinical program can be augmented and eventually substituted by pain-control devices used at home such as TENS, cold packs, or paraffin.

To assist in determining treatment outcome and to be able to reproduce or modify treatment as appropriate, accurate recording of the techniques used and the patient's response to each mode of treatment should be documented for each therapy session. For example, if electrical stimulation is used to control pain, the following should be documented: electrode placement, pulse duration, pulse rate, and duration of stimulation. Appropriate outcome measures should be periodically recorded. For example, if TENS is used as part of a treatment program for pain control, then pain quantity (via visual analog scales or numeral rating scales), location (via body diagrams) quality (via word descriptors), and duration of pain relief would be appropriate measures.

Physical agents and electrical stimulation are used as adjuncts to a total treatment plan. The two case studies that follow emphasize selected techniques (e.g., ultrasound, Fluidotherapy, NMES) in order to link information presented in this chapter. The reader should keep in mind that while the physical agents and electrical stimulation techniques are emphasized for correlative purposes, the role of exercise, splinting, and functional activities should not be underplayed.

CASE STUDY NUMBER 1

Mark, a 45-year-old right hand–dominant machine operator sustained a nondisplaced distal radial fracture on the left secondary to a fall at work. Following 4 weeks of casting, a therapy program for ROM and strengthening was initiated. Because of exacerbation of wrist pain with exercise (10 weeks after injury), the patient was seen by a hand surgeon for consultation. The patient was further diagnosed with radial neuritis and extensor carpi radialis brevis/longus tendinitis. The patient was seen in therapy following the physicians appointment for complete evaluation (Table 8–3).

Chief problems were pain and hypersensitivity over the dorsum of the left hand and wrist and decreased function. Treatment was instituted three times a week. For the first 2 weeks, a wrist resting splint was worn between therapy sessions. Fluidotherapy at 112°F for 20 minutes was used for desensitization, for pain relief, and as a medium in which to exercise (the higher temperature ranges were avoided owing to inflammation around the tendons and the superficial branch of the radial nerve). AROM exercises for the wrist were performed following Fluidotherapy treatment.

At the third treatment session, ultrasound at 3 MHz, 0.75 W per cm^2; pulsed at 20% ERA of 0.5 cm^2 was administered over the extensor carpi radialis tendons (where swelling was also present) for 4 minutes. A low dosage was chosen for nonthermal effects to reduce swelling and inflammation. Ultrasound was discontinued after the burning pain subsided, with 12 treatments administered.

As the pain subsided, resisted exercises with light-grade putty and 2- and 4-lb weights for wrist flexion and extension were initiated. Exercises were progressed to include use of Baltimore Therapeutic Equipment (BTE) Work Simulator with tools for pronation/supination (tools 504 and 601) and wrist flexion/extension (tool 701). After 1 week on the Work Simulator, a tool for upper extremity conditioning (tool 802) using a pushing-and-pulling motion was added.

After 6 weeks of therapy (20 treatment sessions), therapy goals were achieved, and the physician discharged Mark to return to work.

CASE STUDY NUMBER 2

Pam, a 23-year-old right hand–dominant cellular phone saleswoman, fell on her right hand, sustaining a laceration at the wrist level. At the time of the injury the wound was cleansed and sutured. After Pam's complaints of the inability to use her index finger, she was referred by her family physician to a hand surgeon.

TABLE 8–3 Evaluation Findings for Case Study Number 1

	Baseline	Midtherapy	Discharge
Inspection	Slight swelling over extensor tendon insertion	No visible swelling	No visible swelling
Pain location	Dorsum of hand and insertion of wrist radial extensors	Insertion of wrist radial extensors	
Quality	Throbbing on motion; burns on touch	Burning on motion	Throb during resisted pronation/ supination
Quantity			
VAS	90% on motion	50% on motion	25%
Numerical scale	max 10, avg 5	max 8, avg 5	
Girth at wrist	Equal to R	—	—
Pinch strength (lb)	Pad-to-pad 7	NT*	Pad-to-pad 7
Range of motion (wrist)	Flexion: 55 degrees L, 60 degrees R Extension: 60 degrees L, 80 degrees R U.D./R.D. equal to R		Equal to R
Function	Pain on ADL	Exercise against resistance on BTE Work Simulator†	Pain only on resisted supination/ pronation; could exercise in work-simulated activities

†Baltimore Therapeutic Equipment Co., Baltimore, MD.
*NT = Not tested.

Pam underwent a delayed partial repair of the flexor digitorum profundus to the index finger and partial flexor tenolysis. Five days after surgery she was referred to therapy for initiation of treatment. To prevent excessive stress to the partial flexor tendon repair, a dorsal protective splint was fabricated with the wrist at 30° of flexion; 70° of MP flexion; PIPs and DIPs at 0°. Rubberband traction was applied to allow for full active extension and for passive return to flexion. An initial evaluation was performed. Significant objective measurement can be found in Table 8–4.

Three weeks following surgery, the splint was remolded to bring the wrist to neutral, rubberband traction was continued, and controlled ROM exercises were initiated. Four weeks after surgery the splint was discontinued. Fluidotherapy at 112°F for 20 minutes was added to aid with desensitization and superficial heating prior to AROM exercises. An Elastomer pad was placed over the scar to assist with scar remodeling. Cross-friction massage with lanolin was added to improve scar mobility. Tendon gliding exercises were initiated to facilitate tendon glide.

Because Pam was having difficulty with active finger flexion and tendon gliding exercises, the clinician used NMES to assist with flexor tendon gliding

TABLE 8–4 Objective Measurements of Case Number 2

| ROM | Initial Evaluation* | | Discharge | |
	Active ROM	Passive ROM	Active ROM	Passive ROM
MP	NT†	Flexion WNL Extension NT	0–80	WNL
PIP	NT	WNL	0–90	WNL
DIP	NT	WNL	0–50	WNL

Grip Strength (Tested with the Jamar Dynamometer)

| | 8 Weeks after Surgery | | Discharge |
	R	L	R
Level 1	5 lb	30 lb	40 lb
Level 2	10 lb	55 lb	55 lb
Level 3	9 lb	50 lb	53 lb
Level 4	9 lb	35 lb	40 lb
Level 5	6 lb	35 lb	35 lb

Pinch Strength

| | 8 Weeks after Surgery | | Discharge |
	R	L	R
Pad-to-pad	2 lb	7 lb	7.5 lb
Lateral	4 lb	10 lb	17.5 lb
Three-jaw chuck	4 lb	10 lb	10.0 lb

*Active ROM not tested into flexion secondary to repair, extension of PIP, DIP, WNL. Hypersensitivity along incision line.
†NT = Not tested.

exercises (6 weeks after surgery). Stimulation parameters for NMES included 10 sec on, 30 sec off; 4 sec ramp-up. Self-adhesive electrodes were placed, one over the median nerve at the level of the volar wrist just distal to the thumb, and the other just distal to the common flexor origin at the proximal one third of the forearm. Treatment time was 10 minutes initially. An NMES unit was sent home with Pam after four in-clinic treatments and proper patient education. The time of use was gradually increased to use twice per day for 20 minutes each as muscle fatigue diminished.

As ROM and tendon gliding improved, resistive exercises were initiated and progressed (8 weeks after surgery). Included were putty, Hand Helper, and foam squeeze exercises. An exercise program on the BTE was added (10 weeks after surgery) to aid with increasing strength to a fully functional level.

Pam was discharged after 12 weeks of therapy, with only minor strength and ROM deficits. She was able to perform all job and recreational tasks that she desired.

SUMMARY

This chapter guides the therapist through the clinical decision-making process for the careful selection of modalities in a hand therapy program. An understanding of the physiologic and biomechanical effects of physical agents and electrical stimulation is necessary when staging the introduction of modalities into the plan of care. This chapter reviews salient physiologic and biophysical effects, indications, and contraindications and precautions of these modalities as they relate to hand therapy.

REFERENCES

1. Michlovitz, SL (ed): Thermal Agents in Rehabilitation, ed 2. FA Davis, Philadelphia, 1990.
2. Gersh, MR: Electrotherapy in Rehabilitation, FA Davis, Philadelphia, 1992.
3. Rippe, B and Grega, GJ: Effects of Iso prenaline and cooling on histamine induced changes of capillary permeability in the rat hindquarter vascular bed. Acta Physiol Scand 103:252, 1978.
4. Knight, KL: Cryotherapy: Theory, Technique and Physiology. Chattanooga Corporation Education Division, Chattanooga, TN, 1985, p 15.
5. Basur, R, Shephard, E, and Mouzos, G: A cooling method in the treatment of ankle sprains. Practitioner 216:708, 1976.
6. Moore, CD and Cardea, JA: Vascular changes in leg trauma. Surg Forum 70:1285, 1977.
7. Farry, PJ and Prentice, NG: Ice treatment of injured ligaments: An experimental model. New Zealand Medical Journal 9:12, 1980.
8. Benson, TB and Copp, EP: The effects of therapeutic forms of heat and ice on the pain threshold of normal shoulder. Rheumatol Rehabil 13:101, 1974.
9. Gammon, GD and Starr, I: Studies on the relief of pain by counter-irritation. J Clin Invest 20:13, 1941.
10. Belitsky, RB, Odam, SJ, and Hubley-Kezey, C: Evaluation of the effectiveness of wet ice, dry ice, and Cryogen packs in reducing skin temperature. Phys Ther 67:1080, 1987.
11. Wright, V and Johns, RJ: Physical factors concerned with the stiffness of normal and diseased joints. Bull Johns Hopkins Hosp 106:215, 1960.
12. Perkins, J, et al: Cooling and contraction of smooth muscle. Am J Physiol 163:14, 1950.
13. Lundgren, C, Muren, A, and Zederfeldt, B: Effect of cold vasoconstriction in wound healing in the rabbit. Acta Chir Scand 118:1, 1959.
14. Collins, K, Storey, M, and Peterson, K: Peroneal nerve palsy after cryotherapy. The Physician and Sports Medicine 14:105, 1986.
15. Drez, D, Faust, DC, and Evans, JP: Cryotherapy and nerve palsy. Am J Sports Med 9:256, 1981.
16. Abramson, DI, et al: Changes in blood flow, oxygen uptake and tissue temperature produced by the topical application of wet heat. Arch Phys Med Rehabil 42:305, 1961.
17. Warren, CG, Lehmann JF, and Koblanski, JN: Heat and stretch procedures: An evaluation using rat tail tendon. Arch Phys Med Rehabil 57:122, 1976.
18. Gersten, JW: Effect of ultrasound on tendon extensibility. Am J Phys Med 34:362, 1955.
19. Lehmann, JF, et al: Effect of therapeutic temperatures on tendon extensibility. Arch Phys Med Rehabil 51:481, 1970.
20. Borrell, RM, et al: Comparison of in vivo temperatures produced by hydrotherapy, paraffin wax treatment and Fluidotherapy. Phys Ther 60:1273, 1980.
21. Gersten, JW: Temperature rise of various tissues in the dog on exposure to ultrasound at different frequencies. Arch Phys Med Rehabil 40:187, 1959.
22. Head, MD and Helms, PA: Paraffin and sustained stretching in the treatment of burn contractures. Burns 4:136, 1977.
23. Toomey, R, Grief-Schwartz, R, and Piper, MC: Clinical evaluation of the effects of whirlpool on patients with Colles' fractures. Physiotherapy Canada 38:280, 1986.
24. Hoyrup, G and Kjorvel, L: Comparison of whirlpool and wax treatments for hand therapy. Physiotherapy Canada 38:79, 1986.
25. Abramson, DI: Physiologic basis for the use of physical agents in peripheral vascular disorders. Arch Phys Med Rehabil 46:216, 1965.
26. Dyson, M: Role of ultrasound in wound healing. In Kloth, LC, McCulloch, JM, and Feedar, JA: Wound Healing Alternatives in Management. FA Davis, Philadelphia, 1990, pp 259–285.
27. Ziskin, MC, McDiarmid, T, and Michlovitz, SL: Therapeutic ultrasound. In Michlovitz, SL (ed): Thermal Agents in Rehabilitation, ed 2. FA Davis, Philadelphia, 1990.
28. Lehmann, JF, et al: Heating of joint structures by ultrasound. Arch Phys Med Rehabil 49:28, 1968.

29. Lehmann, JF, et al: Heating produced by ultrasound in bone and soft tissue. Arch Phys Med Rehabil 48:397, 1967.
30. Williams, AR, et al: Effects of MHz ultrasound on electrical pain threshold perception in humans. Ultrasound in Medicine and Biology 13:249, 1987.
31. Hogan, RD, Burke, KM, and Franklin, TD: The effect of ultrasound on microvascular hemodynamics in skeletal muscle: Effects during ischemic. Microvasc Res 23:370, 1982.
32. Harvey, W, et al: The stimulation of protein synthesis in human fibroblasts by therapeutic ultrasound. Rheumatol Rehabil 14:237, 1975.
33. Dyson, M, et al: The stimulation of tissue regeneration by means of ultrasound. Clin Sci 35:273, 1968.
34. Portwood, MM, Lieberman, SS, and Taylor, RG: Ultrasound treatment of reflex sympathetic dystrophy. Arch Phys Med Rehabil 68:116, 1987.
35. Reid, DC and Cummings, GE: Factors in selecting the dosage of ultrasound with particular reference to the use of various coupling agents. Physiotherapy Canada 63:255, 1973.
36. Fyfe, MC and Chahl, LA: The effect of single or repeated applications of "therapeutic" ultrasound on plasma extravasation during silver nitrate induced inflammation of the rat hindpaw ankle joint "in vivo." Ultrasound in Medicine and Biology 11:273, 1985.
37. El Hag, M, et al: The anti-inflammatory effects of dexamethasone and therapeutic ultrasound in oral surgery. Br J Oral Maxillofac Surg 23:17, 1985.
38. Binder, A, et al: Is therapeutic ultrasound effective in treating soft tissue lesions? Br Med J 290:512, 1985.
39. Lundeberg, T, Abrahansson, P, and Haker, E: A comparative study of continuous ultrasound, placebo ultrasound and rest in epicondylalgia. Scand J Rehabil Med 20:99, 1988.
40. Cameron, MH and Monroe, LG: Relative transmission of ultrasound by media customarily used for phonophoresis. Phys Ther 72:142, 1992.
41. Halle, JS, Franklin, RJ, and Karalfa, BL: Comparison in four treatment approaches for lateral epicondylitis of the elbow. Journal of Orthopaedic and Sports Physical Therapy 8:62, 1986.
42. Stratford, PW, et al: The evaluation of phonophoresis and friction massage as treatments for extensor carpi radialis tendinitis: A randomized controlled trial. Physiotherapy Canada 41:93, 1989.
43. Dyson, M and Suckling, J: Stimulation of tissue repair by ultrasound: A survey of mechanisms involved. Physiotherapy 64:105, 1978.
44. Roche, C and West, J: A controlled trial investigating the effect of ultrasound on venous ulcers referred from general practitioners. Physiotherapy 70:475, 1984.
45. Roberts, M, Rutherford, JH, and Harris, D: The effect of ultrasound on flexor tendon repairs in the rabbit. Hand 14:17, 1982.
46. Enwemeka, CS: The effects of therapeutic ultrasound on tendon healing. Am J Phys Med Rehabil 68:283, 1989.
47. Turner, SM, Powell, ES, and Ng, CSS: Effect of ultrasound on the healing of cockeral tendon: Is collagen cross-linkage a factor? J Hand Surg 14B:428, 1989.
48. Stevenson, JH, et al: Functional, mechanical, and biochemical assessment of ultrasound therapy on tendon healing in the chicken toe. Plast Reconstr Surg 77:965, 1986.
49. Dyson, M, et al: The production of blood cell statis and endothelial damage in the blood vessels of chick embryos treated with ultrasound in a stationary wave field. Ultrasound Med Biol 11:133, 1974.
50. Zarod, AP and Williams, AR: Platelet aggregation in vivo by therapeutic ultrasound. Lancet 1:1266, 1977.
51. Lehmann, JF and deLateur, BJ: Therapeutic heat. In Lehmann, JF (ed): Therapeutic Heat and Cold, ed 4. Williams & Wilkins, Baltimore, 1990.
52. Report of Electrotherapy Standards Committee, Section on Clinical Electrophysiology of APTA. Electrotherapeutic Terminology in Physical Therapy, Section on Clinical Electrophysiology and American Physical Therapy Association, Alexandria, VA, 1990.
53. Melzack, R and Wall, P: Pain mechanism: A new theory. Science 150:971, 1965.
54. Sjolund, BH and Eriksson, MBE: Endorphines and analgesia produced by peripheral conditioning stimulation. Advances in Pain Research and Therapy 3:587, 1979.
55. Freeman, TB, Campbell, JN, and Long, DM: Naloxone does not affect pain relief induced by electrical stimulation in man. Pain 17:189, 1983.
56. Jette, DU: Effect of different forms of transcutaneous electrical nerve stimulation on experimental pain. Phys Ther 66:187, 1986.
57. Eriksson, MBE, Sjolund, BH, and Nielzen S: Long-term results of peripheral conditioning stimulation as an analgesic measure in chronic pain. Pain 6:335, 1979.
58. Melzack, R: Prolonged relief of pain by brief, intense transcutaneous somatic stimulation. Pain 1:357, 1975.
59. Eriksson, M and Sjolund, B: Acupuncture-like electroanalgesia in TNS-resistant chronic pain. Zotterman, Y (ed): Sensory Functions of the Skin. Pergamon Press, Oxford, 1976, p 575.
60. Berlant, S: Methods of determining optimal stimulation sites for transcutaneous electrical nerve stimulation. Phys Ther 64:924, 1984.
61. Waisbrod, H, et al: Direct nerve stimulation for painful peripheral neuropathies. Journal of Bone and Joint Surgery (Br) 67:470, 1985.
62. Mannheimer, JS: Electrode placement for transcutaneous electrical stimulation. Phys Ther 58:1455, 1978.

63. Hansson, P and Ekblom, A: Pain. Elsevier Biomedical Press, London, 1983, p 157.
64. Wolf, SL and Gersh, MR: Applications of transcutaneous electrical nerve stimulation in the management of patients with pain. Phys Ther 65:314, 1985.
65. Quinton, DN, Sloan, JP, and Theakstone, J: Transcutaneous electrical nerve stimulation in acute hand infections. J Hand Surg 12B:267, 1987.
66. Levy, A, et al: Transcutaneous electrical nerve stimulation in experimental acute arthritis. Arch Phys Med Rehabil 68:75, 1987.
67. Kumar, VN and Redford, JB: Transcutaneous nerve stimulation in rheumatoid arthritis. Arch Phys Med Rehabil 63:595, 1982.
68. Baker, L and Parker, K: Neuromuscular electrical stimulation of the muscles surrounding the shoulder. Phys Ther 66:1930, 1986.
69. Kramer, J and Mendryk, S: Electrical stimulation as a strength improvement technique: A review. Journal of Orthopedic and Sports Physical Therapy 4:91, 1982.
70. McMiken, D, Todd-Smith, M, and Thompson, C: Strengthening of human quadriceps muscles by cutaneous electrical stimulation. Scand J Rehabil Med 15:25, 1983.
71. Kramer, J and Semple, J: Comparison of selected strengthening techniques for normal quadriceps. Physiotherapy Canada 35:300, 1983.
72. Moritani, T and DeVries, HA: Neural factors vs. hypertrophy in the time course of muscle strength gain. Am J Phys Med 58:115, 1979.
73. Baker, L: Aspects of muscle strengthening using neuromuscular electrical stimulation. Transcript of seminar, Annual Conference of the APTA, Las Vegas, June 20, 1984.
74. Stanish, W, et al: The effects of immobilization and of electrical stimulation on muscle glycogen and myofibrillar ATPase. Can J Appl Sport Sci 9:267, 1982.
75. Michlovitz, S: Protocol: Neuromuscular electrical stimulation for wrist rehabilitation patient. 3M Company, St Paul, 1985.
76. Herbison, GJ Teng, C, and Gordon, EE: Electric stimulation of re-innervating rat muscle. Arch Phys Med Rehabil 54:156, 1973.
77. Im, MJ, Lee, WPA, and Hoopes, JE: Effect of electrical stimulation on survival of skin flaps in pigs. Phys Ther 70:37, 1990.
78. Thurman, BF and Christian, E: Response of a serious circulation lesion to electrical stimulation: A case report. Phys Ther 51:1107, 1971.
79. Rowley, B: Electrical current effects on E. coli growth rates. Proc Soc Exp Biol Med 139:929, 1977.
80. Barranco, S and Berger, T: In vitro effect of weak direct current on Staphylococcus aureus. Clin Orthop 100:250, 1974.
81. Guffey, SJ and Asmussen, MD: In vitro bactericidal effects of high voltage current vs. direct current against Staphylococcus aureus. J of Clin Elect 1(1):5, 1989.
82. Becker, R: The direct current control system: A link between environment and organism. NY State J Med 62:1169, 1962.
83. Harrington, DB, Meyer, R, and Klein, RM: Effects of small amounts of electrical current at the cellular level. Ann NY Acad Sci 238:300, 1974.
84. Im, MJ, Lee, WPA, and Hoopes, JE: Effect of electrical stimulation on survival of skin flaps in pigs. Phys Ther 70:37, 1990.
85. Kloth, LC and Feedar, JA: Acceleration of wound healing with high voltage, monophasic, pulsed current. Phys Ther 68:503, 1988.

CHAPTER 9

Splinting—A Problem-Solving Approach

Karen Schultz-Johnson, MS, OTR, CVE, CHT

Therapists learning to splint the pathologic hand frequently ask, "What splint do I use with a specific problem or diagnosis?" The answer "No one splint solution exists for any one diagnosis; no protocol or recipe will tell you what to fabricate . . ." often creates frustration and confusion. The splintmaker-in-training invariably wonders, "Then how will I know what to make?"

Therapists developing splinting skills have needed a problem-solving guide. Consistent with the theme of this text, this chapter outlines the thinking process involved in designing and fabricating a splint. Excellent texts already exist in the biomechanics of splinting.[1-4] This chapter cites these references in a review of the basic splinting principles but does not attempt to reiterate their contents fully.

The objectives of this chapter are to conduct the reader through the problem-solving process with a series of questions:

1. What is the etiology and nature of the diagnosis?
2. What are the implications of the diagnosis?
3. What problems exist in the hand?
4. Which of these problems are amenable to splinting?
5. Which splinting approach will best resolve these problems?
6. Which splint corresponds to the patient's individual needs?
7. How many joints need the splint immobilize?
8. What shall be the surface of splint-skin contact?
9. Which material is optimal for splint-base fabrication?
10. How is the splint secured to the patient?
11. Is splint padding indicated and which material is optimal?
12. When applying force to tissue, what is the optimal degree of force and how should I apply it?
13. What will be the frequency and duration of splint wear?

Each of these questions generates other associated questions. The reader may feel surprised at the number of queries one must answer before designing a splint. However, without considering these many issues, the splint cannot meet its goals. Even when the physician has prescribed a specific splint, the person who makes it and places it on the patient must take responsibility for reviewing the physician's recommendation. With their experience and constant review of the literature, therapists working in hand rehabilitation can offer important insight to the physician.

DATA-GATHERING PHASE

"Form follows function." This famous phrase is as true in splint design as in all other aspects of the design world. The splintmaker-in-training wants to know what to make—what *form* the splint must take. When he or she knows the *function* the splint must accomplish, the answer to the question of form becomes more clear. The first six questions listed here constitute the data-gathering phase of splint problem solving. The answers to these questions lead the clinician to a knowledge of the function—the purpose and goal—of the splint.

Clarification of the Diagnosis

WHAT IS THE DIAGNOSIS?

Even before tackling the challenge of splint design, the fabricator must know the presenting pathology. Unfortunately, therapists sometimes find themselves in clinical situations without an adequate diagnosis written on the prescription. When the therapist and physician work in close proximity, the therapist can personally review the medical record, radiographs, and operative report. When these information sources are not readily available, the therapist must call the referring physician. If the physician is not available, the office nurse or secretary may read the diagnosis from the chart or operative report or both. One hand rehabilitation clinic achieved a successful resolution to this recurring problem when it arranged to have *all* operative reports sent directly to the clinic from the physician's office. The therapist should pursue all avenues to learn the diagnosis.

To foster better communication, the therapist should orient each referring physician to the type of information required on the written splint referral. This information includes, but is not limited to

1. Diagnosis
2. Date of injury/onset/surgery
3. Type of splint
4. Goal of splint
5. Frequency and duration of splinting

When all efforts fail to divulge the diagnosis, a dilemma confronts the therapist. He or she must decide whether to defer the fabrication of the splint until further clarification becomes available or to attempt some "clinical sleuthing" to discern the diagnosis. This clinical sleuthing is actually one component of the patient evaluation that the therapist should consistently perform.

A constellation of clues and information obtained from observation and patient interview often sheds enough light to solve the mystery. The therapist should observe the wound or suture site, the configuration of the suture line, and the type of postoperative dressing applied. He or she should consider the patient's report of diagnosis, nature of pathology, and date of onset. At times, this sleuthing process provides enough information to allow the fabrication of, at least, a conservative splint. However, without adequate information, the treating therapist should defer treatment.

Diagnostic Implications

WHAT ARE THE IMPLICATIONS OF THIS DIAGNOSIS?

The hand is a complex organ. Because of the hand's special characteristics and its response to injury, the specialties of hand surgery and hand rehabilitation have evolved. The hand has many structures and systems in proximity to each other which require independent movement and excursions, yet are interdependent. Thus, injury to the hand rarely affects only one system. Coupling the etiology and duration of the pathology with knowledge of anatomy, kinesiology, and biomechanics, the therapist identifies the affected systems and structures.

WHAT TISSUES ARE INVOLVED?

With a diagnosis of acute metacarpal fracture and an etiology of crush injury, the potential associated lesions in addition to the identified fracture include injury to (1) adjacent muscle (interossei and lumbrical), (2) veins, (3) motor and sensory branches of median and ulnar nerves, (4) skin, (5) fat layer, and (6) fascia, as well as (7) laceration or adhesions of extrinsic extensor and/or flexor tendons. These lesions may result in complications such as decreased active metacarpophalangeal joint (MCP) and interphalangeal joint (IP) extension, limited individual joint or composite MCP and IP extension, decreased active MCP and IP flexion, loss of passive intermetacarpal and carpometacarpal joint (CMC) motion, loss of passive MCP flexion, loss of sensation, edema, infection, and decreased tolerance to cold.

HOW DO THESE TISSUES RELATE TO SURROUNDING TISSUES?

The diagnosis of "3 days post repair of ring finger flexor digitorum profundus (FDP)" illustrates the importance of understanding how the injured tissue relates to surrounding tissue and knowing the duration of the pathology. This injury requires immobilization of all three joints of the injured finger and those of at least the two adjacent fingers because of the "one muscle belly — four tendon," or quadriga,* effect. The profundus muscle has only one muscle belly with four tendons attached to it — one for the distal interphalangeal joint (DIP) of each finger. When the profundus muscle contracts, it pulls upon all four tendons.[5] Thus, when a person wishes to bend the DIP of *one* digit, *all* DIPs flex and *all* of the profundus tendons are under tension. In addition, "electromyographic studies have shown that in simple finger flexion from a

---

*"Quadriga" is Latin for "four reins"; it is used to describe the profundus muscle tendon unit by referring to the charioteer who had control of the four reins to his four horses.[7]

position of extension, the primary flexor is the flexor digitorum profundus."[6] As a result of these two characteristics of the profundus muscle-tendon system, a patient's attempt to flex the small or middle finger DIP could result in rupture of the newly repaired ring finger FDP.

HOW DID THIS PATHOLOGY OCCUR?

Knowledge of the mechanism of injury augments the diagnosis and it may shed light on symptoms and signs that may not appear to coexist logically with a given diagnosis. The example of a patient post middle finger tip amputation illustrates this point.

Because the patient presented with diffuse redness, swelling, and pain that was out of proportion for her diagnosis, the treatment team suspected reflex sympathetic dystrophy (RSD). The splinting aspect of the treatment plan had focused on finger protection and on gently increasing passive range of motion (PROM). Investigating the injury's circumstances, one therapist learned that the patient's hand had been forced downward during the injury. The therapist suspected a carpal fracture, which was confirmed by a subsequent radiograph. Upon receiving a circumferential wrist immobilization splint, the patient's symptoms subsided.

Attempting to fit a patient with a splint without knowledge of (1) which tissues are involved, (2) the relationship of injured tissues to surrounding tissues, and (3) the etiology and duration of the pathology can have unfortunate results. These include worsening of the patient's condition and undoing the efforts of an operative procedure. To create the appropriate splint, the clinician must thoroughly comprehend the diagnosis and its implications.

Problem Identification

WHAT PROBLEMS EXIST IN THIS HAND?

With the diagnosis and its implications clearly in mind, the therapist next identifies the problems present in the hand. Problem identification involves both the collection of data and data interpretation. Data collection requires an assessment of one or more of the following: (1) range of motion (ROM), (2) strength, (3) sensation, (4) tendon status, (5) skin status, (6) scar quality, (7) edema, (8) joint integrity, (9) change in tissue length, and (10) the patient's experience of pain. Whenever possible, the assessment consists of objective measurements. Subjective assessment via observation of the part or via results of performance tests, such as Finklestein's test for de Quervain's tendonitis, supplements the objective measurements. The therapist must be certain to employ assessment techniques which are appropriate to the acuity of the patient. The initial assessment of the hand establishes a baseline with which the clinician compares all subsequent measurements.[8]

The collection of information without its interpretation leads to the failure to identify critical problems. Assessment interpretation enables the therapist to: (1) determine the current problem or combination of problems (problem set), (2) determine the possible problems the extremity could experience in the future, (3) estimate the rehabilitation potential of the injured hand, (4) evaluate patient progress, (5) provide incentives to the patient, and, importantly, (6) monitor the effectiveness of the splinting regimen.

Upon performing a goniometric evaluation, the clinician may find normal passive but limited active motion. Simply recording the numbers has no value. The therapist must go a step farther to determine the reason for the difference in passive and active motion such as tendon adhesions or muscle weakness. Pairing appropriate data gathering with knowledge-based interpretation produces accurate problem identification.

The omission of an evaluation will frequently result in a time-consuming effort to redo the splint. Unfortunately, neglecting to perform an evaluation can have even more serious consequences. For example, failing to check the patient's sensory status, the clinician would not note a sensory loss. The result could be a splint design and instructions to the patient about the splint that do not take sensory compromise into consideration. This could lead to skin breakdown and possibly infection.

The therapist should remember that often a few quick measurements will provide the essential information. Brand[9] reminds us, "Measure what is relevant and measure it with precision." In some few instances, the information gleaned from the physician's report of diagnosis, from the patient interview, and from patient observation suffice to establish the current problem set.

Table 9–1 identifies the problems that frequently confront the therapist and breaks them into problem sets. This division of problem identification will help the splintmaker along the road on the "splint problem-solving map."

TABLE 9–1 Problem Sets

Problem Set I: Tissue Status

Are all tissues in continuity?
Will active motion, passive motion, or the engagement of resistance jeopardize tissue continuity?
Are all tissues of normal length, strength, and density?
Is inflammation present?

Problem Set II: Components of Function

Is active motion normal? If not, why not?
Is passive motion normal? If not, why not?
Is strength normal? If not, why not?
Is sensation normal? If not, why not?

Problem Set III: Scar

Is the scar soft and supple?
Is the scar much higher than the surrounding skin?
Does the observable scar move when the tendon beneath it moves?
Are the superficial and deep scars long enough to allow normal motion?
Is the deep scar too attenuated to allow normal motion?

Problem Set IV: Pain

Does the patient experience pain in conjunction with this pathology that compromises function or treatment compliance?

Problem Set V: Function

Can this patient perform ADLs?
Is the patient's ability to prehend and manipulate objects affected?
Is the patient's fine or gross coordination affected?

Purpose of the Splint

Armed with the outline of the comprehensive problem set, the therapist faces the challenge of identifying the problems that splinting can mitigate or solve. The foundation for this determination is the therapist's comprehension of: (1) normal hand balance, (2) the biologic basis of both wound healing, and (3) tissue's response to stress. The therapist must fully grasp the mechanism producing the problem; this understanding prevents the fabrication of inappropriate splints or the setting of unrealistic expectations.

Comprehension of the mechanism also aids in prioritizing problems. In a thorough treatment plan, the therapist incorporates the short- and long-term goals of splinting. Ideally, the therapist envisions not only the original splint but also, when appropriate, the sequential splints that the patient will use on the way to optimum results.

To identify the problems appropriate for splinting, the therapist must be familiar with the *general* purposes of splinting.[10]

1. Prevent deformity—maintain normal tissue length, balance, and excursion
2. Immobilize/stabilize
3. Protect
4. Correct deformity or dysfunction—reestablish normal tissue length, balance, and excursion
5. Control/modify scar formation
6. Substitute for dysfunctional tissue
7. Exercise

Consider the patient with longstanding rheumatoid arthritis who presents with severe ulnar deviation and subluxation of the MCP joints. Observing the deformity, the therapist may propose fabricating a splint to position the MCPs more anatomically. In this patient, the disease process has destroyed the integrity of the MCP joint capsule and ligaments. Understanding this fact, the therapist considers the goal of the splint.

Can the splint reestablish the integrity of the joint capsule and ligaments and so correct the deformity? Unfortunately, the splint cannot accomplish this goal. However, some patients find that stabilization of the fingers in a more anatomic position enhances function or minimizes pain or both. Function enhancement and pain reduction via stabilization are appropriate purposes for this splint. The therapist should not splint the arthritic patient for whom the splint interferes with function and does not reduce pain.

In the face of complex pathology, the therapist must also determine which problems receive priority treatment. For example, in the diffusely stiff hand, all joints may lack both passive flexion and extension. Because of their special anatomy and kinesiology, passive MCP flexion and IP extension are the most difficult motions to reestablish in the hand. In contrast, the hand more readily regains passive MCP extension and IP flexion. Without the timely and intensely focused efforts of the therapist and patient, these joints will never regain full motion even when subjected to further surgery.

The hand may require a series of splints to realize the optimal result. The typical MCP arthroplasty illustrates this point well. Initially, the therapist fits the arthroplasty patient with a dynamic MCP extension splint. As the case progresses, the therapist may note rotation of the digits and add derotation components to the splint. If MCP flexion does not progress to the optimal arc via exercise alone, the therapist adds an MCP flexion assist. When the dynamic extension assist splint is discontinued, the patient leaves the hand free for function and exercise during the day but wears a static resting splint during sleep. By positioning the hand to preserve the alignment achieved in surgery, the patient may wear this splint for up to a year or even longer after the operation. If the patient still lacks significant MCP flexion, the therapist may recommend wearing the flexion assist during the day for several weeks. Monitoring ROM and alignment as the MCP joint encapsulation process proceeds, the therapist responds to the hand's needs for a sequence of appropriately timed and designed splints.

Splint Approach

WHAT TYPE OF SPLINT WILL BEST ACHIEVE THIS PURPOSE?

The purpose of the splint indicates whether a static, serial static, drop-out, articulated, dynamic, or static-progressive splint will best serve the patient (Table 9 – 2). Other factors, such as the characteristics of the patient (see next section), also have an impact on the splinting approach. The therapist may also find that a combination of approaches will achieve results most rapidly or efficiently or both.

Static splints have no movable parts and maintain joints in one position. They can place tissues in a "stressless" state to promote healing and minimize friction. When holding structures at the end of available elongation, static splints may generate tissue tension (Fig. 9 – 1).

Drop-out splints block joint motion in one direction but allow motion in another. In this way, the patient may use active motion to help resolve a passive limitation but cannot regress to a previous posture. Commonly used on elbow flexion contractures, the drop-out splint prevents elbow flexion but allows the triceps to contract to increase ROM in extension (Fig. 9 – 2).

Articulated splints contain at least two static components and are connected in such a way as to allow motion in one plane at a joint. Some articulating components allow the therapist to limit motion at the ends of the movement arc so that the patient can use a specific arc of motion (Fig. 9 – 3).

Dynamic splints have self-adjusting resilient or elastic components such as spring wire, rubberbands, or springs that create "a mobilizing force on a segment, resulting in passive or passive-assisted motion of a joint or successive joints."[11] In addition, dynamic splints often allow active-resisted motion in the direction opposite of their line of pull. The dynamic splint may exert tension upon one or more anatomic structures. The dynamic tension generated continues even when the shortened tissue reaches the end of its elastic limit (Fig. 9 – 4).

Static-progressive splinting involves the use of inelastic components such as hook-and-loop (Velcro) tapes, dacron line, progressive hinges, turnbuckles, and screws. These components allow progressive changes in joint position as PROM changes without changing the structure of the splint. A static-progressive splint holds shortened tissue at its maximum length. Because the components lack the resilience or elasticity of those used in dynamic splinting, the appropriately set tension of the splint does not continue to stress tissue beyond its elastic limit (Fig. 9 – 5).

Serial static splinting differs from static-progressive splinting. Serial static splints require the therapist to remold the splint to accommodate increases in mobility. Nonremovable, circumferential serial static splints require no cooperation from the wearer except to leave them on. Thus, compliance is usually 100%. Serial casting of proximal

TABLE 9−2 Indications for Splint Approaches

Static

Immobilization:
  To minimize inflammation
  To promote vascularization of skin or bone grafts
Protection for healing bone
Protection for newly repaired structures
Position:
  To shorten or lengthen scar
  To gain mechanical advantage of a given joint
  To support a painful, arthritic joint for function
Pressure on scar for softening and bulk reduction

Serial Static

Decrease PROM limitation with hard "end feel" when therapist wants to maximize control of
  forces generated
Lengthen adhesions

Static-Progressive

Decrease PROM limitation with hard "end feel"—therapist has option of allowing patient to
  have control over forces generated or of maintaining control over forces
Lengthen adhesions

Drop-out

Decrease PROM limitation when active motion can assist in improving PROM

Articulated

Allow motion of joint in one plane while protecting:
  Bone proximally and distally
  Joint capsule and ligaments in the perpendicular plane
Provide specific arc of motion at a joint especially for ligament avulsion fractures

Dynamic

Decrease PROM limitation with soft "end feel"
Substitute for weak or denervated musculature
Provide strengthening of specific muscles while controlling:
  Proximal joints
  Length of muscle tendon unit during contraction
  Force magnitude
  Line of pull
Lengthen adhesions proximally and distally
Provide controlled excursion of healing tendons

---

interphalangeal joints (PIPs) and serial wrist cock-up splints exemplify serial static splinting (Fig. 9−6).

These choices challenge the clinician to choose the one that best serves the patient. While the indications for drop-out and articulated splints are generally apparent, the choice between dynamic splinting and one of the static approaches is often less clear. A full appreciation of the benefits and limitations of each option will assist the therapist in making the final decision.

Consistent motion benefits the hand patient in many ways, including preventing adhesions from shortening or becoming more dense, promoting nourishment of carti-

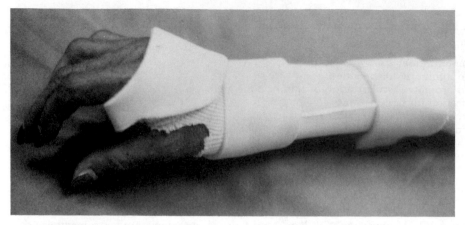

FIGURE 9-1. Palmarly based, static, wrist cock-up splint.

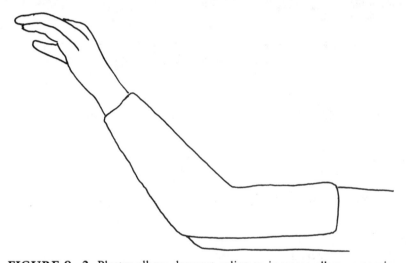

FIGURE 9-2. Plaster elbow dropout splint to increase elbow extension.

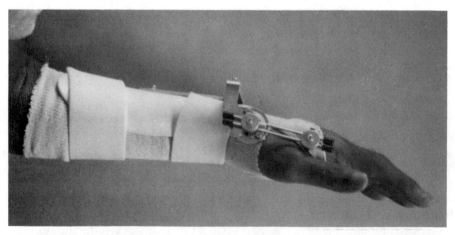

FIGURE 9-3. Articulated wrist splint combines a circumferential palmar portion and a dorsally based forearm portion.

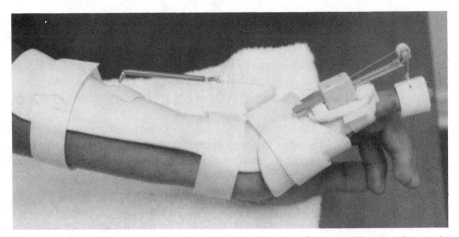

FIGURE 9–4. Dorsal, dynamic splint designed following flexor tendon repair to place the flexor muscle-tendon unit at maximum length. This position optimally directs active flexion exercise force at the tendon adhesion to lengthen the adhesions and maximize active range of motion.

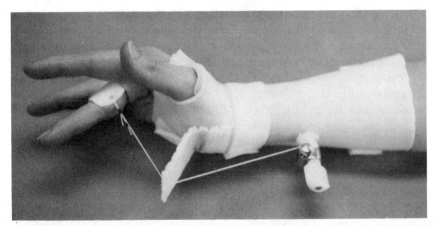

FIGURE 9–5. Circumferential, static-progressive splint to increase passive MCP flexion.

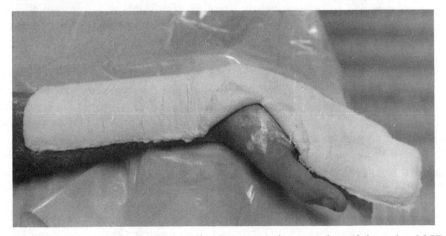

FIGURE 9–6. Plaster slab, serial static splint for composite extension of the wrist, MCPs, and IPs.

lage and minimizing edema. Importantly, a mobile part is one that can more readily participate in function. Dynamic splinting is the approach of choice when muscle imbalance impairs normal hand function but an entirely static splint prevents any hand use. Dynamic splinting of a radial nerve palsy demonstrates this last principle well. The dynamic splint can also provide a special environment for exercising the hand. When these considerations come to the forefront of patient management, the therapist must choose dynamic splinting.

Many therapists have found serial static, and static-progressive splinting to be the technique of choice when faced with PROM limitations. Fess and Phillips state that "application of a small constant force has been shown to be much more beneficial than the intermittent application of large forces."[12] In most cases, low torque load over long periods of time effectively resolves PROM limitation.[13] Describing the benefits of serial plaster casting of joint contractures, Bell-Krotoski states, "the gentle positioning of contracted soft tissue at the end of its elastic limit by the use of plaster casting has a real advantage over 'dynamic splinting,' which supplies intermittent positioning of the contracted soft tissue."[14] Thus, key elements to reducing a PROM limitation include *high time doses* of *low, low load* adequate to *position the shortened tissue at or near the end of its elastic limit.*

Clinical experience consistently demonstrates that patients tolerate static splinting better than dynamic. Static splinting may be the only type of splint a patient will be able to wear while sleeping because the static approach avoids taking the contracted tissue beyond its elastic limit. The resilient force component of the dynamic splint exerts a force that does not stop when the tissue reaches its elastic limit; microtrauma to the tissue will result if the patient keeps the splint on. Thus, static splinting offers the required dose of time required to effect a PROM change.

Because of the difficulty tolerating multiple-hour doses of dynamic splinting, this approach becomes characteristically intermittent. In addition, dynamic splints offer the wearer the opportunity to remove stress from the affected tissue, to position it on slack, so that the splint never delivers the adequate dose of end range time. Considering the aforementioned information, the therapist should always choose static splinting for passive limitations. Yet, clinically, dynamic splints do sometimes achieve the sought-after PROM change. How can this be?

Assessment of torque angle – range of motion — the quantification of the amount of torque force required to gain a certain amount of PROM at a joint — will help the therapist decide what type of splint will resolve PROM limitations. If a joint requires a significant amount of torque in order to gain maximum PROM and has a rapidly rising slope when plotted (as that on the right in Fig. 9 – 7), then the joint will have a hard end feel and serial static or static-progressive splinting will probably be the only means to increase PROM. However, if a joint requires only a low amount of torque to gain maximum PROM and a slowly rising slope (as on the left in Fig. 9 – 7), then the joint will have a soft or springy end feel and dynamic splinting will probably offer a satisfactory, although more time-intensive, result.

The slowly rising slope, the joint with the soft end feel, is indicative of either (1) relatively young scar tissue that has not yet formed significant cross-linking; or (2) a situation in which transient physiologic changes such as swelling or malnourished cartilage have produced the contracture and the body has not yet proceeded to absorb cells required for normal ROM.[14] The rapidly rising slope, the joint with a hard end feel, indicates (1) mature scar tissue with advanced cross-linking, (2) the presence of a "check rein,"[14] or (3) the absorption of tissue required for normal passive motion (as in a PIP flexion contracture when the body absorbs volar skin and joint capsule).

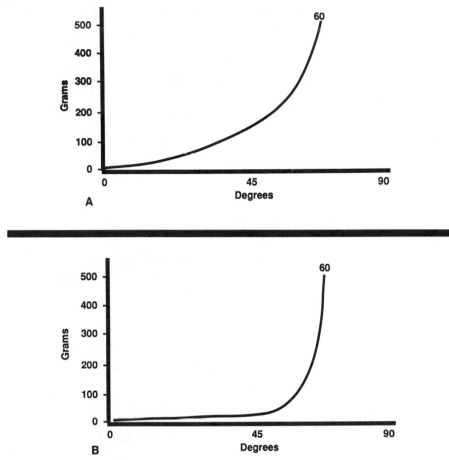

FIGURE 9–7. *A*, The joint with the torque-angle curve has a slowly rising slope and will have a soft end feel. Many types of splinting can resolve the soft limitation. *B*, The joint with the torque-angle curve has a rapidly rising slope indicative of a hard end feel. This joint requires either serial static or static-progressive splinting to resolve the PROM limitation.

Static approaches to PROM limitations will offer the fastest results without additional tissue trauma. However, when optimal results require tissue excursion and the joint limitation feels soft, dynamic splinting embodies the best solution. The analysis of the duration and nature of the contracture coupled with the information gained from torque angle ROM measurements will help the therapist select the appropriate splint.

Considering the Characteristics of the Patient

HOW WILL THIS PATIENT INTERACT WITH THIS SPLINT?

The most innovative and efficient splint becomes worthless when the patient cannot or will not wear it. To maximize splint compliance, the therapist rapidly assesses the patient's physical and cognitive abilities, the patient's financial and geographic status, and the attitudinal and motivational factors. The characteristics of the patient will have an impact on choice of splinting approach, as well as the splint design and materials used in the splint. The answers to the following questions will guide the therapist to a viable splinting solution.

WHAT IS THE PATIENT'S ABILITY TO PAY FOR CARE?

In the case of the patient with few financial resources, the therapist may need to alter the splinting approach. While possibly compromising efficiency or cosmetic appeal, use of less expensive and sturdier materials will offer financial relief to the patient. The therapist may wish to focus on training the patient or family member in splint repair and adjustment to minimize return visits.

WHAT IS THE PATIENT'S ACCESSIBILITY TO A SPLINTING FACILITY?

When geography complicates the patient's care, the therapist must once again consider alternatives that allow maximum benefit from splinting while minimizing the need for return visits for adjustment or repair or both.

WILL THIS PATIENT ASSUME RESPONSIBILITY FOR COMPLIANCE?

Young children and patients with diminished cognitive status will probably require the supervision of a family member, nurse, or aide. Patients who suffer from short-term memory loss may need the splint directions written directly on the splint. To enhance the compliance of adolescents who suffer from "chronic apathy," the therapist may strive to provide an element of patient control to the splinting program and to provide cosmetic appeal to the splint.

CAN THIS PATIENT FUNCTION INDEPENDENTLY WHILE WEARING THE SPLINT?

Patients who must wear a splint continuously, such as following an MCP arthroplasty, may find that the splint compromises their ability to perform activities of daily living (ADLs). Sensitive to the patient's ADL needs, the therapist designs a splint facilitating maximum ADL independence. In many instances, a low-profile approach resolves such problems.

CAN THIS PATIENT DON AND DOFF THIS SPLINT INDEPENDENTLY?

The therapist must assess several aspects of patient function to answer this question. Of tremendous importance is the patient's ability to use the unsplinted hand. In the case of the patient with rheumatic disease or spinal cord injury, this ability may be severely impaired. Such a patient will benefit from special adaptations that allow independence in splint wear (Fig. 9–8). Complex strap-and-loop designs may prove a barrier to the patient with memory and problem-solving deficits. Without adequate perceptual skills, the patient cannot apply the splint properly to the hand.

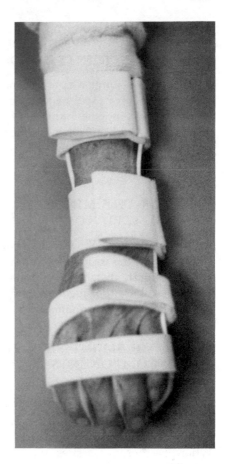

FIGURE 9–8. Splint with strap adaptations—in this case, loops—to aid donning and doffing for a patient with severe bilateral rheumatoid involvement.

CAN THE PATIENT RETURN TO GAINFUL EMPLOYMENT WITH THE SPLINT?

A work splint must meet many criteria. To minimize the reaction of workers and supervisors, the splint should be as inconspicuous as possible. The splint should be low profile and designed with a clear understanding of the hand function required for the job so as not to hinder work performance or place the worker in danger of having the splint caught in machinery. Finally, the splint must be durable enough to tolerate the stresses of the work place.

DESIGN-FABRICATION PHASE

The answers to these first six questions take the clinician to the halfway point along the course of splint problem solving. They prepare the therapist for the design-fabrication phase. In the planning and construction of a splint, the therapist translates the understanding of the needs of the patient obtained during the data-gathering phase into a three-dimensional object. With the *function* of the splint firmly established, the next seven questions help determine the *form* of the splint.

Joint Immobilization

HOW MANY JOINTS NEED THE SPLINT IMMOBILIZE?

The more joints a splint immobilizes, the more difficult hand function becomes. Thus, the therapist seeks a splint design that achieves the treatment goals of the splint while minimizing the number of joints involved. But how does one arrive at this "minimum number"? Once the therapist establishes the problem set and purpose of the splint, the answers to the following questions guide the decision about joint immobilization.

WHAT IS THE MINIMAL NUMBER OF JOINTS THAT MUST BE IMMOBILIZED TO PROVIDE SPLINT STABILITY?

This number will vary depending on the purpose and surface of application of the splint and on the traction forces involved in the splint. For example, MCP flexion splints tend to migrate distally as a product of the traction forces involved. The use of circumferential splints that incorporate the wrist and sometimes the CMC and MCP of the thumb significantly enhances the stability of this splint (see Fig. 9–5).

DOES THE SPLINT SEEK TO INCREASE PROM BY AFFECTING JOINT COMPONENTS?

When the therapist wishes to affect a specific joint and the splint exerts forces over several joints, the design must incorporate stabilization of the nontargeted joints. To illustrate this point, consider a dynamic extension outrigger based at the metacarpal level with the loop placed on the middle phalanx which seeks to exert force on the PIP. When the therapist desires isolated PIP mobilization, the splint must stabilize the MCP joint. Without MCP stabilization, the forces will be dissipated across the *two* joints — the MCP *and* the PIP. The tissue of least resistance will absorb the force. In the case of a normal MCP joint and a contracted PIP joint, the resilient tissue of the MCP joint will lengthen but the PIP will change minimally or not at all. Such a splint will fail to resolve the PIP flexion contracture and may deform and destabilize the previously normal MCP joint (Fig. 9–9).

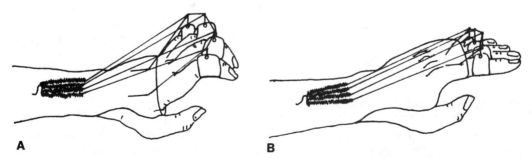

A   **B**

FIGURE 9–9. When a splint exerts forces over several joints, the design must incorporate stabilization of the nontargeted joints. *A*, With the PIP joints targeted, the splint on the left fails to stabilize the MCP joint and dissipates the force across both joints. The splint may destabilize the normal MCP and has little effect on the PIPs. *B*, This splint stabilizes the MCP and directs the force to its target, the PIP.

DOES THE SPLINT SEEK TO INCREASE PROM BY AFFECTING EXTRINSIC TISSUES?

PROM limitations due to tightness of soft tissues that cross more than one joint, such as muscle-tendon units or scar bands, require attention to the position of each joint that the targeted soft tissue crosses. Some situations necessitate the use of proximal joint stabilization while others allow the splint to exert forces across multiple joints simultaneously.

The case of injury to the extensor digitorum communis (EDC) with limited excursion of the muscle-tendon unit illustrates the situation where the splint exerts forces across multiple joints at the same time. Because the fibers of the EDC cross dorsally to the wrist, MCP, PIP, and DIP joints, shortening of the EDC results in decrease of composite passive flexion of these joints. The therapist often finds normal passive flexion of an individual joint but impairment of passive motion when flexing more than one joint simultaneously. To improve excursion and increase the ability to flex more than one joint at a time, the appropriate splint flexes two or more joints simultaneously to stress the EDC muscle-tendon unit (Fig. 9–10,A).

In contrast, the case of intrinsic tightness requires proximal joint stabilization to lengthen a target tissue that crosses more than one joint. The finger that exhibits a passive motion deficit because of intrinsic tightness requires stabilization of the MCP joint in extension while the splint gently flexes the IP joints (Fig. 9–10,B). This approach effectively increases PROM because the intrinsics pass volarly to the axis of motion of the MCP joints and dorsally to the IP joints.

The therapist must keep in mind that healing tissues cannot be stressed prior to achieving adequate tensile strength to tolerate such stress. In addition, the therapist must monitor splinted joints to avoid iatrogenic joint contractures.

DOES THE BONE REQUIRE PROTECTION?

Fracture care has undergone a revolution in recent years, and the approach to protection of healing bone will vary with the referring physician. A well-established axiom for fracture care states that immobilization of the joint above and below the fracture facilitates bone healing.[15] However, the use of a fracture brace, which circumferentially protects healing bone and allows adjacent joint motion, has demonstrated its efficacy.[16] The following factors influence the choice of the method of immobilization: (1) the type of fracture; (2) the location of the fracture; (3) whether internal fixation was used, and if so, what type; (4) the age of the fracture; (5) the age and general health of the patient; and (6) the likelihood that the patient will comply with treatment.

DO SOFT TISSUE STRUCTURES REQUIRE PROTECTION?

When injury disrupts soft tissue structures that cross one or several joints, the splint must control the motion of each crossed joint to avoid overstressing the involved tissue. When injury is to muscle-tendon units having a single muscle belly but multiple tendons (such as the FDP), the splint should also control the motion of the joints of the fingers adjacent to the injured digit.

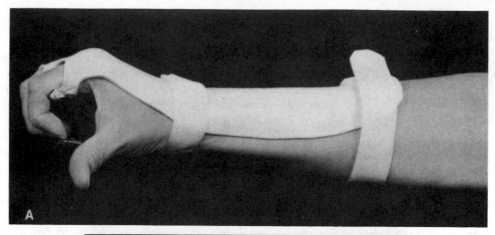

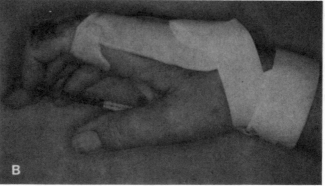

FIGURE 9–10. Splinting to resolve PROM limitations resulting from tightness of soft tissues that cross more than one joint, such as muscle-tendon units or scar bands, requires attention to the position of each joint that the targeted soft tissue crosses. Illustrating a splint to resolve *extrinsic* tightness via lengthening of the EDC, *splint A* controls the wrist position and holds the MCP in flexion while flexing the IP joints. Designed to resolve *intrinsic* tightness, *splint B* leaves the wrist essentially free and positions the MCP joint in extension. (From Fess and Phillips,[2] p 287, with permission.)

DO TREATMENT GOALS REQUIRE CONTROL OF MUSCLE-TENDON UNIT LENGTH?

Even with the continuity of the injured muscle-tendon unit secure, the control of its length can influence the patient's final result. Because muscle contraction has a much greater effect on tendon adhesions when the muscle-tendon unit is held at length, a splint maintaining this position will often be the splint of choice. An exercise splint can take advantage of muscle-tendon unit length to achieve lengthening of adhesions and optimal strengthening of weakened musculature (see Fig. 9–4).

Surface of Application

OVER WHAT SURFACE SHALL I APPLY THE BASE OF THE SPLINT?

Most commonly, splints occupy either the dorsal (see Fig. 9–4) or palmar surface (see Fig. 9–1) of the hand or arm or both. Other surface application alternatives offer yet other options for splinting. The radial "gutter" splint (Fig. 9–11) encompasses the

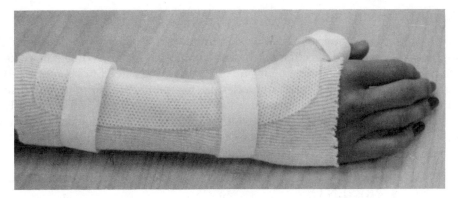

FIGURE 9–11. Radial gutter splint.

dorsal, radial, and palmar surfaces on the radial aspect of the part, and the ulnar "gutter" splint (Fig. 9–12) offers the same approach on the ulnar aspect. The circumferential splint (see Fig. 9–5), or total contact splint, provides a splint base that encloses the part.

Innovative splintmakers have combined these base designs (see Fig. 9–3) as needed to achieve their treatment goals. After deciding on the surface for splint application, the therapist also determines the amount of surface area each component of the splint base comprises. Many factors help to determine the surface of splint application. The following questions will guide the therapist to the final decision.

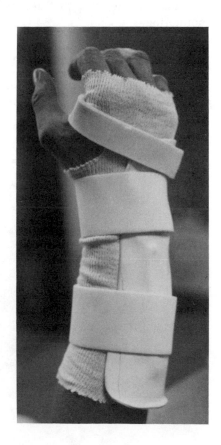

FIGURE 9–12. Ulnar gutter splint.

ARE WOUNDS PRESENT?

In the presence of open wounds or skin grafts, the therapist must consider their location and status before deciding on the surface of application. While some wounds tolerate and indeed benefit from splint pressure, others may need to be kept free from pressure, from moisture that builds up under plastic splints, and from potential splint-generated sheer forces. Close communication with the physician will help with this determination. Important to note is that wounds tolerate plaster of Paris extremely well and that circumferential plaster splints or casts can assist in wound healing.[17]

ARE PINS, BUTTONS, CASTS, EXTERNAL FIXATORS, OR OTHER APPLIANCES PRESENT?

The presence of internal and external fixation devices often requires unique splinting surface applications. The patient need not wait until the physician removes the fixation to enjoy the benefits of splinting. Thermoplastic constructions over and around casts (Fig. 9 – 13) as well as internal and external fixators can function to achieve initial treatment goals such as prevention of PROM limitation or lengthening of adhesions.

To locate the subcutaneous fixation devices, the therapist will benefit from the aid of radiographs, palpation, surgical report, and patient cooperation. The therapist must take particular care to identify the position of subcutaneous pin ends, plates, and screws because the skin adjacent to them may not tolerate splint pressure or may become sensitive to splint pressure if pin migration occurs. Splint migration may also result in skin irritation adjacent to fixation devices. Respect for possibility of pin tract infections prompts the therapist to leave all percutaneous pin sites exposed for cleaning and monitoring.

WHAT IS THE STATUS OF THE PATIENT'S SKIN?

The therapist determines if steroid use, vascular impairment, dermatitis, denervation, or other factors have compromised skin status. Because compromised skin has

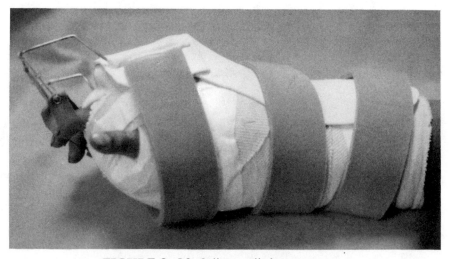

FIGURE 9–13. Splint applied over a cast.

much more difficulty tolerating pressure, the therapist may need to avoid placement of a splint over areas of impaired skin or to use techniques that optimally distribute pressure. Although atrophic skin may not tolerate splint contact from a three-point pressure splint, a circumferential or total contact splint distributes pressure and limits sheer forces enough to allow splint tolerance.[17]

Generally, palmar hand skin has more subcutaneous tissue (fat and muscle) and tolerates pressure better than dorsal hand skin. The therapist must constantly balance the need for adequate pressure distribution with the wish to minimize the amount of skin covered by a splint. Although no one likes having an arm covered in plastic and straps, a minimal contact splint is often poorly tolerated because of its poor pressure distribution.

DOES THE PATIENT HAVE PROBLEMS WITH HYPERSENSITIVITY?

Hypersensitive areas may not tolerate any pressure or sheer from a splint. As with compromised skin, the therapist may circumvent the hypersensitive area by forming a hollow over the area or by avoiding contact with the involved surface. A total contact application may distribute pressure and limit sheer enough for the patient to tolerate the splint. The use of padding, elastomers, or interfaces such as dermal pads and gel sheets may enhance the patient's splint tolerance.

DOES THE PATIENT HAVE CURRENT OR POTENTIAL PROBLEMS WITH EDEMA?

The patient may present with an obviously edematous extremity or may have a diagnosis with great potential for developing edema such as a dorsal hand laceration or wrist fracture. The dorsal or circumferential applications are optimal for minimizing formation of edema. The therapist must avoid creating edema with narrow bands of circumferential pressure and avoid creating windowpane edema by allowing spaces between straps or pieces of thermoplastic.

WHAT SURFACE OF APPLICATION WILL EASE SPLINT CONSTRUCTION?

Strategic selection of the surface of application may speed splint fabrication. When a splint base contacts bony prominences or areas with minimal subcutaneous padding, or both, the therapist must then take additional time to contour and pad the splint. Surface of application takes on greater importance when the therapist plans to use outriggers or attachments designed for a particular surface of application. For example, the attachment of a prefabricated dynamic MCP extension assist outrigger becomes impossible when the therapist has constructed a palmarly based splint. Usually, the therapist should volarly base a flexion splint, and dorsally base an extension splint.

IS SCAR PRESENT THAT AFFECTS HAND FUNCTION?

When the answer to this question is yes, the therapist considers incorporating pressure and elongating tension to the scarred areas into the splint design. Both pressure and tension modify scar.[18] The patient status after Dupuytren's release offers an excellent example. The splint for this patient should exert pressure against the palmar scar and hold the scar at the end of its available elastic length.

WILL A PARTICULAR SURFACE APPLICATION ENHANCE FUNCTION?

The palmar surface of the hand participates actively and constantly in object prehension. The ulnar aspect of the hand and forearm rest against the table when writing. The palmar surface of the hand and forearm are replete with sweat glands and require air circulation for sweat evaporation. For these reasons, the therapist should attempt to keep the palmar and ulnar surfaces of the hand and forearm free of splint materials. Unfortunately, with many splint designs, this is simply not possible. The therapist may need to develop special surface applications to allow functional use of the hand while adhering to the treatment plan and following the principles of splinting.

Splint Base Materials

WHAT MATERIALS SHALL I USE FOR THE SPLINT BASE?

Currently, therapists have a wide range of materials for splint bases from which to chose:

- High-temperature plastics
- Plaster of Paris
- Thermoplastic mesh rolls
- Metal strips and wire
- Neoprene
- Low-temperature plastics
- Fiberglass
- Leather
- Elastomer
- Fabric

Each of these categories contain several subsets. Each material has characteristics that make it more or less appropriate for a given treatment setting or a given application. With the list of materials increasing annually, the therapist must read, network, and attend workshops to maintain a high degree of familiarity with options available for splint fabrication.

Now more frequently used by orthotists than therapists, high-temperature thermoplastic possesses several desirable qualities. High-temperature thermoplastic will probably be the material of choice when the splint design remains a constant and the patient will wear the splint for the long term. The therapist will choose high-temperature thermoplastics or thicker, more rigid low-temperature thermoplastics when the patient requires splint durability and rigidity. For the patient with limited financial resources, the therapist must balance the expense of the materials against the expense of fabrication time. High-temperature thermoplastics may cost less but involve a time-consuming and therefore costly positive-negative mold-making process. A plaster splint may cost a little at the outset but may disintegrate before it has achieved its goal. Bielawski and Bear-Lehman[19] describe an excellent high-temperature wrist gauntlet splint designed for returning the injured person to work. This wrist splint offers comfort, durability, and low cost.

The therapist must carefully consider the relationship of the splint base material to the skin. When the patient's skin reacts to a given material, the therapist must seek alternatives. Sometimes, stockinette or other types of splint liners will resolve the problem. However, because so few patients react dermatologically to pure plaster of Paris, the use of this material can provide a well-tolerated splint base. Optimal ventilation of the skin occurs with plaster and highly perforated thermoplastic. However, perforations can pose obstacles to fabrication when they overstretch or become part of the splint edge. If the hand is well padded with a dressing, a mesh plastic such as Hexelite (Kirschner Medical Corp, Timonium, MD 21093) also becomes an option. However, the mesh plastics can create problems with pressure distribution and with roughness against the skin. In the presence of open wounds, plaster again provides the safest material for direct application.

With the weight of the splint as a major consideration, the therapist should consider thin thermoplastics and fabric. Orthotic weight has an impact on anyone who must wear a splint for long periods of time, and particularly on the patient who must wear one over the long term. The arthritis patient who has a lifelong partnership with a wrist support will appreciate minimal bulk and weight. The combination of fabric and a thermoplastic support offers stability and minimal weight. These splints are commercially available or can be custom fabricated.

The composition of the thermoplastic affects its properties. Should the splint design necessitate close conformity to the hand, thermoplastic with a higher plastic content becomes the material of choice. If the splint requires frequent remolding, the thermoplastics with a higher rubber content are desirable. Circumferential, univalved splint designs such as fracture braces require a flexibility that allows the patient easily to put on and take off the splint. The thermoplastic chosen for this purpose must maintain this flexibility and not crack from fatigue with repeated applications of the splint.

The therapist who makes splints without access to splint pans and heat guns must carefully choose materials. Mesh, plaster, and fiberglass rolls offer the advantage of "low-tech" application and eliminate the need for such splinting equipment. At times, the ease of strap attachment may take precedence over other issues. Fortunately, most materials bond easily to pressure-sensitive hook-and-loop tapes. However, attachment of the straps to plaster, Elastomer, or leather require more time and can challenge the ablest splintmaker.

Securing the Splint

WHAT SHALL I USE TO HOLD THE SPLINT IN PLACE?

As with base materials, therapists now have a wide range of strapping materials from which to choose. Many variations have been developed within each category:

- Hook-and-loop tapes
- Webbing
- Self-adhesive tapes
- Loop tape composites
- Ace wrap
- Elastic

Strategic strap placement ensures splint stability; the therapist must carefully check to see that the strap secures the part it is meant to secure (Fig. 9–14). The therapist

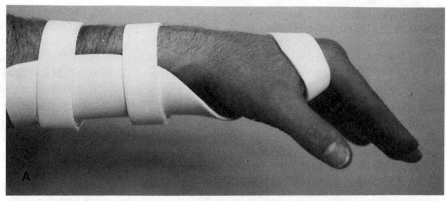

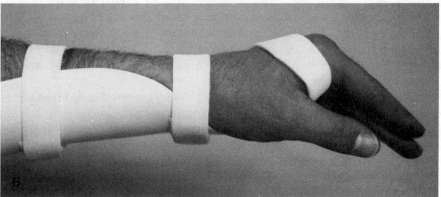

FIGURE 9–14. *A*, The hand gaps away from this splint because the wrist strap is not placed strategically at the wrist. *B*, Correct strap placement ensures proper wrist position and splint conformity.

should avoid the use of soft straps when the splint requires rigid thermoplastic pieces for stability. For example, the palmar bar of an MCP arthroplasty dynamic extension splint must be rigid to isolate the action of the finger flexors to the MCP joints and not allow wrist flexion.

The choice of strap width can significantly affect the splint. Wider straps distribute pressure, enhance splint stabilization on the arm, minimize edema formation, and provide warmth. Narrower straps may allow more joint motion and may avoid cutting into sensitive areas such as the first web space. A thick, padded strap provides more cushioning for the patient. However, the increased bulk may discourage splint wear. As many patients react to strap texture, the therapist must also take this into account. Skin that reacts to poor air exchange or heat will find relief in air-permeable strapping materials.

The number of hook-to-loop connections varies significantly with different types of loop-strapping materials. When the patient adjusts the straps frequently, the life of the loop becomes an important factor. Some loop products offer excellent pressure distribution and skin tolerance but only a short life of hook-to-loop connections. The therapist may enjoy the best of all worlds by sewing a more durable loop material to the end of the softer strapping material where contact with the hook occurs.

Attachment of the strap to the splint varies according to many variables. A circumferential strap, one that extends all the way around the splint and arm, affords better splint security than straps that span only part of the splint. With greater surface area of the hook-and-loop interface, the more secure the strap will be. When inadequate splint base surface area prevents a hook-to-loop attachment, the therapist can use rivets. Splints may also wrap onto the part with Ace wrap or self-adhesive tapes such as Coban (3M Medical-Surgical Division, St. Paul, MN 55144), thus avoiding the need for strap attachment. When elastic wraps are used, the patient must demonstrate (1) the ability to use the optimal amount of compression with the wrap and (2) understanding of precautions for compromise of circulation. Some hook-and-loop products interlock with great force and provide excellent securing of the splint. However, these can challenge even the strongest person to release the strap.

Patients with bilaterally impaired hand function benefit from strap adaptations such as loops (see Fig. 9–8) and D rings, which increase mechanical advantage and allow adapted prehension patterns for strap attachment and release.

To control costs, the therapist may have to compromise cosmesis, bulk, or comfort when choosing the strap material. The more durable loop tape tends to abrade sensitive skin. The patient may have to live with a soiled strap that still functions, rather than buying a clean replacement. Neoprene composite straps provide warmth and have long lives but take up more space underneath clothing. While minimizing the cost component, the temperature and bulk factor may make this material less desirable.

Padding

SHALL I PAD OR LINE ANY PART OF THE SPLINT? WITH WHAT?

Like splint base and strapping materials, each type of padding has unique characteristics. Familiarity with the family of padding products facilitates proper and strategic use. Each material has advantages in specific applications. Distributors' tendency to attach different trade names to identical materials complicates the therapist's effort to identify padding. The table of padding materials in Shafer's *Common Problems, Useful Solutions in Hand Rehabilitation*[20] helps the therapist cross-reference products. However, the types and names increase faster than publications can keep up with them.

Padding usually falls into the category of either closed- or open-cell. Describing the difference, Shafer states, "An open-cell material is one that will absorb fluids, whereas a closed-cell material allows fluids to roll across the surface without penetration."[20] Fabric-surfaced padding such as Alicover (Alimed, Dedham, MA 02026) and moleskin comprise another classification. The elastomers have joined the family of padding materials. Other properties such as heat formability; texture; presence of adhesive backing; and ability to adhere in water, color, thickness, and drapability distinguish padding materials. The therapist should assess the padding's ability to absorb shock, reduce shear stress, and minimize splint migration.[20]

Appropriate use of splint padding can significantly improve the comfort of splint wear. Enhancing pressure distribution, padding protects bony prominences and areas with minimal subcutaneous tissue. Unfortunately, therapists frequently add padding to the splint only after carefully forming the base to the patient. The addition of the padding takes additional room in the splint, causing the splint to fit improperly. Instead of distributing pressure, the padding actually increases the pressure problem. The use of padding to attempt to rectify poor splint fit constitutes yet another abuse of cushioning material. When the splint base conforms poorly to the patient, the therapist must accept the responsibility of remolding it.

Padding materials are available in a variety of thicknesses. Those measuring ⅛ in or less seem to function optimally for most splinting situations. Often, the splint requires only a liner such as stockinette or moleskin to interrupt an uncomfortable skin-plastic interface.

The ability to clean padding materials affects compliance with splint wear. Who can blame the patient who lacks enthusiasm for a splint that appears soiled or has an unpleasant odor? Closed-cell foams minimally absorb perspiration and are cleanable. One foam, Alicover, has a nylon lining and is actually scrubbable. Absorbing perspiration that occurs under the splint, stockinette offers an inexpensive and easily changeable alternative. Some therapists fabricate a custom liner from an athletic tube sock for their patients. Stitching over the cut edges creates a washable and long-lasting liner.

The therapist must scrutinize the density and resiliency of the padding. To test these factors, the therapist may place a thumb and a finger on opposite sides of the padding and pinch forcefully. If the fingers almost touch, then the padding will quickly "bottom out" and will not provide protection. Padding that provides a viscous cushion upon the thumb-and-finger pinch test will offer the best pressure distribution.[21]

Splint liners can minimize splint migration. The therapist should identify materials with higher friction coefficients. The use of such liners to stabilize a splint requires the therapist and patient to monitor the skin carefully.

The therapist must analyze the ease of padding application and removability to appropriately choose the material. Many foams have an adhesive backing that allows easy application to the splint; however, they can be impossible to remove. This can result in the need to fabricate an entire new splint when the time comes to modify the existing splint. Padding the splint with more extreme contours requires a high degree of drapability from the padding material.

Padding color may enhance splint cosmesis. The addition of bright colors to the padding spectrum has added an element of fun to the splinting regimen. Obscuring discoloration, dark colors are acceptable to the patient for longer periods of time. Because the therapist can leave the padding in the splint for a significant duration, dark-colored padding is time and cost effective.

Stress Application to Tissue

HOW MUCH STRESS SHOULD THE SPLINT APPLY TO TISSUE?

In upper extremity rehabilitation, clinicians frequently use splinting to direct and control stress to tissue. As previously described, this can be accomplished via static, static-progressive, serial static, or dynamic splinting approaches. Problem solving comes into play when considering three issues: (1) degree or amount of stress, (2) means of distributing pressure and eliminating shear stress, and (3) components to deliver the stress (Table 9–3).

According to Brand,[22] the determination of the amount of torque needed to overcome a contracture rests on (1) the nature, length, and density of the structures to be mobilized or lengthened; and (2) the distance of the structure from the axis of the joint—the moment arm. Brand refers to the length-tension curves he has generated in the laboratory and suggests that splints should generate enough torque to hold the soft tissues in the section of the curve in which the flat reorientation section is curving up the steep elastic section (Fig. 9–15). Simply stated, this is the amount of stress required to place tissues safely at the end of their elastic limit. Brand goes on to explain that:

TABLE 9–3 Considerations in Applying Force to Tissue

1. How much stress shall I incorporate in the splint?
   Consider: Joint stability and gliding
                Lever arm
                Soft tissue tolerance to sling pressure
2. How shall the splint distribute forces to maximize tissue stress while avoiding pressure and shear?
   Consider: Finger cuff design
                Point pressure in circumferential design
                Splint conformity
3. What components are best for stress delivery?
   Consider: Dynamic
                Static-progressive

In most cases in which continuous external force is applied to a digit with the idea of affecting the angle of the joint, the limitation in the amount of force that can be used is entirely a result of the limited ability of skin and soft tissue to accept pressure without ischemia and pain. The joint and the contracted tissue might safely and usefully accept much more force if it could be applied. Therefore the therapist should usually apply as much force as the surface tissue will accept without ischemia and apply the force as far as possible from the axis of the joint so that the torque is maximized by a long lever arm.[23]

Brand[23] also points out that, in the joint with compromised stability or a block to free gliding, the long lever may further damage or dislocate the joint (Fig. 9–16). In this situation, the splint should apply to force close to the joint to facilitate gliding rather than tilting or angulation. Unfortunately, the short lever arm creates an even greater impediment to generating adequate torque at a joint without causing ischemia and pain in soft tissues. To apply stress to tissue effectively, the splint must generate as much safe torque as possible while spreading the force to avoid pressure and shear stress.

To maximize stress delivery, the splint must direct the force in a line perpendicular to the segment being mobilized. If the splint fails to do this, the joint(s) proximal to the mobilized segment will be either distracted or compressed, and the forces will be dissipated, resulting in these undesired effects (Fig. 9–17).[24] In addition, the splint must

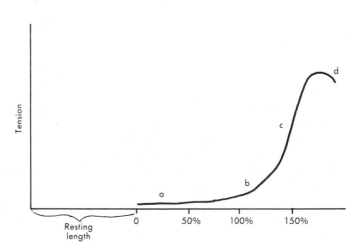

FIGURE 9–15. Length tension curve for typical biologic tissue (e.g., skin). (From Brand,[1] p 106, with permission).

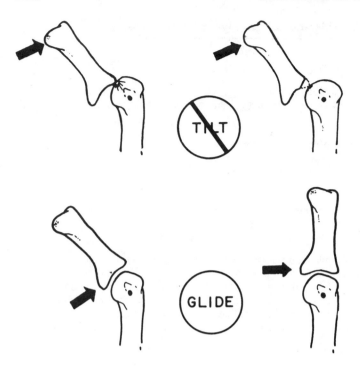

FIGURE 9–16. The heavy arrows demonstrate force applied to a joint that has a partial subluxation, a block to free gliding, or both. In the upper row the force is applied with a long moment arm, resulting in tilting without gliding and finally in absorption of the lip of the phalanx. In the lower row the force is applied with short moment arm, close to the joint, resulting in restored gliding. (From Brand,[1] p 107, with permission.)

also direct forces perpendicularly to the plane of the fingernail or to the rotational axis of the joint. Failure to achieve proper alignment in this plane creates deviating forces and will compromise joint stability (Fig. 9–18).[25]

HOW WILL THE SPLINT DISTRIBUTE THE STRESS?

When the splint functions to direct stress to tissue, the splint-tissue interface must effectively distribute forces. This interface takes on various forms depending upon the splint approach. Finger cuffs or slings, circumferential splints, and three-point pressure splints must successfully meet the challenges of pressure and shear.

Finger Cuffs

Both dynamic and static-progressive approaches employ finger cuffs when directing forces to the fingers. The cuff material and design determines the degree of pressure and shear stress that the soft tissues receive.[26] Cuff materials vary from very soft and flexible (e.g., suede) to the most rigid (e.g., thermoplastic).

Even with low-load application, soft, flexible materials usually fail to exert pressure evenly along their surface. Generating pressure from side to side as the two halves of the sling converge, the soft cuff compromises the function of the neurovascular bundle (Fig. 9–19). With any alteration of the perpendicular angle of pull, such as improvement in the contracture, the resultant tilting of the cuff generates uncomfortable and ultimately dangerous shear stress (Fig. 9–20). Figure 9–21 illustrates Brand's plaster cuff solution, which distributes surface pressure, prevents side-to-side pressure, and minimizes shear stress.

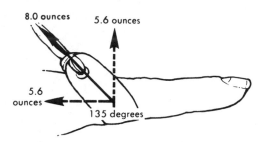

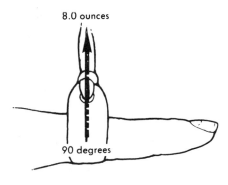

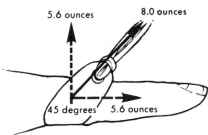

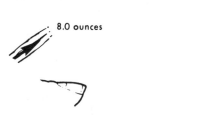

FIGURE 9–17. At 90 degrees the translational force is zero, resulting in no element of joint compression or distraction; at 90 degrees, the line of pull maximizes stress delivery. *Dotted lines* = rotational force; *dashed lines* = translational force; *solid arrows* = traction assist force. (From Fess and Phillips,[2] p 137, with permission.)

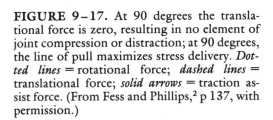

In specific applications, soft loops are safe and effective. The MCP arthroplasty dynamic extension assist splint requires minimal tension to maintain the MCP joints in neutral. In addition, many arthroplasty patients have sensitive skin and live in warm climates. The soft, absorbent suede material frequently used for this splint usually does not cause significant problems with pressure distribution or sheer and is compatible with the requirements of rheumatoid skin.

The soft cuff also works well over the dorsum of the distal phalanx. When splinting over this area, the nail provides a rigid shield against sheer and helps to distribute pressure. The soft loop conforms over the end of the finger and helps to hold the loop in place.

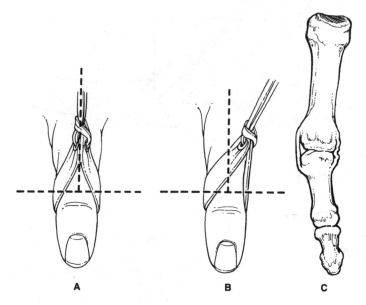

FIGURE 9–18. Correct alignment (*A*). A nonperpendicular pull to the rotational axis of the joint (*B*) will produce unequal stress on the collateral ligaments (*C*). (From Fess and Phillips,[2] p 234, with permission).

Circumferential Splints

Circumferential splinting with plaster offers the ultimate in pressure distribution and shear elimination. When creating serial casts, therapists often think they must generate significant amounts of force against the restricting tissue while molding the cast. The earlier section in splint approach introduced the rationale for the use of low load and the means by which tissue responds to the stress of being placed at the end of its elastic limit. Thus, when molding the cast, the rule remains the same as for dynamic and static-progressive splints: use only enough force to place the tissue at the end of its elastic limit and maintain it.

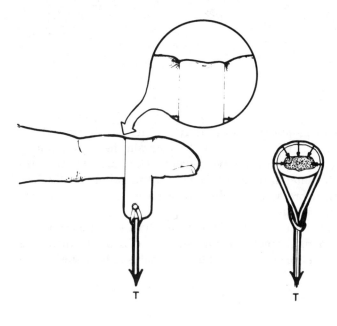

FIGURE 9–19. A flexible sling at right angles to a digit results in (1) pressure under the sling in the line of pull, (2) pressure from side to side because of the convergence of the two halves of the sling, and (3) some shear stress at both edges of the sling. The greatest discomfort arises from the second result listed here. (From Brand,[1] p 97, with permission.)

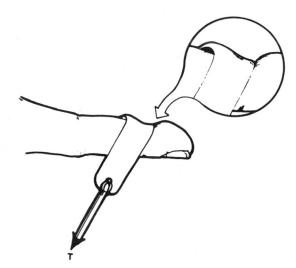

FIGURE 9–20. When a sling is tilted because the angle of pull has changed, the pressure and shear stress are localized to one edge of the sling and are therefore greatly increased. (From Brand,[1] p 97, with permission.)

Three-Point Pressure Splints

Noncircumferential static and serial-static splints may also attempt to position soft tissue at the end of its elastic limit. These splints generally depend on a three-point pressure approach.[27] Success will depend on the conformity of the splint and its ability to distribute pressure.

HOW WILL THE SPLINT APPLY THE STRESS?

Dynamic Force Generators

In dynamic splinting, the therapist uses dynamic elements—self-adjusting resilient or elastic components—such as:

- Rubberband
- Wrapped elastic

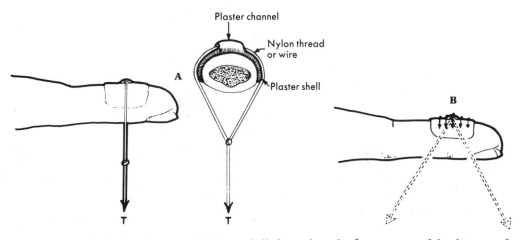

FIGURE 9–21. *A,* By using a small plaster shell, formed on the finger, most of the dangers of a sling are avoided. A loop of thread is passed around the rigid shell, and there is no side-to-side compression. *B,* If the angle of pull on the thread is changed, there is no tilting of the shell because the change of direction occurs at the top of the convexity of the plaster shell. Only the thread changes direction. (From Brand,[1] p 98, with permission.)

- Elastic thread
- Rubber strips
- Springs
- Spring wire
- Coils

Each element has a role to play based on its properties, characteristics, and cost.

Inexpensive and readily accessible, rubberbands have long been the dynamic element of choice. However, repeated stretch and atmospheric changes alter both the force rubberbands can exert and the amount they can elongate. Because testing has revealed that rubberbands of the same make and grade vary in their characteristics, the clinician cannot depend on their consistency.

Only slightly more expensive, wrapped elastic, elastic thread, and graded rubber strips seem less prone to force inconsistencies but will still alter their ability to generate force and elongate with stress and atmospheric change. Offering a special advantage, these latter three examples allow the clinician to determine their length.

The common failing of the four examples examined so far is the difficulty in finding a piece of elastic or rubber that will both generate the amount of force desired and possess the ability to elongate adequately, even with control of length and thickness.

The Kleinert and Weiland[28] approach to flexor tendon repair management illustrates this problem. Many therapists have encountered difficulty in finding a rubberband or elastic that will hold the finger IP joints in adequate flexion and allow the patient to extend the IP joints fully to the limits of the dorsal block. Another example is the dynamic, dorsal PIP extension splint fabricated to generate enough extension torque to resolve PIP flexion contractures while also allowing full ROM exercise of the PIP in flexion. Here again, the element that has the power to hold the joint at the end of its elastic limit in extension may not have the ability to elongate enough to permit full ROM in flexion.

Graded springs entered the treatment arena in 1985. Representing a significant improvement over rubberbands and elastic, research indicated "that springs can give a consistent and controlled force. They are durable and gradable within specific parameters."[29] In addition, the springs demonstrated more success with both generating force and possessing adequate excursion. With experience, therapists recognized that not all springs had the same properties of consistency as the particular brand of springs studied. In addition, the springs lent themselves much more readily to forearm-based splints than to hand-based splints because of their length. If the therapist used a shorter spring, the advantage of excursion was usually lost. Finally, the high-quality springs represented a significant financial investment to the patient.

Spring wire offers yet another dynamic alternative. The major drawback is the high degree of skill with the wire required to achieve the desired results. Several commercially available prefabricated designs circumvent the need for hours of practice before providing a spring wire splint to patients.

The newest element on the scene, the coil, may eventually provide the best of all worlds to the therapist and patient. The coil is compact and can generate both consistently gentle tension and excursion,[30,31] but its current limited applications have proven costly.

Static-Progressive Force Generators

Static-progressive splinting involves the use of inelastic components such as:

- Progressive hinges
- Turnbuckles
- Gears
- Hook-and-loop tape

Some of these components have special application to a specific joint (e.g., elbow hinge). Other components combine with outriggers to generate progressively higher or lower amounts of force at any joint. In static-progressive splinting, turnbuckles, gears, and hook-and-loop tape replace the dynamic component such as the spring. Factors to consider in choosing static-progressive components include (1) joint being splinted, (2) time to fabricate, (3) axis of joint rotation, (4) cost, (5) adjustability, and (6) bulk.

Splinting Regimen

HOW MUCH TIME SHALL THE PATIENT WEAR THE SPLINT?

Splinting regimens vary as much as therapists and patients do. Experienced therapists acknowledge several axioms that guide their decision making.

1. Light tension splinting over many hours yields better results than high tension splinting over a shorter period of time.
2. Joints with PROM limitations with a hard "end feel" require many more hours of splinting than do those with a soft "end feel."
3. During sleep, most patients tolerate static better than dynamic splinting.
4. Active motion and functional use of the hand facilitate achievement of many treatment goals.

The actual splinting regimen varies with (1) the diagnosis and problem set of the patient, (2) the acuity or chronicity of the problem, (3) the goals of the splint, (4) the splint tolerance of the patient, (5) the importance of active motion and/or spontaneous hand use in the patient's program, (6) the number of splints involved in the treatment plan, and (7) the patient's need for unobstructed use of the hand. Therapists must clearly instruct the patient to monitor for changes in color, temperature, sensation, pain, and edema during or directly following splint wear. In addition, the therapist directs the patient to limit the initial use of the splint until skin tolerance is established and then to increase the length of time in the splint gradually.

Before leaving the clinic with a splint, the patient must demonstrate the ability to put it on and remove it properly. Providing written instructions to the patient maximizes compliance with a splinting program. The inclusion of a spouse, relative, or friend during a splint instruction session adds further insurance for proper splint wear.

SUMMARY

This chapter offers a series of guiding questions which, once answered, provide the therapist with the majority of information required to implement an appropriate splinting program. The optimal splint design results when the therapist first asks "What does this hand need?" rather than "What splint goes with this diagnosis?" Splint fabrication does require significant technical skill. Yet, to develop an appropriate splinting treatment plan, the therapist must demonstrate a high level of problem-solving ability that is grounded in data analysis and biomechanical principles.

At the time of this writing, new materials and components are being invented or discovered and added to the therapist's splinting armamentarium. These new materials can and should alter some of the splinting solutions that are currently considered state of the art. In addition, an ever-increasing body of research will continue to direct the decision-making process essential to splinting.

REFERENCES

1. Brand, PW: Clinical Biomechanics of the Hand. CV Mosby, St Louis, 1985.
2. Fess, EE and Phillips, C: Hand Splinting: Principles and Methods, ed 2. CV Mosby, St Louis, 1987.
3. Cannon, NM, et al: Manual of Hand Splinting. Churchill Livingstone, New York, 1985.
4. Malick, MH: Manual on Static Hand Splinting, ed 2. Harmarville Rehabilitation Center, Pittsburgh, 1972.
5. Fahrer, M: Interdependent and independent actions of the fingers. In Tubiana, R (ed): The Hand. Vol 1. WB Saunders, Philadelphia, 1981, p 400.
6. Idler, RS: Flexor tendon anatomy and biomechanics. In Strickland, JW (ed): Symposium on Flexor Tendon Surgery Hand Clinics. Vol 1, No 1. WB Saunders, Philadelphia, 1989, p 9.
7. Verdan, C: Syndrome of the quadriga. Surg Clin North Am 40:425, 1960.
8. Schultz-Johnson, KS: Volumetrics: a Literature Review. Upper Extremity Technology, Glenwood Springs, CO, 1988.
9. Brand, PW: Clinical Biomechanics of the Hand. CV Mosby, St Louis, 1985, p 166.
10. Gribben, MG: Splinting principles for hand injuries. In Moran, CA (ed): Hand Rehabilitation: Clinics in Physical Therapy. Vol 9. Churchill Livingstone, New York, 1986, p 166.
11. Fess, EE and Phillips, C: Hand Splinting: Principles and Methods, ed 2. CV Mosby, St Louis, 1987, p 86.
12. Fess, EE and Phillips, C: Hand Splinting: Principles and Methods, ed 2. CV Mosby, St Louis, 1987, p 59.
13. Light, KE, et al: Low-load prolonged stretch versus high-load brief stretch in treating knee contractures. J Am Phys Ther 20:93, 1976.
14. Bell-Krotoski, JA: Plaster casting for the remodeling of soft tissue. In Fess, EE and Phillips, C: Hand Splinting: Principles and Methods, ed 2. CV Mosby, St Louis, 1987, p 453.
15. Smith and Nephew: Functional Bracing. Smith and Nephew, Hull, England, p 2.
16. Sarmiento, A: Fracture bracing. Clin Orthop 102:152, 1974.
17. Bell-Krotoski, J: Plaster casting for the remodeling of soft tissue. In Fess, EE and Phillips, C: Hand Splinting: Principles and Methods, ed 2. CV Mosby, St Louis, 1987, p 455.
18. Miles, WK: Remodeling of scar tissue in the burned patient. In Hunter, JM, et al (eds): Rehabilitation of the Hand, ed 2. CV Mosby, St Louis, 1984, p 596.
19. Bielawski, T and Bear-Lehman, J: A gauntlet work splint. Am J Occup Ther 40:199, 1986.
20. Shafer, AA: Common Problems, Useful Solutions in Hand Rehabilitation. Alimed, Dedham, MA, 1987, p 26.
21. Bell-Krotoski, J: Personal communication, May 1988.
22. Brand, PW: Clinical Biomechanics of the Hand. CV Mosby, St Louis, 1985, p 106.
23. Brand, PW: Clinical Biomechanics of the Hand. CV Mosby, St Louis, 1985, p 107.
24. Fess, EE and Phillips, C: Hand Splinting: Principles and Methods, ed 2. CV Mosby, St Louis, 1987, p 137.
25. Fess, EE and Phillips, C: Hand Splinting: Principles and Methods, ed 2. CV Mosby, St Louis, 1987, p 234.
26. Brand, PW: Clinical Biomechanics of the Hand. CV Mosby, St Louis, 1985, p 97.
27. Fess, EE and Phillips, C: Hand Splinting: Principles and Methods, ed 2. CV Mosby, St Louis, 1987, p 146.
28. Kleinert, HE and Weiland, AJ: Primary repair of flexor tendon lacerations in zone II. In Verdan, C (ed): Tendon Surgery of the Hand. Churchill Livingstone, London, 1979, p 71.
29. Roberson, L, et al: Analysis of the physical properties of SCOMAC springs and their potential use in dynamic splinting. J Hand Ther 1:110, 1988.
30. May, E and Silfverskiold, KL: A new power source in dynamic splinting: Experimental studies. J Hand Ther 2(3):164, 1989.
31. May, E and Silfverskiold, KL: A new power source in dynamic splinting: Clinical experience and results. J Hand Ther 2(3):169, 1989.

BIBLIOGRAPHY

Bell-Krotoski, JA, Breger, DE, and Beach, RB: Application of biomechanics for evaluation of the hand. In Hunter, JM, et al (eds): Rehabilitation of the Hand, ed 3. CV Mosby, St Louis, 1989, p 139.

Brand, PW: The forces of dynamic splinting: Ten questions before applying a dynamic splint to the hand. In Hunter, JM, et al (eds): Rehabilitation of the Hand, ed 2. CV Mosby, St Louis, 1984, p 847.

Breger-Lee, D, Bell-Krotoski, J, and Brandsma, JW: Torque range of motion in the hand clinic. J Hand Ther 3(1):7, 1990.

Clinical Treatment by Diagnosis

CHAPTER 10

Skeletal Injuries

Susan L. Mannarino, OTR, CHT

This chapter discusses the skeletal injuries to the wrist and hand that most often require therapeutic intervention and outlines the options for evaluation and treatment. Because of the complexity of the structures involved and the many different kinds of injuries possible, the treatment options are many and diverse. Therefore, this chapter does not aim at presenting every treatment possibility. The goal, rather, is to provide insight into treatment of skeletal injuries through an understanding of the several possible diagnoses, their applicable methods of medical management, and the implications of the diagnoses and treatments on rehabilitation.

The objectives of this chapter are

1. To discuss the factors that influence fracture management, including fracture classification, methods of reductions, and how fractures heal
2. To present the general principles of treatment as they relate to fracture healing
3. To discuss the therapeutic management of

   - Distal radial fractures
   - Carpal fractures
   - Metacarpal fractures
   - Proximal and middle phalangeal fractures
   - Distal phalangeal fractures
   - Dislocations of the wrist and hand

FACTORS INFLUENCING FRACTURE MANAGEMENT

Fracture Classification

Several sets of terms can be used to describe and classify fractures. A complete description should include the mechanism of injury, anatomic location, line of fracture, and the relationship of the fragments to each other and the surrounding soft tissues (Fig. 10–1).

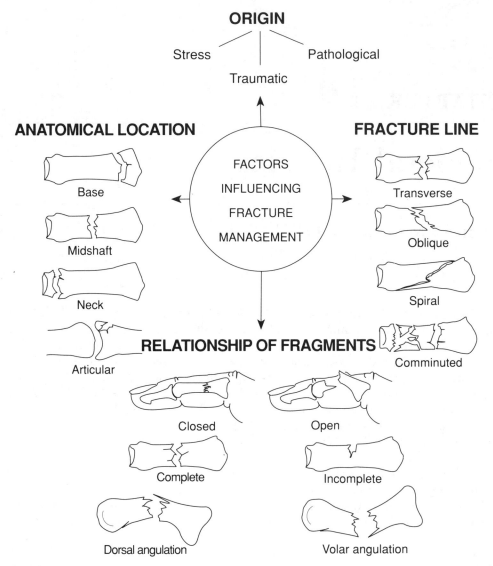

FIGURE 10–1. Many factors influence the method of fracture reduction, the length of immobilization, and the subsequent rehabilitation program.

The major factors that affect the type of fracture produced are the mechanism of injury and the deforming forces acting on the bone.[1] The mechanism of injury determines the line of the fracture. For instance, a torquing force would most likely yield a spiral fracture, whereas a direct blow would produce a transverse or comminuted fracture.[1] Deforming forces in the hand are produced by both the intrinsic and extrinsic muscle systems. These forces will produce a dorsal or volar angulation of the proximal fragment in relationship to its normal alignment.[2] (Specific forces that typically cause deformation in fractures of the hand are discussed in subsequent sections.)

The fundamentals of fracture classification give the therapist a wealth of information with which to design appropriate and individual treatment regimens. These factors will dictate the type of fixation and external stabilization used, the expected rate of healing, and the relative timetable for initiation of various treatment methods. As therapists, full knowledge of the characteristics of a particular fracture is essential in planning a treatment program, but the physician's judgment ultimately determines when the fracture is healed and what primary methods of management are indicated (e.g., when motion can be initiated).

Methods of Reduction

Skeletal fractures can be reduced by closed, open, or distraction techniques. Closed methods of reduction are those that do not require surgical opening of the soft tissues, thereby minimizing soft tissue damage. They generally include manipulation of the fracture followed by application of some type of device to maintain the reduction.[1] The reduction may be maintained using casts, splints, percutaneous pinning (placing of pins through the skin), or other external fixation devices that provide distraction in order to prevent collapse of the reduction.

Open reduction and fixation is primarily performed when closed techniques fail to maintain adequate fracture alignment and stability. Common forms of internal fixation in the hand include Kirschner's wires, interosseous wires, screws, and plates with screws (Fig. 10-2). Fractures with irreducible rotational deformities, and articular, spiral, oblique, and comminuted fractures are often unstable and require open reduction and internal fixation. Multiple fractures and those with associated soft tissue damage benefit from open reduction[1,3-5] to allow the postoperative treatment program to be structured to the requirements of the soft tissues.[3] Segmental bone loss may also require internal fixation to maintain digital length while awaiting a secondary procedure such as bone grafting (Fig. 10-3). Distraction techniques can be performed with or without surgical exposure of the fracture site. The distraction is typically created by using internal pins placed on either side of the fracture and an external apparatus attached to the pins which prevents the fracture or joint from collapsing (Fig. 10-4). This technique may be necessary to maintain a joint space, as with a proximal interphalangeal joint (PIP) fracture dislocation, or to prevent a collapse deformity as can occur in a Colles' fracture.

The therapeutic ramifications of fixation devices lie in their relative stability. Those that provide compression forces to the fracture, such as lag screws with or without plates and tension band wiring, are more stable and require less external support than those that merely hold the fragments in approximation, such as Kirschner's wires. For instance, a proximal phalanx fracture with screw fixation may withstand early composite motion, whereas one with crossed Kirschner's wire fixation may require a proximal phalanx blocking splint to support the fracture during PIP joint motion.

Fracture Healing

"Fracture repair is a unique body process since normal bone is regenerated, rather than healed by scar."[5] The rate of healing, as well as the quality of bone repair, depends on adequate revascularization of the bone. Factors such as age, fracture characteristics, and presence of disease can influence the speed and effectiveness of the repair process.[5]

The rate of healing is directly proportional to the total volume of damaged bone and the width of the defect. For instance, impacted fractures may heal in a few weeks,

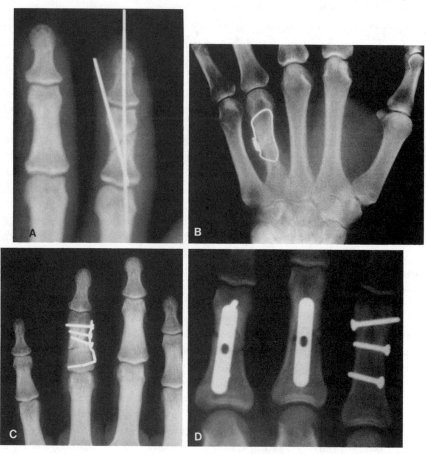

FIGURE 10–2. *A*, Middle phalanx fracture reduced with crossed Kirshner wires. *B*, Metacarpal fracture reduced with interosseous wire. *C*, Middle phalanx fracture reduced with a laterally placed plate and screws. *D*, Proximal phalanx fractures of the index and long fingers reduced with dorsally placed plates and screws and the ring finger reduced with screws.

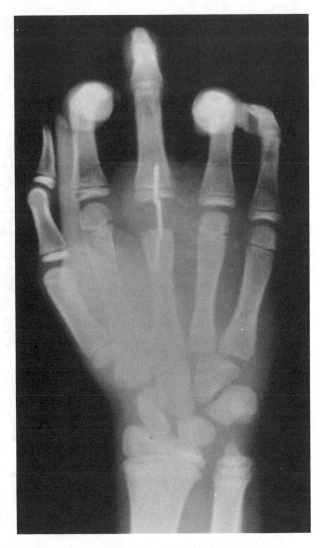

FIGURE 10-3. A spacer wire maintains digital length while the patient awaits a secondary procedure.

whereas displaced fractures may require many months to heal.[6] The rate of union is also influenced by the type of fracture, the particular bone involved, the location of the fracture within that bone, the method of fixation, and the patient's age and general health. Infants heal most fractures in 4 to 6 weeks, adolescents in 6 to 10 weeks, and adults more slowly. After puberty, relatively little difference in healing time is attributable to age.[5-7] Table 10-1 describes typical healing rates for wrist and hand fractures.

Because fracture healing is a process, various terms are used to describe the relative strength of the repair at different points in time. As healing progresses, stability increases, as does the amount of force that can be withstood at the fracture site. For the purpose of this chapter, a fracture is stable when it can withstand at least the forces of active joint motion. Stability can be achieved by bone healing or through an internal or external fixation device, or both. A clinically healed fracture is one that possesses the clinical findings of lack of motion occurring upon gentle stressing of the fracture site and lack of tenderness with direct pressure over the fracture site.[5] A fracture is healed or united when there is roentgenographic evidence of bone healing and/or when the

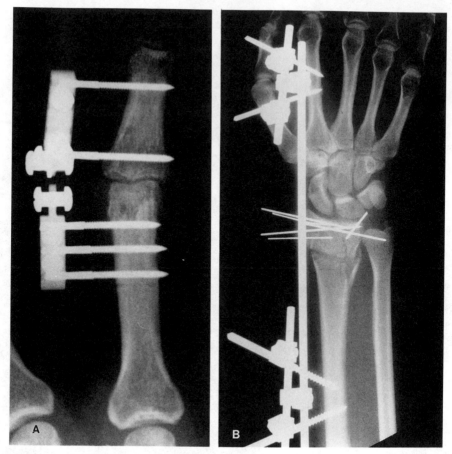

FIGURE 10–4. *A*, "Mini" external fixator used for a proximal interphalangeal joint dislocation. *B*, External fixation of a Colles' fracture.

physician believes the fracture to be stable enough to withstand passive, normal, and resistive stress (e.g., dynamic splinting and hand strengthening).

Familiarity with relative healing times is very important in the hand because radiographic evidence of healing is often not found for many weeks after stability and clinical healing are achieved.[5] Smith and Rider[8] demonstrated that the average healing time on roentgenographic examination for phalangeal fractures is 5 months, and ranged from 1 to 17 months. Clinical healing is often evident in 3 to 4 weeks.

Exceptions to the average rates for healing also make judgments difficult. Union is delayed in areas such as the diaphysis, where there is little cancellous bone; healing there will take two to three times longer than in other areas. Displaced fractures and fractures with marked soft tissue damage also heal more slowly because of decreased blood supply. Open reduction of fractures, because of disturbances of the vascular supply and periosteum, doubles the time for union (although stability is often achieved immediately through internal fixation). Percutaneous fixation with Kirschner's wires may in fact reduce the time needed for union by increasing fracture stability and compression.[5,6,9]

TABLE 10-1 Fracture Healing Rate

Type of Fracture	Rate of Healing
Fractures of the distal radius	
Colles'	
Undisplaced	4 wk
Displaced	6 wk or 4-7 wk
Smith's	6 wk
Carpal fractures	
Scaphoid	3 mo or more
	(needs union on roentgenogram)
Tubercle of scaphoid	8-10 wk
Hamate	4-6 wk
Capitate	(needs union on roentgenogram)
Triquetrum	6 wk
Metacarpal fractures	3-5 wk
Neck	3-4 wk
Shaft	3-5 wk or 4-7 wk
Base	3-5 wk or 4-6 wk
Proximal phalanx fractures	
Base	3-5 wk
Shaft	5-7 wk or 3-4 wk
Head and neck	3-5 wk
Middle phalanx fractures	
Base	3-5 wk
Shaft	10-14 wk
Head and neck articular	3-5 wk
Distal phalanx fractures	
Articular	3-5 wk or 2 wk
Thumb fractures	
Bennett's	6 wk or 4-6 wk
Rolando's	3-4 wk or 4-6 wk

From Sorenson,[17] page 192, with permission.

The therapist must rely on the physician's judgment regarding the ability of the fracture site to withstand the forces produced by various forms of treatment. For example, a fracture may be able to tolerate manual passive motion exercises before it can withstand a dynamic traction force. For this reason, it is important to be very specific in gathering information from the physician. Prompt initiation of the most aggressive, but safe, forms of treatment will hasten recovery and maximize function.

GENERAL PRINCIPLES OF TREATMENT

The treatment of skeletal injuries focuses on obtaining an adequate reduction and maintaining fracture stability while preventing complications such as joint stiffness, tendon adhesions, and edema formation. The most effective therapy program is one that is individualized to address the special problems associated with each injury. To develop such a program the therapist should have a working knowledge of normal anatomy, mechanics of the injury, the method of reduction and fixation as well as the characteristics of bone healing. The information acquired directly effects the appropri-

TABLE 10–2 Referral Flow Chart

Required Information	Treatment Implications
Location of fracture (within the bone)	Position of immobilization, rate of healing, and exercise program affected
Type of fracture A. Open vs closed	A. Special attention to wound healing, dressing changes, and monitoring for infection needed with open fractures
B. Fracture line (comminuted vs spiral, and so on)	B. Can provide information regarding inherent stability, expected healing time, and amount of soft tissue damage
Pertinent medical history A. Mechanism of injury	A. More forceful injury (e.g., crush) more likely to produce associated soft tissue damage, increased edema, stiffness, and tendon adherence
B. Patient's age and medical complications	B. Predictor of potential for rehabilitation and possible problems with healing (bone and/or soft tissue)
Associated soft tissue damage (tendon, nerve, ligament)	Position of immobilization and exercise program may be altered for protection of soft tissue repairs
Reduction A. Date of reduction	A. To monitor progress and carry out a logical progression of treatment in accordance with healing time
B. Method (closed vs. ORIF)	B. Closed — will generally need to wait longer before initiating ROM; less soft tissue damage involved with reduction Open — will often be able to begin motion sooner; can expect increased edema and possibility of tendon adherence

ateness of the therapy program. This information can be gathered from the surgical report, roentgenography, the referring physician, and the patient. Table 10–2 offers some guidelines regarding the type of information that should be obtained and its implications in the development of a treatment program.

Deciding where to begin and how to progress a therapy program following a skeletal injury can be difficult, considering the many types of skeletal injuries that occur and the differing opinions on, and methods of, medical management. Structuring the rehabilitation process around the phases of bone healing offers some guidelines regarding the strength of the fracture site and its ability to withstand various forms of treatment. With this approach, the therapy program can be developed in three phases: (1) phase I — prior to stability or clinical healing, when joint motion may cause movement at the fracture site; (2) phase II — when the fracture is determined to be stable (either through clinical healing or surgical fixation) and can withstand at least active joint motion; and (3) phase III — when the fracture is considered to be healed or united and can withstand passive joint motion and, finally, normal and resistive hand use.

GENERAL TREATMENT TECHNIQUES

The following areas need to be assessed and addressed to varying degrees in all skeletal injuries: edema control, pain management, immobilization, and restoring joint motion. Specific treatment techniques will be discussed as they relate to the management of skeletal injuries.

Edema Control

Continuous, light, and even compression of an edematous extremity is very effective in controlling edema. A bulky or light compressive dressing or a Jobst splint (see Chapter 6) may be needed if the patient presents with severe and or diffuse edema. These fingertip to proximal forearm applications of compression are useful for directing excess fluid toward the lymphatics for systemic drainage versus displacement of the fluid to an area just proximal or distal to the compression. For example, if the edema is localized to the dorsum of the hand and only this area is compressed, the excess fluid is likely to lodge at the digital and or wrist level with likely reinfiltration of the damaged tissues once compression is removed. Elasticized stockinette, Isotoner gloves, finger socks (digital sleeves sewn from Ace bandages or other elasticized material), or Coban wrap are all good considerations for control of minimal to moderate edema and can be chosen for their particular qualities in a given situation. For example, edema localized to a PIP joint may be effectively managed by digital Coban wrapping, whereas excess fluid lodged at the metacarpal phalangeal (MP) joints may best be resolved with the use of an Isotoner glove. Both methods provide proximal and distal control for the given situation. Caution should be used, however, in the case of an unstable fracture where the movement caused by applying a compressive glove, for instance, could adversely affect the reduction. Some additional treatment methods that are effective for reduction of edema include retrograde massage (with stable fractures), cold modalities, galvanic stimulation, and the Jobst pump (see Chapter 8). When using the Jobst pump with acute fractures, a low amount of pressure should be used and protruding pins should be padded to prevent pressure on them.[4] Elevation of the extremity above the heart is a helpful adjunct to any treatment for edema reduction as it aids the lymphatic drainage process. If edema is allowed to remain significant, the increase in interstitial pressure will intensify stiffness and greatly hinder efforts at increasing range of motion (ROM).

Pain Management

Pain that greatly limits the patient's potential active range of motion (AROM) and appears to stem from soft tissue damage, ligamentous stretching, or the patient's low tolerance should be controlled. Complete elimination of pain is not often desirable, as discomfort can serve as a guide to the aggressiveness of treatment. If the treatment itself is painful, this feedback may be an indication that soft tissue damage is occurring and an increase in edema and a loss of ROM are likely to follow. In conjunction with the physician and the patient, the decision to implement oral medications (over the counter or prescription), transcutaneous electrical nerve stimulation (TENS), or even a digital block may be considered to augment the rehabilitation process. The source of pain needs to be carefully determined before being treated, as pain directly over the fracture site could indicate delayed union or a loss of fracture stability. One should also watch for pain that is seemingly out of proportion to the injury so as not to overlook the possibility of an impending dystrophy (see Chapter 15). Any of these suspicions should be reported to the physician immediately.

Immobilization

Splints are commonly used to help ensure immobilization of the fracture through proper positioning and external support during healing and to help restore joint motion once healing is complete. Splinting of the hand for protection and rest is most often done in the "safe" or intrinsic-plus position. This position maintains the ligaments on stretch during immobilization, reducing the possibility of joint contractures. The "safe" position of immobilization is especially indicated with metacarpal and proximal phalanx fractures and whenever there is significant edema in the hand. Possible exceptions include middle phalanx (P_2) and distal phalanx (P_3) fractures, in which a digital gutter splint may be sufficient to support a stable fracture. Positioning for wrist and thumb fractures can usually be achieved without including the digits. In general, stiff joints, even of the uninvolved digits, should be at least intermittently splinted in a "safe" position, and all noninvolved, limber joints should be left out of the splint. An exception to this rule may be the need to include an adjacent digit in the splint for maximum stability or patient comfort. Splint design should also incorporate any external hardware for protection against bumping or snagging, as this type of impact could jeopardize healing (Fig. 10–5).

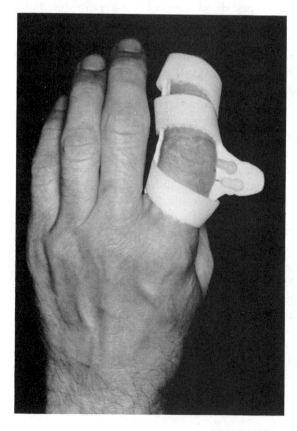

FIGURE 10–5. A digital gutter splint, which incorporates protruding wires for protection.

Restoring Range of Motion

Immobilization, even in the absence of a fracture, produces resorption of bone tissue. Long-axis loading of the bone, as occurs with ROM exercise, increases bone density by deposition of new lamina at the bone surface. In addition, movement of a joint after injury promotes regeneration of articular cartilage.[10] These factors, along with limiting adhesions, increasing circulation, and decreasing edema, make the earliest possible initiation of motion desirable.

ROM exercises may be initiated in several phases. First, the patient should be taught to maintain motion in all joints that, when moved, would not cause stress at the fracture site. For example, a patient with a P2 fracture may be able to perform wrist and MP joint motion (of the fractured digit) immediately following a stable reduction. Second, AROM should be initiated to joints distal and proximal to the fracture site, usually when the fracture is stable. Arthrokinematic or accessory joint motion used in joint mobilization techniques involves movement of joint surfaces on each other. Joint mobilization can sometimes be initiated before traditional passive range of motion (PROM) exercise. The line of application force is directed perpendicular to the joint surface, avoiding stress to nonarticular fractures.[10] PROM exercise (physiologic, or using long levers to move the joint) and therapeutic activities requiring resistance to grip are not indicated until the bone remodeling or healing is evident at the fracture site. Resistive motion not only improves grip strength but can also positively affect healing if the force produced is compressive to the fracture site.[10]

Whether an incision is involved or not, scar formation is inevitable and can often limit the ability to achieve full ROM. Early AROM is most effective to avoid scar adhesions between structures; however, early motion is not always possible. Methods that can be used to alter the normal healing process include deep massage (using caution if the fracture is not yet healed), pressure techniques (Elastomer, Otoform) secured with a pressure dressing, vibration, and tendon gliding exercises.

Deep massage may help to realign collagen fibers, resulting in softening of the characteristic tough random pattern collagen alignment of scar. The use of pressure on the scar provides a stimulus to slow formation and avoid hypertrophy.[10] In theory, the use of vibration disorganizes the scar tissue in preparation for the organizing force provided by active motion.[10] Tendon gliding exercises stress immature adhesions that may adhere tendons to each other, to surrounding soft tissues, or to bone.

Frequent reevaluations of the patient's progress are important to determine the effectiveness of the different aspects of the treatment program. Changes in the treatment program can also be made expediently as the patient's progress, or lack of it, dictates.

The remainder of this chapter deals with specific skeletal injuries. The preceding concepts will be elaborated on as they pertain to clinical decision making in specific areas of treatment. Rehabilitation of each injury will be discussed according to the phases of healing described earlier in this text.

DISTAL RADIUS FRACTURES

Ninety percent or more of all wrist injuries occur as a result of a fall on an outstretched hand. Body weight, age, the distance of the fall, and the position of the wrist and the forearm at impact are all factors in the specific type of injury produced.[1]

Fractures about the distal radius are most commonly categorized into one of three types. Most common by far, not only in the wrist but also in the entire skeleton,[11] is Colles' fracture. Second, accounting for only 5 to 10% of distal radius fractures is Smith's fracture. Last, and more rarely encountered, is Barton's fracture.

Colles' Fracture

Colles' fracture is defined as a complete fracture of the distal radius with dorsal displacement of the distal fragment (Fig. 10–6).[12] This fracture occurs with a lower level of force and less dorsiflexion than most carpal injuries.[1] As many as 70% of these fractures occur in postmenopausal women with osteoporotic bone.[13]

The method of reduction, as well as position of immobilization, is quite variable. Generally, Colles' fracture without comminution or associated carpal injuries, and which remains stable after closed reduction, is treated by cast immobilization. At the other end of the spectrum, a fracture comminuted into more than two fragments, an intra-articular fracture, or one that for other reasons is rendered unstable, is most frequently treated with an external fixation device[4,12] (Fig. 10–7; see also Fig. 10–4). This device works on the principle that a traction force applied to the carpus aligns the fracture fragments via intact ligaments.[12] The medical advantages include the ability for adjustment if displacement occurs, and avoidance of complications commonly caused by circumferential casting.[12] A disadvantage may be the increased healing time required owing to the slight distraction produced at the fracture site. Externally fixed Colles' fractures are usually immobilized for 6 to 8 weeks versus the customary 4 to 6 weeks of casting.[4] Therapeutically, the external fixator allows access to the forearm for edema control and electrode placement for modalities as well as eliminating bulk in the palm which allows for full, composite finger flexion.

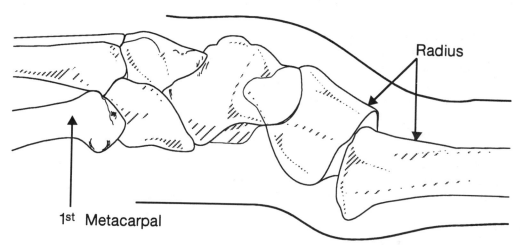

FIGURE 10–6. A Colles' fracture is a dorsal displacement of the distal fragment.

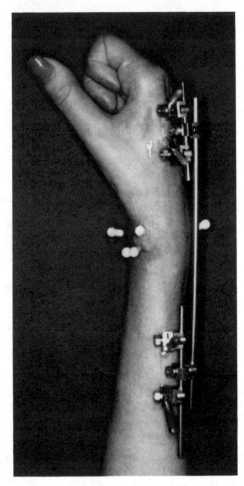

FIGURE 10-7. External fixation of a Colles' fracture.

Smith's Fracture

Sometimes called a reverse Colles', Smith's fracture is a complete fracture of the distal radius with palmar displacement of the distal fragment[4,12] (Fig. 10-8). Customary management is with closed reduction and long-arm casting in supination for 3 weeks, followed by 2 to 3 weeks in a short-arm cast.[4] Smith's fractures are frequently unstable, however, and open reduction and internal fixation are often necessary.

Barton's Fracture

Barton's fracture is a dorsal or volar articular fracture of the distal radius, resulting in subluxation of the wrist[4] (Fig. 10-9). This fracture results from a direct violent injury to the wrist,[13] or dorsiflexion and pronation of the distal forearm on a fixed wrist.[1] Seventy percent of these fractures occur in young men, and the fracture is most often extremely unstable. For this reason, it is usually treated by open reduction and internal fixation and has a 16 week average healing time.[13] However, if stable internal fixation is

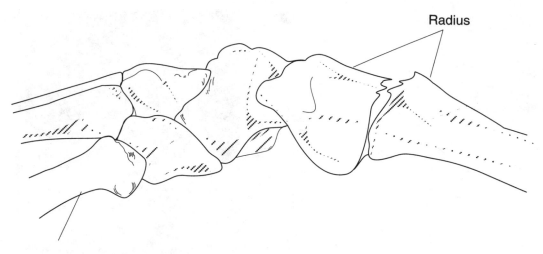

Radius

1ST Metacarpal

FIGURE 10–8. A Smith's fracture is a palmar displacement of the distal fragment.

achieved, AROM and PROM to the digits and wrist may be begun as early as 3 to 5 days after surgery.

Therapeutic Management of Distal Radius Fractures

During phase I of treatment, priorities are edema control, pain control, and ROM of all uninvolved joints. In this acute phase, edema of the hand is often prevalent. Reduction of the edema is of primary concern because of the complications that excess fluid in the hand can create. For the patient with a distal radius fracture these complications include tendon adherence at the wrist, joint stiffness, and carpal tunnel syndrome. If tingling and shooting pains are described in the digits, nerve compression, especially carpal tunnel syndrome, must be considered and evaluation by the physician is recommended.

All edema control techniques discussed earlier that can be used with a cast or external fixator are of potential benefit to the distal radius fracture patient. Trial and error, with frequent reevaluation, is usually the best method in determining the most appropriate treatment for a particular case. Some guidelines, however, would be helpful in deciding where to start. While in the cast, compression to the digits with finger socks or Coban wrap must be accompanied with compression at the metacarpal head level to prevent pooling of fluids there (Fig. 10–10). With external fixation devices, light compressive dressings can be applied to the entire forearm with careful and intricate maneuvering around the pins (Fig. 10–11). Extra precautions should be taken to keep the pin sites free from infection. Daily cleaning with hydrogen peroxide and or mercurachrome is usually adequate to keep the wounds clear of necrotic tissue and to prevent adherence of the skin to the pins.

Proper treatment of pain depends on its source. If the pain is basically confined to the fracture site and is severe, roentgenographic evaluation should be considered to determine if a loss of reduction has occurred. Most commonly, the pain stems from swollen and stiff joints resulting from the original trauma and medical management.

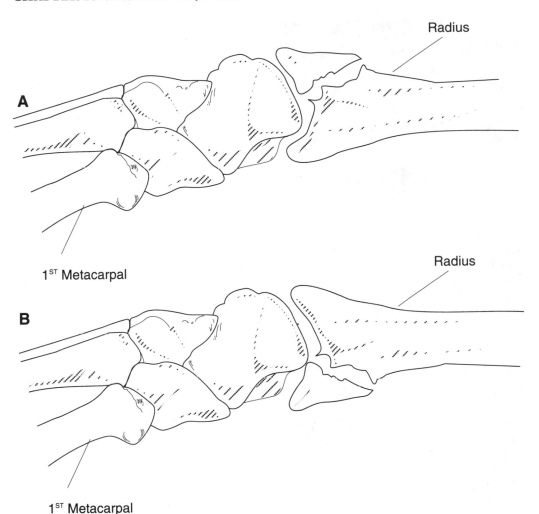

Radius

A

1ˢᵀ Metacarpal

Radius

B

1ˢᵀ Metacarpal

FIGURE 10–9. A Barton's fracture is articular and produces either *A*, a dorsal or *B*, a volar fragment.

This type of pain can be treated with medications, TENS, heat or cold modalities (see Chapter 8), and joint mobilization techniques (see Chapter 7). Whenever the amount of pain described by the patient appears to be grossly out of proportion to the injury, an impending reflex sympathetic dystrophy (RSD) must be considered. Common signs of RSD that may accompany the severe pain are profuse edema, lack of motion, and various vascular and trophic abnormalities[4] (see Chapter 16).

When the patient is referred for treatment prior to removal of the cast, ROM exercises are directed toward the uninvolved joints, including the elbow and shoulder. The most common limitations encountered during casting are flexion of the MP joints and decreased flexion and opposition of the thumb. In treating these areas, it must first be determined if the cast is physically blocking motion of the joints. If full MP motion is not allowed the cast should be cut down below the distal palmar flexion crease of the digits and as far proximal around the thumb as possible, while still maintaining stable fracture positioning.

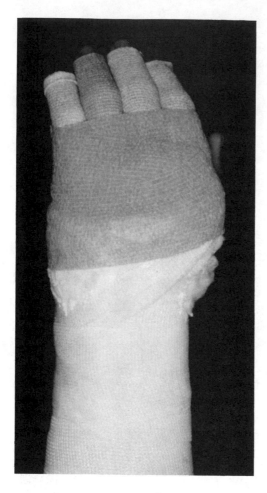

FIGURE 10–10. Appropriate edema control during casting.

Range of motion may also be limited by intrinsic or extrinsic extensor tendon tightness, especially in cases when there has been an excessive amount of dorsal edema. The intrinsic musculature can be stretched through passively attempting full PIP and distal interphalangeal (DIP) joint flexion with the MP joint extended. The extrinsic extensors are maximally stressed through full, passive composite flexion, whereas the MP joint is maintained in maximum flexion while the interphalangeal (IP) joints are brought into flexion. The effectiveness of the extrinsic stretch can be intensified by flexing the wrist simultaneously with the fingers (once wrist motion is allowed). If there is an inability to obtain, or substantial resistance is encountered in order to achieve, the aforementioned passive positions and the digit is absent of other pathology (e.g., arthritis, direct injury), then tendon tightness should be suspected.

If the joints lack full flexion because of joint stiffness and or tendon tightness, various other methods of treatment may be employed in addition to exercise. Taping of the digits into flexion for 20-minute sessions several times a day is beneficial for resolving extrinsic tendon tightness as well as capsular limitations (Fig. 10–12). If motion is severely limited, immobilization between exercise sessions in an intrinsic plus position may be indicated so that gains made during exercise are not totally lost through

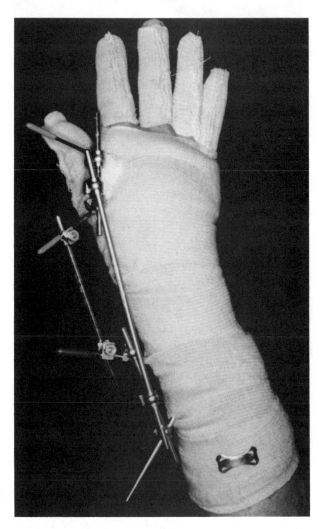

FIGURE 10-11. A light compressive dressing used with an external fixator.

rebound of the tissues to their shortened position while at rest. Dynamic splints for MP flexion, composite flexion, or IP flexion can be employed as appropriate according to the specific source of the limitation (see Chapter 9). Dynamic splinting can safely be applied to the digits in phase I if the distal radius fracture is well stabilized by a cast or external fixator.

If AROM is lacking despite good PROM, then tendon excursion is most likely compromised by adhesions or muscle weakness or both. These may be addressed by concentrated efforts at sustained, active exercise and augmented with use of functional electrical stimulation or biofeedback (see Chapter 8).

Phase II of treatment begins once the fracture is stable and the cast or external fixator is removed. If edema persists, use of an Isotoner glove may be beneficial—especially if the edema is localized to the MP level, or the digits or both. Digital and thumb motion will now have maximum freedom and the emphasis should be on composite motion (see Chapter 7). A splint may be worn for protection, proper posi-

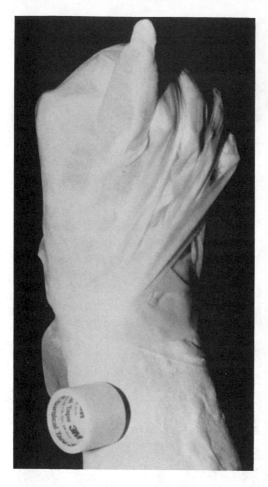

FIGURE 10–12. Paper tape is used over a cotton glove to stretch the digits into flexion compositely and serially.

tioning, and comfort of the wrist until the fracture is healed and the muscles have been strengthened (Fig. 10–13).

The primary focus of phase II is restoring ROM to the wrist. AROM is stressed and should include dorsiflexion, palmarflexion, radial and ulnar deviation, supination, and pronation. Having the patient hold a light object (e.g., a nerf ball) while performing wrist dorsiflexion exercises will help encourage use and strengthening of the wrist extensors in isolation of the digital extensors. Encouragement of normal use and incorporation of therapeutic activities into the treatment plan will be beneficial in eliciting functional motion. The degree and distribution of stiffness often depends on the position and length of immobilization, and the patient's age. For example, restoring ROM in a 68-year-old woman with a Colles' fracture that was casted for 6 weeks is likely to be more difficult than in a 20-year-old man who sustained a Barton's fracture and was able to begin AROM 5 days after surgery.

Phase III should begin when the fracture is healed and can withstand passive stress. Initially, gentle active assisted and PROM exercises should be added to the treatment program and gentle resistance to grip may be instituted using a Hand Helper or soft Therapy Putty to begin hand strengthening and to encourage full excursion of the flexor tendons. Passive motion and/or strengthening should not be continued or progressed if

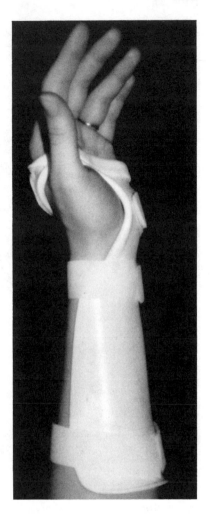

FIGURE 10–13. A wrist immobilization splint.

it exacerbates pain in the wrist. Short exercise sessions of 2 to 3 minutes each are advised initially so that pain and edema are not produced from overactivity of weak musculature. This early use of resistance can help overcome the complication of weak grip strength that is often encountered after wrist fracture.

As the patient's tolerance to passive motion increases, methods such as more aggressive joint mobilization and continuous passive motion devices can be introduced to increase ligamentous extensibility about the wrist and forearm. Weighted stretch exercises may be used to increase wrist palmar and dorsiflexion. If progress is slow, initiation of dynamic splinting to the wrist should help to hasten the process. Dynamic splinting for forearm rotation can also be beneficial, especially in the more acute contractures that have a springy "end feel." If severe extrinsic extensor tightness is present, taping of the digits into flexion along with application of a weight or dynamic splint, to passively palmar flex the wrist, is effective to resolve the tightness and improve composite motion (Fig. 10–14).

The ultimate goal of treatment is to restore normal ROM, which is determined by comparison to the contralateral side. Because of the many factors surrounding a particu-

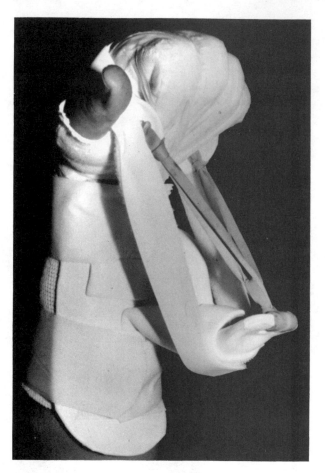

FIGURE 10–14. A dynamic wrist flexion splint applied with the hand taped into flexion to stretch the extrinsic extensor mechanism.

lar fracture (severity, articular involvement, patient's age, and so on), "normal" range is often unrealistic, and functional or potential pain-free range should be the goal. The patient's potential range can often be predicted by the physician, based on findings in surgery and the appearance of the fracture on roentgenographic examination. A general rule is to continue treatment until a plateau is reached that cannot be surpassed with an aggressive treatment program that is adhered to by the patient. Continued, although often less frequent, reevaluation is necessary to determine if the patient has actually reached his or her potential or if an unchangeable factor such as a bony block is preventing further progress.

The second part of phase III, and the final aspect of rehabilitation, is strengthening of the wrist. If the patient has good PROM but limited AROM, muscle weakness may be the problem, therefore, longer rehabilitation time with a focus on strengthening may be required. The program should be carefully geared toward the patient's needs, expectations, and abilities. For instance, a homemaker would have vastly different needs than a construction worker. As with the digits, the strengthening program should be started slowly, with minimal weight and repetitions. Strengthening exercises should not cause significant pain. Pain that continues for more than 20 to 30 minutes following the exercise session is an indication that the program may be too aggressive. If such a program is continued, it could result in a chronically painful, and therefore functionally limited, extremity. The therapist should keep in mind that the wrist extensors are much weaker than the flexors, and the strengthening program should be individualized to each. Progressive resistive exercises, regressive resistive exercises, weight well, and dowel rod exercises are all beneficial means of strengthening the wrist (see Chapter 7). A home program of flexibility and strengthening exercises and gradual weaning to normal activities should be emphasized in order to maximize function and prevent reinjury from overuse.

Complications

Complications in distal radius fractures are common. From the therapist's standpoint, the complications can be divided into those requiring medical management and those that can be addressed therapeutically.

Among the complications that may require either immediate or late medical management are carpal tunnel syndrome, malunion, distal radioulnar joint dysfunction, radiocarpal arthritis, and rupture of the extensor pollicis longus tendon.[11] Of these complications, it is disruption of the distal radioulnar joint that most commonly causes persistent pain and limits forearm rotation after a distal radius fracture.[13] The therapist should be aware of the presence of any of these conditions, as they could all ultimately affect the patient's potential result from rehabilitation.

Complications that can be addressed therapeutically include stiffness of the entire upper extremity, intrinsic contracture from prolonged edema, RSD, and shoulder-hand syndrome.[11] These complications are much easier to prevent than they are to correct after the fact through the use of good early exercise programs, avoidance of using a sling to support the arm, and adequate edema control.

CARPAL FRACTURES

Carpal fractures occur one tenth as often as distal radius fractures, with scaphoid fractures accounting for 60 to 70% of all carpal fractures.[1,6,11] The literature disputes the incidence of the second and third most frequently fractured carpal bone between the lunate and the triquetrum, respectively.[1,6,11,14] The remaining five wrist bones account for only 7 to 10% of all carpal fractures.[1] Up to 90% of carpal fractures occur from a force applied with the wrist in dorsiflexion.

Scaphoid Fractures

The scaphoid's relationship to the radius and its position in both the distal and proximal rows of the carpus make it a bony block to extreme dorsiflexion and very vulnerable to injury.[11,14] The notoriety of scaphoid fractures stems from the difficulty in their diagnosis and the extremely variable healing times characteristic to various fracture sites within the bone.

The fracture is often imperceivable on roentgenogram, when the patient first presents for treatment. Diagnosis is usually made on clinical signs of local pain and swelling in the region of the scaphoid and the history of injury.[1,11,15]

Healing time for scaphoid fractures ranges from 5 to 20 weeks or more, depending on the level of the fracture and the obliquity of the fracture line. Most scaphoid fractures occur in the middle two thirds, or the waist, and heal in 10 to 12 weeks. Fractures in the proximal one third have a poor vascular supply, and may require 12 weeks or more to unite. Fractures of the distal one third are rare but heal within 4 to 8 weeks owing to a rich blood supply in that area.

Healing time depends also on the direction of the fracture line. A horizontal line tends to be compressed with finger motion, and will heal more quickly than a more vertically oriented line which experiences shearing forces from finger motion.[1,6,11,13–15] Treatment most often consists of immobilization in a cast that includes the thumb. Internal fixation, usually with compression screws, is also used. Radiographic signs of healing are usually evident before ROM is initiated because of the large variability of healing times and high rate of nonunions found in scaphoid fractures. Once the cast is removed, rehabilitation is similar to that of other carpal fractures; this is discussed in a later section.

Other Carpal Fractures

Because of the infrequency with which these fractures are encountered, and the similarities in their treatment, they are discussed collectively here.

Fractures of the lunate are more likely to result from repeated compression or stress than from a single force. The lunate is also known to develop an avascular necrosis, known as Kienböck's disease, which is caused by interruption of the blood supply. This diagnosis is treated with prolonged casting and may require salvage procedures such as bone grafting or arthroplasty if fracture union is not achieved.[1,11,14]

Triquetral fractures usually occur when the hand is in ulnar deviation as well as dorsiflexion, and they consist most often of a dorsal chip fragment.[14] Pisiform and hamate fractures may occur from a direct fall on the palm of the hand or a blow from the handle of a racket, golf club, or baseball bat. Pisiform and hamate hook fractures may be treated with excision or immobilization.[11,14] Trapezial fractures are most commonly associated with fracture dislocations of the thumb metacarpal base, or Bennett's fracture.[11] Capitate fractures are very rare because of the central and protected position in the wrist.[11]

Most carpal fractures are treated with cast immobilization and heal within 6 to 8 weeks if they are nondisplaced and have a good blood supply. If the fracture is unstable, open reduction and internal fixation may be necessary.[1]

Therapeutic Management of Carpal Fractures

During phase I of treatment, the patient should be instructed in ROM to all uninvolved joints of the upper extremity to minimize stiffness and reduce edema. If digital stiffness is severe, composite taping can be used and or dynamic splints may be fabricated to fit over the cast, but refitting is essential after cast changes to maintain proper function. Edema and pain control measures should also be taken as appropriate, remembering the principles discussed under general treatment techniques.

Phase II of treatment should commence when the fracture is stable enough for the cast to be removed. Areas of focus should now be the wrist, thumb, and composite flexion, as all will be affected by the prolonged immobilization. Generally, active assisted exercise can be added when the patient's AROM has reached a plateau and is pain free. During this phase, a static or dynamic wrist splint is often needed between exercise sessions for support and protection against additional injury. Light normal use and therapeutic activities can be introduced to encourage motion.

Phase III is initiated when the fracture is fully healed. Dynamic splinting for wrist flexion and/or extension or for composite flexion may be necessary. Usually, the longer the immobilization and the more complex the injury, the greater the need for aggressive techniques to regain motion. Grip strengthening should be initiated immediately, and wrist strengthening should follow once a pain-free passive range has surpassed the active potential. Depending on the patient's occupation and length of immobilization, a formal work hardening program may be needed in addition to a home strengthening program. Once the fracture is clinically healed and the pain and weakness have been resolved, protective splinting may be discontinued.

Complications

The possibility of refracture always exists in the carpal bones. The wrist absorbs a tremendous amount of stress during normal activities and is a frequent site of injury. To provide optimal protection against reinjury, prolonged splinting, at least with heavy or uncontrolled activities, is recommended.[1] Perhaps one of the most common complications seen clinically is persistent pain. In the rehabilitation process it is important for the therapist to respect the patient's discomfort and emphasize the goal of achieving a pain free arc of motion over achievement of maximum range. Non-union, malunion, and delayed union are all common in carpal fractures because of the insufficient blood supply in many areas. Difficulty in maintaining immobilization and difficulty in making early diagnosis also create complications in management of carpal fractures.[1,6]

METACARPAL FRACTURES

Metacarpal fractures most commonly involve the first and fifth rays. Being border digits, they are anchored securely on only one side, leaving them highly mobile and more susceptible to injury. As a result, they are also more difficult to treat.[16] Because first metacarpal (thumb) fractures differ greatly in etiology and treatment from fractures involving the other four digits, these will be discussed separately.

Most fractures of metacarpals two through five tend to be stable because of the numerous ligaments and muscles that attach to these bones. However, given the right conditions, the same ligaments and muscles, along with the extrinsic tendon systems, become deforming forces causing dorsal angulation at the fracture site (Fig. 10–15).

Many metacarpal fractures heal within 3 to 7 weeks, depending on the location of the fracture.[17] The anatomic locations most often used for description of metacarpal fractures are the base, shaft, neck, and head.

Base Fractures

These fractures are generally the result of a direct blow or crushing injury, in which case several metacarpals are often involved. They may also occur with an avulsion of the wrist flexors or extensors resulting from a direct blow or torsional injury.[16]

A single base fracture, especially of the second and third metacarpals, is rare.

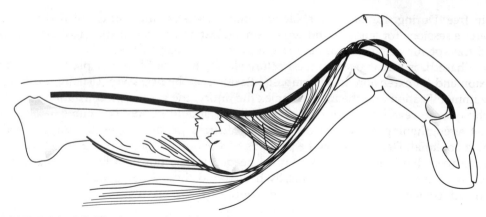

FIGURE 10–15. The interossei and long flexors cause dorsal angulation of a metacarpal neck fracture.

Because of the lack of motion at these carpometacarpal joints, when fractures do occur they are usually stable and of little consequence.[1] However, in the more mobile fourth and fifth rays, a minimal amount of rotation at the base will be magnified many times at the flexed fingertip. Rotational malunion in these digits can cause overlapping of the fingers, functionally limiting grasp.[16,18] In addition, inadequate reduction of the fifth ray can result in decreased grip strength.[1]

Shaft Fractures

Metacarpal shaft fractures are produced by longitudinal compression, torsion, or direct impact. They can be further categorized into comminuted, transverse, or oblique types. They are somewhat slower to heal than the more distal or proximal locations because of the predominantly cortical bone found there.[19]

A comminuted fracture that is impacted, usually as a result of a compression force, is stable and can often withstand guarded motion in 12 to 14 days. An unstable comminuted shaft fracture will most often require open reduction and internal fixation or percutaneous pinning.[20] Significant soft tissue damage and edema often accompany these fractures.[16]

Transverse fractures are usually stable, but the deforming forces of the interossei and the long flexors can cause dorsal angulation. These fractures will generally withstand active motion by 3 weeks.[18]

Oblique fractures are treated similarly to transverse, except shortening and malrotation are more common than angulation.[16] They frequently require open reduction or percutaneous pinning.[20]

Neck Fractures

The neck is the most common location for metacarpal fractures because it is the weakest portion of the bone. Metacarpal neck fractures result from a compression force such as a direct blow with a closed fist. This type of impact causes comminution of the distal metaphysis and palmar angulation of the metacarpal head (or dorsal angulation at the fracture site).[4,18] These fractures most often occur in the fourth and fifth metacarpals and are sometimes called boxer's fractures.[1,16] Although the fracture is impacted, the bone is often unstable due to comminution of the volar cortex.[16]

Unlike a rotation deformity in the fourth and fifth metacarpal base fractures, angulation of metacarpal neck fractures is of little functional consequence. Here, the mobility of the carpometacarpal joints provides compensation for dorsal angulation by increasing the potential for digital flexion.[18,20,21] Problems that occur if the angulation is too great include loss of normal joint contour, pain in the palm with tight grasp, hyperextension at the MP joint (claw deformity) caused by loss of balance of the extensor mechanism,[16] and a cosmetic result that may be unacceptable to the patient.[1] Any angulation of the index and long metacarpals will cause disability in grasp because of the lack of compensatory motion available at the carpometacarpal joints of these digits.[16,18,22]

Head Fractures

Metacarpal head fractures also result from direct impact and extensive comminution is common. These fractures are usually intra-articular, with realignment of the joint surfaces of primary importance. They most often will require open reduction and fixation.

Therapeutic Management of Metacarpal Fractures

Therapeutic management of metacarpal fractures is similar for all anatomic locations. Phase I of treatment is characterized by edema control and immobilization. This phase usually lasts 2 to 3 weeks for closed reductions and 2 to 7 days for internally fixed fractures. Dorsal hand edema is often pronounced and compressive dressings along with elevation are very important. For head and neck fractures, compression should be provided in the web spaces to better control edema at the metacarpophalangeal joint level. Using Kling between the fingers in a light compressive dressing or an Isotoner glove can be very effective in controlling pooling of edema at the MP joints.

Immobilization should be in an intrinsic plus position for most metacarpal fractures.[4,6,8,13,16–18,20] This position not only minimizes the potential for joint contracture but, in many cases, also helps to maintain the reduction. Splints should be carefully molded to incorporate and maintain the transverse and longitudinal arches of the hand. Splinting should be protective as well as positional, incorporating protruding wires and providing dorsal protection against impact as needed.

Phase II is initiated when the fracture is stable. Active and passive exercises can be performed at the interphalangeal joints, but only active motion should take place at the metacarpophalangeal and wrist joints. In anticipation of potential problems such as limited metacarpophalangeal flexion, extensor tendon adherence over the metacarpal and intrinsic and extrinsic tendon tightness, the treatment program should be designed to emphasize exercises that address these areas. These may include active intrinsic plus exercise for metacarpophalangeal flexion, isolated extensor digitorum communis and hook exercises with scar retraction to enhance extensor and differential flexor tendon glide, passive intrinsic-minus exercise for intrinsic contracture, and active composite fisting with wrist flexion for extrinsic tightness. If these problems are not prevented or resolved with exercise, more aggressive forms of treatment, as described in the section on complications, may become necessary.

All digital exercise should be performed in a well-molded wrist splint to support the metacarpals. Use of either the wrist splint (for mid to proximal fractures) or the "safe" position splint (for distal fractures) should be continued for protection between exercises until the fracture is healed.[23]

Phase III is begun when the fracture is healed well, as determined by the physician. PROM at all joints, dynamic splinting for joint and or tendon tightness, and joint mobilization techniques (see Chapter 7) can be added to the treatment program as indicated to restore motion when less aggressive attempts have failed. Caution should continue in order to prevent increased edema or pain that can accompany overly aggressive attempts at increased motion and thus be counterproductive to the end result. Light normal use and therapeutic activities can now be encouraged. Progressive resistive exercises (see Chapter 7) for the hand and wrist can be added at about 8 weeks, providing the fracture is well healed.[23]

Complications

Complications, other than those caused by angulation and rotation, include tendon adherence and intrinsic contracture. The latter two can and should be addressed at the onset of therapy, as previously described, especially when certain predisposing conditions exist.

Extensor tendon adherence is most likely to occur in open fractures in which the periosteum is disrupted, or when a dorsal incision is used for open reduction. Plate and screw fixation applied dorsally may cause a greater potential for adherence than when a lateral application can be achieved. Besides limiting digital flexion and extension, adherence may cause secondary development of a boutonnière deformity. Gradual attenuation of the extensor tendon and subsequent volar displacement of the lateral bands may occur if the digit is compositely stretched into flexion, while there is adherence over the metacarpal.[22] To avoid this problem, the treatment program should include scar remodeling techniques such as friction massage, scar retraction, silicone molds (see Chapter 6), and frequent active exercise. These may be augmented with functional electrical stimulation for maximum stress to the scar. If conservative management does not restore tendon excursion, surgical release may be necessary. The therapist needs to recognize when aggressive passive flexion is creating a PIP extension lag so that continued attenuation of the tendon can be avoided.

Intrinsic contracture is commonly seen with metacarpal fractures, especially those resulting from crush injuries. Because of massive edema from soft tissue damage and immobilization in their shortened position (i.e., the intrinsic-plus or "safe" position), fibrosis of the intrinsic musculature is not uncommon.[16,17,20] Frequent passive exercise in the intrinsic minus position (metacarpal extension and interphalangeal flexion) and, in severe cases, dynamically splinting the hand in this position (Fig. 10–16) is necessary to restore normal muscle-tendon unit length. If not resolved, intrinsic tendon tightness will severely limit grip strength.

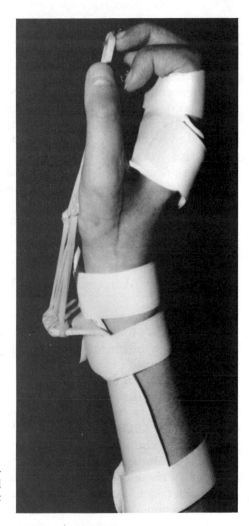

FIGURE 10-16. An interphalangeal joint dynamic flexion splint with the metacarpalphalangeal joints blocked in extension to stretch the intrinsic musculature.

FRACTURES OF THE FIRST METACARPAL

Fractures of the first metacarpal occur less frequently than other metacarpal fractures because of the dissipation of forces possible through this highly mobile ray. For this reason, dislocations of the metacarpophalangeal joint will generally happen before a fracture.[16] These fractures are also distinctly different from other metacarpal fractures, in that most occur at or near the base.[1,8]

Thumb metacarpal fractures are often classified as extra-articular or intra-articular. Extra-articular or shaft fractures can be either transverse or oblique, and intra-articular fractures are most often Bennett's fracture dislocations or, secondarily, Rolando's fractures.[20] The distinction between intra-articular and extra-articular fractures is important in terms of prognosis. The thumb metacarpal will tolerate up to 30 degrees of angulation in an extra-articular fracture without functional loss. However, inadequate reduction of an intra-articular fracture can cause substantial disability.[13]

Bennett's fracture dislocation is the most common intra-articular fracture of the thumb. The mechanism of injury is an axial blow against a partially flexed metacarpal (e.g., as in a fist fight),[20] which produces a volar lip fragment that remains attached to the anterior oblique ligament.[16]

Nineteen different treatment approaches have been described in the literature, all with good results.[17,20,21] Treatment is aimed at perfect realignment of articular surfaces. Reduction is initially attempted through closed methods and percutaneous pinning followed by 4 weeks of cast immobilization. AROM is begun at 4 weeks and PROM not until 6 to 8 weeks, or when union occurs and the pins are removed.[13,16,20] If accurate reduction does not appear likely by this method, open reduction and internal fixation with small cancellous screws and immediate ROM may be the treatment of choice.[20,24]

Rolando's fracture is similar to Bennett's except that there are multiple intra-articular fragments and anatomic reduction is frequently impossible.[13] Fortunately, these fractures are uncommon.

Therapeutic Management of First Metacarpal Fractures

Proper treatment of injuries to the thumb is especially crucial because of its contribution of 50 to 60% of total hand function.

Phase I of treatment should consist of ensuring full ROM to all upper extremity joints not included in the cast or splint. This phase may last only a few days, as with a screw fixation, or 6 weeks with closed reduction and casting.

Phase II treatment protocols vary greatly, depending on the medical management used. Generally, a stable fracture (internally fixed or 4 to 6 weeks following reduction) can withstand AROM and gentle PROM to the thumb and wrist. If the thumb's PROM is found to be considerably greater than its AROM, tendon adherence may be the cause. Limited tendon excursion is not an uncommon complication, especially after open reduction. Functional electrical stimulation can be used to augment excursion of the extensor or flexor tendons, or both. Scar massage and silicone molds are also effective in maintaining tendon glide at the incision site. The exercise and splinting program should also address thumb abduction and opposition as immobilization may cause a first web space contracture. Light activities that require fine motor pinch, abduction, and opposition should be stressed. During phase II, splint protection should be continued between exercises and at night.

Phase III (generally between 6 and 8 weeks) may include more aggressive techniques such as taping, dynamic flexion (Fig. 10–17), and joint mobilization. These methods are used to increase the PROM when there is significant impairment as compared with the contralateral thumb. Gentle resistance, such as Therapy Putty, can be used for pinch and opposition as long as the fracture is healed and the thumb is pain free. Between 8 and 10 weeks, strengthening and a gradual return to normal activities without splint protection should begin.

Additional variables in treating thumb metacarpal fractures relate to their medical management. For instance, Kirschner's wire fixation may be limited to the first metacarpal or may go through the first metacarpal and into the second metacarpal for greater stability. In the first case early circumduction exercises may be appropriate, but in the second case these would be impossible. Another variable to be aware of is the increased likelihood of severe thumb and wrist joint stiffness, as well as extrinsic extensor tendon tightness with a fracture that is held for 6 weeks versus one that is allowed AROM at 3

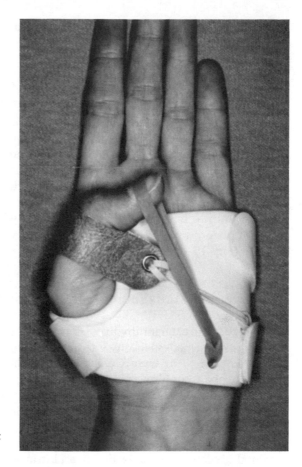

FIGURE 10–17. A composite, dynamic thumb flexion splint.

weeks. With prolonged immobilization, dynamic traction and an overall more aggressive treatment program can be anticipated.

Complications

Complications that may occur after a first metacarpal fracture include malunion, which in turn may result in chronic subluxation of the metacarpal trapezial joint.[20] Joint instability or post-traumatic arthritis, or both, are not uncommon, especially following an intra-articular fracture. Pain and instability will lead to loss of pinch strength and may necessitate a metacarpophalangeal arthrodesis.[17]

FRACTURES OF THE PROXIMAL AND MIDDLE PHALANGES

Fractures of the proximal and middle phalanges tend to be of similar type and require similar management. However, a great difference of opinion does exist with regard to the best method of treatment for a given fracture situation.[23] Proximal and middle phalanx fractures are more difficult to treat than those of the metacarpals and distal phalanx because of frequently associated tendon injuries and instability resulting from lack of soft tissue support.[4]

Proximal Phalanx Fractures

Proximal phalanx fractures are more common than those of the middle phalanx.[4,17,26] They occur with the greatest frequency on the radial side of the hand, involving the thumb and index finger. The proximal or midshaft areas are most frequently involved, with a fall or direct blunt trauma being the leading cause of injury.[4]

The deforming forces are the bony insertion of the interossei at the base of the proximal phalanx, which flexes the proximal fragment, and the central extensor tendon inserting on the base of the middle phalanx, which extends the distal fragment. This force couple produces a characteristic volar angulation of the unstable proximal phalanx fracture (Fig. 10–18).[4,16,25]

Therapeutic Management of Proximal Phalanx Fractures

Phase I of treatment involves attention to edema, pain reduction, and immobilization. Digital edema, especially when accompanied by external Kirschner's wires, is best controlled with 1-in wide Coban wrap applied in a distal-to-proximal loose spiral fashion. Coban conforms nicely around the pins without leaving gaps and is easily separated without removal for pin care. Pain can usually be controlled through immobilization and oral medications as needed. Immobilization of the joints distal and proximal to the fracture site is necessary in order to maintain the reduction and to protect the finger from further injury. In fractures that involve the base or shaft of the proximal phalanx, immobilization in an intrinsic-plus position is recommended not only to maintain the reduction but also to prevent extension contractures from forming at the metacarpophalangeal joints. Proximal phalanx head or neck fractures that have maintained full MP motion and well-stabilized middle phalanx fractures can be sufficiently immobilized in a digital gutter splint.[23] Stable, nondisplaced fractures can be treated with buddy taping and active motion to discourage tendon adherence to callus formation.[16]

With phase II of treatment, mobilization is usually begun between 3 and 15 days after reduction for extra-articular, nondisplaced, stable, and internally fixed fractures,[4,16] and between 3 and 4 weeks after reduction for all other fractures.[4,16,17] A study by

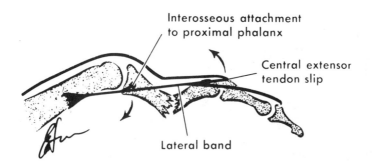

Interosseous attachment to proximal phalanx

Central extensor tendon slip

Lateral band

FIGURE 10–18. The intrinsics and the extrinsic extensor mechanism exerting deforming forces at the level of the proximal phalanx. (From Hunter et al,[4] p 287, with permission.)

Strickland and colleagues[27] showed that fractures immobilized more than 4 weeks would cause a rather large decline in performance, but the difference between starting at 3 weeks versus 4 was negligible.

Problems encountered with therapeutic management of proximal phalanx fractures are many, and primarily result in limited PIP joint flexion. This is especially true with a distal head or neck fracture. Proximal or base fractures tend to involve the flexor tendons or the MP joints, or both. Midshaft fractures, especially spiral or oblique, are likely to produce rotational deformities in the digit. Immobilization is a prime source of joint stiffness, particularly with transverse fractures of the proximal and middle phalanges where slow healing time necessitates prolonged immobilization.

Tendon involvement is a serious problem, especially with displaced fractures that disrupt the overlying tendon sheath.[4] For limited excursion of the FDS or Flexor digitorum profundus (FDP), or both, treatment should emphasize isolated gliding exercises such as blocking and differential gliding exercises (see Chapter 7) to maximize excursion of the two tendons with respect to each other. Extensor tendon adherence will cause a PIP joint extensor lag as well as limit passive PIP flexion. Isolated exercise for the extensor mechanism should be performed by passively flexing the MP joint while attempting active extension of the PIP joint. Scar massage and retraction may also be useful to increase and maintain flexor and extensor tendon excursion during healing. Electrical stimulation can be used by about 4 weeks following most fracture reductions,[23] and is indicated when PROM is considerably greater than AROM. If the fracture is at the insertion of a tendon, good healing must be present prior to using electrical stimulation to that muscle tendon unit.

When a patient has difficulty performing exercise on their own and PROM is physiologically allowed, continuous passive motion supplied by a continuous passive motion (CPM) device is a treatment modality available for use by the therapist. Because PROM has been shown to assist in healing cartilage and reduce pain and edema, it may be useful for an injury in which heavy scarring is anticipated and lack of motion, pain, and swelling are exhibited, especially when seen in an intra-articular fracture.[10,28]

Limited passive flexion at the MP and PIP joints, and PIP flexion contractures are also common problem areas. Unfortunately, they cannot be aggressively treated until phase III of treatment is initiated. The fracture must be clinically healed or held rigidly stable, before aggressive PROM and dynamic splinting can be used. At this point, taping the digits into flexion several times a day for 20-minute sessions, may be adequate to restore supple passive flexion.

Dynamic flexion splinting is often the most efficient and effective method of restoring passive flexion to the more severely limited joints. Caution should be used, however, in considering dynamic flexion when adherence of the extensor tendon over the proximal phalanx is suspected. In this case, overstretching may create a functionally limiting PIP extensor lag through attenuation of the extensor tendon between the site of adherence and its insertion.

Intrinsic tightness is a common occurrence and should be avoided with frequent intrinsic stretching exercises (see Chapter 7). A wrist and proximal phalanx blocking splint with dynamic traction is useful for more severe cases that do not respond to exercise.

Flexion contractures of the proximal interphalangeal joints are best avoided with static extension splinting between exercises during fracture healing. When contractures do occur, joint mobilization and passive exercise are often not enough to restore full extension. Prefabricated dynamic extension splints such as the Safety Pin, Capener, and

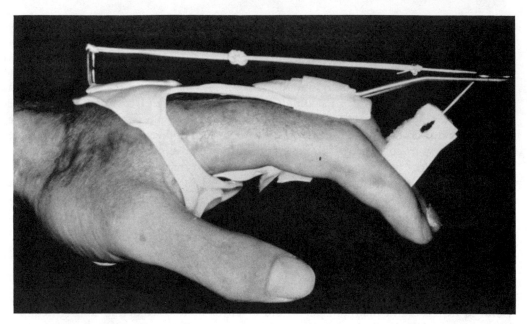

FIGURE 10–19. A dynamic proximal interphalangeal joint extension splint.

LMB are most effective with contractures that have a soft or springy "end feel" of approximately 30° or less. For contractures with a hard "end feel" or those greater than 30°, a short dorsal outrigger with a lumbrical bar (to maintain the MP joints in flexion) tends to achieve better results with its 90° angle of traction and custom fit (Fig. 10–19). Serial casting of the joint into extension may also be very effective. Caution should be used, however, with application of dynamic extension splinting to a proximal phalanx fracture that has been plated dorsally. The force created may loosen or dislodge the screws. Intermittent dynamic splinting needs to be augmented with static extension splinting to maintain the improvements acquired.

Middle Phalanx Fractures

Fractures of the middle phalanx are much less common than in the other phalanges because of the tendency for the PIP joint to dislocate before a fracture will occur.[16] They are most often caused by a crushing injury and the distal shaft is the most frequent portion of the bone to be affected.[4] The deforming forces here are more variable. A neck fracture will angulate volarly because of the pull of the superficialis. A base fracture, which is proximal to the FDS insertion, will angulate dorsally, owing to the extending force of the central slip on the proximal fragment, as well as the flexion force of the FDS on the distal fragment. A midshaft fracture may angulate in either direction or not at all.[23] Shaft fractures also have the slowest healing time of any hand fracture (10 to 14 weeks). Because of the slow healing time and the fact that these fractures are often open and comminuted, obtaining union and maintaining motion at the PIP joint are difficult to achieve.

Therapeutic Management of Middle Phalanx Fractures

The same principles of phase I treatment used with proximal phalanx fractures may be used here. The methods discussed for correction of tendon adherence and PIP joint stiffness also apply. With this level of fracture, however, the additional problems of altered DIP joint function can be expected because of its proximity to this joint.

As mobilization begins in phase II, emphasis will be on FDP blocking and differential glide exercises. Functional electrical stimulation to the FDP may also be beneficial (see Chapter 8).

When clinical healing is achieved, phase III of treatment may include the use of resistance. Flexing into Therapy Putty increases the force used on the muscle tendon unit, helping to increase FDP excursion as well as to restore grip strength.

Active DIP flexion cannot be adequately addressed, however, unless supple passive range is available. Dynamic flexion splinting (Fig. 10–20) for 30- to 45-minute sessions, and IP joint taping with Coban for 15- to 20-minute sessions, are two effective methods for increasing passive suppleness of the DIP joint. Before using IP taping, it is very important that the middle phalanx fracture be well healed. The torque created at the middle phalanx by this method could cause displacement of an unstable fragment.

Splinting for protective purposes can usually be discontinued at 3 to 5 weeks following reduction when the majority of phalangeal fractures are healed. Some excep-

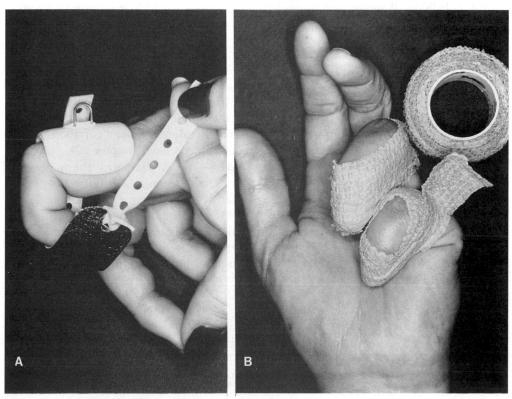

FIGURE 10–20. *A*, Dynamic flexion splinting of a distal interphalangeal joint. *B*, Use of Coban to increase passive flexion of the distal interphalangeal joint.

tions are midshaft, comminuted, and internally fixed fractures, which require prolonged protection.[2]

Complications

Major complications include tendon adherence, joint stiffness, post-traumatic arthritis (generally with articular fractures), and malunion (nonunion is uncommon).[17,25] Some interesting studies have been done on factors that influence digital performance following phalangeal fractures. Huffaker, Wray, and Weeks[29] found that crush injuries, damage to flexor or extensor tendons, and skin loss in the fractured finger caused significantly decreased ROM of the unfractured fingers. Associated flexor tendon injuries had the greatest effect. Related joint injury, multiple fractures, crush, flexor or extensor tendon injuries, and skin loss each significantly decreased final ROM in the fractured digit.[29] In other words, the extent of the injury markedly affects the final ROM of the entire hand.

The study by Huffaker, Wray, and Weeks[29] found damage to the flexor tendon to be more detrimental to ROM in the fractured digit than did damage to the extensor tendon. A study by Strickland and associates[27] found the opposite to be true. In addition, Strickland's study lists increasing patient age as having a greater negative influence on outcome than comminution and displacement. This information is helpful in formulating the prognosis for recovery of motion following a given fracture and in setting realistic goals for treatment.

FRACTURES OF THE DISTAL PHALANX

Distal phalanx fractures account for half of all hand fractures because the fingertips are exposed more to trauma than other parts of the hand. The long finger, not surprisingly, is the most frequently involved digit, with the thumb being second.[25] Intra-articular fractures, which involve avulsion of the extensor tendon, are most commonly of the dorsal lip. These fractures are classified as mallet injuries (see Chapter 12).

The remainder of this section focuses on extra-articular fractures, the majority of which occur at the distal end or tuft of the bone. The mechanism of injury is usually a crush, with comminution, nailbed injuries, extensive soft tissue damage, and hematomas often associated with the fracture.[4,16,25,26] Even though comminution is often severe, fractures of the tuft do not significantly displace. Their inherent stability is due to the dense network of connective tissue present in the fingertip, preventing the insertions of the flexor and extensor tendons from creating a significant deforming force on the fracture.[16,25] Reduction is usually not necessary and treatment is directed to the soft tissues.[16,30]

Therapeutic Management of Distal Phalanx Fractures

Phase I of treatment consists of wound management with appropriate dressings (see Chapter 6), digital edema control, and splinting for pain relief and protection. Allowance for full motion of the proximal joints is important during the period of immobilization. Patients should be instructed in exercises to obtain and maintain full

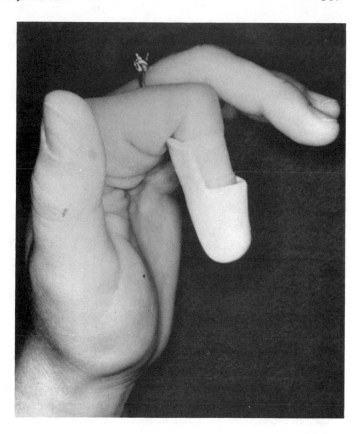

FIGURE 10–21. A "tip protector" splint.

motion in the uninvolved joints as the patient will typically posture the finger in full extension because of pain or the fear of pain with motion. A splint that protects the dorsal aspect of the fingertip is usually indicated with these injuries, especially when the nailbed has been repaired (Fig. 10–21). Care must be taken to keep the wounds dry and clean. Frequent dressing changes and adequate ventilation in the splint are necessary to prevent maceration and skin breakdown. Complete immobilization of the DIP joint is recommended for 1 to 3 weeks[16,23,25] to allow wounds to heal and pain from acute edema and hematoma to subside.

Phase II, mobilization, begins with gentle AROM with emphasis on blocking to the FDP. By 3 weeks, gentle-passive or active assisted motion can be performed within the patient's tolerance. Protective splinting between exercises is still recommended.[23]

Desensitization exercises are very important, especially with tuft fractures, and should be initiated as soon as wounds are healed (see Chapter 11). Fluidotherapy may be a helpful modality for the hypersensitive fingertip (see Chapter 8). Activities requiring fine motor skills and manual desensitization techniques, including tapping, should be emphasized.

Phase III can be initiated as soon as the fracture is healed and the soft tissues can withstand the force produced by these more aggressive therapy techniques. If a lack of passive DIP flexion continues to be a significant problem, the use of Coban for IP taping (discussed under P2 fractures) is often beneficial. The unyielding DIP joint may better respond to dynamic traction. If full PIP motion is present, a distal phalanx (P3) blocking

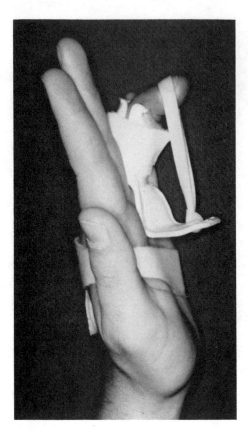

FIGURE 10–22. A dynamic distal interphalangeal joint flexion splint with the proximal joint blocked in extension.

splint with isolated traction to the DIP joint is most effective in restoring extensibility to the dorsal capsule (Fig. 10–22).

If the fingernail was destroyed or removed, a nailbed splint, fabricated from silicone rubber with a plastic overlay secured to the fingertip with Coban, can be used to help remodel and flatten the nailbed in preparation for new nail growth (Fig. 10–23).

Therapy Putty is again useful in achieving maximum FDP excursion and for regaining strength. In this case, it can also be used for desensitization of the fingertip to pressure. As normal hand use is resumed, it may be beneficial to use buddy tapes to secure the injured finger to an adjacent digit in order to assist the patient with incorporation of a sensitive finger into activities, as avoidance can become a habit instead of a necessity.

Complications

In addition to prolonged pain and hypersensitivity, tuft fractures can progress to non-unions. Interposition of fat and soft tissue between the fragments is frequently the cause. These non-unions are often asymptomatic, but, if pain does persist, removal of the fragments is necessary.[22]

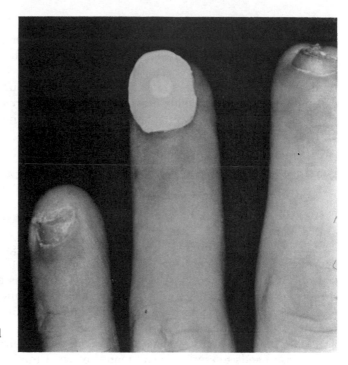

FIGURE 10–23. A nailbed splint.

DISLOCATIONS

A dislocation is the temporary displacement of a bone from its normal position in a joint. For the scope of this chapter, discussion will be confined to the most frequently occurring dislocation of the wrist and that most often treated in the hand. The references used in this section provide a wealth of information on many additional dislocations that may be encountered in rehabilitation.

Dislocations in the Wrist

Dislocations of carpal bones is not extremely common, but failure to recognize them occurs frequently.[13] They are produced by mechanisms similar to those that cause most wrist injuries; a fall or other impact on an outstretched hand, with hyperextension of the wrist. The intensity of the impact is one of the major factors that dictates the resultant injury.[31] For example, tripping on the driveway and catching your fall on an outstretched hand would most likely result in a distal radius fracture, whereas falling from a platform at 15 feet on an outstretched hand with your body weight all behind you would more likely produce a dislocation, with or without a fracture. Carpal dislocations are difficult to diagnose because typical views on roentgenogram can appear normal. The damage can be confined to the ligaments and the carpal bones may spontaneously realign after the injury. Careful examination is needed to detect the presence and the extent of instabilities in the wrist.

The most common carpal dislocation is of the perilunate type.[32] The lunate is the bone around which the rest of the carpus dislocates. The carpus may dislocate in a dorsal or palmar direction with respect to the lunate. For a dislocation of this magnitude to occur, the rupture of many ligaments is required.[14] Closed reduction and casting for a 6- to 8-week period may be the treatment of choice, if the dislocation is diagnosed within the first 1 to 3 weeks after the injury. If the reduction cannot be maintained by casting, percutaneous pinning may be necessary. For gross instability, which is likely to be accompanied by extensive ligamentous damage, open reduction and internal fixation with repair of the ligaments is indicated.[11]

THERAPEUTIC MANAGEMENT OF DISLOCATIONS IN THE WRIST

The general principles of rehabilitation for wrist dislocations are the same as those for carpal fractures. During phase I of treatment, edema control and exercise to all distal and proximal joints are required.

Exercises during phase II should begin slowly and gently, using pain as a guide for aggressiveness. The goal of treatment here is to regain maximum motion and strength, but only within a stable and pain-free range. If pain is allowed to persist or increase through exercise, it may very well become a chronic, functionally limiting complication just as with a wrist fracture. A static wrist support is often necessary for comfort and protection between exercise sessions.

When the ligaments are healed sufficiently, as determined by the physician, phase III exercise needs to emphasize all planes of wrist motion. Continuous passive motion devices, weighted stretching and dynamic splinting may be used as needed to regain passive motion.

The final phase, which is strengthening, should include all muscles that cross the wrist. Therapy Putty and Hand Helper exercises will increase grip strength. Progressive resistive, weight well, and dowel rod exercises are all appropriate strengthening tools for the well-healed, pain-free wrist (see Chapter 7). Work simulator and work hardening protocols may be indicated for patients who have been casted for prolonged time periods and will be returning to heavy and/or repetitive activities.

COMPLICATIONS

Complications that are encountered mainly involve persistent pain and stiffness, which may require a partial wrist fusion. Undiagnosed or misdiagnosed dislocations can result in various instability patterns in the wrist and post-traumatic arthritis. These problems again lead to pain and stiffness, and often require surgical intervention.[13,31]

Dislocations in the Hand

The most frequently encountered acute dislocation in the hand is a dorsal displacement at the PIP joint.[32] The mechanism of injury is usually a longitudinal compression force directed at the tip of an extended finger.[32] Patients frequently state that they "jammed" the finger while playing volleyball, basketball, or softball. The magnitude of the force will influence the complexity of the injury.[31] To dislocate the PIP joint, at least one—and sometimes all three—of the supporting structures must be damaged. These structures are the volar plate and the ulnar and radial collateral ligaments. Initial treatment, duration of immobilization, and prognosis are directly related to the postreduction stability of the joint. The degree of ligament disruption is primarily determined by testing the integrity of the joint during active and passive motion. The most appropriate form of treatment can then be determined.[33]

THERAPEUTIC MANAGEMENT OF DISLOCATIONS IN THE HAND

Stable Dislocations

Most dorsal dislocations are stable following reduction; this includes those with bone fragments that are less than 20% of the articular surface.[33] Treatment regimens described in the literature vary widely. Presented here is a relative consolidation of those views.

Phase I of treatment for this group would include edema control to the digit and immobilization of the PIP joint in 25° to 45° of flexion, depending on the relative stability of the joint[4,23,32,33] (Fig. 10–24).

Phase II, mobilization, would begin as soon as the pain and edema have subsided somewhat, usually within the first 7 to 10 days. Early active motion is extremely important because of the great potential for the flexor tendons to become adherent to the volar plate. Isolated superficialis and profundus exercises should be emphasized and functional electrical stimulation used to enhance tendon glide as needed. All motion is done within the confines of the dorsal blocking splint, as extension beyond the prescribed position could cause redislocation. Passive flexion exercise is usually initiated along with active motion. The inherent edema of the digit will create severe stiffness if passive stretch is avoided for an extended period of time. Dorsal taping or gentle dynamic traction may be indicated if full passive flexion is not achieved by about 3 weeks.

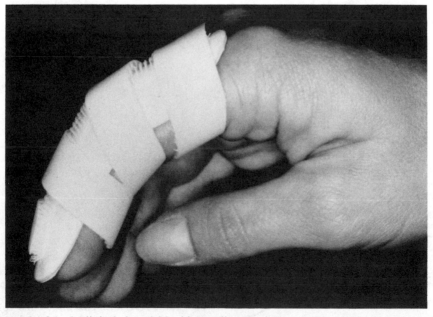

FIGURE 10–24. A digital dorsal blocking splint used to prevent proximal interphalangeal joint extension.

When minimal damage is incurred by the ligaments, the dorsal blocking splint may be discontinued at 3 weeks.[4,31] The digits may then be buddy taped for an additional 3 weeks,[32] or the dorsal blocking splint may be gradually adjusted into extension over a 3-week period (i.e., 10° each week).[23] The latter method discourages formation of a fixed flexion contracture by supporting the digit in extension between exercise sessions, and prevents reinjury while healing is still in progress.

Phase III, unrestricted motion, is usually aimed at restoring full extension to the PIP joint. Passive extension exercises and dynamic extension splinting can often be initiated 6 weeks after reduction.[23] Resistance to the flexor tendons to enhance excursion and increase strength can usually be initiated by 8 weeks after reduction. Therapy Putty is especially helpful in encouraging flexion of the injured digit as well as to provide resistance to a weak extensor apparatus.

Unstable Dislocations

When the joint is unstable, most often because of the presence of a large bone fragment, open reduction and ligament repair are indicated. The most frequently used technique is that described by Eaton,[33] in which the volar plate is advanced into the defect in the articular surface of the middle phalanx and secured by a pull-out wire to a button at the dorsum of the middle phalanx (Fig. 10–25). A Kirschner's wire may be

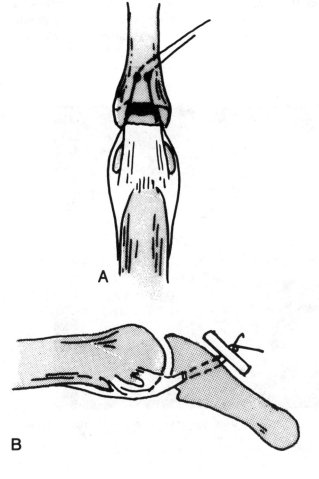

A

B

FIGURE 10–25. Volar plate advancement described by Eaton. (From Neviaser,[30] p 1203, with permission.)

used to maintain the joint in 35° of flexion if the repair is delayed and secondary contracture of the soft tissues resist the reduction.

Phase I of treatment may require splint stabilization, but the digit will most frequently be held in a bulky dressing or cast until the button is removed. The wire or pin, or both, is removed at 3 weeks, when phase II (mobilization into flexion) is initiated within a dorsal blocking splint. The splint may be discontinued at 5 weeks, when gentle active and passive extension of the PIP joint is allowed. Splinting can now be changed to an extension gutter, which should be serially adjusted as extension improves.

Phase III focuses again on achieving full PIP joint extension. Dynamic extension splinting may be initiated between 6[23] and 8[33] weeks. Gentle progressive strengthening may be initiated at 8 weeks after reduction.[23]

COMPLICATIONS

The major problem during rehabilitation is not instability but swollen joints and prolonged stiffness. These complications are due to thickening of the injured joint capsule, which can last up to 1 year,[32] and the pain associated with passive PIP flexion, which may be present for more than 9 months following the injury.[22] The patient should be educated as to the severity of this particular injury and the prolonged course of rehabilitation that is likely to follow.[17] Failure to treat, or inadequate treatment of, a volar plate injury can lead to recurrent dislocations, flexion contracture, swan neck deformity, and traumatic arthritis.[17] Arthrodesis or implant arthroplasty may be indicated as salvage procedures for these unfortunate results.

CLINICAL DECISION MAKING: CASE STUDY

The variety and complexity of skeletal injuries make rehabilitation a real challenge to the therapist. The therapist needs a solid understanding of the anatomic and medical fundamentals of treatment to design safe, effective protocols.

The following discussion of the therapeutic management of a metacarpal fracture illustrates how the therapist integrates the principles of treatment discussed in this chapter into a realistic and logical progression.

HISTORY

M.S. is a 19-year-old, right hand–dominant man who sustained closed, transverse, midshaft, metacarpal fractures of his right ring and small fingers (Fig. 10–26). The fractures were produced by striking a wall with his fist. The patient, who was in good physical health, was employed as a truck driver and delivery man.

SURGICAL REPORT

Closed reduction of the fractures was attempted on the date of injury, without success. Shortening of the ring metacarpal and dorsal angulation at both fracture sites were present upon roentgenogram following the closed reduction. The patient was then scheduled for open reduction and internal fixation of both fractures

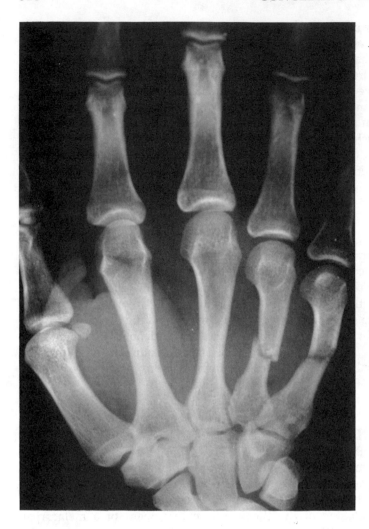

FIGURE 10–26. Preoperative roentgenograms of midshaft fractures of the fourth and fifth metacarpals.

with A.O. plates and screws (Fig. 10–27). This procedure was performed 1 week after the original injury.

THERAPEUTIC MANAGEMENT

Phase I: 0 to 4 Days

During this phase, the patient's hand was immobilized in an intrinsic-plus position in a surgical bulky dressing. Instructions were given to keep the hand elevated above the heart at all times.

Phase II: 4 Days to 2 Weeks

Evaluation

The patient was referred to therapy to begin AROM 4 days after surgery. The bulky dressing was removed and the hand assessed for edema, condition of the wounds, level of pain, and ROM.

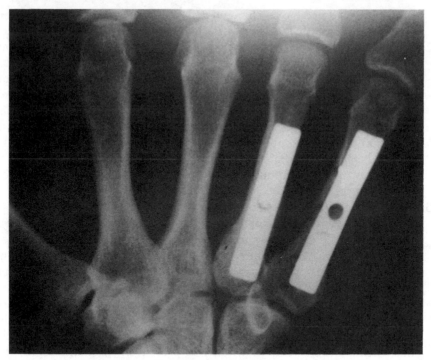

FIGURE 10-27. Postreduction roentgenograms of the fractures described in Figure 10-26.

Edema was minimal throughout the hand and digits but was moderate to severe on the ulnar, dorsal aspect of the hand. A circumferential measurement was taken at the level of the distal palmar flexion crease to monitor the effectiveness of the edema control measures that were chosen.

Slight bloody drainage was present at the incision site, but no signs of infection were noted.

The patient had stopped taking his pain medication and was very comfortable at rest. Considerable pain was present, however, during attempts at motion.

ROM was very limited, especially at the MP joints of the ring and small fingers. The index and long fingers and the thumb demonstrated full passive motion and only minimal active limitations. All other upper extremity joints were within normal limits. Initial active range of motion measurements were as follows:

Ring finger	MP	PIP	DIP
	25/60	0/80	0/40
Small finger	MP	PIP	DIP
	30/55	0/90	0/50

Treatment Priorities

Given the general treatment protocol for rehabilitation of metacarpal fractures, the physician's orders, and the information gathered during the initial evaluation, the following treatment priorities were addressed:

1. Wound management—A sterile gauze dressing was applied over the incision site to absorb drainage and prevent bacteria from entering the wound. The

dressing would need to be changed daily for the first several days to monitor for signs of infection or formation of a hematoma.

2. Edema control—The significant pooling of edema over the fracture and operative site is normal for the extensive disruption of soft tissues that has occurred. Effective control of edema is important to decrease the possibility of heavy scarring, which could greatly compromise motion. A light compressive dressing was applied with extra attention to the web spaces and the ulnar-dorsal aspect of the hand. Finger socks were applied for digital compression. The need for elevation of the hand above the heart was still emphasized. Active abduction and adduction of the digits was incorporated into the exercise program with the goal of creating a pumping action of the intrinsic muscles to help force excess fluid from the hand.

3. Pain control—Once active motion is allowed, it is not unusual for the patient's pain level to increase. The patient was instructed to use the oral medication that was effective after surgery in order to make him more comfortable during exercise sessions. Precautions were given to not progress the recommended exercises while using medications as pain can serve as a guide to appropriate treatment level.

4. Proper positioning—The patient's ring and small fingers were placed in a forearm-based, "safe" position splint, to wear for protection and positioning at all times except during exercise sessions. This decision was based on the minimal edema and good motion that was present in the radial digits, the stable fixation provided by the A.O. plates, and the lack of motion and edema present in the ulnar digits. The wrist was included in the splint because of its articulation with the metacarpals.

5. Regaining ROM—Because of the stable fixation used, composite AROM was initiated to the ring and small fingers 4 days after surgery. A well-molded wrist immobilization splint was used during exercise to provide extra support for the fracture sites and to maintain the palmar arch.

MP flexion was emphasized with intrinsic plus exercises and Velcro trapper assists.

Maintenance of glide of the extensor tendons over the operative sites was addressed with isolated finger extension and intrinsic minus exercises. AROM was performed to the ring and small fingers and the wrist for 10 minutes of each waking hour.

Because the thumb, index, and long fingers were only immobilized for 4 days and were not included in the splint, normal ROM was returned quickly to these.

Phase III: 2 + Weeks

Reevaluation

Edema remained moderate at the ulnar-dorsal aspect of the hand, but circumferential measurements were significantly decreased. The incisions were well healed and the sutures were removed.

Pain was reported as minimal except during finger flexion at the end of the range.

ROM measurements were improved by 50° and 40° of total active motion in the ring and small fingers, respectfully, but significant extensor lags and limited flexion remained problematic at the MP joints.

The lack of motion at the MP joints was brought to the attention of the physician, who determined that the fractures could now withstand PROM.

Revised Treatment Priorities

Priorities now shift from wound management and edema control to scar management and restoration of full AROM and strength. Because of the early initiation of motion, the progression of treatment would be slow and close monitoring was necessary.

1. Scar management—Because of the lack of full active MP extension, formation of adhesions to the extensor tendons was suspected. The patient was instructed in gentle scar massage and retraction to be done with exercise sessions. In addition, a silicone insert of Elastomer was fabricated and secured with Coban over the scar to help control hypertrophy and subcutaneous adhesion formation through pressure. The patient was cautioned against creating pain or increased edema with scar management efforts, as these reactions would be counterproductive.
2. Edema—As the edema was now localized to one area, the method was changed to a Jobst stockinette, fitted over the Elastomer. This method was chosen for its ability to be easily removed for friction and retrograde massage to the scar.
3. Proper positioning—The patient's splint was adjusted for correct fit because of edema reduction, and to increase the MP flexion in accordance with the patient's improving ROM. The patient continued to have difficulties with extension, so an extension resting pan was fabricated to wear between exercises during the day.
4. Regaining ROM—By 2 weeks after surgery the patient was able actively to flex his MP joints to their passive potential. Because the physician's orders had been upgraded to include PROM, the patient was instructed in self-passive exercises. At 3 weeks postoperative, the patient's ROM was as follows:

Ring finger	MP	PIP	DIP
AROM	25/60	0/100	0/60
PROM	0/75	0/105	0/80

Small finger	MP	PIP	DIP
AROM	0/60	0/90	0/85
PROM	0/75	0/100	0/90

The patient had now experienced a week of self-passive motion without increased pain or other adverse effects. As passive MP flexion was still limited, exercises were augmented with composite taping. The taping helped to improve extensibility of the MP joint capsule and resolved the slight extrinsic extensor tightness that had developed in the small finger. These methods were able to produce full flexion without sacrificing extension and without the need for dynamic splinting.

The extensor lag of the ring finger was not responding to exercise and scar retraction alone. Electrical stimulation of the extensor digitorum communis was used during treatment sessions at the 4-week point. After several sessions, the extension lag was greatly improved.

5. Regaining strength—Because of the important role of the ring and small fingers in power grip, this patient's grip strength was significantly decreased. At 6 weeks after surgery, gentle resistive exercises were initiated with Therapy Putty, a Hand Helper with the light resistance of one rubberband, and Progressive Resistive Exercises to the wrist with ½ lb of weight. Gentle mobilization was performed to the transmetacarpal ligament to help restore the natural arches of the hand and the mobility of the fifth ray, which is very important to power grip.

Resistance and repetitions were gradually increased over the next 4 weeks, at which time the patient was released for full duty. The patient did not perceive any difficulties with returning to his prior occupation and avocational interests at that time, so a work hardening program was not pursued.

Discharge Status

By 6 weeks after surgery, the patient had regained full AROM except for a 10° extension lag at the ring metacarpophalangeal joint. Splint protection was continued until 8 weeks after surgery and only light hand use was allowed until 10 weeks after surgery.

Grip strength was decreased by 25% at 10 weeks, and scar maturation was not yet complete. Recommendations for a home program consisted of continuation of resisted gripping exercises and scar massage.

SUMMARY

This chapter has attempted to provide the reader with a working knowledge of a wide variety of skeletal injuries in the wrist and hand. Factors influencing the medical and therapeutic management of fractures and dislocations were discussed. Therapeutic management and common complications were discussed for fractures of the distal radius, the carpals, metacarpals, and phalanges and for common dislocations in the wrist and hand.

REFERENCES

1. Harkness, JW, Ramsey, WC, and Ahmadi, B: Principles of fractures and dislocations. In Rockwood, CA and Green, DP (eds): Fractures in Adults. JB Lippincott, Philadelphia, 1984, p 130.
2. Weinmann, JP and Sicher, H: Bone and Bones Fundamentals of Bone Biology, ed 2. CV Mosby, St Louis, 1959, p 309.
3. Heim, U and Pfeiffer, KM: Internal Fixation of Small Fractures. Technique Recommended by the AO-ASIF Group, ed 3. Springer-Verlag, New York, 1988, p 179.
4. Wilson, RL and Carter, MS: Management of hand fractures. In Hunter, JM, et al (eds): Rehabilitation of the Hand, ed 3. CV Mosby, St Louis, 1990, p 284.
5. Connolly, JF: DePalma's The Management of Fractures and Dislocations. Vol 1. WB Saunders, Philadelphia, 1981, p 200.
6. Jupiter, JB and Silver, MA: Fractures of the metacarpals and phalanges. In Chapman, MW and Madison, M (eds): Operative Orthopaedics. JB Lippincott, Philadelphia, 1988, p 1235.
7. Opgrande, JD and Westphal, SA: Fractures of the hand. Orthop Clin North Am 14:779, 1983.
8. Brahsear, HR and Raney, RB: Shand's Handbook of Orthopaedic Surgery, ed 9. CV Mosby, St Louis, 1978, p 465.

9. Gershuni, DH: Principles of wire fixation. In Chapman, MW and Madison, M (eds): Operative Orthopaedics. JB Lippincott, Philadelphia, 1988, p 141.
10. Saunders, SR: Physical therapy management of hand fractures. J Am Phys Ther Assoc 69 (12):1065, 1989.
11. Frykman, SF and Nelson, EF: Fractures and traumatic conditions of the wrist. In Hunter, JM, et al (eds): Rehabilitation of the Hand, ed 3. CV Mosby, St Louis, 1990, p 267.
12. Szabo, RM: Fractures of the distal radius. In Chapman, MW and Madison, M (eds): Operative Orthopaedics. JB Lippincott, Philadelphia, 1988, p 1279.
13. Connolly, JF: DePalma's The Management of Fractures and Dislocations. Vol. 2 WB Saunders, Philadelphia, 1981, p 1008.
14. Posner, MA: Carpal bone dislocations and fractures. In Chapman, MW and Madison, M (eds): Operative Orthopaedics. JB Lippincott, Philadelphia, 1988, p 1251.
15. Ferlic, DC: Scaphoid fractures. In Strickland, JW and Steichen, JB (eds): Difficult Problems in Hand Surgery. CV Mosby, St Louis, 1982, p 105.
16. Upton, J: Fractures. In Wolfert, FG (ed): Acute Hand Injuries: A Multispecialty Approach. Little, Brown, Boston, 1980, p 125.
17. Sorenson, MK: Fractures of the wrist and hand. Clin Phys Ther 9:191, 1986.
18. Sandzen, SC: Atlas of Wrist and Hand Fractures. PSG, Littleton, MA, 1979, p 227.
19. Elkouri, ER: Review of cancellous and cortical bone healing after fracture or osteotomy. J Am Podiatr Assoc 72:464, 1982.
20. O'Brien, ET: Fractures of the metacarpals and phalanges. In Green, DP (ed): Operative Hand Surgery, ed 2. Churchill Livingstone, New York, 1988, p 709.
21. Green, DP: Dislocations and ligamentous injuries in the hand. In Evarts, CM (ed): Surgery of the Musculoskeletal System. Vol 1. Churchill Livingstone, New York, 1983, p 2:119.
22. Watson, HK and Maglana, W: Complications of fracture management of the hand and wrist. In Gossling, HR and Pillsbury, SL (eds): Complications of Fracture Management. JB Lippincott, Philadelphia, 1984, p 389.
23. Cannon, NM, et al: Diagnosis and Treatment Manual for Physicians and Therapists, ed 2. Hand Rehabilitation Center, Indianapolis, 1985.
24. Dobyns, JH and Linscheid, RL: Fractures and dislocations of the wrist. In Rockwood, CA and Green, DP (eds): Fractures in Adults, JB Lippincott, Philadelphia, 1984, p 411.
25. Green, DP and Rowland, SA: Fractures and dislocations in the hand. In Rockwood, CA and Green, DP (eds): Fractures in Adults. JB Lippincott, Philadelphia, 1984, p 313.
26. Lamb, DW: Fractures. In Lamb, DW and Kuczynski, K (eds): The Practice of Hand Surgery. Blackwell Scientific, Boston, 1981, p 200.
27. Strickland, JW, et al: Factors influencing digital performance after phalangeal fracture. In Strickland, JW and Steichen, JB (eds): Difficult Problems in Hand Surgery. CV Mosby, St Louis, 1982, p 126.
28. Salter, RB and Ogilvie-Harris, DJ: Healing of intra-articular fractures with continuous passive motion. American Academy of Orthopaedic Surgeons Instructional Course Lectures, Vol XXVIII. CV Mosby, St Louis, 1979, p 102.
29. Huffaker, WH, Wray, RC, and Weeks, PM: Factors influencing final range of motion in the fingers after fractures of the hand. Plast Reconstr Surg 63:82, 1979.
30. Barton, N: Fractures of the phalanges of the hand. Hand 9:1, 1977.
31. Neviaser, RJ: Dislocations and ligamentous injuries of the digits. In Chapman, MW and Madison, M (eds): Operative Orthopaedics. JB Lippincott, Philadelphia, 1988, p 1199.
32. Bush, DC: Dislocations of the small joints of the hand—simple and complex. In Cowen, NJ (ed): Practical Hand Surgery. Yearbook Medical, Chicago, 1980, p 295.
33. Eaton, RG: Joint Injuries of the Hand. Charles C Thomas, Springfield, IL, 1971.

CHAPTER 11

Nerve Injuries

Terri Skirven, OTR/L, CHT

Rehabilitation of the individual with a peripheral nerve lesion requires the full repertoire of the therapist's skills and judgment. A nerve injury frequently results in long-term and severe functional limitations. Motor power, sensibility, and sympathetic function may all be disrupted, and, unless managed properly, fixed postural deformities may result. The objectives of this chapter are to (1) discuss nerve anatomy, nerve response to injury and classification of nerve injuries; (2) facilitate an understanding of the treatment goals and priorities during the acute, recovery, and chronic phases following nerve injury; and (3) discuss treatment techniques that are unique to nerve injuries including motor retraining, splinting, sensory reeducation, and desensitization.

ANATOMY REVIEW

The peripheral nerve is an extension of the central nervous system, which is made up of a great number of neurons. The neuron is the smallest functional unit of the peripheral nerve and consists of the following: (1) the nerve cell body; (2) its peripheral extension, the axon or nerve fiber; and (3) the anatomic unit at the synaptic terminal that is the motor or sensory end receptor. The peripheral nerve consists of a combination of motor, sensory, and sympathetic neurons.

The motor neuron cell bodies are located in the anterior column of the spinal cord. The sensory neuron cell bodies are found in the dorsal root ganglia, and the sympathetic neuron cell bodies in the sympathetic ganglia of the autonomic nervous system. Within the nerve cell bodies are manufactured metabolic materials that contribute to the nutrition of the nerve fiber. Axons may be myelinated or unmyelinated and are surrounded by a sheath of Schwann cells. The axon is further encased in a connective tissue sheath termed the endoneurium.[1]

Nerve fibers are grouped together in bundles called fasciculi or funiculi (Fig. 11–1). Each bundle is a combination of motor, sensory, and sympathetic fibers of varying proportions. They are encased in a connective tissue sheath termed the perineurium. The fasciculi, embedded in epineurium, are further arranged in groups with other

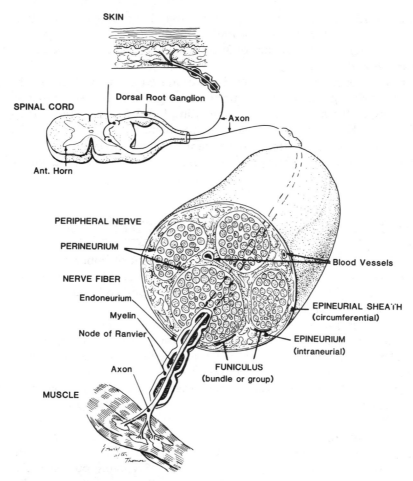

FIGURE 11–1. Schematic anatomy of a peripheral nerve. (From Omer, GE: Acute management of peripheral nerve injuries. In Mackin, EJ [ed]: Hand Clinics: Hand Rehabilitation. WB Saunders, Philadelphia, 1986, with permission.)

fasciculi or they can proceed singly. The epineurium is condensed at the surface of the nerve trunk to form an encasing sheath or the epineurial sheath.

NERVE RESPONSE TO INJURY

Nerve response to injury proceeds in two phases.[2] The first phase involves the disintegration of the axon and the breakdown of its myelin sheath, a process that is referred to as wallerian degeneration. This degeneration occurs distal to the level of injury.

What remains distally are the empty Schwann sheaths and endoneurial tubes that subsequently undergo some degree of shrinkage and collapse with a decrease in the fascicular cross-sectional area. Degeneration also occurs at the motor and sensory end receptors. The second phase of the nerve's response to injury involves neuronal regeneration with sprouting of the axon. For nerve regeneration to be successful, the axon must cross the injury site and enter the same endoneurial tube. The rate of regeneration is 1 to 3 mm per day after an initial latency of 3 to 4 weeks with additional delays at the injury site and at the end organ.[3]

The process of nerve regeneration is complicated by many factors. These factors may include shrinkage of the endoneurial tubes, preventing reentry of the sprouting axons; scarring at the injury site, short-circuiting the progress of the sprouting axons; mismatching of the motor, sensory and sympathetic fibers; and degeneration of the motor or sensory end receptors. Consequently, even under the most favorable of conditions, severance of a peripheral nerve usually results in some degree of residual deficit.

CLASSIFICATION OF NERVE INJURIES

Nerve injuries are classified according to the extent of injury to the axon and the connective tissue sheath. Two systems of classification have been described by Seddon and Sunderland, and have been compared by Bowers and colleagues[4] in their article on nerve suture and grafting (Table 11–1).

The prognosis for recovery of function following a nerve injury and repair is affected by many factors: the nature and level of the injury; the timing and technique of repair; and the age and motivation of the patient. For example, clean, simple lacerations do better than crush injuries because of the lesser degree of tissue reaction and scarring. More proximal lesions do less well because there is a greater combination of motor, sensory, and sympathetic fibers at more proximal levels, resulting in a greater possibility for mismatching during axon regeneration. In addition, proximal lesions take longer to regenerate, allowing more time for degeneration of motor and sensory end receptors. Microsurgical repair by an experienced surgeon, timed appropriately according to the nature and extent of the injury, is essential for a favorable outcome. For example, primary repair may be delayed if wound contamination exists, and secondary repair is done with extensive extremity wounds where the level of nerve injury cannot immediately be determined.[5] Also contributing to a favorable outcome is the surgical technique. Accurate axon alignment and the avoidance of tension at the suture line promotes optimal nerve regeneration. Younger patients do better than older patients because of the adaptability of the nervous system in a younger person with a greater ability to relearn and interpret an altered pattern of sensory impulses following nerve repair.

SPECIFIC NERVE LESIONS

Radial Nerve

Radial nerve injuries may be associated with fractures of the humeral shaft, fracture and dislocation of the elbow, fractures of the upper third of the radius, and compression of the nerve at the level between the radial head and the supinator muscle. The latter type of compression is referred to as radial tunnel syndrome.

Motor, sensory, and functional loss associated with radial nerve lesions depends on the exact site of injury (Fig. 11–2). With forearm level lesions the following muscles are involved:

TABLE 11–1 Comparison of Seddon and Sunderland Classifications of Nerve Injuries

		Clinical Findings				
	Pathology	Motor	Sensory	Treatment	Recovery	Therapy Implications
Neurapraxia (Seddon) First degree (Sunderland)	Anatomic and axonal continuity	Complete paralysis	Minimal loss	Observation	Complete	Short-term, focused
Second degree (Sunderland) Axonotmesis (Seddon)	Transection axon but endoneurium intact	Complete paralysis	Complete loss	Observation	Usually complete	Moderate intervention
Third degree (Sunderland)	Transection axon—loss of endoneurial tube continuity but perineurium intact (traction lesion)	Complete paralysis	Complete loss	Surgical intervention may be required	Incomplete	Moderate intervention
Fourth degree (Sunderland)	Continuity of nerve trunk via epineurium but severe disorganization (neuroma in continuity)	Complete paralysis	Complete loss	Surgical intervention	Incomplete	Long-term comprehensive
Neurotmesis (Seddon)	Loss of nerve trunk continuity, complete disorganization	Complete paralysis	Complete loss	Surgical intervention mandatory	Never complete	Long-term comprehensive
Fifth degree (Sunderland)	Loss of nerve trunk continuity, complete disorganization	Complete paralysis	Complete loss	Surgical intervention mandatory	Never complete	Long-term comprehensive

Adapted from Bowers et al,[4] p 447, with permission.

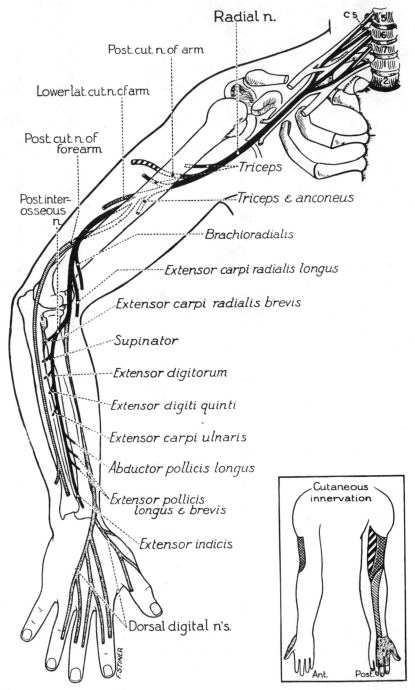

FIGURE 11–2. The course and distribution of the radial nerve. (From Haymaker, W and Woodhall, B: Peripheral Nerve Injuries. WB Saunders, Philadelphia, 1953, with permission.)

- Extensor carpi ulnaris
- Extensor digitorum communis
- Extensor digiti minimi
- Abductor pollicis longus
- Extensor pollicis longus
- Extensor pollicis brevis
- Extensor indicis proprius

The functional deficit includes loss of metacarpal phalangeal (MCP) joint extension of all digits, of thumb radial abduction and extension, and of ulnar wrist extension. The sensory loss involves the dorsal aspect of the thumb and the dorsum of the second, third, and half of the fourth ray to the level of the proximal interphalangeal (PIP) joint. If the posterior interosseous nerve branch is solely involved with forearm level lesions, no cutaneous sensory deficit will occur.

With lesions at the elbow level, the motor loss involves all of the above muscles with the addition of the

- Supinator
- Extensor carpi radialis longus
- Extensor carpi radialis brevis

The functional loss includes loss of ulnar and radial wrist extension and weakened supination, as well as loss of MCP joint extension and thumb extension and radial abduction. The sensory loss is the same.

With lesions just proximal to the elbow, the motor loss will include the brachioradialis as well as all of the above, and the additional functional deficit is weakened elbow flexion. Lesions in the upper arm involve all of the aforementioned, with the addition of the triceps. Functionally, elbow extension is lost. The classic deformity associated with radial nerve lesions is the wrist drop deformity (Fig. 11–3). Hand grip is significantly

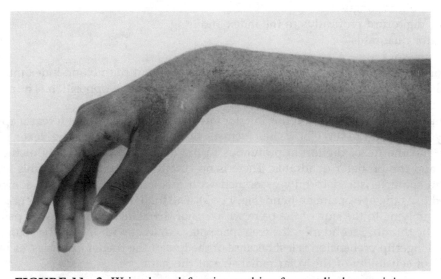

FIGURE 11–3. Wrist drop deformity resulting from radical nerve injury.

compromised due to the loss of wrist extensors which position and help to stabilize the wrist during grasp.

Median Nerve

Median nerve injuries can be associated with humeral fractures, elbow dislocations, distal radius fractures and dislocations of the lunate into the carpal canal, as well as knife and glass lacerations of the volar wrist. Compression of the median nerve can occur at the carpal canal (carpal tunnel syndrome), between the two heads of the pronator teres in the forearm (pronator syndrome), and compression of the anterior interosseous nerve in the forearm.

Deficits associated with median nerve lesions depends on the site of the injury (Fig. 11–4). With a low or wrist-level lesion, the following muscles are involved:

- Opponens pollicis
- Abductor pollicis brevis
- Flexor pollicis brevis (superficial head)
- First and second lumbricales

Functionally, thumb opposition is lost, compromising activities requiring fine prehension. Sensory loss involves the volar surface of the thumb, index and long and radial half of the ring fingers, and the dorsal surface of the distal phalanges of the thumb, index, long, and radial half of the ring fingers with some variations.

With a high-level lesion at the elbow or above, in addition to the aforementioned, the following muscles are also involved:

- Pronator teres
- Flexor carpi radialis
- Flexor digitorum superficialis
- Palmaris longus
- Flexor pollicis longus
- Flexor digitorum profundus to the index and long
- Pronator quadratus

Functionally, pronation and wrist flexion is weakened, and thumb and index interphalangeal (IP) joint flexion is lost in addition to the loss of thumb opposition. The sensory loss is the same with a high-level lesion.

The median nerve gives off the anterior interosseous branch in the forearm approximately 8 cm distal to the elbow. Involvement of this branch affects the flexor pollicis longus and the flexor digitorum profundus to the index and occasionally of the long finger, and the pronator quadratus. There is no cutaneous sensory loss at this level.

The characteristic deformity associated with median nerve injuries is sometimes referred to as the ape or simian hand (Fig. 11–5). The thenar eminence is flattened, with the thumb lying to the side of the palm with loss of the ability to oppose and palmarly abduct the thumb. Secondarily, the web space may contract with loss of the span of the thumb. Fingertip prehension is lost because of the loss of the thenar intrinsics, as well as the loss of sensibility of the volar radial side of the hand.

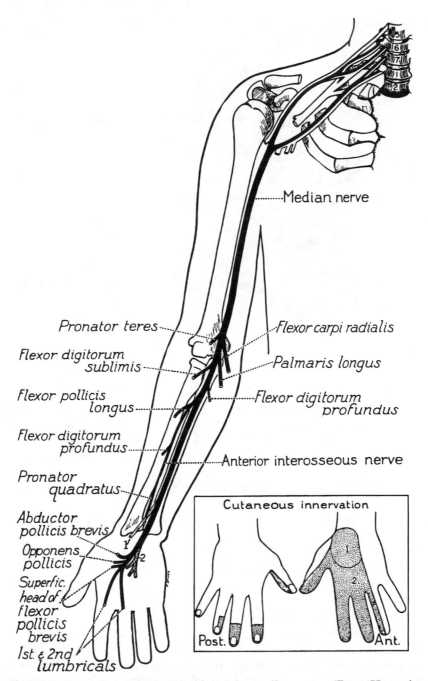

FIGURE 11–4. The course and distribution of the median nerve. (From Haymaker, W and Woodhall, B: Peripheral Nerve Injuries. WB Saunders, Philadelphia, 1953, with permission.)

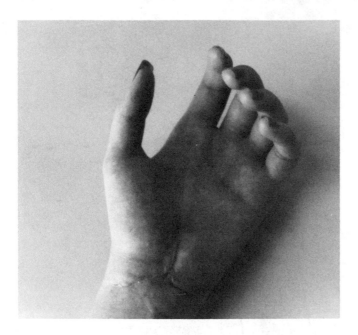

FIGURE 11–5. Median nerve palsy with flattened thenar eminence.

Ulnar Nerve

Ulnar nerve injuries can be associated with fractures of the medial epicondyle of the humerus and the olecranon of the ulna. Glass and knife lacerations of the wrist can involve the ulnar nerve as well. Common sites of compression are within Guyon's canal at the wrist level and within the cubital tunnel proximally.

Deficits associated with an ulnar nerve lesion depends on the site of injury (Fig. 11–6).

With a low or wrist-level lesion, the following muscles are involved:

- Abductor digiti minimi
- Flexor digiti minimi
- Opponens digiti minimi
- Lumbricales to the fourth and fifth digits
- Dorsal interossei
- Palmar interossei
- Flexor pollicis brevis (deep head)
- Adductor pollicis

Functional grip and pinch are affected. With attempts at lateral pinch, the thumb substitutes for the loss of the adductor with the flexor pollicis longus, resulting in flexion of the IP joint during attempts at pinch. This posture is called Froment's sign. Finger abduction and adduction are lost and the ability to actively flex the MCP joints of the ring and small with simultaneous active IP extension is not possible. Because of the loss of the intrinsics, there is a decrease in power grip and a loss of fine prehension. The sensory loss involves the superficial terminal branch of the ulnar nerve which supplies sensation to the volar surface of the ulnar aspect of the palm distally, and the volar surface of the small and ulnar half of the ring fingers.

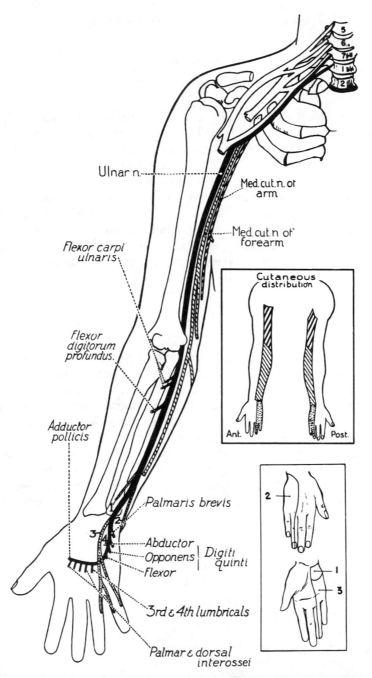

FIGURE 11–6. The course and distribution of the ulnar nerve. (From Haymaker, W and Woodhall, B: Peripheral Nerve Injuries. WB Saunders, Philadelphia, 1953, with permission.)

With a high-level lesion — that is, one at or above the elbow, the following muscles are additionally involved:

- Flexor carpi ulnaris
- Flexor digitorum profundus to the ring and small

Functionally, the clinical picture is the same with hand grip further weakened by the loss of the profundus to the ring and small finger. Sensory loss involves both the palmar and dorsal cutaneous branches of the ulnar nerve in addition to the superficial terminal branch. These branches innervate the dorsal surface of the small and ulnar half of the ring finger, and the proximal palm on the ulnar side.

The characteristic deformity associated with ulnar nerve lesions is the claw deformity (Fig. 11–7). The ring and small fingers rest in a posture of MCP joint hyperextension and IP joint flexion. This posture results from the loss of the balancing influence of the intrinsic muscles on the extrinsic flexors and extensors. In addition, there is atrophy of the interossei with hollowing between the metacarpals and flattening of the hypothenar area.

EVALUATION

Nerve injuries can result in deficits in muscle strength, in protective and discriminative sensibility, and in sympathetic function. Postural disturbances of the hand result from muscle imbalance, and this along with muscle weakness can lead to a loss of joint mobility and the formation of joint and soft tissue contractures. These sequelae have a serious impact on hand function and self-care, work, and leisure activities. Therefore, the essential elements of the therapist's evaluation include manual muscle testing, range of motion (ROM) evaluation, sensibility examination, evaluation of sympathetic function, and an analysis of the impact of the injury on the patient's functional status. A careful evaluation serves to set a baseline from which to gauge the process of reinnervation, as well as to judge the effectiveness of therapy. Ongoing reevaluation allows

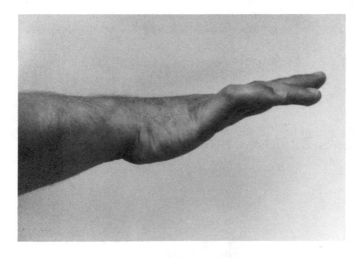

FIGURE 11–7. Claw deformity associated with ulnar nerve injury.

monitoring of the patient's status to ensure that loss of joint mobility does not develop as a result of muscle weakness and to monitor for signs of damage to insensate skin. These evaluations are covered thoroughly in Chapter 3. However, there are specific details in the evaluation of the nerve injured hand that are important to recognize.

In evaluating muscle power, it helps to be familiar with the sequence of innervation for a particular nerve. Muscle reinnervation occurs in the sequence in which they are normally innervated as the nerve travels distally. Knowledge of this sequence allows a more focused evaluation and can help in distinguishing among trick motions, compensatory motions, and weakly innervated muscles.

According to Tubiana[6] trick motions can be produced in four ways: through the effects of gravity, sudden relaxation of the contracting muscle, tenodesis effects, and anomalous innervations. For example, in certain positions of the arm, gravity can cause the elbow to extend, even with paralysis of the triceps. Elbow extension should be tested with the upper arm abducted to 90° and internally rotated to avoid the effects of gravity. With loss of function of the flexor pollicis longus, the patient may quickly contract and then relax the thumb extensor so that the thumb falls back into a slightly flexed posture making it seem as if some voluntary flexion is occurring. Tenodesis may occur when tendons cross more than one joint. For example, active wrist extension produces enough tension on the finger flexor tendons at the wrist to result in finger flexion. This is really a passively produced flexion but can be mistaken for active flexion. Finally, anomalous innervations can be a source of error. A common variation in nerve supply is with the flexor digitorum profundus and with thenar intrinsics and the proportion of median versus ulnar innervation. Compensatory motions are produced by muscles that are not the prime movers but have a secondary action and assist the prime mover. In the absence of the prime mover, motion may still be observed. For example, elbow flexion can be produced by the brachioradialis in the absence of biceps or brachialis function.

Radial Nerve

Common trick motions for the radial nerve include elbow extension using gravity in the absence of triceps function; wrist extension produced by finger flexion (i.e., when the digits flex, pull is exerted on the extensor digitorum communis tendons resulting in wrist extension) finger extension produced through tenodesis action (i.e., with wrist flexion the digits fall into extension). Compensatory motions include extension of the thumb IP joint produced by virtue of the insertion of the abductor pollicus brevis into the extensor expansion of the thumb. In testing, to avoid being misled by these trick motions, the proximal joints must be stabilized to avoid the effects of tenodesis; the extremity should be carefully positioned to avoid the effects of gravity; and in testing thumb extension, extension is required at all three joints simultaneously.

Median Nerve

With median nerve palsy, the flexor pollicis brevis, which is partially ulnar innervated can substitute for palmar abduction. In the absence of the opponens pollicis, the patient may be able to touch the thumb to each of the fingertips using the flexor pollicis brevis, but this is with a lateral approach and is not true opposition, as shown in (Fig.

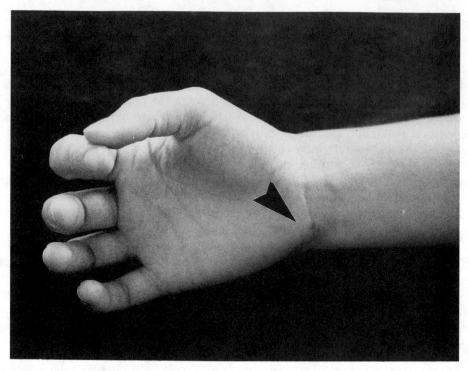

FIGURE 11–8. Attempted opposition with a median nerve palsy. Without the opponens pollicis, the thumb cannot achieve true opposition and makes contact with the lateral aspect of the digit.

11–8). In testing the abductor pollicis brevis the thumb must be truly perpendicular to the palm to avoid substitution by the abductor pollicis longus. In testing for opponens function, the thumb should be positioned in the rotated and opposed position and the patient asked to hold the position. With weakness or paralysis of the opponens, the patient will be unable to hold the position.

Ulnar Nerve

With ulnar nerve palsy, extension of the IP joints can be produced by the extensor digitorum communis in the absence of intrinsic function, but only if the MCP joints are blocked from hyperextending. The extrinsic extensors can produce finger abduction, and the extrinsic flexors can produce adduction in the absence of the dorsal and palmar interossei. During attempts at thumb adduction, the flexor pollicis longus may compensate and produce adduction in addition to IP joint flexion. In testing finger abduction and adduction, the hand must rest on a flat surface and the long finger should be used, with the patient asked to move it from side to side. Tests for thumb adduction should be done with the thumb IP joint straight.

When evaluating ROM, one must be aware of the key contractures and limitations that may occur with each injury so that the evaluating therapist can anticipate these and monitor accordingly. For example, with radial nerve injuries, shortening of the wrist and finger flexors may occur, resulting in loss of wrist and MCP joint extension. Following median nerve injuries, loss of web space span may occur because of loss of thumb abduction, and a loss of pronation is also possible. With ulnar nerve injuries and the claw deformity, there is a vulnerability for the development of flexion contractures of the IP joints of the fourth and fifth digits. ROM monitoring on a regular basis allows the therapist to detect problems early and adjust the treatment program appropriately.

Sensibility testing is particularly relevant with nerve injuries. An initial examination can aid in the diagnosis of a suspected nerve injury or can serve to establish a baseline. Regular reevaluation on a monthly basis allows monitoring of nerve regeneration and can aid in determining readiness for sensory reeducation. Sensibility testing is also included in disability determinations because of the significant functional impact of sensibility loss. Sympathetic function is assessed by observation of the color and temperature of the skin in comparison to an intact area; of the presence or absence of sweating; of any changes of the nails or atrophy of the finger pulps; and observation of skin texture.[7] Tinel's sign is also used to monitor nerve regeneration. This sign is said to represent the advancing terminations of the regenerating sensory axons.

Finally, pain is addressed as part of the therapist's assessment. Severe, burning pain in the distribution of the injured nerve, referred to as causalgia, may be associated with a nerve injury. Neuromas may also be a source of extreme pain when touched and may develop at the site of the injury. Clinical features of the patient's pain are documented such as the time of onset following the injury, the quality of the pain, its distribution, and precipitating factors.

THERAPEUTIC MANAGEMENT

The remainder of the chapter will focus on the rehabilitation of nerve injuries during the acute, recovery, and chronic phases. The acute phase refers to the early postinjury and postsurgery time when the focus is on healing and prevention. The recovery phase refers to the period of reinnervation when retraining and reeducation are stressed. The chronic phase refers to that time when the potential for reinnervation has peaked and the patient is left with significant residual deficits. The emphasis during this phase is on compensatory function.

Acute Phase

The objectives of the therapist's management during the acute phase are primarily protection and prevention; protection of the traumatized or surgically repaired nerve and prevention of joint contracture and further injury secondary to decreased sensibility. Table 11-2 highlights information important for the therapist to obtain at the time of referral and the therapy implications. The types of diagnoses seen during this phase may include an acute nerve compression, postsurgical decompression and release, and postsurgical repair of a lacerated nerve.

PERIOD OF IMMOBILIZATION

The purpose of postoperative immobilization or splinting is to (1) minimize tension at the repair site, (2) protect the nerve from disruption, and (3) in the case of nerve

TABLE 11–2 Referral Information and Treatment Implications

Required Information	Treatment Implications
Nerve Involvement	
A. Specific nerve injured	A. Indicates sensory and motor impairment; provides focus for evaluation
B. Classification and level of injury	B. Indicates prognosis and facilitates goal setting
C. Mechanism of injury; clean vs crush	C. Indicates degree of tissue reaction and scar to anticipate more damage with crush injuries than with clean lacerations
D. Other structures involved	D. Treatment protocols must be integrated to allow appropriate management for all injured structures
Surgical Management	
A. Date of repair	A. Nerve repairs protected from stress for 3–5 wk
B. Position of joints to allow relaxation of the nerve juncture	B. Tension at the nerve juncture can compromise results; relaxation of the nerve juncture achieved by flexing the joints across which the nerve passes
C. Type of repair	C. Early repair is superior to late repair; with nerve grafts, axons must regenerate across two junctures

compression or following decompression, immobilize or splint to minimize and facilitate the resolution of the inflammatory reaction.

Splinting following nerve repair may be done by the attending physician or the therapist with either a plaster cast or a removable plastic splint. The choice is usually made by the physician who considers the reliability of the patient and his or her lifestyle. Positioning, whether with casting or splinting, is done with joints flexed or extended in order to avoid tension at the repair site. For example, with a median nerve repair the wrist may need to be flexed. The specific position of the splint and duration of use is determined by the surgeon and communicated to the therapist. In general, immobilization is maintained for 3 to 4 weeks following nerve repair at which time the tensile strength of the nerve is great enough to withstand stress. An important consideration, when splinting the hand with compromised sensation, is the potential for skin breakdown. Splints must be carefully fabricated to avoid pressure areas, and the patient must be instructed to monitor the skin for any signs of breakdown such as redness or blistering.

Splinting following a nerve compression or contusion is done to rest the involved area to facilitate the resolution of the inflammatory reaction. If applied acutely the splint is worn continuously for 1 to 2 weeks and then intermittently thereafter. The splint is positioned to allow a minimum of pressure on the nerve at the site of compression. For example, with carpal tunnel syndrome, the wrist is positioned in neutral to slight extension, which minimizes pressure on the median nerve.[8]

During the period of immobilization, the therapist must monitor the status of the unimmobilized joints and instruct the patient in ROM exercises to ensure maintenance of joint mobility.

POSTIMMOBILIZATION

The priorities of the therapy program at this stage are to recover ROM lost during the period of immobilization, to enhance function, and to educate the patient in a program of protection and prevention.

Increase of Range of Motion

ROM exercises are directed at recovering the motion lost during the phase of immobilization. For example, with a low median or ulnar nerve repair the wrist is positioned in flexion during the phase of immobilization and the patient may have restricted wrist extension when permitted to begin exercises. Exercises are directed at gradually recovering wrist extension, generally starting with active range of motion (AROM).

Passive and active assisted exercises are introduced depending on the patient's progress as well as on specific precautions relevant to the individual case. For example, if the patient is recovering ROM at a satisfactory rate with the active program, then passive range of motion (PROM) exercises may not be necessary. However, if progress is slow (i.e., less than a 5° gain per week), then PROM exercises may begin. In any case, aggressive stretching exercises are avoided to protect the repaired nerve from a potentially harmful maximum stretch. Occasionally, specific ROM limits will be imposed by the surgeon to protect a nerve repaired under tension or when a nerve gap has had to be overcome with more extensive joint positioning. In these cases the therapy approach may be to increase incrementally the amount of ROM allowed by a specific number of degrees on a week-to-week basis; for example, following median nerve repair under tension, wrist extension may be permitted at a rate of 10° per week. Splints may be serially adjusted to ensure that ROM limits are not exceeded.

Enhancement of Function

Splinting is also used at this stage with the aim to enhance function. When the nerve injury results in muscle paresis or paralysis, and muscle imbalance disrupts the normal resting posture of the hand, soft tissue and joint contractures may result, as well as overstretching of the weakened muscle by the pull of its antagonist. Splinting is used to restore the normal resting posture and to prevent secondary joint contractures. By restoring a more normal posture, the splint may also enhance function. With each nerve injury specific requirements must be fulfilled. The exact style of the splint, the material from which it is made, and the method of construction is, to some extent, secondary as long as the splint resolves the problem and is acceptable to the patient.

Radial Nerve Splints. The critical problem with radial nerve palsy is the loss of wrist extension. The wrist rests in a flexed posture, which puts the wrist extensors at risk for overstretching. In addition, the MCP joints rest in a more extended position when the wrist is flexed due to the tension placed on the extensor digitorum communis across the flexed wrist. This extended MCP joint position, if unrelieved, may result in shortening of the collateral ligaments and, hence, extension contractures.

The splint applied must support the wrist in extension. A simple wrist cock-up splint or a Futuro splint may be used. There is also a loss of MCP joint extension because of the involvement of the extrinsic finger extensors. The wrist splint can be made to include the MCP joints, supporting them in neutral or slight flexion. However, supporting the MCP joints limits full flexion and may result in a loss of MCP joint flexion if not monitored closely. Many patients prefer a wrist splint without MCP joint support and report satisfactory function.

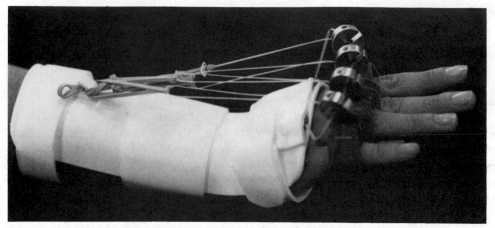

FIGURE 11–9. Phoenix outrigger.

A dynamic splint with an outrigger to assist finger and thumb extension can additionally be used to allow a full arc of finger motion. The splint can be made dorsally with the wrist supported in a slight degree of extension. The commercially available low-profile Phoenix outrigger can be used to provide the extension assist (Fig. 11–9). Colditz[9] has developed a splint for radial nerve palsy that reestablishes the normal tenodesis pattern of the hand. The splint includes a dorsal trough with a low-profile outrigger that extends across the wrist to the level of the proximal phalanges. Finger loops are worn around each proximal phalanx, and nylon cord is directed from these loops through channels on the outrigger and pulled to a proximal attachment point on the dorsal base of the splint (Fig. 11–10A). When the digits are flexed, tension on the cord brings the wrist into extension, and when the wrist is flexed the digits are pulled into extension. (Fig. 11–10A & B)

The specific splint chosen, whether static or dynamic, must be one that is functional for the patient but also cosmetically acceptable, for the splinting program to be successful. Some patients reject a dynamic splint as too bulky or attention getting and will not wear it, preferring a static splint. When the dominant extremity is involved, the functional requirement usually takes precedence and a dynamic splint is frequently the best choice. When the nondominant extremity is involved, the functional requirement may be less, and the patient's concern for cosmesis may lead to the choice of a static splint. At night, a simple wrist splint is sufficient to position the wrist and allow the fingers to fall into a normal resting posture.

Median Nerve Splints. Median nerve injury results in loss of the ability to position the thumb in opposition to the fingers and to palmarly abduct the thumb. Splinting is needed to facilitate thumb and finger prehension and to maintain the thumb web space. A hand-based splint that positions the thumb in palmar abduction and opposition to the index and long fingers can be used (Fig. 11–11).

However, some patients find that they do just as well without a splint and can use compensatory motions to substitute for the absent thenar intrinsics. If the opponens splint is not used, the web space must be maintained either with a web spacer splint worn at night or with conscientious web stretching, or both. If a web space contracture does develop, serial web space splinting would be indicated to restore the web space.

Ulnar Nerve Splints. The loss of the interossei and the fourth and fifth lumbricales

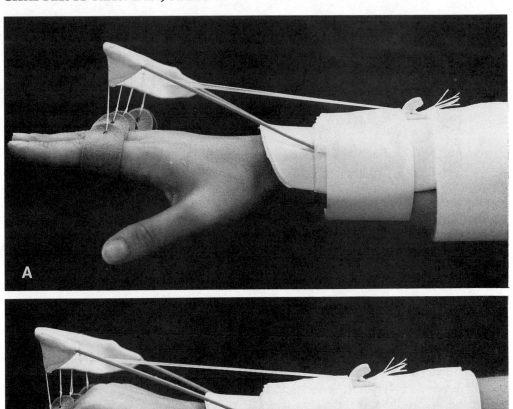

FIGURE 11–10. *A*, Splint for radial nerve palsy designed by Colditz,[9] which reestablishes the tenodesis pattern of the hand. *B*, With digital flexion the wrist is brought into extension.

with ulnar nerve injury results in a claw deformity. The resting position is one of MCP joint hyperextension with PIP and distal interphalangeal (DIP) joint flexion owing to the unopposed action of the extrinsic flexors and extensors. The posture is more pronounced with the ring and small fingers, because the index and long finger lumbricales are median innervated. The deformity may initially be passively correctable, but, left untreated, fixed flexion contractures may result at the PIP and DIP joint levels. Functionally, the patient will have difficulty with grasp, because he or she will be unable to extend the fingers in approaching objects to be grasped. Splinting is needed to provide a counterbalance for the extrinsic muscles that will help prevent the development of flexion contractures, and allow extension at the IP joints to facilitate grasp.

A dorsal hand-based splint that blocks MCP joint hyperextension can be fabricated. With the MCP joint blocked, the extensor digitorum can exert its pull distally, and extension is then possible at the IP joints. The splint is fabricated to allow full digital

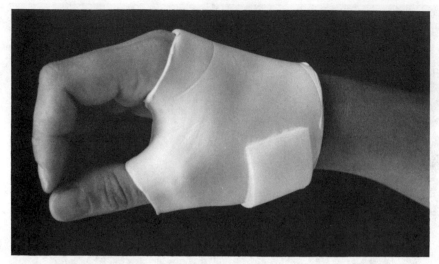

FIGURE 11–11. Opponens splint for median nerve palsy.

flexion (Fig. 11–12). A simple alternative is to limit MCP joint hyperextension using finger cuffs over the proximal phalanges with elastics volarly and proximally attached to a wrist strap or band (Fig. 11–13). When the patient extends, the cuff limits MCP joint hyperextension and then IP joint extension is possible. If PIP flexion contractures have already developed, dynamic, serial static, or three-point extension splinting is needed to correct the deformity and restore passive PIP joint extension.

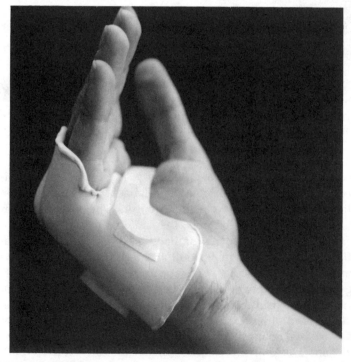

FIGURE 11–12. Splint used to counteract the claw deformity of ulnar nerve palsy.

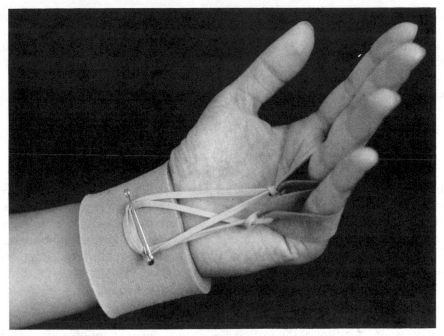

FIGURE 11–13. Alternative method for splinting an ulnar nerve palsy to counteract clawing.

Patient Education

A fully informed and involved patient is one of the most important ingredients for a successful rehabilitation program. The therapist's early sessions with the patient should be focused on education. A simplified explanation of nerve function and the consequences of injury, as well as what outcomes can be expected needs to be covered. Patients must be aware of the slow rate of nerve regeneration and the guarded prognosis with complete and high lesions in order to adjust their expectations accordingly. Communication between the therapist and surgeon is essential to ensure that the same information is being conveyed.

A clear, simple, and realistic home program must also be a part of this early education process. What the patient does outside of the therapy clinic is just as important as the supervised therapy sessions. Patients must know what deformities they are at risk for developing and what measures they need to take for preventing these. The therapist must work with the patient in developing a schedule of exercise and splint use that is reasonable within the context of the patient's lifestyle but that achieves the goals of therapy.

The patient must also know the risks related to the loss of sensation. Callahan[7] describes in detail specific precautions that need to be emphasized. For example, because of the loss of sensation, the patient is susceptible to thermal injuries as well as to those from sharp or abrasive objects. Because of the loss of feeling, the patient may grip objects with more force and may sustain the grip longer, resulting in skin breakdown and blister formation. Once injury has occurred, healing may take longer than usual because of the decreased nutrition and vascularity of denervated skin.[10]

The patient must be instructed to avoid handling very hot, cold, sharp, or abrasive objects. When using tools or other objects, sustained grasp must be avoided, tools should be changed frequently, tool handles built up to distribute pressure, and protective work gloves worn. Regular skin inspection is stressed with prompt treatment of any wounds or blisters that may result from daily activities or from improperly fitting or applied splints. Brand[11] recommends daily soaks and oil massage to compensate for the dryness of the skin and reduced compliancy under pressure that occurs because of the loss of the sweating function of the skin that normally maintains moistness and protects the skin from cracking.

Recovery Phase

Once clinical signs of reinnervation become apparent, the therapy program and treatment goals must be reestablished. With the return of sensory and motor function, retraining and reeducation become important. As muscles are reinnervated, therapy is designed to enhance the recovery of strength and control. As skin receptors are reinnervated, techniques of desensitization and reeducation are applied to normalize and maximize the recovery of functional sensibility.

MOTOR RETRAINING

Motor retraining begins at the earliest evidence of muscle reinnervation. Before this time, passive exercises are important to maintain joint ROM and muscle-tendon length. Some clinicians also advocate the use of electrical stimulation to forestall the deterioration of denervated muscle. The rationale is that the recovery of muscle strength following reinnervation will be more complete if the physiologic muscle integrity is maintained with electrical stimulation. However, research support for this theory is limited, and the use of electrical stimulation for denervated muscle is not a universally agreed on practice. Once reinnervation begins, however, electrical stimulation may be used to give the patient the proprioceptive feedback of the recovering muscle. Active and active assisted exercises are provided for the function the muscle is primarily responsible for. Position and hold exercises are very helpful at this stage. For example, the involved joint or joints are placed in the desired position, and the patient is asked to hold the position through contraction of the desired muscle. During this exercise, electrical stimulation of the muscle can enhance the patient's efforts. Refer to Chapter 8 for a more indepth discussion of electrical stimulation. Biofeedback can also help by increasing the patient's awareness of minute contractions through visual and auditory feedback. Initially, the therapy sessions must be kept short to avoid fatigue. As the patient demonstrates increasing control, isotonic exercises are introduced. Functional activities are incorporated in the program to provide practice in coordinating movement patterns and to further increase strength and endurance. Progressive resistive exercise is also used to increase strength when the target muscle reaches the fair grade.

Key exercises for the radial nerve lesions involve wrist, finger, and thumb extension. Wrist extensor muscle activity is easily monitored using biofeedback, a useful technique during the early stages of motor return. When retraining the finger extensors, intrinsic substitution should be eliminated by preventing IP extension while attempting MCP joint extension. Coban wrap can be used to position the IP joints in flexion when isolating extensor digitorum communis activity (Fig. 11–14). Key exercises for median nerve lesions involve the thenar intrinsic muscles. The thumb is positioned in opposition and the patient is asked to hold it this way. Positioning and holding in palmar abduction

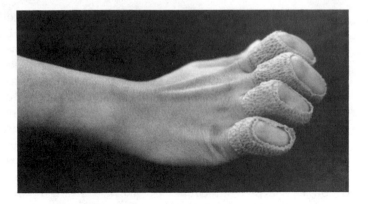

FIGURE 11–14. Exercise for the extensor digitorum communis.

is also practiced. A circular object such as a jar lid can be placed perpendicularly in the palm and the patient can attempt to trace the perimeter of the jar lid with the thumb, a motion that requires the action of the opponens and the abductor pollicis brevis (Fig. 11–15). Finger abduction and adduction exercises are key with ulnar nerve lesions. The patient's hand is placed palm down on a flat surface that can be dusted with powder to eliminate friction, and abduction and adduction of the digits is attempted. Lateral pinching exercises are also important and involve activity of the first dorsal interosseous muscle and the adductor pollicis.

DESENSITIZATION

Regeneration of a sensory nerve is frequently associated with dysesthesia. A light touch of the involved area may range from being mildly irritating to extremely painful in

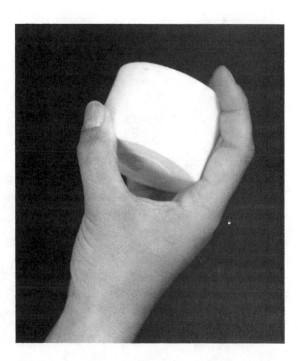

FIGURE 11–15. Exercise used to assist the rotatory action of the opponens pollicis.

the case of neuroma formation. Desensitization has been described by several authors[7,12,13] as helpful in reducing this hypersensitivity. Desensitization refers to the process of lessening reactivity to an external stimulus through the use of a graded series of modalities and procedures. Treatment begins with exposure to a stimulus that is slightly irritating but tolerable, and as tolerance increases, more noxious stimuli are introduced. Barber[12] has developed a structured approach to the evaluation and treatment of hypersensitivity. Three sensory modalities are used in Barber's approach—textures, contact particles, and vibration. In the testing phase, the patient is instructed to rank a series of each of these modalities ranging from the least to the most irritating.

For example, 10 different types of textures fixed to dowels are organized by the patient from the least to the most irritating (Fig. 11–16). Particulate materials, from cotton to sharp-edged cubes, are likewise arranged, in 3-lb coffee cans. Vibratory stimulus is applied with a commercially available vibrator and is ranked according to the cycles per second (cps), the duration of application, and whether the stimulus is intermittent or sustained. After arranging the hierarchy, the patient selects a tolerable but mildly irritating stimulus from each of the three modalities and uses this in treatment to desensitize the involved area. The textures are rubbed, tapped, or rolled over the area; the hand is immersed in the particulate materials; and the vibratory stimulus is applied in either a continuous or an intermittent fashion. Treatment is performed daily, three to four times a day, for 10 minutes a session. When the stimulus becomes tolerable, the next in the series is used. Maximum progress occurs when the most irritating of the series is tolerated. Barber[12] reviewed a series of 124 patients who participated in the desensitization program at the Downey Hand Center between March 1980 and March 1982. The length of treatment averaged 7 weeks and was initiated an average of 8 to 13 weeks after injury. Barber found that all 124 patients improved to the extent that they

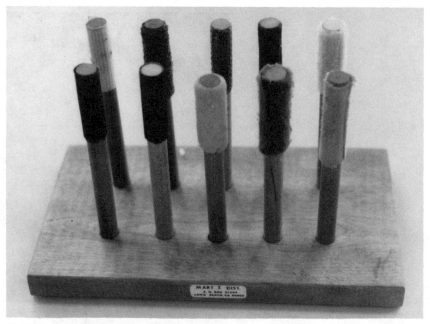

FIGURE 11–16. Graded textures fixed to dowels used in a desensitization program.

were discharged from treatment and were able to return to work. They all showed improvement in some aspect of the hand sensitivity test.

SENSORY REEDUCATION

The prognosis for recovery of discriminative sensibility following nerve injury is generally considered poor. This poor prognosis is because during nerve regeneration, the axon may be blocked by scar at the suture line, a neuroma may form, or the axon may enter a different endoneurial tube or may reinnervate a different end organ. Consequently, when the affected area is stimulated, the patient will be unable to interpret the stimulus correctly because the nerve impulses received by the brain will be altered compared with the preinjury pattern; that is, the stimulus may be applied at one place on the hand and be perceived at another place. Cortical reorganization is needed to improve tactile discriminative ability and sensory reeducation has been proposed by many investigators as an effective approach to the problem.[14-16] As defined by Dellon,[14] sensory reeducation is one or several methods that help the patient with a sensory deficit learn to reinterpret the altered pattern of neural impulses elicited by stimulation of the involved area of skin.

Dellon[14] identified a pattern of sensory recovery following nerve injury. Pain is the first to recover, followed by perception of vibration of 30 cps, the perception of moving touch, constant touch, and vibration of 256 cps.[14] The return proceeds from proximal to distal. When the perception of 30 cps and moving touch have returned to a particular area, the first phase of Dellon's sensory reeducation program can begin. The goal of the first phase is to reeducate the localization of the stimulus and submodality-specific perceptions (e.g., moving versus constant touch). The eraser end of a pencil is used to stimulate the specific area or zone. A moving touch stimulus is used initially and a visual and tactile matching process is used. Stimulation of the affected area of the hand is done with the patient's vision occluded, and patients are asked to localize where they were touched. If the response was incorrect, the stimulation is repeated with the patient's eyes open, and patients concentrate on matching the tactile impression with the visual image. Finally, the stimulation is repeated with the patient's eyes closed and patients concentrate on matching what they are feeling with what they have just seen.

When the patient can perceive constant touch, this same approach is used to reeducate localization of this touch submodality. Once moving and constant touch are perceived at the fingertips with good localization, the second phase of Dellon's program begins. The goal of this phase is the recovery of tactile recognition. Familiar household objects are used that vary in size, shape, and texture. A similar visual-tactile matching process is used during this phase. As recognition improves, the patient is challenged to discriminate more subtle differences.

Callahan[15] divides her sensory reeducation into two types—protective and discriminative. The goal of protective sensory reeducation is to educate the patient in techniques of compensation for the loss of protective sensory input, as discussed under patient education, and begins during the acute phase of management. Discriminative sensory reeducation is similar to Dellon's[14] approach, with training tasks involving localization and graded discrimination of textures, shapes, and objects. Callahan[15] recommends a quiet setting, daily practice, and short sessions of 10 to 15 minutes each, two to three times a day, incorporating the visual-tactile matching process described previously. Discriminative sensory reeducation begins when there is a return of touch perception out to the fingertips within the range measured by Semmes-Weinstein monofilaments numbered 4.31 or lower.[15]

Chronic Phase

When the patient's progress has peaked and there are significant and functionally limiting residual deficits, the focus of the therapy program turns toward compensation. A complete inventory of the patient's functional abilities and limitations is taken.

Adaptive techniques and assistive equipment are suggested when appropriate to allow independent function in self-care, work, and leisure activities. For example, the patient with a median nerve injury may require a buttonhook to fasten buttons. Splinting alternatives are explored that improve function and are practical and cosmetic for long-term use. Splints previously provided during the acute and recovery phases are reevaluated and refabricated or modified as needed. The goals of splinting at this stage are essentially the same as for earlier phases but have a greater emphasis on the splint's ability to improve function and its practicality for long-term use.

Surgical alternatives are considered at this stage, including nerve exploration and grafting, joint fusions, and tendon transfers. If there has been minimal or no nerve regeneration, and satisfactory compensatory function has not developed, then tendon transfers may be appropriate.

TENDON TRANSFERS

Tendon transfer is a technique that involves the application of motor power of one muscle to another weaker or paralyzed muscle by transfer of its tendinous insertion. This procedure does not add to but rather redistributes power in an attempt to improve function. The therapist can play an important role both before and after surgery. Preoperatively, full PROM must be obtained as incomplete PROM may compromise the results of the transfer. Maintaining optimal soft tissue status is also important. Tissues and scars must be supple and mobilized. The donor muscle is strengthened preoperatively, and isolated control is emphasized. This muscle will be performing a new function that can only approximate the lost motion; it must be in optimal condition to maximize results. Finally, a realistic attitude on the patient's part must be fostered. The tendon transfer is a palliative procedure. Return to normal, full ROM is not expected.

Postoperatively, tendon transfers are immobilized for 3 to 5 weeks. During this protected phase, the therapist may be asked to fabricate a splint that places the hand and wrist in a position that minimizes tension on the transfer. In addition, attention is paid to the uninvolved joints to ensure maintenance of ROM, and edema control techniques are used as needed.

Mobilization of the transfer begins after 3 to 5 weeks of splinting or casting. Active movement of the transfer prior to this time could result in elongation or rupture at the site of tendon juncture because there is insufficient strength and maturation of the healing tissue to allow active movement. The patient attempts the desired motion through contraction of the donor muscle.

When first attempting to use the muscle in its new role, the patient should focus on the motion that the donor muscle did before the transfer. For example, with a pronator teres to radial wrist extensor tendon transfer, the patient should attempt wrist extension while at the same time thinking about and initiating pronation. Biofeedback and electrical stimulation of the donor muscle can be used to increase the patient's awareness and isolated control. Overstretching of the transfer can occur at this stage if exercise is done too vigorously in the direction opposite to that of the transfer. For example, after tendon transfer to restore wrist and finger extension is performed, flexion exercises are done cautiously, avoiding simultaneous wrist and finger flexion and postponing passive flexion exercises until later stages of therapy. Protective splinting is continued during this stage to prevent overloading of the tendon junctures that can occur with inadvertent and unsupervised activity of the hand. Splinting also supports the desired position of the hand during this early phase when the tendon transfer may not be fully functioning or strong. The splint is removed only for exercise and hygiene. In addition, massage is begun to mobilize the scars and soft tissue to reduce edema. Adhesions can occur anywhere along the route of the transfer but are most often at the incision and must be treated early with massage to avoid binding of the transfer and compromise of the functional result. The patient is instructed to carry out a home program using all of the aforementioned techniques.

After 6 to 8 weeks, when the tendon juncture sites are strong enough to withstand stress, passive exercises and functional activities can be added to the program and the splint decreased to night use only. Strengthening with putty and other forms of resistive exercise can begin after 8 to 12 weeks. The specific exercises and activities are individualized according to the transfer.

A basic familiarity with the most common tendon transfers for the wrist and hand is essential. This includes knowledge of the purpose of the transfer, the donor muscle used, and the early precautions to be observed. (Table 11–3).

CLINICAL DECISION MAKING: CASE STUDY

B.W. is a 25-year-old right hand–dominant man who sustained a glass laceration of the ulnar, volar aspect of the right wrist, resulting in a complete laceration of the palmar branch, the superficial terminal branch, and the deep terminal motor branch of the ulnar nerve at the level of the pisiform, with loss of a 1-cm segment from the superficial terminal branch. Injury occurred when the patient slipped and fell onto a trash bag filled with wine bottles.

B.W. underwent a primary microsurgical repair of the ulnar nerve with anastomosis of all three divisions. Application of a bulky dressing with a dorsal plaster splint was applied with the wrist flexed at 50° to prevent tension at the repair site of the nerve.

THERAPEUTIC MANAGEMENT, ACUTE PHASE

Evaluation

B.W. was referred for hand therapy and splinting, 5 weeks after repair when his cast was removed. Prior to this time, the cast had been repositioned once in a lesser degree of flexion. Referral was for splinting, exercise, and patient education. The initial evaluation included medical, social, and vocational history; active and passive ROM evaluations; manual muscle test; sensibility examination; and a functional evaluation of activities of daily living (ADLs).

TABLE 11-3 Common Tendon Transfers

Level	Function	Transfer	Early Precautions
Radial nerve	Wrist extension	Pronator teres to extensor carpi radialis longus and brevis	Avoid simultaneous wrist and digital flexion to prevent overstretch of the transfer
	Finger extension	Flexor carpi ulnaris or flexor carpi radialis to extensor digitorum communis	
	Thumb extension	Palmaris longus or flexor digitorum superficialis to extensor pollicis longus	
Median nerve	Opposition	Flexor digitorum superficialis, palmaris longus or extensor digiti minimi	Avoid simultaneous wrist, thumb, and finger extension
	Thumb IP flexion (high lesions)	Brachioradialis to flexor pollicis longus	
	DIP flexion of index (high lesions)	Flexor digitorum profundus of the long, ring, and small to the flexor digitorum profundus of the index	
Ulnar nerve	Correct claw (control MCP joint hyperextension)	Flexor digitorum superficialis, extensor indicis proprius, extensor digiti minimi to intrinsics	Avoid full MCP joint extension; avoid simultaneous finger, thumb, and wrist extension
	Thumb adduction	Flexor digitorum superficialis, or extensor carpi radialis longus to adductor pollicis	
	Index abduction	Abductor pollicis longus, extensor carpi radialis longus, extensor indicis proprius to first dorsal interossei	
	Dip flexion of the long, ring, and small (high lesions)	Side-to-side tenodesis of flexor digitorum profundus of index	

Problems identified included the following:

1. Paralysis of the ulnar nerve innervated intrinsics resulting in loss of active IP joint extension of the ring and the small fingers; loss of thumb adduction, and loss of abduction and adduction of the digits; and resting of the ring and small in a claw posture.
2. Secondary limitations of the wrist in extension because of prolonged positioning in flexion during cast immobilization, with a tight and adherent volar scar.
3. Loss of protective sensibility of the ulnar side of the palm and ulnar volar half of the ring and volar surface of the small finger. Loss of sympathetic function.
4. ADL difficulties secondary to the impairment of the dominant function of the right hand.

Establishing Treatment Priorities

The initial program focuses on recovery of ROM lost during cast immobilization, prevention of a fixed claw deformity, a protective sensory reeducation program, and regular monitoring for the return of ulnar nerve function.

1. Recovery of ROM—Active, active assisted, and passive ROM exercises were provided to recover wrist extension. A volar splint was used initially to support the wrist in maximum extension and was adjusted to increase the position of the wrist toward greater extension as the patient improved.
2. Prevention of deformity—Splinting and patient education were used to prevent the development of a fixed claw deformity. A small, hand-based splint was provided, with a dorsal block limiting hyperextension of the MCP joints of the fourth and fifth fingers but allowing full flexion. Initially, that was worn in conjunction with the wrist splint. IP joint extension was possible with this splint through the action of the extensor digitorum communis. B.W. was thoroughly instructed in the potential for the deformity and the necessity for using splint continuously, and for daily monitoring to ensure that PIP joint flexion contractures were not developing.
3. Protective sensory reeducation—B.W. was instructed to avoid very hot or cold, abrasive or sharp objects; to avoid sustained grasp; to change his grip frequently when working with tools; and to build up handles of tools. Recovery of sensation was monitored regularly, and discriminative sensory reeducation was begun when the perception of moving and constant touch was present. Localization exercises were performed with a visual tactile matching process. B.W. performed these exercises at home four times a day for 5 to 10 minutes each session.
4. Monitoring for return of ulnar nerve function—Periodic sensory and motor tests were performed to allow appropriate upgrading of the program and introduction of more challenging intervention strategies.

THERAPEUTIC MANAGEMENT: RECOVERY PHASE

Reevaluation

Repeated measurements of ROM reflected recovery of full wrist ROM after 4 weeks of therapy. At 5 months, manual muscle test revealed trace to poor strength of the abductor digiti minimi. Protective sensibility had returned to the ulnar aspect of the palm and ring and small digits with localization increasing in accuracy.

Reestablishing Treatment Priorities

The focus of therapy during this phase was on motor retraining and further sensory reeducation.

1. Motor retraining—As strength increased from poor to fair, active and active assisted exercises for the interossei, hypothenars, fourth and fifth lumbricales, and thumb adductor were provided, with progression to light resistance when a fair plus grade of strength was achieved. General putty gripping and pinching exercises, as well as resistance for abduction and adduction of the fingers, was provided. During the earlier phases of reinnervation, biofeedback and electrical stimulation were used to increase B.W.'s awareness of muscle contraction and augment his efforts.
2. Sensory reeducation—Discriminative sensory reeducation exercises included texture, shape, and size discrimination exercises using the ulnar palm and ring and small fingers. Also, discrimination of objects embedded in rice was done, using the ring and small fingers to search for the objects, and the thumb and the ring and small were used to pick the object out of the rice.

FOLLOW-UP STATUS

At 1 year after nerve repair, B.W. demonstrated full ROM of the wrist and hand. Manual muscle test reflected activity of all ulnar innervated intrinsics in the good range of strength.

Grip and pinch strength were still 20% less than on the uninvolved side. Sensibility examination reflected recovery of localization and of protective and light touch sensibility but two-point discrimination was 12 mm at the tip of the small finger and on the ulnar half of the tip of the ring finger. B.W. has resumed his previous work and leisure activities.

SUMMARY

The management of the patient with a peripheral nerve injury challenges the full range of the therapist's knowledge and skills. A thorough understanding of nerve anatomy, nerve response to injury, classification of nerve injuries, and specific nerve lesions is necessary to establish a frame of reference.

A careful assessment is essential to the treatment planning process and includes manual muscle testing, ROM evaluation, sensibility examination, evaluation of sympathetic function, and an analysis of the impact of the injury on the patient's functional status. Goals are set and treatment provided according to the phases of nerve recovery.

During the acute phase, the objectives of the therapist's management include protection of the traumatized or surgically repaired nerve to allow healing, prevention of joint contracture and avoidance of further injury secondary to decreased sensibility.

These objectives are accomplished through the use of protective and functional splints, ROM exercises, and patient education in safety precautions for decreased sensation. During the recovery phase, retraining and reeducation become important. As muscles are reinnervated, exercise, biofeedback, and electrical stimulation are used to enhance the recovery of strength and control. As skin receptors are reinnervated desensitization is used to reduce hypersensitivity and sensory reeducation is needed to improve tactile discrimination. In the chronic stage when progress has peaked and functional deficits remain, the focus of therapy is on compensation for loss of function. Techniques include the use of assistive devices, adapted methods and functional splints. Finally tendon transfers may be performed to redistribute remaining power with hand therapy being important both before and after surgery. Full passive motion, supple and nonadherent tissues, and isolated control and strength of the donor muscle are all preoperative goals. Postoperatively, emphasis is on initial protection of the transfer through splints and reeducation of the tendon transfer to perform its new functions.

REFERENCES

1. Sunderland, S: Nerves and Nerve Injuries. E & S Livingstone, Edinburgh and London, 1968, p 4.
2. Beasley, R: Hand Injuries. WB Saunders, Philadelphia, 1981, p 278.
3. Omer, G: Nerve response to injury and repair. In Hunter, JM, et al (eds): Rehabilitation of the Hand. CV Mosby, St Louis, 1990, p 517.
4. Bowers, WH, et al: Nerve suture and grafting. Hand Clin 5:447, 1989.
5. Omer, G: Nerve response to injury and repair. In Hunter, JM, et al (eds): Rehabilitation of the Hand, CV Mosby, St Louis, 1990, p 519.
6. Tubiana, R: Examination of the Hand and Upper Limb. WB Saunders, Philadelphia, 1984, p 167.
7. Callahan, A: Nerve injuries in the upper extremity. In Malick, MH and Kasch, MD (eds): Manual on Management of Specific Hand Problems. AREN Publications, Pittsburgh, 1984, p 26.
8. Baxter-Petralia, P: Therapist's Management of Carpal Tunnel Syndrome. In Hunter, JM, et al (eds): Rehabilitation of the Hand. CV Mosby, St Louis, 1990, p 641.
9. Colditz, JC: A dynamic radial palsy splint. J Hand Ther 1:3, 1988.
10. Sunderland, S: Nerves and Nerve Injuries. E & S Livingstone, Edinburgh and London, 1968, p 522.
11. Brand, PW: Clinical Mechanics of the Hand. CV Mosby, St Louis, 1985, p 103.
12. Barber, LM: Desensitization of the traumatized hand. In Hunter, JM, et al (eds): Rehabilitation of the Hand. CV Mosby, St Louis, 1990, p 721.
13. Hardy, MA, Moran, CA, and Merritt, WH: Desensitization of the traumatized hand. VA Med 109:134, 1982.
14. Dellon, AL: Evaluation of Sensibility and Re-education of Sensation in the Hand. Williams & Wilkins, Baltimore, 1981, pp 117, 203.
15. Callahan, AD: Methods of compensation and re-education for sensory dysfunction. In Hunter, JM, et al (eds): Rehabilitation of the Hand. CV Mosby, St Louis, 1990, p 611.
16. Wynn Parry, CB: Rehabilitation of the Hand. Butterworth, London, 1973, p 113.

BIBLIOGRAPHY

Basmajian, JV: Biofeedback—Principles and Practice for Clinicians. Williams & Wilkins, Baltimore, 1979.

Beasley, RW: Hand Injuries. WB Saunders, Philadelphia, 1981.

Brand, PW: Clinical Mechanics of the Hand. CV Mosby, St Louis, 1985.

Cannon, NM, et al: Manual of Hand Splinting. Churchill Livingstone, New York, 1985.

Fess, EE: Rehabilitation of the patient with peripheral nerve injury. In Mackin, EJ: Hand Clinics: Hand Rehabilitation. WB Saunders, Philadelphia, 1986.

Fess, EE and Phillips, CA: Hand Splinting: Principles and Methods. CV Mosby, St Louis, 1987.

Haymaker, W and Woodhall, B: Peripheral Nerve Injuries. WB Saunders, Philadelphia, 1953.

Omer, GE: Acute management of peripheral nerve injuries. In Mackin, EJ (ed): Hand Clinics: Hand Rehabilitation. WB Saunders, Philadelphia, 1986.

Peacock, EE: Wound Repair. WB Saunders, Philadelphia, 1984.

Sunderland, S: Nerves and Nerve Injuries. E & S Livingstone, London, 1968.

Toth, S: Therapist's management of tendon transfers. In Mackin, EJ: Hand Clinics: Hand Rehabilitation. WB Saunders, Philadelphia, 1986.

Wynn Parry, CB: Rehabilitation of the Hand. Butterworth, London, 1973.

CHAPTER **12**

Tendon Injuries

Karen M. Stewart, MS, OTR, CHT

The management of the repaired or reconstructed tendon presents a special problem in clinical decision making. Our task is to preserve joint mobility while we encourage development of a strong, healthy tendon that glides freely within the surrounding tissues. This task requires striking a careful balance between protecting the healing tissues and applying controlled stress to increase strength and motion. To plan the appropriate intervention at the appropriate time, the therapist must have a clear understanding of tendon and soft tissue healing, the operative procedures performed, the many factors that differentiate one patient and one injury from another, and the treatment techniques available. As Evans[1] stated, "as hand therapists we are obligated to think in terms of the biologic response and biomechanical properties of the tissues that we treat. Would we expect those who are responsible for applying controlled stress to a healing tendon to know less about their science than those who repair it?" This chapter discusses primary repair of digit flexor and extensor tendons, as well as two types of reconstructive surgery: tenolysis and staged tendon grafts. The case study illustrates clinical decision making in the management of primary repair of both flexor and extensor tendons, as well as flexor tenolysis.

The objectives of this chapter are to (1) describe common approaches to rehabilitation for these patients; (2) discuss the rationale for each approach, with particular attention to how management is dictated by phases of wound healing; (3) delineate precautions, evaluations, and treatment techniques specific to each surgical procedure; and (4) demonstrate how this information is integrated in clinical decision making.

Because sound clinical decisions can be made only by integrating basic knowledge, the reader must have read previous chapters, particularly Chapters 1 to 3 and 6 to 9, before this one. Much of the material that follows is dependent on having read and comprehended these earlier chapters.

SURGICAL OPTIONS

Tendon Repairs

Tendon repairs can be divided into primary, delayed primary, and secondary repairs. According to some authors,[2,3] a *primary repair* is performed within 24 hours after injury, whereas a *delayed primary repair* (delayed direct repair) is performed between 24 hours and 3 weeks after injury. A *secondary repair* is one performed more than 3 weeks after injury. Others[4,5] consider a secondary repair to be one performed more than 2 weeks after injury. The logic of these definitions lies in the ease of end-to-end repair. After 2 weeks the wound can no longer be bluntly dissected but must be incised surgically to perform the repair; after 3 weeks scarring may be extensive and muscle contracture may lead to retraction of tendon ends, making a secondary end-to-end repair potentially much more complex. Additional dissection may be needed to retrieve retracted tendons, and the repair may not be possible except under tension, which increases the risk of rupture, repair elongation, and longstanding muscle shortening with accompanying joint contractures.

Tendon Reconstruction and Secondary Procedures

TENOLYSIS

If a repaired tendon fails to recover adequate excursion secondary to excessive adhesions, the surgeon may elect to perform a tenolysis: surgical excision of the scar tissue that binds the tendon to surrounding tissues.

TENDON GRAFTS

If a tendon is badly damaged or retracted, or if other characteristics of the injury point to a poor prognosis for end-to-end repair, the surgeon may decide to perform a tendon graft. A segment is harvested from a tendon that can be spared (such as palmaris longus or a long toe extensor). The graft is sutured to distal and proximal tendon stumps; distally the graft may be attached to bone instead.

Sometimes scarring or damage to surrounding tissues is so extensive that a conventional tendon graft is unlikely to recover adequate gliding. Pulleys may be destroyed and in need of reconstruction. A reconstructed pulley has a high risk of adherence to tendon or tendon graft.[2,6] In these cases, staged tendon grafts may be performed.[6] In stage I, a flexible silicone rubber rod is placed in the tendon bed. The rod, or implant, is attached distally to bone, at the site of the original tendon insertion, and the proximal end is left free. Before skin closure, pulleys are reconstructed over the implant as needed. The implant remains in place for several months, during which a pseudosheath forms around it. In stage II surgery, the implant is replaced with a tendon graft, which now has a smooth gliding bed and strong, nonadherent pulleys. This procedure, more commonly used for flexor than for extensor tendons, is discussed in greater detail later in this chapter.

TENDON HEALING: IMPLICATIONS FOR REHABILITATION

After repair, tendon healing follows the usual three phases, described in detail in Chapter 2. During the inflammatory phase, little collagen is laid down, and end-to-end tendon repairs are held together only by the strength of the suture material. During fibroplasia scar formation is rapid, but the new scar is extremely weak and the repair is easily disrupted by excessive force. During the scar maturation phase increasing repair strength allows us to apply greater and greater stresses to the tendon, thus influencing the scar remodeling. Based on this knowledge of tendon healing, most rehabilitation protocols for primary tendon repairs prohibit active motion (which imparts greater stress than does protected passive motion) before 3 weeks.

There now exist suture techniques designed to withstand almost immediate active motion,[7-10] and hand specialists are showing much interest in initiating carefully controlled active flexion within the first few days after flexor tendon repair. However, such an approach should be taken only by an experienced hand therapist working closely with a skilled surgeon. Research involving these techniques has been limited, and the methods are not yet widely accepted, so this chapter does not address early active mobilization programs.[11-14]

Factors affecting adhesion formation and rate of healing include patient age, health, and nutritional status, the means of injury and the surgical technique used. Some patients, for no apparent reason, seem to form very heavy tendon adhesions that virtually cement the tendon to the surrounding tissues. Other patients form very few adhesions or thinner, filmier adhesions that seem to elongate more easily and allow the tendon to glide. These latter patients may also run a greater risk of rupture because of insufficient scar formation between tendon ends.

Whatever the reasons, some adhesion formation is inevitable. The challenge of rehabilitation is to encourage development of long, gliding adhesions that do not restrict motion, and at the same time to avoid rupture, gap formation, or attenuation of the repair.

We now have an abundance of experimental evidence that *controlled* passive mobilization during the first few weeks of healing (inflammatory and fibroplasia phases) stimulates an intrinsic healing response and leads to improved gliding and repair strength.[15-22] Reports from clinical studies support the efficacy of controlled early passive mobilization in improving tendon gliding.[22-24] These studies provide scientific evidence that controlled passive motion improves the physiologic response of the healing tendon. Specific early controlled mobilization protocols are described later in this chapter.

PRIMARY REPAIRS

Primary Repair of Flexor Tendons

INITIAL REFERRAL

Therapy may begin from 1 day to 4 weeks after surgery, depending on whether the patient is being treated with immobilization or some form of early protected passive mobilization. Regardless of how much time has elapsed, certain information is vital to successful treatment planning.

TIMING OF REPAIR

How long after injury was the tendon repaired? A long-delayed secondary repair carries the complications of soft tissue contraction and scarring.

MECHANISM OF INJURY AND TECHNIQUE OF REPAIR

What was the mechanism of injury? What was the condition of the tendon and peritendinous structures intraoperatively? Was the laceration a clean cut, leaving healthy, bleeding ends that will heal well, or were the ends crushed and avascular, setting the stage for severe edema and heavy scar formation? Ragged tendon ends must be trimmed before repair, thus sacrificing some tendon length. Loss of tendon length may put excessive tension on the repair and increase the risk of rupture.

IDENTIFYING THE INJURED TENDONS

Because the flexor digitorum profundus (FDP) tendons have a common muscle belly (the index may or may not have an independent muscle belly), all four fingers must be protected together, even if only one FDP tendon is injured. In cases when only the flexor digitorum superficialis (FDS) is injured, the risk of attaining limited excursion of the FDS is high, because a full fist can be attained actively with minimal to no FDS gliding. Normally the FDP is more active than the FDS in active fisting, with the FDS contracting only when resisted[25] or when the wrist is simultaneously flexed.[26] When more than one tendon is injured at the same level, differential gliding may be difficult to recover.

ASSOCIATED INJURIES

Were there any associated injuries? Nerves, for example, are frequently injured along with flexor tendons. Associated nerve injuries need to be carefully handled so as not to result in further complications. For example, an ulnar nerve injury at the wrist may lead to a claw deformity, with proximal interphalangeal (PIP) contractures and limited metacarpophalangeal (MP) flexion, as well as sensory loss. Even when the flexor tendon program is not compromised by these associated injuries, a perfectly gliding and strong tendon is of little use to an insensate hand with stiff joints. Vincular injury (see ''Flexor Tendon Zones, p. 357) will impair the vascular nutrition to the tendon, and has been shown to compromise results in zone 2.[27]

LEVEL OF REPAIR

The level at which the tendon was injured may not always correspond to the location of the original superficial wound, because a given point on the tendon can correspond to different superficial landmarks depending on the position of the hand and wrist. During flexion the tendon glides proximally and the skin folds. Therefore, if the patient was injured when a glass broke in his hand (with his fingers in flexion) the skin may be lacerated over the middle phalanx, overlying zone 2, though the flexor digitorum profundus tendon was cut at the base of the distal phalanx, actually in zone 1. This concept is important to understand, as the level of tendon injury is not always obvious, and yet it carries important implications for treatment. If the tendon was under tension, as occurs in a tight fist, the proximal portion will retract proximally like a stretched rubberband that is suddenly cut. Unless restrained by vincular attachments or other structures, the proximal portion of the tendon will retract proximally every time the patient tries to flex the finger.

FLEXOR TENDON ZONES

Each flexor tendon zone has characteristics that dictate differences in surgical and rehabilitative treatment. The flexor zones are depicted in Figure 12–1.

Zone 5

Zone 5 extends from the musculotendinous junction in the distal forearm to the wrist level. Tendons at this level must be repaired early, as they very quickly retract with muscle contraction. Here the tendons lie very superficially, and can easily become adherent to overlying skin and surrounding structures. Such adhesions are often more yielding than are adhesions in zones 2 through 4. The primary challenges with zone 5

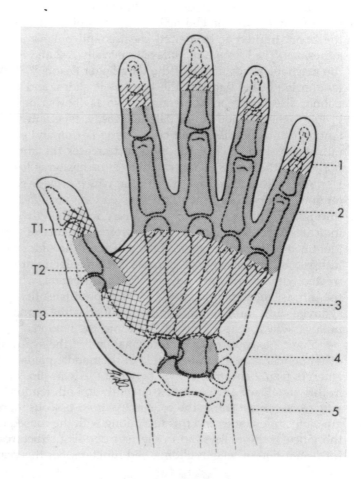

FIGURE 12–1. Flexor tendon zones as defined by the committee on tendon injuries, International Federation of Societies for Surgery of the Hand (IFSSH). (From Kleinert, HE, Schepel, S, and Gill, T: Flexor tendon injuries. Surg Clin North Am 61:267, 1981, with permission.)

injuries are the restoration of differential gliding and prevention of flexor muscle-tendon unit contracture. Median and ulnar nerves and radial and ulnar arteries are also frequently lacerated in these injuries and must be protected and treated appropriately.

Zone 4

In Zone 4 the tendons pass through the narrow carpal tunnel, within which they are enclosed in a synovial sheath (one for the flexor pollicis longus [FPL] and one for the FDS and FDP). In this zone injuries are usually to more than one tendon, and are often accompanied by injury to nerves or blood vessels. Intertendinous adhesions are highly likely here, given the proximity of tendons to each other.

Zone 3

Here the tendons of the fingers emerge from the carpal tunnel and the lumbricals take their origin from the FDP. Injuries at this level usually heal well, with few complications and good recovery of excursion. However, intrinsic muscle contractures can result from adhesions and protective positioning during the first few weeks of healing, if the therapist is not careful to perform gentle passive intrinsic-minus and MP range of motion (ROM) in this period.

Zone 2

In Zone 2, the tendons enter the synovial sheaths. These sheaths provide lubrication for smooth tendon gliding beneath the pulleys that hold the tendons firmly down to the bone. Injured and repaired sheaths and pulleys are potential sites for restrictive adhesions. The loss of any pulleys (especially A-2 and A-4) has been shown to decrease the mechanical advantage of the long finger flexors.[28-30] When a pulley is missing, the tendon is not held against the bone as it glides, and pulls away from the bone in a palmar direction, a phenomenon known as "bowstringing." This phenomenon is often visible to the eye, and can be palpated easily, especially within the phalanges, where the tendon stands out like a taut cord during flexion and stretches the overlying skin. The outward, palmar pull of the tendon decreases the angular rotation of the joint, so a portion of the active flexion or strength of flexion is lost.

Also within zone 2 lie the vincula, which provide segmental vascular supply to the tendons. Injury to the vincula impairs tendon nutrition by eliminating extrinsic nutrition through vascular perfusion; such injury may thereby compromise healing (research[27] indicates vincular injury does compromise results of repair). However, studies have identified a rich source of intrinsic nutrition through synovial fluid diffusion.[31,32] This intrinsic nutrition may compensate for vincular injury, particularly if the patient is treated with an early passive mobilization program, which has been shown to increase the intrinsic healing response.[22] Weber[33] postulates that passive mobilization improves synovial diffusion through a milking effect as the tendon passively glides beneath the pulleys, which propel synovial fluid into the tendon.

Zone 2 extends from the proximal end of the synovial sheaths (at the level of the distal palmar crease) to the middle of the middle phalanx, just distal to where the FDP emerges from beneath the FDS, between the twin slips of the FDS insertion. Therefore, in this zone, laceration is very frequently to both tendons, at a point where they lie in very close contact within the constrictive fibro-osseous tunnel. Intertendinous adhesions are almost inevitable, and this fact, along with the consequences of injury to the sheath, the vincula, the pulleys, and other surrounding structures, poses significant problems for restoration of tendon gliding and function. For this reason zone 2 is also known as "no man's land," where for many years primarily repaired tendons in this zone were expected to fail or to regain little or no motion.[34]

Zone 1

Zone 1 includes only the FDP, as it passes through the distal portion of the sheath to its insertion at the base of the distal phalanx. Injuries at this level are often ruptures, with or without bony avulsion at the tendon insertion, and may be repaired under tension. These repairs require careful handling to prevent failure of a repair performed under tension, development of distal interphalangeal (DIP) flexion contractures secondary to protective positioning, or poor gliding under A-4 and A-5 pulleys. Taking into account these problems and their anatomic and biomechanical causes, Evans[35] has developed a well-reasoned early passive mobilization protocol for the zone 1 injury.

Zones in the Thumb

In the thumb T-1, T-2, and T-3 correspond roughly to zones 1 to 3 in the fingers. The anatomic considerations are not as complex as in the fingers. Because the FPL is the only extrinsic flexor tendon lying within its synovial sheath, intertendinous adhesions are not a consideration distal to the carpal tunnel.

Treatment Approaches and Rationale

There are two fundamental approaches to management of primary tendon repairs: initial immobilization and early controlled mobilization. The rationale for each method is based on the phases of wound healing. During the inflammatory and early fibroplasia stages, when excessive stress will stretch or rupture the repair, the tendon is usually protected against active motion. Approximately 3 weeks after repair, the scar remodeling phase begins. Active motion is initiated during this phase, on the well-accepted principle that controlled stress strengthens scar and influences orientation of collagen fibers to allow increased gliding. By 3½ to 4 weeks the immobilized tendon probably has formed sufficient scar to tolerate active motion. However, canine studies by Gelberman[19] revealed that at 3 weeks the strength of an immobilized tendon repair was no greater than its strength immediately after suture. In contrast, a passively mobilized tendon showed two to three times the strength of an immobilized tendon. Hitchcock and colleagues[20] indicate that early controlled mobilization increases resistance to rupture (rupture or breaking strength, which for practical purposes can be equated with tensile strength). Other studies have shown improved gliding, stimulation of an intrinsic healing response, and decreased adhesion formation with early passive mobilization.[16-20]

Early controlled passive mobilization initiated during the inflammatory and fibroplasia stages, must be applied very carefully to avoid elongating or rupturing the fragile scar forming between tendon ends. A more comprehensive discussion of the rationale for early mobilization can be found in articles by Gelberman and Woo[21] and Strickland[36] in the special issue on tendons in the *Journal of Hand Therapy*.

In my opinion no single method is always appropriate, and none should be used in "cookbook" fashion. At every stage of rehabilitation, the program should be modified according to the actual status of the patient, the tendon, and the surrounding tissues, and *not* according to a formula.

The immobilization and early controlled passive mobilization approaches to flexor tendon management are now discussed, using the phases of wound healing as a framework. Thus, stage I includes the inflammatory and fibroplasia phases, and stage II consists of the scar remodeling phase.

STAGE I: PROTECTIVE PHASE

The goal of therapy in this stage is to ensure development of a strong tendon repair and minimize restrictive adhesions. Therefore, the tendon is protected against active flexion and excessive passive extension, both of which could place unacceptably large stresses on the repair site.

Immobilization

Although other methods are now widely used with excellent results, the classic treatment by early immobilization is still preferred by some surgeons, and is always the treatment of choice for the noncompliant patient or patients under age 10. Therefore, the hand therapist must be ready to treat these patients appropriately.

Following surgery, the hand is immobilized with the wrist in 10° to 30° of flexion, with the MP joints in 40° to 60° of flexion and the interphalangeal (IP) joints in neutral. Immobilization may be through casting or splinting, depending on the comfort and compliance of the patient (splints may be too easy for a noncompliant patient to remove but are more comfortable and do not soften if they become wet). The child who is too young to cooperate in wearing a cast should be casted from fingertips to above the elbow to ensure that the cast cannot be removed. No wrist or finger motion at all is allowed.

If joint stiffness is expected (e.g., if the PIPs are immobilized in some flexion to protect repaired digital nerves or joint structures and therefore run a risk of developing flexion contractures, or if the patient is arthritic or elderly) the splint should be removed during therapy sessions at least once a week for gentle protected passive range of motion (PROM). When performing protected passive extension, adjacent joints are held in flexion to allow gentle passive extension of each joint individually. This technique stretches the joint structures while avoiding stretch to the tendon juncture. This maneuver should be performed only with extreme delicacy or avoided completely for joints at the level of the actual repair.

Early Controlled Mobilization

Early mobilization refers to various forms of early *passive* mobilization of the repaired tendon, rather than active motion. These techniques were originally developed for injuries in "no man's land." They are widely used, however, for injuries both distal and proximal to zone 2. Because such protocols call for a high degree of patient compliance, their use should be carefully considered and patients monitored closely. These protocols are well-supported in the literature by the studies cited earlier.[16-20,22]

In stage I of controlled early mobilization programs patients are seen in therapy one to five times a week for wound care, edema control, evaluation of passive flexion and active extension, and monitoring and updating of the home program. Frequency of exercise sessions and number of repetitions of each exercise are adapted to the needs of the patient. A patient with a persistent inflammatory response or particularly stiff fingers needs frequent sessions with a low number of repetitions, whereas fewer sessions with more repetitions are appropriate for a patient who quickly develops full passive flexion and active extension to the limits of the splint. A recent study by

Gelberman and associates[37] indicates that the greater the number of repetitions and the longer the daily duration of passive mobilization, the better the results will be. This study concerned the use of continuous passive mobilization (CPM) but has implications for any form of passive mobilization in management of tendon repairs.

Within a day or two of suture removal the superficial scar may tolerate gentle massage, as described in Chapter 6. Often tendons and peritendinous tissues become tightly bound to the superficial scar; massage is a form of controlled stress that gently stretches the adhesions as they form.

Early controlled passive mobilization protocols can be divided into two basic types: Duran and Houser's controlled passive motion technique,[38,39] and Kleinert and colleagues' dynamic flexion technique.[40,41] Many therapists use a combination of the two approaches. In both protocols, the patient must not actively flex the digits or extend beyond the limits imposed by the splint. Passive extension is also prohibited except in certain instances as indicated below.

Duran and Houser's Controlled Passive Mobilization Technique. This approach was originally developed for repairs in zones 2 and 3.[38,39]

Postoperative Splinting. After tendon repair, a dorsal cast or splint is applied, maintaining the wrist in 20° of flexion, with the MPs in a relaxed position of flexion (Duran and his colleagues[38,39] do not specify the number of degrees), and allowing full IP extension. A suture is placed in the nail intraoperatively for attachment of a rubberband running from fingertip to just proximal to the volar wrist crease. The rubberband holds the digits lightly in flexion, to protect the tendon against inadvertent active flexion and to ensure that the repair is not under any tension.

Exercise Program. This technique assumes restrictive tendon adhesion formation can be prevented by passively moving the tendon juncture through 3 to 5 mm of excursion. Passive flexion and extension of the DIP joint with the MP and PIP joints held in flexion moves an FDP repair distally away from an FDS repair. Passive motion of the PIP joint with the MP and DIP joints held in flexion moves both repairs away from the site of injury and thus from other injured tissues (Fig. 12–2). Six to eight repetitions of each exercise are performed twice a day for the first 4½ weeks, until about 1 week into the scar remodeling phase.

Kleinert Method. This approach was also developed for primary repairs in zone 2.[40,41]

Postoperative Splinting. After surgery, the patient is placed in a dorsal protective splint holding the wrist in 45° of flexion and the MPs in 40°, with the IPs allowed to extend to neutral. Rubberband traction is applied to the fingernail for protective flexion as in the Duran protocol, but in this case the rubberband is also used to resist active extension to the limits of a dorsal protective splint. The rubberband then pulls the finger passively into flexion (Figs. 12–3 and 12–4). Lister and co-workers[42] have published electromyographic (EMG) studies showing that the flexors relax during sustained resisted digit extension, thus supporting Kleinert's contention that the technique is a relatively low-stress means of achieving passive glide of the tendon to prevent adhesions.

In recent years, the Kleinert splint has been modified in two basic ways. One of the greatest concerns in management of primary flexor tendon repairs is the control of adhesions both between FDS and FDP and between the tendons and their surrounding sheath and other structures. To prevent such adhesions, postoperative rehabilitation aims to achieve the best possible passive gliding of the two tendons in relation to each other and to other structures (differential tendon gliding).

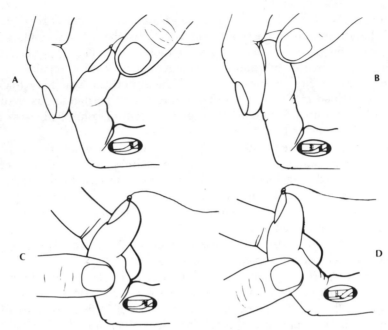

FIGURE 12–2. Duran and Houser's controlled passive mobilization exercises. *A,B,* Passive extension of the DIP (with PIP in flexion) moves the FDP repair distally, away from the FDS repair. *C,D,* Passive extension of the PIP (with DIP in flexion) moves both repairs distally, away from other healing structures at the site of injury. (From Duran, RJ, et al: Management of flexor tendon lacerations in zone 2 using controlled passive motion postoperatively. In Hunter, JM, et al [eds]: Rehabilitation of the Hand: Surgery and Therapy, ed 3. St Louis, CV Mosby, 1990, p 410, with permission.)

Excursion studies have found that complete passive differential flexor tendon excursion is achieved only by passive flexion of the joints distal to the repair, making passive DIP flexion essential in mobilization of an FDP repair.[43] Horibe and associates[44] noted also that PIP flexion elicits the greatest amplitude of FDP excursion within zone 2. The standard Kleinert splint flexed the MPs more than the IPs, with very little DIP flexion at all. Therefore, dynamic traction is now often directed through a palmar pulley instead of from proximal to the wrist, to more fully flex the PIP and DIP joint,[41,45,46] as shown in Figure 12–5.

In the thumb, flexor pollicis longus (FPL) repairs between MP and IP joints can be more effectively mobilized through isolated IP flexion.[47] This fact suggests that the MP should be immobilized to allow isolation of IP flexion. I suggest immobilization in 10° to 20° of thumb MP flexion.

A more recent cadaver study has provided findings somewhat contradictory to those of early excursion studies,[48] indicating that the original Kleinert splint may attain satisfactory differential tendon gliding. There is still much to be learned about how best to attain optimum tendon excursion in early passive mobilization programs.

Another change is in the magnitude of resistance to extension. It has been experimentally shown that increasing the force of rubberband tension does not increase reciprocal relaxation of the flexors and only increases the risk of flexion contractures.[49] Clinical experience has shown that PIP flexion contractures may develop when the

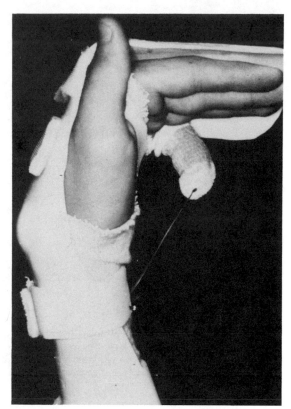

FIGURE 12-3. This splint, similar to the traditional Kleinert splint, holds wrist and MPs in flexion. The rubberband is attached to a moleskin tab instead of to the fingernail, as this zone 1 injury was repaired with a pullout suture and button that covered the nail. Dynamic traction holds the finger in flexion, with greatest flexion at the MP. Similar splinting is used by Duran, with the splint extending only to PIP level.

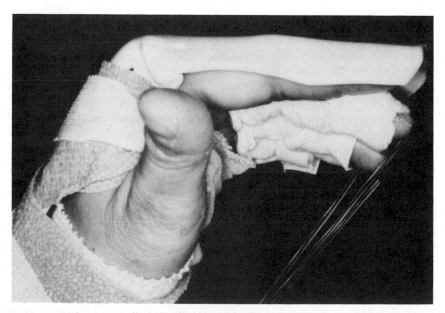

FIGURE 12-4. Patient extending IPs against rubberband traction in a traditional Kleinert type of splint. Note this patient is unable to extend his IPs completely. To prevent development of flexion contractures, either the traction force must be decreased or the IPs must be intermittently splinted in extension.

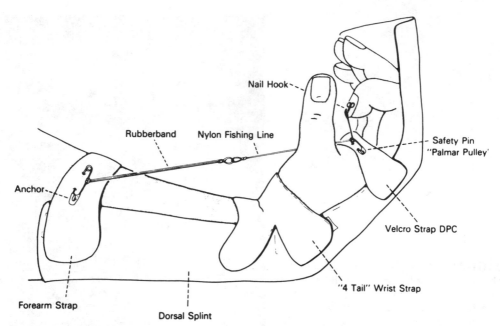

FIGURE 12–5. The splint designed by Thomes and used by Chow and associates. Note the palmar pulley that redirects dynamic traction to increase IP flexion. Although not illustrated here, this splint also incorporates variable dynamic traction, as described in the text. (From Chow, JA, et al: A combined regimen of controlled motion following flexor tendon repair in "no man's land." Plast Reconstr Surg 79:447, 1987, with permission.)

finger rests in PIP flexion as it does with both Duran and Kleinert approaches. Some clinicians therefore prefer to strap the IPs in extension at night[50]; a foam wedge placed behind the proximal phalanges will increase MP flexion and protect against excessive stretch when the fingers are held in extension.

As the finger reaches full extension against standard dynamic traction, the force exerted by the dynamic traction increases dramatically. This force may increase the difficulty of achieving full extension and contribute to the development of flexion contractures. The splint now in use by Chow and associates[46] and developed by therapist Linwood Thomes (Fig. 12–5) uses a double rubberband, half of which is removed during exercise to decrease resistance.[46,51] The splint used by Werntz and associates,[41] shown in Figure 12–6, incorporates more constant light resistance through a coiled lever that rotates to allow easy full extension.

Exercise Program. The patient extends the finger to the limits of the splint 20 times every hour, working against the resistance of the rubberband, and allowing the rubberband to flex the finger passively between repetitions. When using any protocol involving dynamic flexion splinting, I prefer to add protected passive extension of individual IP joints by the therapist, and passive flexion of both individual joints and the entire finger by the patient, four times a day (Fig. 12–7).

My Preferred Method. My preferred approach (sometimes referred to as a "modified Duran" approach) uses active extension without rubberband resistance, to decrease the risk of flexion contracture. The protocol is based on clinical experience[52,53] and the already cited research, and is similar to protocols used by many other therapists who have found drawbacks in the "pure" Kleinert or Duran and Houser techniques.

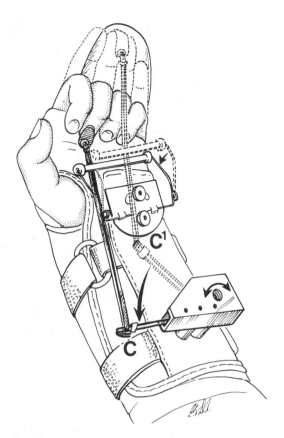

FIGURE 12–6. The postoperative flexor tendon traction brace (PFT), now used by Kleinert and associates, incorporates constant resistance to active extension. The roller bar (which also acts as a palmar pulley to increase passive IP flexion at rest) moves away from the palm during extension; the proximal coiled lever swings distally to decrease resistance during extension and then springs back proximally when the finger relaxes. (From Werntz, JR, et al: A new dynamic splint for postoperative treatment of flexor tendon injury. J Hand Surg 14A:559, 1989, with permission.)

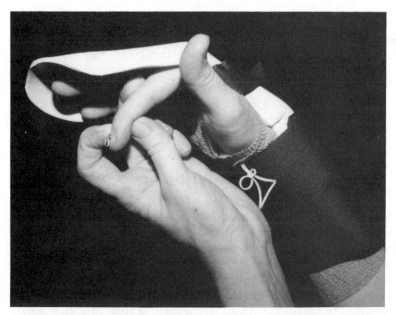

FIGURE 12–7. Protected passive extension of PIP (DIP and MP held in flexion). Protected extension should be performed only by the therapist or by reliable patients. Protected passive extension of the MPs should be performed at least once a week by the therapist, when the splint is removed in the clinic.

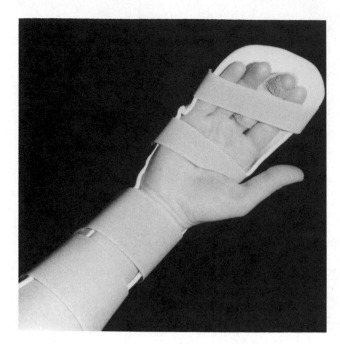

FIGURE 12–8. Splinting for zone 1 repairs as proposed by Evans. Dorsal protective splint is similar to that used in other protocols, but without dynamic flexion. The DIP is also held in flexion with a dorsal static splint. For a complete explanation of the protocol, readers are referred to Evans.[35]

Postoperative Splinting. Although the dorsal protective splint is similar, the degree of wrist and MP flexion is smaller and dynamic flexion is not used. The wrist is immobilized in 30° of flexion (more comfortable than a greater degree of flexion) and the MPs in 40° of flexion, with the IPs strapped into extension. The Evans protocol for zone 1 injury,[35] mentioned earlier, uses a similar dorsal splint without rubberband traction, but adds static DIP flexion splinting and other exercises addressing zone 1 problems (Fig. 12–8).

Exercise Program. Finger straps are removed every 1 to 2 hours for passive flexion and active extension to the limits of the splint—5 to 20 repetitions, depending on the patient's degree of pain and stiffness. The patient also performs 5 to 10 repetitions of protected passive flexion and extension exercises at each IP joint as in the Duran protocol, four to six times a day.

STAGE II: ACTIVE MOBILIZATION

This stage begins approximately at the beginning of the scar remodeling phase, and extends to the end of therapy. Scar remodeling continues for months or years: in order to achieve maximum strength and tendon glide, patients usually need to continue some form of exercise or splinting even after completion of formal therapy.

During this stage, programs are progressed in a roughly similar fashion in all flexor tendon protocols, regardless of whether immobilization or early controlled mobilization was used in the first stage. However, the level and type of injury and other factors should be taken into account in determining the rate at which the program is progressed. The following discussion covers all approaches, with notations about important differences.

Initiation of Active Range of Motion

At the end of 3 to 4 weeks, gentle active motion may be initiated. The determination as to when to start motion is made not on the basis of rigid timeliness, however, but should be made according to the quality of tendon gliding observed when active flexion is first attempted. This determination is usually made by the attending physician, but therapists should understand the basis of the decision and may be called upon to make the decision independently.

If on first attempting active flexion the patient demonstrates fluid, easy flexion to within 1 or 2 cm of the palm, there are probably only very few, fine, filmy adhesions supporting the healing tendon. This good tendon gliding may be due to a predominance of intrinsic healing, and the tendon juncture may be strong enough to withstand active motion. However, we cannot be sure, because the tendon may also have a high risk of rupture. Given the quality of motion demonstrated, there is certainly no harm in delaying active flexion exercise. In that case the tendon should be protected against active motion for at least an additional week, and active motion should start very gently, with place-hold exercises (see farther on).

The tendon may instead develop dense, inelastic adhesions and glide very poorly, as shown by minimal, jerky active flexion, occurring mainly in joints proximal to the site of the repair. In that case, isolated glide can be assessed by *gently* blocking the proximal joint in extension while the patient attempts to flex the DIP. In some cases, motion may not be visible but can be perceived through careful palpation. For instance, the therapist or physician may feel some tendon gliding by placing his or her finger over the course of the tendon in the patient's hand. In the same way, slight joint rotation can be perceived with the therapist's finger placed distal to the joint in question. When even careful palpation reveals no motion, the therapist faces one of two conclusions: (1) the tendon has ruptured, in spite of the protective steps taken; or (2) the tendon is exceptionally adherent, and more vigorous attempts to move it are necessary. *This decision must be referred to the physician.* Moreover, the inexperienced hand therapist should *not* attempt to test tendon function at all.

In the Duran and Houser approach active flexion is delayed until 5½ weeks. At 4½ weeks the splint is removed, and the patient now wears a wrist band to which the rubberbands are attached. When the patient extends the wrist, the fingers (or thumb) are brought into flexion passively, and when the fingers are extended the wrist is brought into flexion (Fig. 12–9). The patient performs active extension exercises (similar to those used in the Kleinert approach) in addition to the passive mobilization exercises described earlier. At 5½ weeks the wrist band is removed and the patient begins active flexion, including blocking, FDS gliding, and fisting.

According to Kleinert[41] active flexion is initiated at 4 to 6 weeks, depending on the quality of flexion demonstrated initially. Many therapists who follow the Kleinert or the "modified Duran" approach use Duran's wrist cuff as an intermediate means of protection.[39]

Progressing Active Range of Motion

For the inexperienced therapist, progression of active flexion exercises is perhaps the most difficult aspect of flexor tendon management. The decision to progress a patient's exercise program is dependent upon the quality of tendon glide. Tendon glide is assessed through ROM measurements, visual observation, and palpation. Both location and quality of tendon adhesion can be identified by palpating while testing tendon glide with the hand and wrist in varying positions. Active extension limitations are

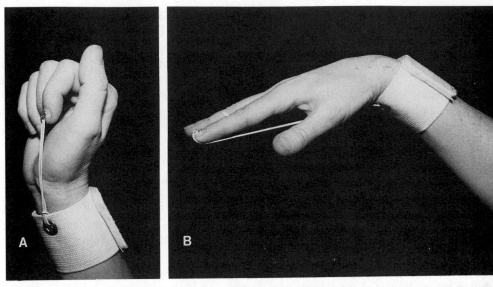

FIGURE 12–9. Dynamic traction with a wrist band. *A*, When the patient extends his wrist, the fingers are passively flexed, thus preventing simultaneous extension of wrist and fingers. *B*, When the patient extends his fingers, his wrist is passively flexed.

another clue. For example, if the patient can extend the PIP to neutral with the MP and wrist held in flexion, and can repeat this with the wrist extended, but extends the PIP much less with the MP extended, then we know that tendon adhesions are restricting glide in zone 2 or 3 (Fig. 12–10). Tendon glide should be constantly reevaluated to progress the program quickly enough without overstressing the healing tendon.

Active flexion exercises may begin with place-hold fisting, to protect a tendon that is gliding moderately well. This technique, described in Chapter 7, is designed to place less stress on the juncture by requiring only a gentle muscle contraction to maintain flexion instead of a greater contraction to pull the tendon through its full excursion.

In a week or less, exercise should be progressed to tendon gliding, as described by Wehbe and Hunter[54] (see Chapter 7). Some patients have difficulty performing the straight fist, but all patients should perform hook fisting, which provides maximum differential gliding between the two tendons. Differential gliding is also provided by blocking exercises for FDP and FDS. Blocking exercises should be initiated with caution, as they involve some resistance to flexion.

Strengthening

Flexion against resistance elicits a strong muscle contraction, which stresses existing adhesions and helps prevent further formation of dense, restrictive adhesions. Much controversy surrounds the question of when to initiate resistance to the healing tendon. A recent study[55] examined the use of resistance in immobilized repairs, beginning as early as 4 weeks. The authors developed guidelines to determine when resistance was both safe and necessary to elicit a greater muscle contraction in the presence of tendon adhesions.

Although immobilized tendons may be more severely adherent, they are also theoretically less able to withstand resistance than are tendons that have been subjected to the controlled stress of early passive mobilization. By 3 weeks, even mobilized

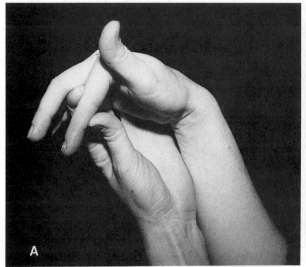

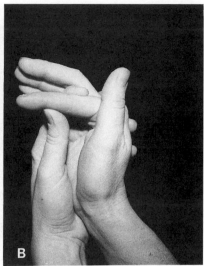

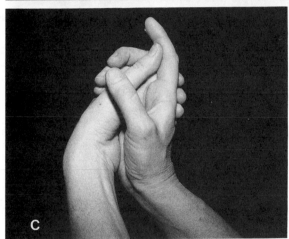

FIGURE 12–10. Testing for cause of limited extension. *A*, The PIP can be extended completely with wrist and MPs flexed. The restriction is not due to articular or periarticular PIP contracture. *B*, The PIP can be extended with the wrist extended and the MP flexed. *C*, The PIP cannot be extended when both MP and wrist are extended. We have seen that each joint crossed by the flexor tendon has passive extension within normal limits, so tendinous rather than articular or periarticular adhesions or contractures are implicated. Adhesion is probably in zone 2 or 3 between PIP and wrist, since MP extension pulled the PIP into flexion.

tendons had reached only 20% of their ultimate tensile load in Gelberman's canine study.[19] Although stronger than immobilized tendons in early stages, mobilized tendons, too, were still substantially weaker than normal. These findings point out the need for using extreme caution in applying resistance to the healing tendon.

Resistance is initiated gently at 7 or 8 weeks, depending on the strength of the repair (if the surgeon has provided this information), the quality of gliding, and the adherence of the tendon to surrounding tissues. Resistance should be delayed for a week or more if the tendon is gliding freely, as there are fewer adhesions to provide support. However, a severely adherent tendon may begin very lightly resisted exercise as early as 4 to 5 weeks, and the program should be progressed more quickly.

Resistance to lacerated FDS tendons should be initiated as early as possible, as FDS does not pull through strongly in the full fist unless resisted.[25] Because lacerations of FDS and FDP tendons in zone 5 are very well nourished and heal well, they are often ready to withstand blocking as early as 3 weeks and very lightly resisted exercise as early as 5.

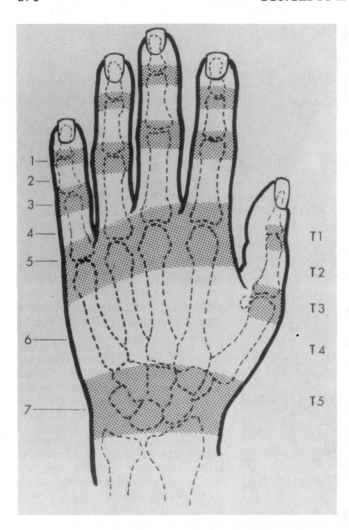

FIGURE 12–11. Extensor tendon zones as defined by the committee on tendon injuries, IFSSH. (From Kleinert, HE, Schepel, S, and Gill, T: Flexor tendon injuries. Surg Clin North Am 61:267, 1981, with permission.)

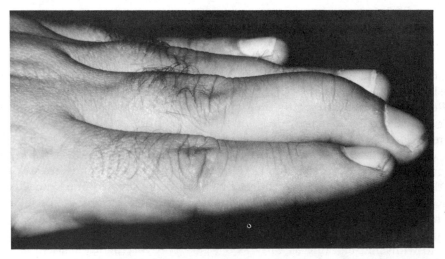

FIGURE 12–12. Mallet deformity caused by a zone 1 extensor tendon injury.

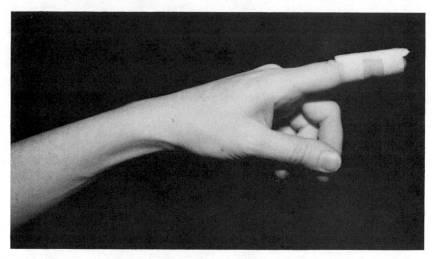

FIGURE 12–13. Dorsal splint for DIP extension.

Resistance can start with light prehension, isometric strengthening and sustained grasp activities, which provide low stress to the tendon repair, and use of the hand as a light assist in activities of daily living (ADLs). Suggested activities include lightweight pegboards and jigsaw puzzles, tissue crumpling, and transferring handfuls of packing "popcorn" from one bowl to another. In a week or two, if adhesions are a problem, the patient can begin sanding (using sanders with adapted handles to facilitate sustained grasp).

Graded resistance may be added within a week or two, starting with transferring beans instead of packing "popcorn" and progressing to gentle putty squeezing. Patients should be taught not to squeeze with excessive force, as even the softest putty can provide excessive resistance when squeezed too vigorously. There is also the risk that the patient will perform too many repetitions. Patients enjoy this exercise and may find themselves squeezing putty for long periods of time while watching television or while otherwise distracted. The price they pay is inflammation, with resultant pain, swelling, and stiffness.

To eliminate unnecessary and expensive splinting, dynamic extension splints should only be used for resistive exercise if the patient has simultaneous muscle-tendon unit adherence or shortening, or is unable to grasp putty or other exercise equipment.

The program is gradually progressed to provide greater strengthening with the use of grip exercisers and heavy-resistance activities. Progressive or regressive resistive exercise increases the strength of the wrist and entire upper extremity, which is vital to sustain a functional grasp. Unrestricted use is usually allowed at 12 weeks.

SPECIFIC PROBLEMS

Joint Flexion Contractures

Joint flexion contractures can develop very easily if patients are not followed closely. When limited extension is noted in any joint, one must determine whether the limitation is due to joint contracture, tendon adhesions/tightness, or both. To evaluate limitations in PIP extension, for example, the adjacent joints and the wrist should be held passively in flexion while the PIP is gently extended passively and actively. If the PIP extends more easily with the adjacent joints flexed than extended, the limitation is at least partly due to tendon tightness or adherence. Often joint contractures develop secondary to longstanding tendon adherence or muscle shortening that prevents active extension. Established or developing contractures can be addressed through splinting and ROM exercise; however, they are much easier to prevent than to correct, so our efforts at achieving full joint mobility should begin in the protective stage of therapy.

Muscle-Tendon Unit Contracture

In zone 4 or 5 injuries, flexor muscle-tendon tightness may develop secondary to prolonged positioning in combined wrist and MP flexion or to flexor tendon adhesions. This tendon tightness restricts simultaneous passive extension of wrist and fingers. A serially remade plaster or thermoplastic splint can be worn at night, gradually bringing wrist and fingers into further extension as it becomes available. This type of splinting is very gentle and can therefore be initiated as early as 4 or 5 weeks after repair, when dynamic splinting would place too much stress on the repair. The patient can then be progressed into dynamic splinting if tightness persists.

Multiple Lacerations in Zones 4 and 5

A multiple tendon laceration at the wrist level is almost always a candidate for dynamic extension splinting. Adhesions are generally heavy at wrist level owing to the proximity of so many structures. In addition, if not carefully handled, PIP flexion contractures may result from median or ulnar nerve injury that upsets the mechanical balance of the hand. As already noted, dynamic extension splinting can provide not only stretch to tight or adherent extrinsic flexor tendons and to joint flexion contractures, but also resistance to flexion to promote better tendon pull-through. Ultrasound may be useful for severely adherent tendons, subject to the precautions outlined in Chapter 8. Neuromuscular electrical stimulation (NMES) may also be helpful, to elicit stronger contractions. NMES is appropriate when resistance is initiated.

Primary Repair of Extensor Tendons

DIFFERENCES BETWEEN FLEXOR AND EXTENSOR TENDONS

Whereas the flexor tendons are bound closely to each ray by a strong pulley system from the distal palm to the DIP joint, the extensors lack a complex pulley system. The extensor tendons are vulnerable to "bowstringing" with pulley damage only in cases when the extensor retinaculum, which acts as a pulley at the wrist, is stretched or injured and not repaired.

Just proximal to the MP joint the juncturae tendinum connect the extensor digitorum communis (EDC) tendons of the small, ring, long, and sometimes index finger. These intertendinous slips assist extension of adjacent fingers; they may also prevent retraction of a lacerated EDC. The extensor indicis proprius (EIP) and extensor digiti minimi (EDM) are not connected to any other tendon through juncturae.

For a large proportion of their total length the flexor tendons travel through sheaths. In contrast, the extensor tendons are enclosed in a sheath only where they travel beneath the extensor retinaculum. Thus, for most of their length they are extrasynovial.

Blood supply to the extensor tendons is provided by vascular mesenteries, which can be compared with the vincula supplying the flexor tendons within the digits. The vascular contribution is much less where the tendons are synovial, deep to the extensor retinaculum; here synovial diffusion is probably the chief source of nutrition.[56]

Because they lie superficially, extensor tendons are often involved in complex injuries to the dorsum of the hand. The extensors closely overlie the periosteum and are therefore likely to form adhesions in the presence of bony or periosteal injury.

The healing extensor tendon must be carefully protected against excessive stretch during the first weeks of active motion, for two reasons. The first reason is that even the uninjured extensor tendon is considerably weaker than its flexor counterpart because of different functional demands. The strength required for the flexor tendons to exert the forces of power grasp is far greater than that required for the extensors to open the hand for grasp or to provide the balance of forces needed for prehension. An uninjured flexor system can overpower an unprotected extensor tendon that has recently undergone repair, leading to stretching and weakening of the extensor.

The second reason to carefully protect the extensor tendons is that they are also relatively flatter, broader, and thinner than the flexors. These characteristics contribute to the relatively greater susceptibility to stretch or rupture as compared with the flexor tendons, particularly in extensor tendon zones 1, 2, and 3 (Fig. 12–11).

This vulnerability explains why simple repaired extensor tendon lacerations have been traditionally treated with immobilization. We can easily get away with immobilization in many cases because extensor tendons do not have to glide through sheaths except at the wrist, and adhesions, though restrictive, may be less of a functional problem than for flexor tendons, particularly in the extrasynovial zones (1 through 6). However, this traditional view is now being challenged in the literature. Although the extensor tendons have a shorter excursion to recover than do the flexors, any loss of excursion is potentially a proportionately greater functional loss. Extensors must also recover lateral mobility, which can be eradicated by tendon adhesions. Clinical experience shows that the traditional prolonged immobilization in zones 1 through 4 can cause significant extensor contractures and that extensor tendon adhesion formation can be extremely restrictive in complex injuries.[56-58] These observations have prompted a trend toward earlier mobilization, as explained later in this chapter.

A further anatomic difference is that the extensor system within the digits (zones 1, 2, and 3) is not a discrete tendon as with the flexors, but rather a complex interweaving of intrinsic and extrinsic tendons whose delicate balance must be preserved to maintain functional extension and avoid deformity. A detailed discussion of all the complexities of the extensor apparatus is beyond the scope of this book. Readers are encouraged to consult the references cited at the close of this chapter for further, essential detail.

INITIAL REFERRAL

As with all tendon injuries, initial referral information should include individual patient characteristics, level and means of injury, associated injuries, any time lag between injury and repair, intraoperative status of involved tendons, and surgical procedures performed. Injury or repair of the tendon sheath is a factor only at the wrist level, and tendon retraction is a less significant problem than for flexor tendons. Delayed repair is more risky with extensor tendons given the severe deformities that can result from disruption of the delicate balance of the extensor mechanism.

TREATMENT APPROACHES AND RATIONALE

The level of injury is the primary determinant of treatment for extensor tendons (see Fig. 12–11). Injuries distal to the MP joint (zones 1 through 4) are treated similarly by most surgeons and therapists. Surgical repair is not always needed; many injuries are responsive to simple immobilization (or very cautious passive mobilization), followed by gradual active, passive, and resistive exercise and splinting to regain motion. The protective stage of treatment not only includes the inflammatory and fibroplasia phases but also extends a week or more into the remodeling phase. This extended protective phase is necessary given the extreme delicacy of the extensor mechanism within the digit. Proximal to the MP (zones 5 through 7) immobilization is the classic method preferred by many due to the relative vulnerability of extensor tendons to rupture in the first few weeks. In recent years, however, early controlled mobilization of zone 5 through 7 injuries has gained wide acceptance.[57–64]

Zones 1 and 2 — DIP and Middle Phalanx

Injuries at this level are to the terminal extensor tendon and are frequently closed injuries caused by ruptures rather than lacerations. Following injury the DIP droops into flexion, in the so-called mallet deformity (Fig. 12–12). The original injury, left untreated, can lead to a further deformity in some patients. No longer tethered by its distal insertion, the entire extensor mechanism slides proximally, exerting excessive force on the PIP. If the volar plate is lax, a swan neck deformity (PIP hyperextension and DIP flexion) could result.

These injuries are sometimes repaired surgically, but often simple reapproximation of the tendon through immobilization allows the tendon to heal without surgical repair.

Splinting. The DIP should be immobilized in neutral to very slight hyperextension, leaving the PIP free to maintain mobility. It is essential to immobilize in sufficient extension to prevent development of a DIP extensor lag. Caution should be used, however, as excessive hyperextension has been shown to cause local ischemia and skin necrosis over the dorsum of the joint.[65] Immobilization may be via cylinder cast, Kirschner's wire (K-wire) — particularly if there is an associated fracture — or splint. A dorsal splint (Fig. 12–13) leaves the palmar surface free for sensory input and is less likely to block PIP motion, but in some patients a palmar splint may immobilize more effectively on the three-point pressure principle. As with other splints that lie so closely contiguous to the skin during prolonged immobilization, this splint should be lined to prevent excessive perspiration and resultant skin maceration. The patient attends therapy weekly to have the splint monitored and to perform ROM exercises to uninvolved joints. At those times the splint is adjusted to allow for decreases in edema, and the lining can be changed.

Exercise. At 6 to 8 weeks, gentle active range of motion (AROM) exercise is initiated, emphasizing full extension. Flexion exercises are very gentle at first, to prevent overstretching the newly healed terminal extensor tendon. Evans[66] advocates allowing 20° to 25° for the first week, increasing to 35° the next week, and increasing gradually thereafter. The splint is worn at night and between exercises for the first 2 weeks, and gradually discontinued during the day thereafter. After another 2 weeks it can be discontinued completely. If an extensor lag develops, the finger should be returned to full-time splinting for an additional week or two. Occasionally, a DIP extensor lag may have to be accepted ultimately, in the interest of regaining functional flexion, but in most patients, carefully supervised exercise and splinting can protect against attenuation of the tendon while flexion is regained. All extensor tendon injuries, at whatever level, pose this problem of balancing functional needs with protection against extensor lag, and splint schedules must be monitored and adjusted accordingly.

Zones 3 and 4 — PIP and Proximal Phalanx

At this level, as in zones 1 and 2, both closed injuries and lacerations are common. The central slip is usually involved, with or without involvement of lateral bands or other parts of the complex extensor mechanism. A PIP extensor lag results, and with repeated PIP flexion, the transverse retinacular ligament and triangular ligament stretch (if they were not already injured) and allow the lateral bands to migrate to a position palmar to the axis of PIP flexion. The displaced lateral bands increase PIP flexion, and at the same time direct all the intrinsic extensor strength to the DIP. The muscular imbalance results in what is called the boutonnière deformity (Fig. 12 – 14). This deformity, characteristic of untreated central slip injury, is marked by PIP flexion and DIP hyperextension, both aggravated by attempted extension of the PIP.

Splinting. These injuries are treated by immobilization with or without surgical repair. Using K-wires, cast, or splint, the finger is held in full PIP extension (Fig. 12 – 15). K-wires may be removed at 3 weeks and the joint supported by a splint alone. If the lateral bands are repaired, the DIP may be immobilized as well. In the established boutonnière deformity (from an old injury), serial casting may be necessary to recover lost passive extension before attempting splinting or surgical repair to maintain functional extension. In these cases, surgical repair has a guarded prognosis.[56,67]

After 6 weeks of immobilization, the extensor apparatus may become severely adherent and the PIP joint very stiff, but if adequate immobilization is not maintained, the delicate extensors may stretch, leading to a PIP extensor lag and flexion contracture. It is usually much easier to increase PIP flexion than to increase PIP extension, given the anatomy of the PIP joint and the superior strength of the flexors (see Chapters 1 and 10). Nonetheless, the current trend among experienced hand therapists is to begin careful mobilization earlier, especially when there is associated soft tissue or bony injury that increases the risk of tendon adhesions, capsular tightness, and residual deformity.

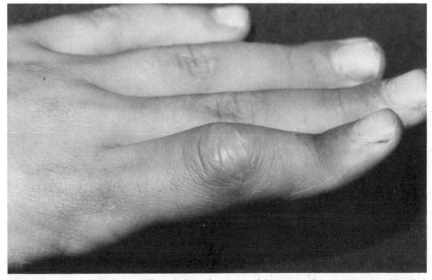

FIGURE 12–14. Boutonnière deformity caused by zone 3 extensor tendon injury.

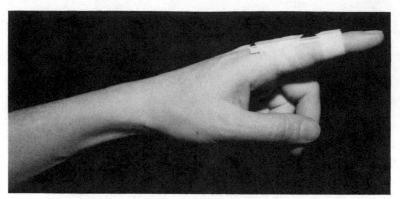

FIGURE 12-15. Dorsal PIP extension splint.

Exercise. In a conservative program, isometric active extension may begin at 3 weeks within the splint, but active flexion is delayed longer. At 4 to 6 weeks the therapist may begin supervised gentle active PIP flexion exercises with assisted extension. If any extensor lag develops the patient should be returned to immobilization for another week. A static splint is worn at night and between exercises for 2 to 4 weeks, and night splinting should be continued until at least 10 weeks after injury.

In early mobilization programs active flexion may begin as early as 3 to 4 weeks after injury with dynamic extension splinting to protect extensors and resist flexors. In this case, a static PIP extension splint should be worn at night initially, and protection continued until 10 weeks after injury.

Exercises emphasize active extension to 0°. This can include composite extension and PIP extension with the MP blocked in flexion. At 7 to 8 weeks, if there is no extensor lag, the extensors can tolerate gentle passive flexion and resisted extension, with dynamic flexion splinting waiting until 8 to 10 weeks.

PIP level injuries can be very difficult to manage. A balance must be maintained between extensor lag and flexion contracture on the one hand, and a functionally limiting extension contracture on the other.

Zones 5, 6, and 7

Immobilization. Although the extensor tendon exhibits several different anatomic characteristics as it travels from the distal forearm to the MP joint (tendon sheaths at wrist level, juncturae tendinum on the dorsum of the hand, the beginnings of the extensor hood at the MP level), the variations do not dictate substantial variations in treatment. The classic approach is immobilization, usually lasting 3 to 4 weeks, until the scar remodeling phase is established. The tendons here lack the intricate interdependence of the extensor apparatus in the digits; therefore, they can withstand earlier motion with less risk of deformity.

Splinting. Following repair, the hand is splinted for 3 weeks at all times, and then between exercise sessions for an additional 2 to 3 weeks, with night splinting usually for 2 or 3 weeks thereafter. The splinting timetable must be altered to respect such complications as joint stiffness and extensor lags. Immobilization is in 30° to 45° of wrist extension, MPs and IPs at 0. For extensor pollicis longus (EPL) repairs, the thumb is immobilized in complete extension at the carpometacarpal (CMC), MP, and IP joints with the wrist also held in extension. Because there is little extrinsic extensor tendon glide over the metacarpals with IP flexion,[68] the IPs may be left free following a zone 5 to 7 repair, if the juncture is secure. At rest the patient can wear a removable palmar support to hold the IPs in extension and prevent a PIP extensor lag.

With isolated injuries to the extensor indicis proprius, extensor digiti minimi, or the thumb extensors only the affected digit need be immobilized. If the common extensor tendon is injured proximal to the juncturae tendinum, all four fingers should be immobilized in full MP extension, because flexion of adjacent fingers would increase tension on the repair. If the injury is distal to the juncturae, the injured finger should be immobilized at 0°, with adjacent fingers in 30° of flexion. This position protects the repair by passively gliding the proximal tendon distally through the pull of the juncturae, thus reducing tension on the suture site.

Zone 7 injuries that include only the wrist extensors can be immobilized in wrist extension alone (40° to 45°), but if the finger extensors are involved, the MPs should also be held in extension. Because they lie so closely adjacent within a synovial sheath at this level, extensor tendons need careful handling to recover differential gliding. Evans[66] has proposed a program of splinting and mobilization designed to create shear between adjacent tendons through individual digit flexion with the other digits held in extension. This consideration is important given the severe restrictions imposed by scar tethering over the dorsum of the wrist.

Exercise. Active mobilization begins at 3 weeks. Exercise begins gently, with the wrist maintained in extension, to protect against excessive stretch while promoting tendon gliding. The program emphasizes active and active-assisted MP extension, followed by limited active flexion (to only 30° or 40° initially) with IPs extended. Hook fist–making (IP flexion with full MP and wrist extension) maintains IP motion while eliciting an isometric EDC contraction.

In all zone 5 to 7 injuries night splinting should continue for an additional 2 to 4 weeks after beginning mobilization, to help counterbalance the pull of the stronger flexors and prevent stretch of the extensors in the early remodeling phase.

By 4 weeks the patient can begin individual finger extension exercises, and by 5 to 6 weeks the program may be progressed to include full fist-making and EDC gliding exercises (starting in a gentle fist and extending the MPs while maintaining IP flexion, to form a hook fist). This exercise is particularly important for zone 5 injuries, to stress junctures gently and promote gliding over the dorsum of the hand. For injuries in zones 5 and 6 the splint may now be modified to include only the wrist.

By 6 weeks resisted flexion will not place excessive stress on the extensor tendons, and the patient can begin combined wrist and finger flexion. The tendons are sufficiently well healed at 6 to 7 weeks to withstand gentle passive flexion, dynamic flexion splinting, and resisted extension.

Once again, a balance must be maintained between the healing extensors and the stronger flexors. MP extensor lags are an all-too-common problem. A minimal lag, however, can be far less functionally limiting than an extension contracture. The latter may develop if the MPs were immobilized in full extension for too long a time. MP extension contractures develop easily because of the anatomic configuration of the articulating bones and the collateral ligaments.

If the wrist extensors are involved, great care must be taken not to overstress these vital structures, which are placed under an extremely heavy load during normal hand use. They should be protected with intermittent splinting up to 2 months, and active motion should be carefully supervised, beginning with active extension and relaxation, and then slowly progressing to active flexion. Evans[66] suggests limiting active wrist flexion to 0° at 4 to 5 weeks, and delaying full wrist flexion until 7 or 8 weeks.

Controlled Early Mobilization. Early mobilization following extensor tendon repair proximal to the MP joint is essentially the reverse of the early controlled passive motion technique used for flexor tendons. Dynamic extension splinting for early passive mobilization of extensor injuries has been used by many hand specialists for years, but there has been little in the literature until recently. This approach is supported by EMG studies by Allieu, Asencio, and Rouzaud[60] showing that if the wrist is maintained in extension, resisted flexion produces EMG silence in the digit extensors.

I have had good results from several approaches. Published accounts do not always specify splinting positions and other important variables; all agree, however, that early mobilization programs must start within days of the surgery and can be used only with patients from whom compliance can be dependably expected.[60-64]

One of the most appropriate approaches for inexperienced therapists is that described by Evans and Burkhalter.[64] The protocol for this approach (described in the next few paragraphs) includes very clear guidelines for avoiding excessive stress to tendon junctures.

At 3 to 5 days following tendon repair, a custom-made splint is applied to the hand, maintaining the wrist in 40° of extension. Dynamic traction holds the MPs at 0°, and a removable palmar block prevents MP flexion beyond 30° for the index and middle fingers, and 38° for the ring and small fingers. (Fig. 12–16). Through intraoperative measurement and calculations using radians and moment arms at the metacarpal head, Evans and Burkhalter have determined that this degree of flexion produces excursion of 3 to 5 mm at the tendon repair site. This excursion is recommended by Duran and Houser for early passive flexor tendon mobilization. The patient flexes to the palmar block 10 to 20 times each waking hour, allowing the dynamic traction to return the fingers to full extension. In therapy protected passive flexion of individual IP joints is performed, with the wrist and MPs held in full extension.

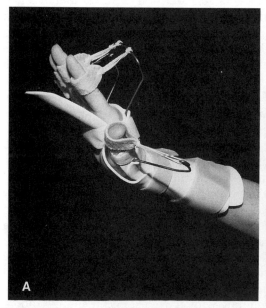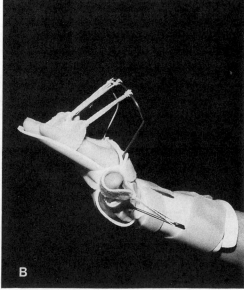

FIGURE 12–16. Dynamic extension splint used by Evans and Burkhalter for complex extensor tendon injuries in zone 5–7 and T-4 and T-5. *A*, MPs rest at 0°. *B*, The removable palmar component prevents MP flexion beyond a safe range.

For EPL lacerations the dynamic traction is applied to the distal phalanx. The wrist is held at 40° of extension, the CMC in a neutral position, and the MP at 0°, with the IP free to flex to 60° against the dynamic traction.

At 21 days, the palmar block is removed from the finger extensor splint, and the traditional extensor tendon program is followed from this point on. However, the patient continues to wear the dynamic splint during the day, with a static extension splint at night, for another 2 to 3 weeks.

SECONDARY PROCEDURES

General Concepts

Even after the most meticulous tendon repair and rehabilitation, further surgery may be needed to restore function. In extreme cases secondary surgery may involve amputation of a nonfunctional digit; other options include arthrodesis (surgical joint fusion) or procedures to release or rebuild restrictive joint structures. Procedures for restoration of tendon glide include tendon grafts, tenolysis, and tendon transfers. Two of these procedures will be discussed: tenolysis and staged tendon graft.

PREOPERATIVE CONSIDERATIONS

A patient is not a candidate for either procedure until he or she has reached a plateau in PROM and AROM. Waiting until a plateau is reached ensures that the surgery is performed only in those patients for whom it is needed. The *minimum* time elapsed between primary repair and secondary reconstruction is 3 months, according to most authors, although many would wait until 4 to 6 months.[69,70] Waiting this period of time allows adequate time for scar remodeling and for reestablishment of adequate vascular and sensory status, both of which are crucial for a successful functional result. Preoperatively the muscle powering the tendon must be at optimum strength, joints and other soft tissues must be supple, and any other health problems or systemic disorders such as diabetes must be well controlled.

Another prerequisite for secondary procedures is a compliant and well-informed patient. Postoperative therapy demands close adherence to a rigorous program, and may be painful. Patients must understand this and be prepared to undertake the responsibility. They must consider how well the ultimate functional result will meet their needs and goals. Some patients may be better served, for example, by an arthrodesis to provide joint stability and give increased strength to a stiff and painful finger. Surgical and nonsurgical options should be thoroughly discussed with patient and surgeon.

INTRAOPERATIVE PARTICIPATION

When possible, the therapist should be present during reconstructive surgery, to observe the condition of the involved tissues, the exact procedures performed, and the intraoperative range of motion. If, for example, tendon pulleys are excised or reconstructed the therapist can visualize them exactly as they are, and thus be better prepared for planning therapy that will adequately protect the pulleys and take into account the postoperative biomechanics of the tendon system. If the therapist cannot be present, he or she should ask for detailed operative notes from the surgeon.

The patient may be awake during tenolysis, if performed under sedation and local anesthesia or regional block, and in some cases, the surgeon will request that the patient move the hand during surgery, to test the available tendon excursion. If planning to make such a test, the surgeon should inform the patient before surgery.

Tenolysis

Tenolysis is surgical excision of adhesions that limit tendon glide. One indication for tenolysis is PROM that markedly exceeds AROM. For example, full passive extension and an extensor lag of 40° at MP and PIP may indicate need for extensor tenolysis. Another indication is tendon adhesions that restrict passive motion (extensor adhesions limiting passive flexion, or flexor adhesions limiting passive extension).

After tenolysis, new tendon adhesions will form at the site of surgery. The goal of postoperative therapy is to reinstitute active motion as quickly as possible to apply controlled stress and ensure that any new adhesions are long, filmy, and elastic, allowing the tendon to glide. This means beginning therapy *within* 24 hours. The only reasons to delay therapy are signs of infection, poor vascularity, or excessive inflammation.[71]

Edema should be quickly controlled through elevation and gentle compressive Coban wrapping to each finger. The use of continuous passive motion (CPM), as discussed subsequently, may also help in control of edema.[71] One must bear in mind that surgery cuts through not only scar but also surrounding tissues, inevitably interrupting the vascularity of this recently healed tendon. Therefore, during the first few weeks, the tendon is vulnerable to rupture, and great caution should be exercised in passive mobilization and early resisted motion.

Motion will be painful as it involves moving the tendon through a fresh wound. The degree of pain and pain tolerance varies tremendously from patient to patient, and pain control methods vary accordingly. Some patients are fine with no pain medication at all. Others benefit from transcutaneous electrical nerve stimulation (TENS), and others from pain medication. Using a local anesthetic injected by the patient through a catheter placed in the surgical incision at the time of tenolysis is possible. This technique requires a high degree of patient compliance, and carries with it the risk of infection, so must be used with caution.[70]

For the first week or so, patients are seen daily. The quality of exercise is extremely important, with the patient working to achieve the greatest possible flexion and extension with each repetition of each active exercise. However, if the surgeon reports that the tendon quality is questionable, only place-hold active exercises should be performed for the first week.

FLEXOR TENOLYSIS

Splinting

If preoperative flexion contractures were corrected in surgery, the fingers should be splinted in extension between exercises, and passive extension exercises should place special emphasis on the released joints. If the transverse carpal ligament was released to perform tenolysis at wrist level, the patient's wrist should be supported in 10° to 20° of extension for the first 2 to 3 weeks.

CPM devices can be a useful adjunct to therapy, especially after a tenolysis that involves release of joint contractures, or in a patient who is known to be unusually apprehensive of pain and cannot be expected to exert adequate force in immediate postoperative exercise. CPM should begin within 24 hours of surgery for maximum effectiveness. The device is disconnected from the fingers every hour for active exercise, as passive motion does not elicit the tendon excursion so crucial to the success of tenolysis. If the patient can tolerate its use during sleep, the device can be very helpful in maintaining passive motion, thus decreasing or eliminating the characteristic postoperative morning stiffness.

Exercise

Beginning on day one, the patient performs place-hold fist-making, blocking, and (if applicable) individual FDS tendon gliding exercises, 5 to 10 times hourly. Fewer repetitions may be performed only if there is a pronounced inflammatory response or if exercise causes an increase in pain that persists more than 15 minutes. All joints are ranged passively three to four times a day, 10 times each. Within a few days, tendon gliding exercises (hook, fist, and straight fist) should replace or supplement place-hold fist-making. Wrist flexion and extension should be incorporated into full fist exercises to attain complete flexor tendon excursion: the patient moves from a position of full finger and wrist extension to full finger and wrist flexion 10 times. This exercise is contraindicated initially if the transverse carpal ligament was released. Active wrist flexion can overstress a healing transverse carpal ligament in the first few weeks after surgery.

After suture removal and adequate healing of the incision, scar massage helps to prevent recurrence of adhesions between the skin and underlying tissues. Retrograde massage can begin even earlier for edema control, with care to avoid suture lines.

At 2 to 3 weeks the frequency of supervised therapy appointments can be decreased for patients who demonstrate good ROM and perform their home program well. Because collagen formation is nearing its peak, it is important to keep home exercises frequent to maintain tendon gliding. Daytime splinting may be phased out if joint contractures appear to be under control, but problem areas should be carefully monitored and the splinting schedule adjusted as needed. A patient can begin light prehension activities and use his or her hand as an assist at home.

At 3 to 4 weeks, patients may actually feel increased internal resistance to active flexion, as tendon adhesions form. They must persist in aggressive and frequent exercise to maintain or increase tendon glide. Lightly resistive exercise, beginning with sustained grip activities, promote tendon gliding in this difficult stage. Progressive strengthening should wait until 6 to 8 weeks, with full resistance at 12 weeks. By waiting until this time reestablishment of vascularity and decreased danger of tendon rupture is allowed. Patients can return to sedentary jobs or light duty at about 8 weeks, but a longer delay is appropriate for heavy manual labor.

Some patients are heavy scar formers and must begin light resistive exercise much earlier, with gentle manual resistance applied by the therapist within the first week. This technique requires a delicate touch and should be performed by an experienced hand therapist in close communication with a skilled hand surgeon.

EXTENSOR TENOLYSIS

Extensor tenolysis is handled similarly, with a few variations. Initially, the finger may be splinted in extension if the delicate extensors need support following an extensive lysis. If this extra support is not needed, then the finger can be left free and, indeed, may need passive flexion exercises or dynamic flexion splinting within a few days of surgery if capsulotomies were performed. CPM may also be indicated in such cases.

Initial exercises include hourly active and place-hold extension (as well as EDC gliding, if the lysis was proximal to the PIP joint), active fisting, and PROM. The patient can be progressed quickly into light hand use, as no resisted extension is involved. Resisted flexion exercises will assist in achieving a full fist, but extension should be carefully monitored, as an extensor lag could result from overly aggressive flexion. Usually, the patient can return to work sooner after extensor tenolysis than after flexor tenolysis. In some cases, the patient can return to work within a month after surgery.

Staged Tendon Reconstruction

Sometimes a tendon is so weak, or is severely adherent and lying in a bed that is so badly scarred, that tenolysis will not be sufficient to restore functional motion to the finger. If any pulleys must be excised to free a tendon, the tendon will lose vital power unless at least the A-1, A-2, and A-4 pulleys are preserved or reconstructed surgically.[28-30] Tenolyses involving pulley reconstruction have a poor prognosis because of the potential for postoperative adherence between pulley and tendon, and the risk of stretching out the newly reconstructed pulley in the aggressive postoperative therapy program.[2] In such cases, staged tendon reconstruction can provide, in two subsequent procedures, a functional tendon graft that glides well in a smooth bed, with strong reconstructed pulleys. In stage 1 a flexible silicone rubber tendon implant is put in place of the damaged tendon, and left for at least 3 months. During this time a pseudosheath forms around the implant. This pseudosheath provides an optimal bed for the tendon graft that replaces the implant in stage 2.[6]

A staged tendon graft is a salvage procedure, involving much time and effort for a functional result. This procedure is not appropriate for cases in which the tendon would benefit from a simple tenolysis.

The following discussion will cover only flexor tendons (usually FDP), but the same principles apply to therapy following staged extensor tendon grafting. The reader should also be aware that at times the DIP is fused and a staged tendon graft used to flex the PIP only. This procedure, producing what is known as a "superficialis finger," is a useful alternative for some fingers in which the usual staged FDP tendon graft is not appropriate.[72]

STAGE 1

Surgery

In the first procedure, the scarred tendon is removed, along with other scar tissue that would impede later gliding. Any necessary joint releases are performed at this time. If pulleys can be preserved, they are left intact. A Hunter silastic implant (Hunter Tendon Implant, Holter-Hausner International, Box 1, Bridgeport, PA 19405) is threaded through the pulleys. This implant is a flexible, flat silicone rubber rod fixed distally with a screw. The rod usually extends from the distal phalanx to the forearm, with the proximal end left unattached.

Any pulley reconstruction is done at this point. The proximal end of the implant is pulled to observe both the strength of the pulleys, and the passive potential of the system.

Splinting

The patient is placed in a postoperative dressing and cast as for early passive mobilization following primary flexor tendon repair (without rubberband traction), and sent to therapy in several days to 1 week, depending on the anticipated joint stiffness or complications.

In therapy, the cast can be left on and the dressing debulked to allow full passive flexion, or a dorsal protective splint may be made. Splinting in 30° wrist flexion and 60° to 70° MP flexion is maintained for the first 3 weeks to keep the proximal end of the tendon well within the forearm and encourage formation of the pseudosheath during the fibroplasia phase. Splinting to correct flexion contractures may be incorporated.

Exercise

Passive flexion and active and passive extension to the limits of the splint are performed four to six times a day, to encourage gliding of the implant.

A possible complication is synovitis due to overexercise or to poor handling of the implant during surgery.[6] The hand should be monitored for signs of synovitis: increased redness, swelling, heat, and pain over the course of the implant. If these signs occur, the hand should be rested in the splint until inflammation resolves, and then exercises should be resumed slowly. When synovitis cannot be controlled conservatively, the implant must be removed surgically.

Edema control measures including elevation, Coban wrapping, and careful retrograde massage begin in the first few days, and scar massage as soon as the incision is well healed and sutures are removed.

At 3 weeks the splint is discontinued and the patient is given a trapper, or buddy strap, that passively flexes the involved finger when the adjacent finger flexes actively (Fig. 12–17). AROM and PROM exercises continue as before.

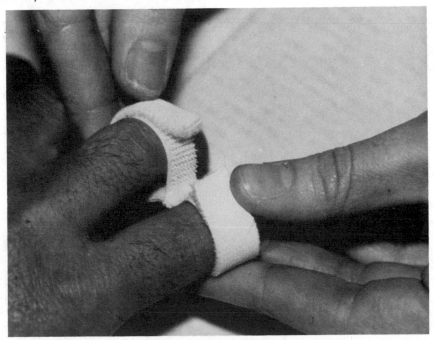

FIGURE 12–17. Buddy strap. When this patient makes a fist, the involved finger is passively flexed by its attachment to the uninvolved finger.

By 6 weeks most patients can return to work. Usually 3 months elapse before stage 2, to allow scar maturation and recovery of optimal joint mobility.

STAGE 2

Surgery

In stage 2, the implant is replaced with a tendon graft taken from either plantaris or a toe extensor. The graft is fixed distally to the stump of the tendon or directly to the bone (as in an avulsion of the FDP insertion). The proximal end of the graft is attached to a "motor" tendon that will power the graft. The motor is usually the FDP, but may be FDS.[6]

Splinting

The postoperative cast or splint is in 30° to 40° of wrist flexion and 60° to 70° of MP flexion, with IPs allowed to extend completely.

If any of the reconstructed or damaged pulleys appears intraoperatively to be weak or vulnerable to stretch, a pulley ring is constructed of Velcro and felt, to be replaced later with a thermoplastic ring when edema subsides and firm circumferential pressure is appropriate (Fig. 12–18).

This pulley ring is placed over the weak pulley as reinforcement, and may be worn by the patient for weeks or months, depending on whether any "bowstringing" is noted at the pulley site.[6] When active flexion is initiated, the pulley should be reinforced by manual pressure to the digit during exercise, as a pulley ring alone is a poor substitute for the actual pulley, lacking the necessary combination of strength, close fit, and flexibility provided by the pulley.

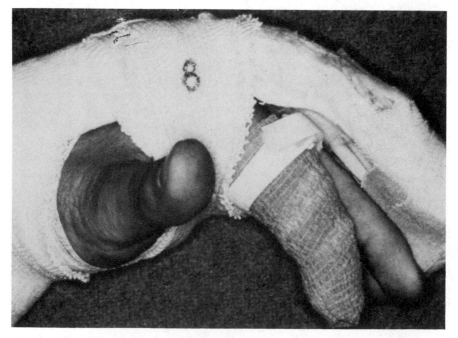

FIGURE 12–18. Pulley ring worn to reinforce a flexor tendon pulley reconstructed over a tendon implant.

Exercise

Within 1 or 2 days therapy begins, with debulking of the dressing to allow complete passive flexion and active extension as allowed by the cast. Elastic traction into flexion may be applied, and therapy follows a flexor tendon early controlled mobilization protocol with a few variations.

Because there are two junctures to protect, proximal and distal, and because the vascularity of the involved finger is at greater risk following two or three surgical procedures, the protective splint is maintained and active flexion is not allowed until well into the scar remodeling phase (as early as 4 weeks for a poorly gliding graft, but as late as 6 weeks if the graft glides well). Bear in mind also that because the graft itself has no intrinsic circulation, it is dependent on adhesions for nutrition needed for healing. For another 2 weeks after splint removal, protection is provided by a dynamic traction from a wrist cuff as described by Duran and Houser[39] for primary repairs. Active flexion begins with place-hold fisting, and progresses through active tendon gliding exercises and blocking by 8 weeks.

Light resistance is introduced at 10 weeks, with progressive resistive exercises at 12 weeks, and return to work shortly thereafter. Patients such as ironworkers, whose work places unusually heavy demands on their hands, should return to work no earlier than 4 months after surgery.

COMPLICATIONS

PIP flexion contractures are often a preoperative as well as a postoperative problem for these patients. These should be prevented as far as possible through careful ROM and splinting as for primary repairs, bearing in mind that these may be longstanding contractures and that the graft should be protected more carefully for the reasons just outlined.

Passive DIP flexion must be performed with care, because DIP flexion contractures, too, often develop in stage 2. The implant is often attached at the FDP insertion by a screw and the graft is attached at the same site, producing potentially restrictive scarring at that point. The prolonged positioning in marked flexion following the two surgical procedures may lead to attenuation of the terminal extensor tendon, thus increasing the extensor lag.[6]

Staged Grafting with the Active Tendon Implant

An active tendon implant has been developed by Hunter and associates,[6,72,73] but this is not in wide use and therefore will not be discussed here. In brief, the active tendon implant is attached proximally to the muscle that is to motor the graft. Thus, the implant begins to function immediately as a tendon graft, allowing conditioning of the muscle during stage 1 therapy.[6,72,73]

CLINICAL DECISION MAKING: CASE STUDY

A case study discussing the management of flexor tenolysis in replanted digits was selected to illustrate the need to modify the rehabilitation program carefully according to tissue status, rates of healing, associated injuries, and the patient's ability to carry out the program at home. This patient was treated in Italy, where some of the techniques I prefer could not be used.

REPLANTATION

History/Surgery

L. C., a 20-year-old male operator of heavy farm machinery, amputated his nondominant left index and long fingers at the base of the proximal phalanges. Injury was by a clean cut from an axe, which the patient was using to cut firewood. The fingers were replanted within a few hours, with bony fixation via crossed K-wires, repair of all digital nerves, both digital arteries to the index, the radial artery of the long finger, the principal veins, the extensor apparatus, and both FDPs. FDS was not repaired. The K-wires did not immobilize any joints.

Therapy

At 28 days, the patient was referred for therapy, which concentrated on edema control, pin and wound care, and AROM, as well as isolated passive flexion and extension of each IP and MP joint. Although I prefer to see patients within a few days of replantation, to initiate edema control and wound care and protected ROM, the attending surgeon chose to delay therapy. He instructed the patient in edema control measures and performed all wound care. One pin was removed from each digit at 2 months, and the others remained in place until 3 months, as they did not impede joint motion and served to reinforce the healing bone.

By the start of therapy the FDP tendons were markedly adherent, but some glide was apparent. The picture was complicated, however, by a troubling phenomenon known as paradoxical extension (or lumbrical plus). In the literature this problem is more commonly recognized following unrepaired FDP injury distal to the lumbrical origin or in cases of flexor tendon grafts of excessive length. In those cases, the FDP glides too far proximally, transmitting its force to the extensor mechanism via the lumbricals (which take their origin from the FDP) and thereby extending the interphalangeal joints.[26,74-76] However, paradoxical extension can occur in the presence of heavy FDP adhesions or adhesions of the lumbricals to a repaired FDP[77] and has been noted by Silverman, Willette-Green, and Petrilli[58] in a series of replants proximal to the FDS insertion. Although this patient's lumbricals had not been repaired in surgery, they had apparently healed in some fashion and scarred to surrounding tissues including the FDP. When the patient attempted to make a fist, the adherent profundus tendons had such a restricted excursion that after flexing the MPs they acted as a fixed origin for the lumbricals. Although the lumbricals are normally electromyographically silent during fisting,[26] in this case either they contracted in an effort to assist MP flexion (and thereby extended the IPs) or they were scarred to the profundus and mechanically transmitted the profundus contraction to the extensor mechanism. The result was very strong IP extension with attempted fisting (Fig. 12–19).

Fisting is very frustrating and difficult for a patient whose fingers go into paradoxical extension with attempts at flexion. However, when the MP is blocked in extension, the lumbricals are at a mechanical disadvantage and the short

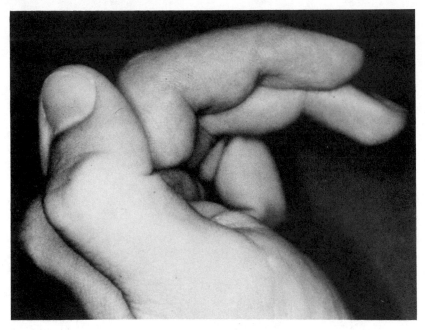

FIGURE 12–19. Case study: paradoxical extension (lumbrical plus). Attempted flexion produces MP flexion and IP extension. Although not shown here, the IPs actually resist passive flexion during attempted fisting but can be completely flexed passively when relaxed (see Fig. 12–21).

excursion of the FDP is sufficient to flex the IPs. Therefore, we addressed the problem by emphasizing blocking exercises. Blocked IP flexion very quickly returned, showing that the FDP was indeed gliding, albeit within a restricted range (Fig. 12–20).

In our efforts to gain sufficient flexion we anticipated a loss of extension, so we were careful to emphasize active extension, to increase extensor strength and counterbalance the pull of the flexors.

Gentle passive flexion began at 6 weeks with dynamic splinting to individual joints, and proceeded to overall stretch to the extensors using Coban wrapping in a fist (Coban, Medical Products Division/3M, St. Paul, MN). Gentle resisted flexion also began at 6 weeks, given the extreme adherence of the FDP in both fingers. Resisted exercise, PROM, and functional hand use were graded in accordance with healing and as appropriate to progress in strength and ROM measurements.

Isometric grasp exercise, putty exercises, and grasping activities were nearly impossible for this patient, given the paradoxical extension. In lieu of these he wore a dynamic PIP extension splint that blocked the MPs in extension and simultaneously provided to the FDP gentle passive stretch and resistive exercise in the most mechanically advantageous position.

By 4½ months the patient demonstrated PROM within normal limits (Fig. 12–21), active extension lacking only a few degrees at the PIP joints, and full active flexion at the DIPs with blocking exercises (see Fig. 12–20). Paradoxical extension was still strong: attempted fisting produced MP flexion and IP extension (see Fig. 12–19).

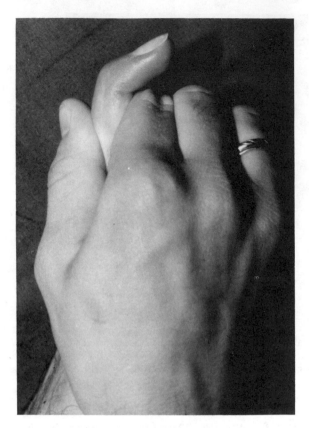

FIGURE 12-20. Case study: FDP gliding with finger blocking is very strong.

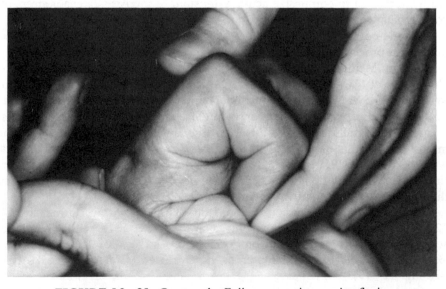

FIGURE 12-21. Case study: Full preoperative passive flexion.

TENOLYSIS

Flexor tenolysis was indicated for this patient because passive flexion was within normal limits but active flexion was severely limited and, in fact, had reached a plateau by 3 months after repair in spite of increasingly aggressive therapy. In a replanted digit, tenolysis is normally delayed until at least 6 months after surgery, in order to allow sufficient scar maturation and recovery of vascularity.[78] For this patient, however, several factors prompted an early tenolysis, at 4½ months after replantation. For various reasons, this patient had limited time available for hand therapy, and he was willing to take the risk of early surgery. In addition, his vascularity was excellent, and this was an exceptionally compliant, healthy patient who had healed well and quickly after replantation.

Intraoperative Findings

Tendons were found to be very healthy but markedly adherent. Following extensive flexor tenolysis, all pulleys were preserved, with the exception of portions of A-3 of the index finger and A-2 and A-3 of the long finger (Fig. 12–22). No pulleys were reconstructed or repaired. In surgery proximal traction on the tendons produced flexion to 2.5 cm from the distal palmar crease.

Postoperative Therapy

Therapy was initiated the day after surgery. This patient did not have much difficulty with pain and, in fact, chose to discontinue his pain medication within 2 days. Edema was addressed with elevation and Coban circumferential wrapping. Sterile wound care was performed in therapy, beginning with debulking of the postsurgical dressing. The nonstick antibiotic-impregnated gauze was left undisturbed, to minimize the risk of infection. Dressings were changed every few days in therapy.

The patient was instructed in the standard post-tenolysis exercises described earlier. Although no effort had been made to free the lumbricals in surgery, it was immediately apparent that the paradoxical extension had been eradicated by the tenolysis: on the first day the patient achieved active flexion to about 3.5 cm from the distal palmar crease in spite of postoperative edema.

Extension showed a minor lag. Given the history of extensor tendon injury and mild preoperative PIP extensor lag, the patient also immediately began isolated active and passive PIP extension exercises, and the fingers were supported in a serially adjustable static extension splint between exercises and at night, with traction applied at the DIP joint. Resisted extension exercises were initiated within a week.

The patient was seen daily until 10 days after surgery, at which time he demonstrated flexion *exceeding* that obtained intraoperatively. Frequency of therapy was decreased to three times a week.

At 12 days, sutures were removed, and gentle scar and retrograde massage were initiated. The incision was very well healed at this point, and skin condition was good, with minimal erythema and no ecchymosis. In view of the excellent AROM, exercise frequency was cautiously reduced to every 2 hours, and the splint schedule was decreased to nights and three times a day for 2 hours. The patient

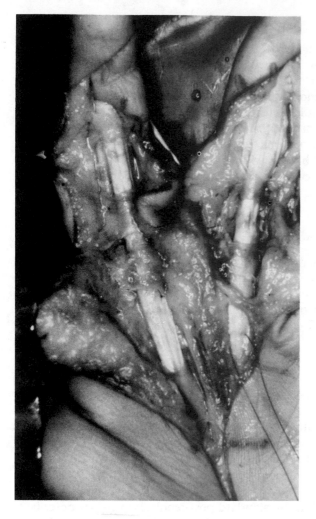

FIGURE 12–22. Case study: Extensive flexor tenolysis was performed, preserving as many pulleys as possible.

monitored his motion at home using a template, with instructions to increase exercise frequency if AROM decreased or stiffness increased.

At 3 weeks, the patient began to use his hand very lightly at home. At 4 weeks very gentle resisted exercise began with light pickups and sustained grasp activities, progressing to squeezing and pinching lightly resistive putty at 6 weeks. If recovery of active flexion had not progressed quickly, manual resistance could have been started earlier by the therapist and daily therapy visits would have continued. If the vascularity had appeared poor or the flexor tendons had not appeared so healthy intraoperatively, resistance would have been delayed until at least 7 weeks.

Although they are beyond the scope of this chapter, desensitization and sensory reeducation programs formed an important part of this patient's rehabilitation. Patients typically have great difficulty regaining functional use of fingers with limited or absent sensibility. In spite of returning sensibility, this patient needed much encouragement to use the fingers, even after he achieved virtually a full fist (index finger lacking 15 mm from the distal palmar crease; long finger lacking 5 mm) and almost complete extension (Fig. 12–23).

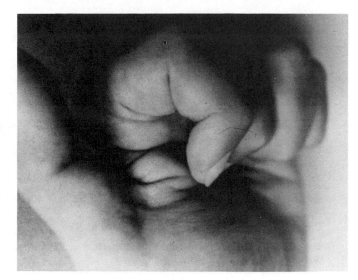

FIGURE 12–23. Case study: At 7 weeks following flexor tenolysis, patient attained an almost complete fist. Active extension lacked 20° at PIPs, but passive extension and flexion were both within normal limits.

RESULTS

At 10 weeks the patient was discharged and returned to work on light duty, having achieved a grip strength of 50 lb compared with 96 lb in the dominant hand. Pinch strength was proportionately lower, which is not surprising given the lack of intrinsic muscle power to the index and long fingers.

This case was selected because it *did not* represent a typical patient followed in a typical manner: it presented some unusual features including an extremely good candidate for both surgery and therapy. Therapy after tenolysis was quite aggressive, and was described to illustrate the importance of adapting the program to the patient's needs.

SUMMARY

The rehabilitation of the injured or reconstructed tendon is complex, demanding, and extremely rewarding. This chapter has reviewed the surgical management of tendon repairs, tendon reconstruction, and secondary surgical procedures. Concepts in tendon healing and the implications for rehabilitation were also presented. A detailed discussion of the therapeutic management of flexor and extensor tendons, as well as the management following tenolysis and staged tendon reconstruction, provided the reader with a comprehensive overview of tendon management. The case study illustrated the clinical decision making relevant to the management of a flexor tenolysis in replanted digits.

The therapist must understand fully the myriad factors affecting tendon healing and restoration of gliding, and must work closely with both patient and surgeon to design a program that will produce maximum recovery of function. The therapist who is just beginning to explore the exciting specialty of hand management is urged to study the literature cited in the references.

REFERENCES

1. Evans, RB: Management of the healing tendon . . . what must we question? J Hand Ther 2:61, 1989.
2. Schneider, L: Flexor Tendon Injuries. Little, Brown, Boston, 1985, p 77.
3. Kleinert, H and Verdan, C: Report of the committee on tendon injuries. J Hand Surg 8:794, 1983.
4. Kleinert, H, Schepel, S, and Gill, T: Flexor tendon injuries. Surg Clin North Am 61:267, 1981.
5. Cash, S: Primary care of flexor tendon injuries. In Hunter, J, et al (eds): Rehabilitation of the Hand, ed 3. CV Mosby, St Louis, 1990, p 379.
6. Hunter, J, Singer, D, and Mackin, E: Staged flexor tendon reconstruction using passive and active tendon implants. In Hunter, J, et al (eds): Rehabilitation of the Hand, ed 3. CV Mosby, St Louis, 1990, p 427.
7. Brunelli, G and Monini, L: Technique personnelle de suture des tendons flechisseurs des doigts avec mobilisation immediate. Ann Chir Main 1:92, 1982.
8. Mantero, R and Bertolotti, P: La mobilisation precoce dans le traitement des lesions des tendons flechisseurs au canal digital. Ann Chir 30:889, 1976.
9. Becker, H and Grossman, JA: The bevel (Becker) technique for flexor tendon repair. In Tubiana, R (ed): The Hand. Vol. III. WB Saunders, Philadelphia, 1988, p 213.
10. Lee, H: Double-loop locking suture: A technique of tendon repair for early active mobilization. Part I: Evolution of technique and experimental study. J Hand Surg 15A:945, 1990.
11. Allen, B, et al: Ruptured flexor tendon tenorrhaphies in zone II: Repair and rehabilitation. J Hand Surg 12A:18, 1987.
12. Cullen, K, et al: Flexor tendon repair in zone 2 followed by controlled active mobilisation. J Hand Surg 14B:392, 1989.
13. Small, J, Brennen, M, and Colville, J: Early active mobilisation following flexor tendon repair in zone 2. J Hand Surg 14:383, 1989.
14. Lee, H: Double-loop locking suture: A technique of tendon repair for early active mobilization. Part II: Clinical experience. J Hand Surg 15A:953, 1990.
15. Mason, J and Allen, H: The rate of healing of tendons: An experimental study of tensile strength. Ann Surg 113:424, 1941.
16. Gelberman, R, et al: Flexor tendon healing and restoration of the gliding surface: An ultrastructural study in dogs. J Bone Joint Surg 651:583, 1980.
17. Gelberman, RH, et al: The influence of protected passive mobilization on the healing of flexor tendons: A biochemical and microangiographic study. Hand 13:120, 1981.
18. Woo, SL-Y, et al: The importance of controlled passive mobilization on flexor tendon healing. A biomechanical study. Acta Orthop Scand 52:615, 1981.
19. Gelberman, R, et al: Effects of early intermittent passive mobilization on healing canine flexor tendons. J Hand Surg 7:170, 1982.
20. Hitchcock, T, et al: The effect of immediate constrained digital motion on the strength of flexor tendon repairs in chickens. J Hand Surg 12A:590, 1987.
21. Gelberman, R and Woo, SL-Y: The physiological basis for application of controlled stress in the rehabilitation of flexor tendon injuries. J Hand Ther 2:66, 1989.
22. Gelberman, R and Manske, P: Effects of early motion on the tendon healing process: Experimental studies. In Hunter, J, Schneider, L, and Mackin, E (eds): Tendon Surgery in the Hand. CV Mosby, St Louis, 1987, p 170.
23. Strickland, J and Glogovac, S: Digital function following flexor tendon repair in zone 2: A comparison of immobilization and controlled passive motion techniques. J Hand Surg 5:537, 1980.
24. Strickland, J: Flexor tendon injuries, flexor tenolysis, rehabilitation and results, Part 5. Orthop Rev 16:137, 1987.
25. Backhouse, K and Catton, W: Experimental study of the function of the lumbrical muscles. J Anat 88:133, 1954.
26. Long, C and Brown, M: Electromyographic kinesiology of the hand: Muscles moving the long finger. J Bone Joint Surg 46A:1683, 1964.
27. Amadio, P and Junter, J: Prognostic factors in flexor tendon surgery in zone 2. In Hunter, J, Schneider, L, and Mackin, E (eds): Tendon Surgery in the Hand. CV Mosby, St Louis, 1987, p 138.
28. Barton, N: Experimental study of optimal location of flexor tendon pulleys. Plast Reconstr Surg 43:125, 1969.
29. Doyle, J and Blythe, W: The finger flexor tendon sheath and pulleys: Anatomy and reconstruction. In American Academy of Orthopedic Surgeons: Symposium on Tendon Surgery of the Hand. CV Mosby, St Louis, 1975, p 81.
30. Hunter, J and Cook, J: The pulley system: Rationale for reconstruction. In Strickland, J and Steinchen, J (eds): Difficult Problems in Hand Surgery. CV Mosby, St Louis, 1982, p 94.
31. Manske, P and Lesker, P: Nutrient pathways of flexor tendons in primates. J Hand Surg 7:436, 1982.
32. Manske, P and Lesker, P: Diffusion as a nutrient pathway to the flexor tendon. In Hunter, J, Schneider, L, and Mackin, E (eds): Tendon Surgery in the Hand. CV Mosby, St Louis, 1987, p 86.
33. Weber, E: Nutritional pathways for flexor tendons in the digital theca. In Hunter, J, Schneider, L, and Mackin, E (eds): Tendon Surgery in the Hand. CV Mosby, St Louis, 1987, p 91.

34. Bunnell, S: Surgery of the Hand, ed 3. JB Lippincott, Philadelphia, 1956.
35. Evans, R: A study of the zone 1 flexor tendon injury and implications for treatment. J Hand Ther 3:133, 1990.
36. Strickland, J: Biologic rationale, clinical application, and results of early motion following flexor tendon repair. J Hand Ther 2:71, 1989.
37. Gelberman, R, et al: Influences of the protected passive mobilization interval on flexor tendon healing: A prospective randomized clinical study. Clin Orthop Rel Res 264:189, 1991.
38. Duran, R and Houser, R: Controlled passive motion following flexor tendon repair in zones 2 and 3. In AAOS Symposium on Tendon Surgery in the Hand. CV Mosby, St Louis, 1975, p 105.
39. Duran, R, et al: Management of flexor tendon lacerations in zone 2 using controlled passive motion postoperatively. In Hunter, J, et al (eds): Rehabilitation of the Hand, ed 3. CV Mosby, St Louis, 1990, p 410.
40. Kleinert, H, Kutz, J, and Cohen, M: Primary repair of zone 2 flexor tendon lacerations. In AAOS Symposium on Tendon Surgery in the Hand. CV Mosby, St Louis, 1975, p 91.
41. Werntz, J, et al: A new dynamic splint for postoperative treatment of flexor tendon injury. J Hand Surg 14A:559, 1989.
42. Lister, G, et al: Primary flexor tendon repair followed by immediate controlled mobilization. J Hand Surg 2:441, 1977.
43. McGrouther, D and Ahmed, M: Flexor tendon excursions in "no man's land." Hand 13:129, 1981.
44. Horibe, S, et al: Excursion of the flexor digitorum profundus tendon: A kinematic study of the human and canine digits. J Orthop Res 8:167, 1990.
45. Slattery, P and McGrouther, D: A modified Kleinert controlled mobilisation splint following flexor tendon repair. J Hand Surg 9B:34, 1984.
46. Chow, J, et al: A combined regimen of controlled motion following flexor tendon repair in "no man's land." Plast Reconstr Surg 79:447, 1987.
47. Brown, C and McGrouther, D: The excursion of the tendon of flexor pollicis longus and its relation to dynamic splintage. J Hand Surg 9A:787, 1984.
48. Cooney, W, Lin, G, and An, KK-N: Improved tendon excursion following flexor tendon repair. J Hand Ther 2:102, 1989.
49. Citron, N and Forster, A: Dynamic splinting following flexor tendon repair. J Hand Surg 12B:96, 1987.
50. Stegink Janson, C and Minerbo, G: A comparison between early dynamically controlled mobilization and immobilization after flexor tendon repair in zone 2 of the hand. J Hand Ther 3:20, 1990.
51. Dovelle, S and Heeter, P: The Washington regimen: rehabilitation of the hand following flexor tendon injuries. Phys Ther 69:1034, 1989.
52. Stoddard, C: Personal communication, May, 1982.
53. Rosenthal, E: Personal communication, October, 1984.
54. Wehbe, M and Hunter, J: Flexor tendon gliding in the hand. Part II. Differential gliding. J Hand Surg 10A:575, 1985.
55. Cifaldi, D and Schwarze, L: Early progressive resistance following immobilization of flexor tendon repairs. Presented at 13th Annual Meeting, American Society of Hand Therapists, Toronto, 1990.
56. Rosenthal, E: The extensor tendons. In Hunter, J, et al (eds): Rehabilitation of the Hand, ed 3. CV Mosby, St Louis, 1990, p 458.
57. Rosenblum, N and Robinson, S: Advances in flexor and extensor tendon management. In Moran, CA (ed): Hand Rehabilitation. Clin Phys Ther 9:17, 1986.
58. Silverman, P, Willette-Green, V, and Petrilli, J: Early protective motion in digital revascularization and replantation. J Hand Ther 2:84, 1989.
59. Allieu, Y, et al: Suture des tendons extenseurs de la main avec mobilisation assitée: À propos de 120 cas. Rev Chir Orthop 70 (Suppl 2): 69, 1984.
60. Allieu, Y, Asencio, G, and Rouzaud, J: Protected passive mobilization after suturing of the extensor tendons of the hand: A survey of 120 cases. In Hunter, J, Schneider, L, and Mackin, E (eds): Tendon Surgery in the Hand. CV Mosby, St Louis, 1987, p 344.
61. Evans, R: Therapeutic management of extensor tendon injuries. In Mackin, E (ed): Hand Rehabilitation. Hand Clin 2:157, 1986.
62. Evans, R and Burkhalter, W: A study of the dynamic anatomy of extensor tendons and implications for treatment. J Hand Surg 11A:774, 1986.
63. Browne, E and Ribik, C: Early dynamic splinting for extensor tendon injuries. J Hand Surg 14A:72, 1989.
64. Evans, R: Clinical application of controlled stress to the healing extensor tendon: a review of 112 cases. Phys Ther 69:1041, 1989.
65. Rayan, G and Mullins, P: Skin necrosis complicating mallet finger splinting and vascularity of the distal interphalangeal joint overlying skin. J Hand Surg 12A:548, 1987.
66. Evans, R: Therapeutic management of extensor tendon injuries. In Hunter, J, et al (eds): Rehabilitation of the Hand, ed 3. CV Mosby, St Louis, 1990, p 492.
67. Burton, R: Extensor tendons: Late reconstruction. In Green, D (ed): Operative Hand Surgery, ed 2. Churchill Livingstone, New York, 1988, p 2073.
68. Brand, P: Biomechanics of tendon transfers. Orthop Clin North Am 5:205, 1974.

69. Strickland, J: Flexor tenolysis: A personal experience. In Hunter, J, Schneider, L, and Mackin, E (eds): Tendon Surgery in the Hand. CV Mosby, St Louis, 1987, p 216.
70. Schneider, L and Mackin, E: Tenolysis: Dynamic approach to surgery and therapy. In Hunter, J, et al (eds): Rehabilitation of the Hand, ed 3. CV Mosby, St Louis, 1990, p 417.
71. Cannon, N: Enhancing flexor tendon glide through tenolysis . . . and hand therapy. J Hand Ther 2:122, 1989.
72. Hunter, J, Blackmore, S, and Callahan, A: Flexor tendon salvage and functional redemption using the Hunter tendon implant and the superficialis finger operation. J Hand Ther 2:107, 1989.
73. Hunter, J, et al: Active tendon implants for flexor tendon reconstruction. J Hand Surg 13A:849, 1988.
74. Parkes, A: The "lumbrical plus" finger. J Bone Joint Surg 53B:236, 1971.
75. Kilgore, E and Graham, W: The Hand: Surgical and Non-Surgical Management. Lea & Febiger, Philadelphia, 1977, p 326.
76. Zancolli, E: Structural and Dynamic Bases of Hand Surgery, ed 2. JB Lippincott, Philadelphia, 1979, p 305.
77. Burkhalter, W (moderator): Panel discussion 4: Rehabilitation: Flexor and extensor tendons. In Hunter, J, Schneider, L, and Mackin, E (eds): Tendon Surgery in the Hand. CV Mosby, St Louis, 1987, p 558.
78. Steichen, J and Idler, R: Surgical aspects of replantation and revascularization. In Hunter, J, Schneider, L, Mackin, E, and Callahan, A (eds): Rehabilitation of the Hand, ed 3. CV Mosby, St Louis, 1990, p 801.

CHAPTER 13

Rheumatoid Arthritis

Helen Marx, OTR, CHT

Rheumatoid arthritis (RA) is a disease that affects the whole body and the whole person. For the patient with RA, the pain, deformity, and loss of functional independence that accompanies manual restrictions can be devastating. For the therapist, the evaluation and treatment of this chronic disease present a complex challenge, because the disease involves not just the joints but all the tissues of the hand.

The objectives of this chapter are to: (1) review the basic pathology and pathomechanics contributing to hand dysfunction in rheumatoid arthritis, (2) present a systematic approach to patient evaluation, (3) correlate patient evaluation and treatment, and (4) discuss treatment modalities including thermal agents, splinting, therapeutic exercise, and joint protection.

ETIOLOGY/INCIDENCE

Rheumatoid arthritis is a chronic, systemic, inflammatory disorder that affects primarily the synovial tissues of diarthrodial joints. Prolonged synovitis within joints or tendon sheaths results in secondary changes of articular structures including articular cartilage, bone, joint capsule, ligaments, and tendon. Fascia and muscle may be affected as well as internal organs, eyes, and skin.

The cause of RA remains unknown.[1] There are currently two theories that describe the histologic changes observed with RA. The first theory proposes that an interaction of antigens and antibodies in synovial tissues, cartilage, and synovial fluid produces the changes associated with RA. This theory is referred to as the *extravascular immune complex hypothesis*.[2] A second theory proposes that rheumatoid joint disease results from cellular hypersensitivity.[2]

Rheumatoid arthritis affects both sexes and can occur at any age. The disease process is characterized by periods of exacerbation and remission. With RA, there are five basic patterns of progression (Table 13–1).[3] About 35% of patients experience

TABLE 13–1 Types of Progression of Rheumatoid Arthritis

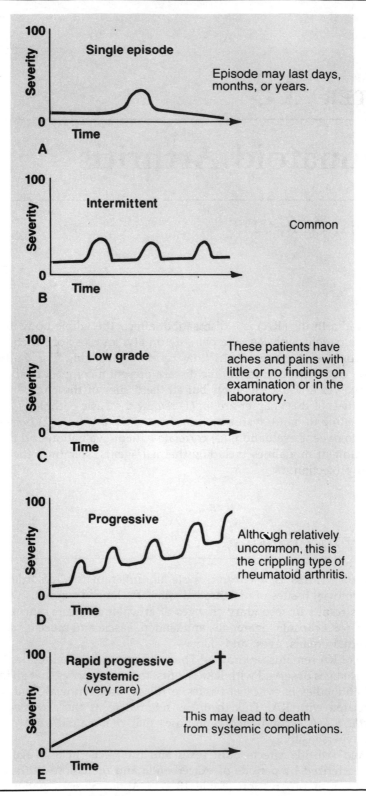

From Fritz, Paxinos, and Gall,[3] with permission.

monocyclic disease, which is a single episode lasting days, months, or years. With a monocyclic disease process, a complete spontaneous recovery is expected. A polycyclic course, one of intermittent exacerbations, occurs in 50% of patients with RA, whereas a progressive unremitting course is seen 15% of the time.[4]

PATHOMECHANICS

In the normal synovial joint, a bony end plate of dense subchondral bone is covered by a smooth layer of articular cartilage. The periosteum, a fibrous membrane carrying blood vessels and nerves, covers the surface of the bone that is not covered by cartilage. A sleeve of fibrous tissues, the joint capsule, connects bone to bone. Fibrous extensions of ligaments and tendons join the joint capsule and contribute to its strength.

The capsule is lined with a thin synovial membrane that produces synovial fluid. The joint surfaces are nourished and lubricated by this synovial fluid. Rheumatoid arthritis initiates a complex biochemical response of the immune system causing inflammation of the synovium. This inflammatory response produces an increase in the amount of synovial fluid as well as a change in the composition of the fluid. As a result of these changes, the fluid no longer drains from the capsule efficiently so pressure within the capsule is increased. With prolonged inflammation, there is a destructive overgrowth of the synovial tissue, called pannus, which extends into the articular surface.

If there is early remission of the inflammation, the episode will have caused pain but no permanent joint damage. With prolonged inflammation, there is destruction of joint tissues as a result of impaired nutrition, erosion by powerful enzymes in the altered synovial fluid, and mechanical injury of compromised supporting periarticular structures.

The integrity of the skeletal hand arches and efficiency of movement depend on the preservation of joint tissues. Abnormal posture and motion of the hand and wrist in patients who have RA result from changes in the balance of forces across multiple joints. For example, the wrist deformities associated with RA contribute to the ulnar deviation and subluxation deformity that can occur at the MP joint.

Based on an understanding of the pathomechanics of the rheumatoid process, the following concepts form the foundation of any therapy program to manage RA of the hand.

- *Control the inflammation*: Synovitis of the wrist, digital joints, and tendon sheath linings initiates the structural changes that impair hand function. Evaluating and controlling inflammation becomes a primary treatment concern.
- *Consider the status of all the tissues in the hand*: The destructive process goes beyond the joint capsule to affect soft tissues including tendon, muscle, and nerve. The therapist should seek to preserve the integrity of these tissues and to maintain their function.
- *Focus on joint systems rather than isolated joints*: Structures of the hand are interdependent in providing the stability and mobility necessary for function. Forces act across multiple joints, with changes at one joint (whether by disease or therapeutic intervention) altering the forces acting on the adjacent joints. Therefore, treatment cannot be isolated to an individual joint and should address joint systems.

EVALUATION

Treatment of the patient with RA begins with a comprehensive evaluation including medical and social history and physical and functional assessments. The physical evaluation involves a systematic examination of skin, joint stability and mobility, muscle-tendon function, as well as sensibility, in order to identify and categorize according to priority problems related to this complex disease. A significant portion of the text is devoted to evaluating the characteristic patterns of hand deformity associated with RA.

Medical-Social History

Hand problems must be seen in perspective with the patient's medical and social history as well as functional status. Critical information should be obtained from the referring physician, through review of the medical records, or during the patient interview. Table 13–2 provides an outline that can be used as a guide for the initial interview of patients. The patient interview is particularly important for the therapist to gain an understanding of the patient's perception of the disease and its treatment. Because RA is

TABLE 13–2 Medical/Social History: Guideline for Patient Interview

Medical history
   Diagnosis
   Disease progression
   Systemic involvement
   Date of onset
   Joints affected
Social history
   Age
   Marital status
   Home environment
   Vocation
   Avocation
Medical management (past–present–anticipated)
   Medication
   Education
   Surgery
   Therapy
   Home program
Current symptoms
   Recent changes observed
   Remission/exacerbation of inflammation
Reason for seeking medical treatment
   Decreased function
   Cosmesis
   Environmental/social change demanding increased function
   Pain
Expectations
   Patient's
   Referring health professional's
   Family's

a chronic disease, decisions regarding the management of present problems must be made in context with the information obtained from the medical-social history.

Physical Assessment

Objective measurements, as outlined in Chapter 3, should be assessed and recorded including edema, active range of motion (AROM) passive range of motion (PROM), grip, and pinch. Because RA effects all the tissues of the hand, the physical assessment should include evaluation of each system involved, including skin, muscle, tendon, nerve, and joint. Particular attention should be paid to the effects of synovitis on each of the systems of the hand.

SKIN

Physical assessment of the hand begins with examination of the skin. Acute inflammation is indicated by areas of redness and warmth that may be tender to palpation. Abnormal skin color may also indicate vasculitis, Raynaud's phenomenon, or ischemic skin lesions, all of which are problems sometimes associated with RA.

Atrophic skin, commonly described as "tissue paper skin," and ecchymosis are often seen after prolonged use of steroid medications. Signs of fragile skin and blood vessels warn the therapist that extra care must be taken in using modalities of heat and cold, massage, and adhesives on the skin. Care must also be taken to avoid trauma to the skin; do not apply splints with unfinished edges or improper fit.

Data from clinical observations suggest atrophic skin may be an indication that the individual is less likely to form dense scar following surgery. As a result, the time of immobilization for healing following reconstructive procedures may need to be lengthened. For these patients, achieving stability may take priority over increasing range of motion (ROM). The location and size of subcutaneous nodules should be noted. When possible, their width and height should be measured or estimated in centimeters. Usually nodules are not painful, but if they are in an area where pressure is applied (by activity or splinting) they may become painful or enlarged. For example, nodules on the ulnar border of the forearm may be affected by weight bearing on the forearms. Nodules at the lateral aspects of the digits may be affected by pinch activities.

TENDON

Tenosynovitis is inflammation of the synovial tendon sheath lining. Occurring in both the extrinsic flexors and extensors, tenosynovitis creates swelling that impairs tendon glide. Prolonged tenosynovitis may result in tendon adherence or destruction of tendon tissue by synovial invasion or ischemia. Tendons are subjected to additional mechanical injury and are at high risk for rupture when they must move over bony prominence such as the distal ulna or Lister's tubercle. The most common tendon ruptures associated with RA involve the extensor tendons of the ring and small fingers, the extensor pollicis longus, and the flexor pollicis longus.[6]

Acute tenosynovitis is indicated by swelling, tenderness, and pain on active motion. Tendons are palpated at rest and with active motion. Swelling, crepitation, and tendon nodules are noted. "Triggering," which is a snapping or actual locking of the tendon with active motion, may also be present.

MUSCLE

Muscle weakness can result from the rheumatoid pathology directly involving the intrinsic and extrinsic muscle tissue. Muscle weakness can also occur as a result of disuse when pain and joint limitations restrict function for a prolonged period of time.

Muscle wasting may produce visible atrophy. Strength is measured in several ways: dynamometer, pinch meter, and manual muscle testing. Adapted methods for measuring very weak or painful grip and pinch include use of an adapter sphygmomanometer or gauges that have soft rubber bulbs.[5]

Both ROM and strength measures may vary considerably from day to day or at different times of the day. Therefore, recording the circumstances under which testing was performed including the presence, location, and description of pain; the time of day; presence of stiffness or fatigue; and the time, type, and dosage of medications is useful.

NERVE

Loss of muscle function, weakness, and atrophy can also result from neuropathy. Peripheral neuropathy in rheumatoid disease is believed to be caused by arteritis and impairment of the neural blood supply.

Compressive neuropathies also occur. Tenosynovitis of the digital flexors may cause median nerve compression within the carpal tunnel. Flatt[6] estimated that one quarter of all patients with RA have carpal tunnel syndrome. Ulnar nerve compression at the wrist is less common but may occur when synovitis extends from the carpal canal. Compression of the posterior interosseous branch of the radial nerve may result from synovitis extending from the elbow joints.

Sensory testing is indicated when cursory examination suggests deficits. When sensory and/or motor deficits indicate cervical spine involvement, appropriate cervical evaluation and treatment should be initiated.

JOINT

The evaluation of joint deformity is based on an understanding of normal anatomy, the structural changes created by RA, and the effect of both internal and external forces acting on involved joints.

General Considerations

Synovitis. Localized enlargement of a joint or tendon area is an indication of synovitis. Synovitis within a joint is first apparent as the joint capsule distended with synovial fluid. As shown in Figure 13–1, in the finger, swelling is of the "fusiform" (spindle-shaped) type. Initially the area is soft and fluctuant, or boggy. If the inflammation is prolonged, the fluid thickens. The synovial tissue proliferates. Pannus grows within the joint space and the area feels firmer. In the late stages, the synovium may herniate the joint capsule and appear as a firm mass. Boggy synovitis indicates the need for rest splinting. Swollen joints that feel firmer indicate the need for rest splinting alternated with cautious exercise to maintain mobility.

Joint Integrity. Whereas PROM measurements quantitate motion, gentle palpation and joint mobilization are used to evaluate joint integrity. With RA, the joint may be fused owing to fibrous or bony ankylosis, or passive motion may be decreased because of secondary joint contractures. Excessive joint motion may be present because the

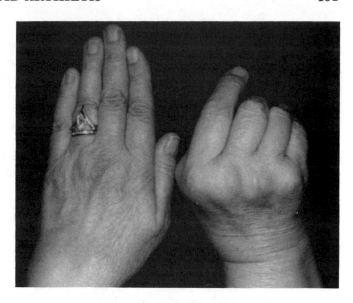

FIGURE 13–1. Synovitis present at MCP joints of the right hand.

capsule and ligaments have become lax. Such a joint would be described as unstable, indicating that the joint's ROM goes beyond its normal limits. As the disease progresses, unstable joints may become subluxed or dislocated. When a joint is subluxed, the articular surfaces are still in contact but the joint surfaces are no longer in their normal alignment. In the evaluation it should be noted whether a subluxed joint can be manually reduced to its normal anatomic position. When a joint is dislocated, the articular surfaces of the joint are no longer in contact.

Crepitus. Crepitus is a palpable or audible grating or grinding sensation that occurs with motion. Crepitus is sometimes painful. The location of the crepitus should be identified. At a joint, crepitus may indicate a partial destruction of the articular surface. Along the tendon, crepitus indicates tenosynovitis. The crepitus is described as palpable or audible, constant or intermittent, and occurring with active or passive motion.

Active Versus Passive Motion. AROM measurements are compared with PROM measurements. In the presence of good passive range, diminished active motion may indicate decreased tendon gliding (i.e., trigger finger) or actual tendon rupture. In some cases the tendon may be displaced or overstretched, as occurs with the ulnar displacement of the extensor tendons at the MP joints. Decreased active motion may also be a sign of muscle weakness or motor nerve compression.

Specific Joint Evaluation

Wrist. Flatt[6] states that 75% of patients with rheumatic disease show involvement at the wrist. With persistent rheumatoid disease this joint will become involved bilaterally in 95% of patients.[9] Instability of the radioulnar joint and associated "ulnar head syndrome" are the most commonly observed wrist deformities.[6,10] Radial deviation deformity at the wrist contributes to ulnar deviation at the metacarpophalangeal (MP) joints, commonly termed the "zigzag effect."

The normal wrist positions the hand for function. The position of the hand in relationship to the forearm affects the balance of tension of extrinsic hand muscles, which is determined by their relative lengths. The power and direction of forces in the digits is influenced by wrist position. Slight extension of the wrist allows stronger grasp.

Five to 10° of ulnar deviation at the wrist allows the index finger to rest in line with the radius for function.

When the wrist is examined the presence of acute inflammation must be determined. The therapist observes and palpates the wrist, noting the presence of warmth, tenderness, and synovial swelling. Both intra-articular synovitis and tenosynovitis of flexor and extensor tendons produce swelling at the wrist. Strong dorsal and palmar ligaments of the wrist contain and conceal early intra-articular synovitis. Palpable swelling may be noted near the radial and ulnar styloid processes where the wrist joint capsule is thinner. More diffuse swelling bulging distal to the extensor retinaculum is one sign of tenosynovitis of the extensor digitorum communis. Localized swelling at the volar aspect of the wrist is a sign of tenosynovitis of the digital flexors. Pain at the extremes of ROM and diminished grip strength secondary to wrist pain also indicate inflammation of joints and tendons at the wrist.

Examination of the wrist then continues with evaluation of joint integrity and muscle-tendon function. With prolonged synovitis, instability or loss of motion may result at the intercarpal, radiocarpal, and radioulnar joints. Table 13–3 outlines problems that are initiated by synovitis at the wrist, the changes occurring at the involved joints, and their effect on adjacent joints.

The posture of the wrist both at rest and during power grip should be observed. Frequently the hand moves into radial deviation as unstable carpals shift ulnarly. The lateral stability of the wrist is tested by gentle passive mediolateral mobilization. Anteroposterior stability is also tested by gentle passive mobilization. Volar subluxation of the carpus is tested by resting the forearm in pronation and the wrist in neutral. If a hollow or step-off is felt at the dorsum of the wrist just distal to the radius, the wrist has subluxed volarly.

The most common wrist deformity, ulnar head syndrome, results from involvement of the extensor carpi ulnaris tendon and the triangular fibrocartilage complex. The ulnar head becomes dorsally prominent and unstable. Radioulnar joint stability is tested by supporting the radiocarpal joints with the forearm resting in pronation. With gentle passive mobilization, an unstable distal ulna shifts anterioposterior, resembling a piano key. The prominence of the distal ulna may appear exaggerated by a volar displacement of the ulnar-carpal bones.

Thumb. The thumb is the most mobile digit of the normal hand. Whereas the MP and interphalangeal (IP) joints move in flexion and extension, the unique anatomy of the carpometacarpal (CMC) joint provides mobility as well as stability in all planes of motion. Opposition and rotation allow dexterous pad-to-pad pinch. Thumb deformities associated with RA occur in patterns of longitudinal collapse (i.e., boutonnière deformity) and in patterns of lateral instability.

Each joint of the thumb is examined for signs of acute inflammation. The CMC joint is palpated volarly and at the dorsal radial aspect to evaluate warmth, tenderness, and swelling. CMC joint pain and crepitus are tested by passive circumduction of the thumb while axial compression is applied. Ligamentous stability of the CMC joint is tested by applying axial compression while the thumb is held in adduction. The base of the metacarpal can be felt to move radially if stability has been compromised.

The MP and IP joints are palpated mediolaterally and anterioposteriorly. Circumferential measures at the MP and IP joints may be recorded. The MP joint is positioned in full flexion to test joint stability. Intact collateral ligaments are taut in this position and should limit radial and ulnar deviation. Lateral motion of the IP joint should be limited in both flexion and extension.

TABLE 13-3 Wrist—Characteristic Deformities

Joints	Problem Initiated by Synovitis	Changes at Involved Joint(s)	Effect on Forces Acting on Other Joints
Intercarpal joints	Loss of ligament support Erosion of bone	Loss of capacity of carpals to accommodate changes in hand position and therefore decreased ROM Instability and pain Dislocation of carpals (scaphoid and lunate)	Longitudinal arch is disturbed Mobility of 4th and 5th metacarpals is decreased Radiocarpal joint changes
Radiocarpal joint	Loss of ligament support Erosion of bone	Fibrosis and/or fusion Ulnar shifts of carpus *or* Palmar subluxation and radial rotation of the carpals	Radial deviation of the wrist and metacarpals with ulnar deviation of MPs Zigzag collapse at more distal joints; inefficient tendon force
Distal radioulnar joint	Loss of ligament support Erosion of bone Weakening and/or displacement of tendon	Ulnar head syndrome Dorsal prominence and instability of ulnar head Loss of supination, pronation, and dorsiflexion Increased flexion of 4th and 5th metacarpals ECU tendon displaced to act as wrist flexor and ulnar deviator	Sometimes rupture of extensor tendons of digits 3, 4, and 5 Wrist instability limits spread of distal arch for grasp

The posture of the rheumatoid thumb is observed at rest as well as during tip and lateral pinch. The most common thumb deformity resembles the boutonnière (Fig. 13-2). MP joint synovitis causes the dorsal capsule to become lax. The extensor pollicis longus (EPL) moves ulnarly. The extensor pollicis brevis insertion is compromised and, in extreme cases, completely ruptured. When the proximal phalanx subluxes volarly, the dislocated EPL and intrinsics move the IP joint into hyperextension. Initially the joint will remain passively flexible, but with time the deformity may become fixed.

Synovitis at the CMC joint is a factor in other thumb deformities. For example, dorsal radial subluxation of the head of the first metacarpal may reduce the first web space. When the first metacarpal does rest in flexion, adduction, and supination, compensatory MP joint hyperextension and IP joint flexion occur, resembling a swan neck posture. If there is lateral instability of the MP joint secondary to synovitis, the ulnar collateral ligament of the MP may be further injured in pinch activities. A deformity of

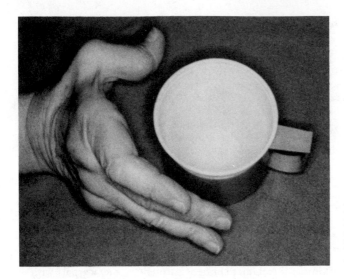

FIGURE 13–2. Boutonnière deformity of the thumb with MCP joint flexion and IP joint hyperextension limits the patient's ability to grasp and pinch.

adduction with radial deviation at the MP joint may result. CMC joint subluxation with the boutonnière type deformity previously described also occurs but is less common.[11,12]

Metacarpophalangeal Joints. The normal anatomy of the MP joint influences the changes that occur with pathology. The shape of the joint surfaces at the MP joint allows some rotation, abduction, and adduction. The metacarpal heads are characterized by an ulnar slope, which is especially evident at the second and third metacarpals. The phalanges rest in slight ulnar deviation and tend to shift in an ulnar direction during flexion.

The collateral ligaments at the MP joint normally are lax in extension, allowing lateral motion. Unequal length of the radial and ulnar collateral ligaments allows greater ulnar deviation. Differences in the insertions of the radial and ulnar intrinsic muscles into the extensor mechanism also favor ulnar deviation in the normal hand.

The flexor tendon is restrained at the MP joint by a retinacular system that forms a fibrous sling. In the normal hand, there is an ulnar bend in the flexor tendon at the MP joint, which places greater stress on the ulnar side. The force required on the flexor tendon during tip pinch is estimated to be six times the pinching force at the fingertip. With the MP flexed at 30°, the force placed on the volar portion of the ligament is approximately three times that of the pinch force; the force toward ulnar deviation, approximately twice as great.[13]

At the MP joints, ulnar deviation and volar subluxation or dislocation are the most common deformities. (Table 13–4 lists the common deformities; Fig. 13–3 illustrates several.) Inflammation weakens the supporting structures that normally resist ulnar deviating forces. Displacement of the extensor and/or flexor tendons and abnormal intrinsic muscle tone increase the force toward ulnar deviation. When there is destruction or lengthening of the collateral ligaments, flexion forces of the intrinsic muscles as well as the extrinsic flexors cause volar subluxation and later dislocation at the MP joint.

The evaluation begins by observing and palpating the MP joints for synovitis. To test for volar subluxation, the proximal phalanx is held in a neutral position. The dorsal and volar surfaces are palpated, starting distal to the MP joint and moving proximally. A step-off indicates subluxation. To test collateral ligament stability, the proximal phalanx

TABLE 13–4 Fingers — Characteristic Deformities

Characteristic Deformities	Changes at Involved Joints	Collapse pattern
Ulnar deviation	MP joint capsule(s) become lax Collateral ligaments become lax Extensor and flexor tendons move ulnar to MP joint axis (increased by radial deviation of the wrist) Intrinsic muscles become tight	Instability and ulnar deviation of digits Volar subluxation, later dislocation at MPs
Boutonnière	PIP joint capsule becomes lax Central extensor tendon is stretched Lateral bands move volar to PIP joint axis Oblique retinacular ligaments shorten	MP hyperextension PIP flexion DIP hyperextension
Swan neck	Flexor tenosynovitis PIP joint capsule, volar, plate, and accessory collateral ligaments become lax Lateral bands move dorsal to PIP joint axis Oblique retinacular ligaments lengthen	Increased MP flexion PIP hyperextension DIP flexion
Mallet	DIP joint capsule becomes lax Extensor tendon insertion is stretched or ruptured	DIP flexion

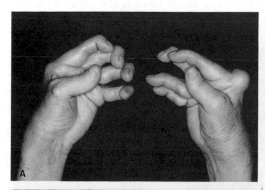
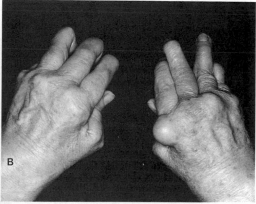
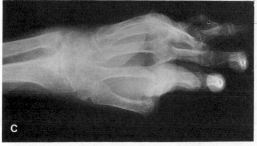

FIGURE 13–3. *A* and *B*, Severe rheumatoid arthritis with MCP joint subluxation, mallet deformities of the left DIP joints, swan neck deformities of the right ring and little fingers, and boutonnière deformities of the thumb. *C*, Roentgenogram confirms the MCP joint destruction and subluxation.

is held in full flexion, while gentle radial and ulnar stress is applied. Pain and lateral motion are noted.

The evaluation should also test for intrinsic tightness, which is frequently a contributing factor to the formation of volar subluxation and dislocation deformities of the MP joint (see Chapter 3). If volar subluxation limits MP extension it may not be possible to test for intrinsic tightness. Similarly, if proximal interphalangeal (PIP) flexion is limited by joint or tendon problems, intrinsic testing may not be possible.

Interphalangeal Joints. Synovitis at the PIP and distal interphalangeal (DIP) joints is also evaluated by observation and palpation. When the joint capsule is distended by synovial fluid, a fusiform, or spindle shape, is apparent. Firmer asymmetrical swelling indicates involvement beyond the joint capsule.

Joint stability is tested by gentle mobilization, in both an anteroposterior and a lateral direction, as the joint is held in extension. The IP joints differ from the MP joints in that lateral motion does not normally occur. Collateral ligaments provide lateral stability during flexion and extension. Radial and ulnar deviation can result when synovitis damages joint surfaces and supporting structures. However, flexion and extension collapse deformities are more common. These collapse deformities include the boutonnière deformity (PIP flexion with DIP hyperextension) and the swan neck deformity (PIP hyperextension with DIP flexion) (Table 13–4).

Boutonnière Deformity. The boutonnière deformity occurs when synovitis weakens the extrinsic extensor at the PIP joint and the fibers that secure the lateral bands. The lateral bands move volar to the axis of the joint so that, instead of extending the PIP joint, they become PIP joint flexors. The name "boutonnière" refers to the resemblance of the lateral bands to a buttonhole, as the PIP pushes upward and increases their separation. The force of the lateral bands increase at their insertion, resulting in hyperextension at the DIP joint (Fig. 13–4).

Swan Neck Deformity. The swan neck deformity most frequently begins as synovitis of the flexor sheaths and limits PIP flexion.[10] The flexor force is therefore increased

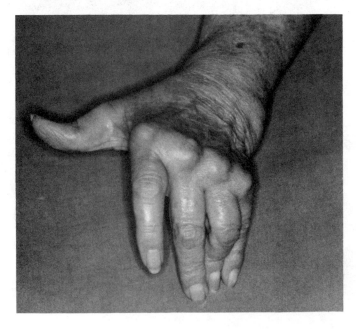

FIGURE 13–4. Boutonnière deformity of the ring finger with MCP joint flexion and DIP joint hyperextension. MCP volar subluxation and ulnar deviation are also shown.

at the MP joint. Intrinsic muscle contraction, lacking the balancing flexion force, extends the PIP joint. Synovitis weakens the supporting structures at the PIP joint. The lateral bands move dorsal to the axis of the joint, further aiding hyperextension at the PIP joint with flexion at the DIP joint.

The development of the swan neck deformity may also be initiated by synovitis at the PIP causing rupture of the flexor digitorum superficialis, or synovitis at the DIP joint causing lengthening or rupture of the insertion of the extensor digitorum communis.

Mallet Finger. Lack of DIP extension due to lengthening or rupture of the insertion of the terminal extensor tendon without PIP joint deformity is called mallet finger.

Mutilans Deformity. Mutilans deformity, also called opera glass hand, refers to severe joint destruction with resorption of articular bone. With loss of bone length, tendon function becomes ineffective and the joints become unstable and floppy.

Functional Assessment

The ultimate goal of arthritis treatment is to maintain or improve function in activities of daily living (ADLs), whether the treatment approach is medical, rehabilitative, surgical, or psychosocial. Functional assessment of the rheumatoid hand may be thought of as a description of the use of the hand in ADLs. Objective testing provides one part of this description. The subjective findings and the clinical judgment of the therapist, which are difficult to quantify, are equally valuable.

For example, Phillips provided a guideline that 20 lb of grip and 5 to 7 lb of pinch strength are necessary for most ADLs.[7] However, many individuals with arthritis can maintain their independence despite even more limited prehension strength. Over time these people develop skilled substitution patterns. Although objective measures of grip and pinch strength are important, the therapist must analyze the adaptive patterns of hand use before reconstructive surgery to ensure that function is not compromised.

Rancho Los Amigos Hospital's "Arthritis Hand Assessment"[8] offers a helpful guideline for functional assessment of the patient with RA. The assessment form includes a checklist for observations of selected tasks, grip and pinch measurements, timed writing, skin care, as well as the patient's ratings of pain, cosmesis, and function.

The status of the proximal upper extremity joints as well as the lower extremity joints must be considered in functional assessment. Hand placement as well as prehension and dexterity determine the person's ability to use the hand. Lower extremity limitations that cause difficulty in rising from a seated position or in ambulation affect the weight-bearing demands placed on the upper extremities.

TREATMENT

The general goals of conservative management of the rheumatoid hand are to alleviate inflammation and pain, maintain the stability and mobility of joints by preserving articular and periarticular structures, and maintain or improve muscle-tendon function and balanced patterns of motion. Synovitis, the inflammation of joint and/or tendon linings, which results in the secondary changes of articular structures including articular cartilage, bone, joint capsule, ligaments, and tendons. As a result, the underlying principle in the management of the rheumatoid hand is to control inflammation. In the natural course of this systemic disease, periods of exacerbation and remission occur.

TABLE 13–5 Progression of Symptoms

1. Acute inflammation with increased blood flow and increased production of synovial fluid
2. Proliferation of synovial tissue and subsequent formation of pannus
3. Consolidation of synovial fluid and the formation of fibrinous adhesions
4. Structural changes that create deformities

Acute inflammation localized at a particular joint may or may not recur during an active phase of the disease. When planning a treatment program, one must constantly reevaluate the patient, monitoring the progression of synovitis (Table 13–5) and subsequent articular changes, and alter the treatment program accordingly.

The treatment techniques to be discussed include modalities, splinting, exercise, and joint protection. In the presence of acute synovitis, priorities include modalities that reduce pain and help control inflammation, including local rest and joint protection. As the symptoms progress, preservation and/or restoration of motion as well as compensation for the mechanical changes affecting the joints become appropriate. During this later phase, the program incorporates modalities such as thermal agents, therapeutic exercise, splinting, and continued joint protection.

Patients with RA may be referred for care of the hand early or late in the progression of their disease. The ideal situation is for the patient to be referred early so that problems can be identified and therapy can begin to decrease pain, control inflammation, and reduce the mechanical injury to affected joint structures. Preoperative and postoperative therapy is essential for achieving the best possible functional results from complex reconstructive surgeries and salvage procedures.

Modalities

Heat provides comfort and reduces muscle spasm. Superficial heat modalities including moist heat packs, paraffin, and electric heating pads or mitts are convenient for home use. Cold also provides temporary comfort, relieving pain and muscle spasm. Some patients prefer home use of ice packs and cold compresses over use of heat. As a modality to control discomfort, the choice of superficial heat or cold is made according to the patient's preference. However, when a joint is hot and swollen, heat application may increase symptoms whereas application of cold or electrical stimulation (or both) may be more effective in reducing pain and inflammation.[14,15]

In a summary of studies relevant to the use of heat and cold, Banwell[14] and Michlovitz[15] indicated that neither heat nor cold modalities have been shown to affect the basic joint pathology or provide long-term benefit. Heat is believed to aid in stretching exercises by relaxing muscle spasms and increasing the elasticity of ligamentous structures. Deep heat modalities—ultrasound and diathermy—have been shown to increase intra-articular temperatures.[14] Superficial heat modalities are preferred in the treatment of RA because of their relative safety and because they are economical for home use.

Electrical stimulation using conventional transcutaneous nerve stimulation is useful to some patients for pain control.[16] Biofeedback aids pain control through muscle relaxation and can be helpful in muscle reeducation. Electrical stimulation done to achieve muscle contraction for strengthening or muscle reeducation involves risks of overloading fragile joints and tendons. The result can be increased inflammation or tissue damage.

When selecting modalities, the therapist should keep in mind that RA is a chronic disease. Modalities selected should take into consideration discharge plans, long term use and home program needs.

Splinting

With RA, controlling inflammation is the first priority. Local rest provided by static splinting is beneficial and reduces further trauma to the involved area(s). Static splints do *not* prevent deformity when the disease is progressive but provide support and protection to involved joints. Splints also aid in alleviating pain that occurs with motion and therefore assist function. Table 13–6 lists the indications and provides brief descriptions of the static splints frequently useful for RA patients.

There are a number of precautions that should be considered when splinting the rheumatoid hand. In selecting the splint to be used, one should think in terms of joint systems. For example, immobilizing one joint increases stress at adjacent joints. For patients whose skin show atrophic changes, extreme care must be taken to avoid pressure points or shearing forces.

An important consideration is that the splint may be needed for long-term care. In these cases, splint materials and straps are selected that are adjustable and can accommodate changes in swelling and position.

When dynamic splints are used, they should provide gentle, prolonged, passive stretch. Application of excessive force can increase inflammation or cause mechanical injury to fragile tissues. Dynamic splints are used selectively and cautiously to reduce joint contractures and to control motion following surgery. Dynamic splinting is not appropriate during acute inflammation.

Exercise

The goals of an exercise program are to maintain and/or increase strength and endurance, as well as passive and active motion. Repetitive or resistive motion can aggravate synovitis of joints and tendon sheaths. Therefore, caution must be used to balance local rest and active exercise in order to control inflammation.

Progressive resistive exercise is contraindicated when inflammation is present. When joint changes have altered the direction of forces exerted by muscles, the exercise can produce deforming forces and be counterproductive. For example, repetitive and forceful pinch and grip exercises are contraindicated when there is MP joint involvement because of the role of flexor forces in contributing to the ulnar deviation deformity.[13] Atrophy resulting from pathology of the muscle tissue in RA cannot be reversed by resistive exercise. In fact, resistance may be traumatic and accelerate muscle tissue destruction and scarring.[6] Active, nonresistive, or light resistive exercise is useful in maintaining muscle strength. If atrophy is a result of disuse, some gains in muscle bulk and strength will be seen.

Isometric exercises are important in arthritis care because they can be performed with the joints supported in proper alignment and, therefore, with less pain and joint stress. Isometric exercise is especially useful in providing motion to intrinsic muscles.[17]

TABLE 13–6 Static Splints

Splint	Indication(s)	Description
Full hand resting splint	Acute inflammation at multiple joints	Volar splint fits over distal two thirds of forearm and extends to fingertips; thumb C-bar optional Generally wrist is positioned a 5° to 10° ulnar deviation, at neutral or slight extension MPs rest at 0° deviation in slight flexion, usually 30°. PIPs rest at slight flexion; if C-bar used, thumb rests in abduction
Volar wrist or gauntlet	Wrist inflammation, grip weakness secondary to pain, carpal tunnel syndrome (used with caution if inflammation or instability is present at the MPs)	Fits volar to distal two thirds of forearm and extends proximal to the distal palmar crease so that full MP flexion is possible; area cut out at the thenar eminence allows full thumb opposition Gauntlet is fit as volar wrist splint but extends dorsaly around the full circumference of the UE; area over the ulnar head is relieved to avoid pressure area; gauntlet provides more rigid fixation when radioulnar joint is unstable
Metacarpal-phalangeal support	Inflammation and/or instability at MPs joints	Generally the wrist is positioned at 5° to 10° ulnar deviation; at neutral or slight extension; fits volar to metacarpal heads (may or may not have individual finger separators that provide support on the ulnar aspect of the proximal phalanges); may be palmar piece that leaves wrist free or may extend past wrist Support MPs in extension or slight flexion and 0° deviation; PIP flexion in this splint stretches tight intrinsics
Ulnar drift positioning splint	Ulnar drift deformity	Cuff or hinged splint fit at the MPs to block ulnar deviation; is fit to aid function

TABLE 13–6 (*continued*)

Splint	Indication(s)	Description
Thumb spica	Inflammation or instability at thumb CMC joint	Fits over radial aspect of wrist and extends proximal to thumb IP; thumb positioned in abduction; splint immobilizes wrist, CMC, and MP joints Used to alleviate pain; short opponens may be used, but generally wrist motion must be restricted to alleviate CMC pain
Figure-eight splint	Flexible swan neck deformity	Fits volar to PIP and dorsal to proximal and middle phalanges; limits motion to −20 or −30 extension; allows full PIP flexion; may also be fit at thumb IP and MP
Mallet splint	DIP extension lag, DIP lateral instability	Fits volar or dorsal to DIP joint; maintains distal joint extension and lateral stability
PIP extension splint	Boutonnière	Fits volar to PIP or circumferentially; maintains maximum PIP extension; allows full MP and DIP motion

Wickersham and Schweidler[18] recommend a combination of AROM and isometric exercises to maintain muscle strength and improve ROM. They cite studies that show that three to four daily repetitions of moving a joint through its ROM will usually maintain that ROM and that a single daily brief, maximal, isometric contraction lasting from 1 to 10 seconds is sufficient to stimulate an increase in static muscle strength.

Understanding the characteristic patterns of deformity previously described aids in identifying the muscle tendon functions most likely to be affected by RA. Motions that are especially important to maintain in early RA include supination, wrist extension (with balance of radial and ulnar extensors), extension at the MP joints by the extensor digitorum communis, radial deviation of the fingers by the intrinsics, thumb IP flexion, as well as independent flexor digitorum superficialis and profundus function. Maintaining intrinsic muscle length with intrinsic stretching exercises should also be initiated early in the rheumatoid process.

When RA has progressed to the extent that joint integrity has been impaired and muscle-tendon function compromised, patterns of motion are analyzed and exercises selected with caution to minimize joint stress and restore balance. Exercise cannot correct deformities that result from structural changes.

Objective measurements of swelling, joint range, and strength are necessary to monitor an exercise program. Aggressive stretching of the delicate structures of the hand is destructive. PROM exercises, if used at all, must be gentle. Gentle, active-assistive exercise is preferable to PROM exercise. The joint protection principle, "Respect pain," is especially important in exercise. Increased pain or discomfort that lasts longer than 1 hour after exercise indicates that the exercise has been too stressful.[5]

Joint Protection

Joint protection is the process of reducing internal and external stress on the joints during functional activity. Observing inflammation and body mechanics during activity and understanding the mechanical changes that occur in the involved joints guide decision making. Changes in tools or methods, or both, are used to redistribute the forces according to the strength or vulnerability of the joints. Published data suggest that forces applied during activity can produce deformity.[5,13,19-21] However, the value of joint protection in altering deformity when there is progressive tissue destruction by the disease is not proven. Advising patients that practicing joint protection techniques will prevent deformity is not appropriate. The practice of joint protection techniques is generally accepted and is believed to reduce internal and external joint stress, assist in managing inflammation, increase comfort in activities, and slow the progression of the deformity.[5,19-21] Cordery[19] described the principles of joint protection listed in Table 13-7.

Joint protection techniques include the reduction of forces, elimination of activity, rest, work simplification, and energy conservation.[5,19-21] Table 13-8 discusses methods of joint protection as they could be applied to two common activities.

For the individual, practice of joint protection becomes a problem-solving process. First, patients must be able to identify stressful activities. Although the elimination of all joint stress would be impossible and certainly undesirable, protecting inflamed or unstable joints is a priority. Activities that are repetitive and those that involve greater weight or force are the ones most important to consider. A choice must be made to either eliminate or change the activity (altering method or equipment). The therapist can provide instruction, guidance, and supervised practice. The patient must learn to identify stressful activities and choose the appropriate changes.

Many helpful resources exist for patient education (see the chapter appendix). Self-help courses offered by local Arthritis Foundation chapters reinforce clinic teaching.

SURGERY

Upper extremity surgery is a rapidly growing and changing area of arthritis care. Factors in the dramatic progress in upper extremity rehabilitation include improvements in the techniques and materials available and the development of hand surgery and hand therapy as specialty areas.

TABLE 13-7 Joint Protection Principles

1. Maintain muscle strength and joint ROM.
2. Avoid positions of deformity.
3. Use the strongest joints available for the job.
4. Use each joint in its most stable anatomic and functional plane.
5. Avoid holding joints or using muscles in one position for any undue length of time.
6. Avoid any activity that cannot be stopped immediately if it proves beyond the power of the patient to complete the task.
7. Respect pain.

TABLE 13–8 Examples of Applications of the Principles of Joint Protection

| | | | Alternatives | | | |
| | | | Reduce the Force | | | |
Activity	Problem	Avoid Weight	Change Method	Use Equipment	Eliminate Activity	Rest Pacing	Conserve Energy
Pouring milk from carton to glass	Synovitis at MP joints; tenosynovitis of flexor tendons or fingers; weak grip and pain	Buy milk in small cartons. Pour into smaller containers after purchase.	Use two hands.	Plastic handles; tiltboard for support.	Another person performs task; use refrigerator container with spigot	—	Wheeled cart for moving carton to counter
Writing	Synovitis at MP joints; tenosynovitis of flexor tendons or fingers; weak grip and pain	Reduce pinch force on pen.	Use tripod pinch; shorthand or notehand; type	Enlarged barrel on pen; Felt-tip pen; low-friction tip pen; typewriter	Another person performs task; taperecorder; dictation	Frequent brief rest periods; shorter periods of writing	—

Surgery is a therapeutic tool to be used in addition to medication and nonoperative management of arthritis. Although older texts refer to surgery as a "last resort" indicated to salvage function after advanced joint destruction, the current practice of hand surgery includes procedures that are useful in the earlier stages of the disease. In fact, delaying evaluation for surgery until late-stage deformity may allow joint destruction so extensive that results for reconstructive surgery are compromised. Procedures may be categorized as preventive, reparative, or reconstructive. In practice, surgery provides some combination of delay, repair, and/or correction of deformity. The general goals of surgery are to prevent or delay further joint destruction, relieve pain, increase function, and improve cosmesis. Procedures that are useful in RA are listed in Table 13–9.

There are procedures, such as distal ulna resection, for which the postoperative care is simple and usually performed independently by the patient. Other procedures, such as MP joint implant arthroplasties[22–25] require careful rehabilitation and close communication among surgeon, patient, and therapist. The therapist must have direct guidance by the surgeon. In a general hospital or clinic setting, this may require that the therapist initiate contact with the surgeon to understand clearly the procedures performed, the precautions, and the goals of treatment.

The previously mentioned manual published by Rancho Los Amigos[8] is available as a guide for treatment following surgery. However, it must be emphasized that, as stated in the introduction to that manual:

TABLE 13–9 RA Surgeries

Wrist	Synovectomy
	Nerve decompression
	Resection of distal ulna
	Implant resection arthroplasty
	Arthrodesis
Extensor tendons	Tenosynovectomy
	Tendon repair
	Tendon transfer (i.e., extensor indicis proprius to extensor digitorum communis)
	Tendon relocation (i.e., centering extensor digitorum communis at MPs)
	Tendon graft
Flexor tendons	Tenosynovectomy
	Carpal tunnel, digital tendon sheath release
	Tendon repair
	Tendon graft
MPs	Synovectomy (with reconstruction of ligaments, capsule, intrinsic transfer)
	Implant resection arthroplasty (with tendon relocation, capsule and ligament repair, intrinsic transfer)
IPs	Synovectomy
	Intrinsic release
	Ligament reconstruction, release
	Implant resection arthroplasty
	Arthrodesis
Thumb	Synovectomy
	Contracture release
	Capsulodesis
	Implant arthroplasty
	Interpositional arthroplasty (CMC)
	Arthrodesis

. . . this document is to be used only as a guide, not an established routine that is followed in every surgical case. Since no two patients are alike, each case needs to be discussed with the surgeon in order that exception to the routine regimen can be explained to and understood by the therapist managing the postoperative occupational therapy care.

CLINICAL DECISION MAKING: CASE STUDY

Sally L. is a 34-year-old righthanded mother of two, who has had RA since age 27. Onset of her disease was sudden with multiple joints involved. The disease progression has been intermittent. At present, symptoms are controlled with nonsteroidal anti-inflammatory medications.

MEDICAL AND SOCIAL HISTORY

She was referred to her hand surgeon for evaluation by her rheumatologist at her own request. Her concerns were wrist pain and loss of grip strength. Acute synovitis was noted at the wrist, signs of chronic inflammation at the MPs, and flexor tendons. Roentgenography revealed osteoporosis but no subchondral bone destruction. Surgery was not indicated at this time. She was referred to therapy by the surgeon for instruction in a home program of exercise, splinting, and joint protection instruction.

Sally indicated that she is a homemaker and that 18 months ago she and her husband became parents of two foster children, ages 7 and 9. She had previously worked as a legal secretary but did not wish to resume employment outside the home. She grew roses and belonged to a gardening club.

She described past episodes of extreme fatigue with severe pain in her knees, feet, shoulders, wrists, and hands. She stated that symptoms were much improved at present, but her knee pain, wrist pain, and limited grip strength continued to limit her activities. She was concerned by changes in the appearance of her hands and wished to prevent deformities. She stated that she had both physical and occupational therapy as a hospital inpatient at the onset of her disease, but none recently. She discarded her full resting splints when they no longer fit comfortably. She walked without ambulation aids and was able to sit and rise from a chair without upper extremity assistance.

PHYSICAL ASSESSMENT

Physical assessment of her hands revealed swelling at MP joints and along the flexor tendons in the palms bilaterally. These areas were not warm or tender. Crepitus was palpable along flexor tendons. Intrinsic tightness was noted.

On the right, passive finger flexion exceeded active flexion. At the MPs, collateral ligaments were lax. At the wrist, swelling could be palpated distal to the radial and ulnar styloid processes. Supination and wrist extension were limited actively and passively. The distal ulna was prominent but not lax. She described pain at the wrist at extremes of motion and during grip. No limitations were noted in elbow flexion and extension or shoulder motion.

On the left, findings were the same, with two exceptions. Passive and active finger flexion were equal. Additionally, she described the left wrist as less painful than the right.

Measures were recorded, including circumference measures for wrist and digits, AROM and PROM, Jamar dynamometer tests of grip strength, and B & L pinch gauge measures of tip, lateral, and three-point pinch strength.

TREATMENT

Treatment goals were discussed with Sally including the following:

1. Control of inflammation—symptoms indicated acute synovitis at the wrist; a later phase of inflammation at MPs and flexor tendon sheaths
2. Maintenance of joint integrity at involved wrist and MP joints
3. Increase in AROM of the fingers on the right and in tendon gliding bilaterally

To control inflammation, bilateral rest splints were provided. Because of involvement at the MPs and intrinsic tightness, splints immobilized both MP and wrist joints. IPs were left free, allowing active flexion for tendon glide and intrinsic stretching. She was advised to wear these at night and during the day as much as her activities would reasonably allow at present. The practical problems in doing this were acknowledged.

Basic concepts of joint protection were introduced. She was advised to prepare a list of activities that were particularly difficult or uncomfortable for her hands and wrists. This list would be used in later treatment sessions for discussion and practice of joint protection principles.

Moist heat was applied to increase comfort and reduce muscle spasm before exercise. She was instructed in doing this at home and was cautioned to discontinue if the use of heat caused any increase in discomfort. She then practiced a home program of gentle active exercises selected to improve tendon gliding and active finger flexion including blocking to isolate flexor digitorum superficialis and profundus tendons and intrinsic stretching. She was advised to limit each exercise to five slow, gentle repetitions and to do this in four brief exercise periods during the day.

In 2 weeks, the patient's wrist comfort was significantly improved bilaterally. There was minimal change at the MPs. Active and passive finger flexion was increased on the right. At this time, gentle active exercises to improve wrist extension and supination were added to the home program. Isometric exercises for strengthening both intrinsic and extrinsic muscles were also added.

The emphasis of treatment at this time shifted to discussion and practice of joint protection methods. Using her list of difficult activities, alternate methods and adaptive equipment were introduced. She attended a group session on joint protection in the clinic and was encouraged to participate in the Arthritis Foundation's self-help classes.

At 1 month, she demonstrated full finger flexion. Wrist motion was increased. She had chosen to make significant changes in her home activities, reducing the demands for powerful and repetitive grip. She described discomfort at the wrist as intermittent and of short duration. As a result, grip strength was increased. She was advised to continue her home program of gentle ROM exercises. She was advised to continue using her resting splints when discomfort indicated increased inflammation.

Regular treatment was discontinued. Recheck was scheduled in 2 months. She was encouraged to phone for an earlier appointment as needed. Her history of recurrent flareups involving multiple joints suggests that this is likely to occur. Periodic reassessment is indicated.

SUMMARY

Rheumatoid arthritis is the cause of complex hand problems that must be identified and set in order of priority. Treatment plans are based on systematic evaluation and periodic reassessment of inflammation, joint integrity, and muscle-tendon function. When there is progressive destruction of tissues by active disease, therapy will not prevent or reverse deformities.

REFERENCES

1. Arnett, FC (ed): Bulletin on the Rheumatoid Diseases, Revised Criteria for the Classification of Rheumatoid Arthritis. Vol 38, No 5, 1989.
2. Schumacher, HR (ed): Primer on the Rheumatic Diseases, ed 9. Arthritis Foundation, Atlanta, 1988.
3. Fritz, W, Paxinos, J, and Gall, E: Rational use of new nonsteroidal anti-inflammatory drugs. Drug Therapy 1978.
4. Ferlic, DC, Smyth, CJ, and Clayton, ML: Medical considerations and management of rheumatoid arthritis. J Hand Surg. Vol 8 (5):85–86, 1983.
5. Melvin, J: Rheumatic Diseases—Occupational Therapy and Rehabilitation. FA Davis, Philadelphia, 1983.
6. Flatt, AE: Care of the Rheumatoid Hand. CV Mosby, St Louis, 1983.
7. Phillips, C: Hand therapy in early stages of rheumatoid arthritis. In Hunter, JM, et al (eds): Rehabilitation of the Hand. CV Mosby, St Louis, 1978.
8. The Professional Staff Association of the Rancho Los Amigos Hospital: Upper Extremity Surgeries for Patients with Arthritis, A Pre- and Post-Operative Treatment Guide. RLAH, Downey, CA, 1979.
9. Wilson, RL: Rheumatoid arthritis of the hand. Orthoped Clin North Am 17(2):315, 1986.
10. Swanson, AB: Pathomechanics of deformities in hand and wrist. In Hunter, JM, et al (eds): Rehabilitation of the Hand. CV Mosby, St Louis, 1990.
11. Nalebuff, EA: Diagnosis, classifications and management of rheumatoid thumb deformities. Bull Hosp Joint Dis 24:119, 1968.
12. Nalebuff, EA and Philips, CA: The rheumatoid thumb. In Hunter, JM, et al (eds): Rehabilitation of the Hand, ed 2. CV Mosby, St Louis, 1984.
13. Smith, EM, et al: Flexor forces and rheumatoid metacarpophalangeal deformity. JAMA 198(2):150–154, 1966.
14. Banwell, BF: Therapeutic heat and cold. In Riggs, GK and Gall, EP: Rheumatic Diseases, Rehabilitation and Management. Butterworth, Boston, 1984.
15. Michlovitz, S: The Use of Heat and Cold in the Management of Rheumatic Diseases. In Michlovitz, S (ed): Thermal Agents in Rehabilitation, ed 2. FA Davis, Philadelphia, 1986.
16. Mannheimer, JS, Lund, S, and Carlsson, C: The effect of transcutaneous electrical nerve stimulation on joint pain in patients with rheumatoid arthritis. Scand J Rheumatol 7:13–16, 1978.
17. McBain, KP, Galbraith, B, and Brady, F: Non-operative Management of Adult-Onset Rheumatoid Arthritis. The Arthritis Society, Vancouver, 1981.
18. Wickersham, B and Schweidler, H: Arthritis—Self Study Guide for Physical and Occupational Therapists. Southwest Arthritis Center, Tucson, 1983.
19. Cordery, JC: Joint protection—a responsibility of the occupational therapist. Am J Occup Ther 19:285–293, 1965.
20. Chamberlain, ME, Ellis, M, and Hughes, D: Joint protection. Clin Rheum Dis 10 (3):727–742, 1984.
21. Brattstrom, M: Principles of Joint Protection in Chronic Rheumatic Diseases. Lund, Sweden, Student Literature, 1973.
22. Carter, MS and Wilson, RL: Post Surgical Management in Rheumatoid Arthritis. In Hunter, JM, et al (eds): Rehabilitation of The Hand. CV Mosby, St Louis, 1978.

23. DeVore, G: Preoperative Assessment and Post Operative Therapy and Splinting in Rheumatoid Arthritis. In Hunter JM, et al (eds): Rehabilitation of the Hand. CV Mosby, St Louis, 1978.
24. Madden, JW, DeVore, G, and Aren, AJ. A rational postoperative management for metacarpophalangeal joint implant arthroplasty. J Hand Surg 5:358–366, 1977.
25. Swanson, AB, Swanson, GD, and Leonard, J: Postoperative Rehabilitation Program in Flexible Implant Arthroplasty of the Digits. In Hunter, JM, et al (eds): Rehabilitation of the Hand. ed 2., CV Mosby, St Louis, 1984.

APPENDIX: PATIENT EDUCATION RESOURCES

PUBLICATIONS

Arthritis Foundation, Atlanta: Taking Care: Protecting Your Joints and Saving Your Energy. December, 1985. AF Patient Services Dept, 1314 Spring St NW, Atlanta, GA 30309.

Arthritis Health Professions Association: Guide to Independent Living for People with Arthritis. Arthritis Foundation, Atlanta, GA, 1988.

Bingham, B: Cooking with Fragile Hands. Creative Cuisine, Inc, PO Box 518, Naples, FL 33939, 1985.

Brattstrom, M: Joint Protection and Rehabilitation in Chronic Rheumatic Disorders. Aspen Publishers, Inc, Rockville, MD, 1987.

Feinberg, J: Principles of Joint Protection and Work Simplification for Persons with Rheumatoid Arthritis. Indiana University Medical Center, Occupational Therapy Dept, Long Hospital, Room 399, 1100 W Michigan St, Indianapolis, IN 46223.

Furst, G, Gerber, L, and Smith, C: Rehabilitation Through Learning: Energy Conservation and Joint Protection—A Workbook for Persons with Rheumatoid Arthritis. US Dept of Health and Human Services, Public Health Service, National Institutes of Health, Bethesda, MD, 1984.

Haviland, N, Kamil-Miller, L, and Silva, S: A Workbook for Consumers with Rheumatoid Arthritis. American Occupational Therapy Association, 1978.

Klinger, J: Self-Help Manual for Patients with Arthritis. Arthritis Foundation, Atlanta, GA, 1980.

Lorig, K and Fries, J: Arthritis Helpbook. Addison-Wesley Publishing Co, Reading, MA, 1980.

Ocone, L and Thabault, G: Tools and Techniques for Easier Gardening. Gardens for All, Inc, 180 Flynn Ave, Berlington, VT 05401, 1984.

Watkins, R and Robinson, D: Joint Preservation Techniques for Patients with Rheumatoid Arthritis. Northwestern University—Rehabilitation Institute of Chicago, 345 E Superior St, Chicago, IL 60611, 1974.

VIDEOTAPES

Arthritis Foundation: Self Help with Robin May. Video One, Inc, 10304 S Dolfield Rd, Owings Mills, MD 21117.

Marx, H, Lumsden, R, and Miller, E: Arthritis: Best Use of the Hands—Rheumatoid Arthritis. Video Education Specialists, 1309 E Northern, Phoenix, AZ 85020, 1988.

CHAPTER 14

Cumulative Trauma

Patricia Baxter-Petralia, MS, OTR/L
Veronica Penney, OTR/L

Cumulative trauma disorders are a major cause of lost work time in hand-intensive industries. As a result, the rehabilitative management and prevention of these injuries has become increasingly important to the employer, as well as the injured employee. Statistics from the National Safety Council[1] indicate 90,000 hand injuries occurred in the workplace in 1989. Cumulative trauma, also referred to as repetitive trauma disorders, overuse syndrome, and repetitive strain injuries, is an inflammatory response to the overuse of anatomic structures. The disorder develops from repeated movements occurring over an extended period of time. Structures such as muscle, tendon, synovial sheath, and nerve may be affected, resulting in problems such as tendonitis, tenosynovitis, and nerve entrapment. Diagnoses frequently attributed to cumulative trauma injury include trigger finger, lateral epicondylitis, carpal tunnel syndrome, and de Quervain's disease.

The objectives of this chapter are to (1) explore the etiology of cumulative trauma disorders; (2) discuss the implications of wound healing in the management of cumulative trauma disorders; and (3) present the evaluation, conservative, and postsurgical management of three different cumulative trauma disorders—carpal tunnel syndrome, lateral epicondylitis, and de Quervain's disease.

ETIOLOGY OF CUMULATIVE TRAUMA

The etiology of cumulative trauma disorders varies. Factors such as repetition, force, mechanical stress, posture, vibration, and temperature extremes can be associated with the development of cumulative trauma. For example, work performed in sustained, unnatural postures such as wrist flexion, deviation, and hyperextension has been shown to be a risk factor for the development of cumulative trauma disorders.[2-4] Barnhart and Rosenstock[5] reported cases of carpal tunnel syndrome in grocery checkers who were required to perform repeated wrist flexion and extension while handling items and packing bags. Jobs requiring repetitive high-speed motions have been implicated in the etiology of cumulative trauma disorders.[6] Silverstein and colleagues[2] studied 574 workers exposed to varying amounts of repetitive motion and concluded that high-repetition jobs with assembly rates of 30 seconds per assembly positively correlated with hand and wrist cumulative trauma disorders. The combination of two or more factors in a single work setting appears to increase the possibility of cumulative trauma disorders. For instance, one study[7] showed carpal tunnel syndrome to be strongly associated with high force–high repetition work and to a lesser degree with high-repetition work alone.

Many of the diagnoses frequently associated with cumulative trauma can also occur as a result of post-traumatic, systemic, or idiopathic injuries. For example, carpal tunnel syndrome may accompany wrist and forearm fractures. De Quervain's disease may be seen in conjunction with the systemic changes of pregnancy. The treatment of each injury may vary depending on the etiology. This chapter presents the management of diagnoses attributed to overuse syndromes.

RELATIONSHIP OF WOUND HEALING TO CUMULATIVE TRAUMA

An understanding of the concepts of wound healing is significant to the management of cumulative trauma in both the conservative and postsurgical stages. Overuse may result in microscopic muscle tears, soft tissue injury, or irritation of gliding structures, which in turn produces a localized inflammatory response. The longer the insult is allowed to occur, the greater the chance for the development of chronic inflammation and resultant scar formation.[8] Therefore, the concepts of wound healing apply to cumulative trauma even though no visible wound is present. If surgery is necessary, wound healing must again be addressed within the context of surgical repair. The remainder of the chapter presents the conservative and postsurgical management of three cumulative trauma disorders: carpal tunnel syndrome, lateral epicondylitis, and de Quervain's disease. The development of each rehabilitation program will be based on the stages of wound healing and will be divided into phases 1 and 2. The patient is considered to be in phase 1 during the acute inflammatory stage, when the treatment focuses on minimizing the effects of the inflammatory process. When the inflammatory phase is controlled, the patient moves to phase 2, but is monitored for recurrence of acute symptoms. Goals in phase 2 focus on strengthening, increasing motion, and returning the patient to work.

CARPAL TUNNEL SYNDROME

Anatomy and Etiology

Carpal tunnel syndrome (CTS) is compression of the median nerve as it passes through the carpal tunnel.[9] Located in the proximal palm, the carpal tunnel is composed of an arch of bones dorsally and the transverse carpal ligament volarly, as illustrated in Figure 14–1. At this level, the median nerve innervates the thenar muscles responsible for opposition and supplies sensation to the volar aspect of the thumb, index, long, and radial aspects of the ring finger and palm.[10] When compression occurs, the resulting symptoms may include decreased sensation in the median innervated areas of the hand, complaints of pain and paresthesia, and decreased strength and coordination. As the

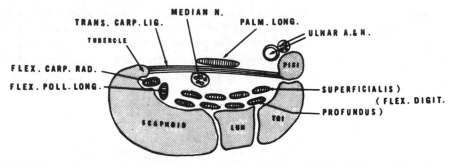

FIGURE 14–1. Anatomy of the carpal canal. (From Calliet, R: Hand Pain and Impairment, ed 3. FA Davis, Philadelphia, 1982, p 13, with permission.)

condition progresses, atrophy as well as sympathetic changes, such as dry or shiny skin, may be noted in the median innervated portion of the hand.

According to the work of Sunderland,[11] compression alters the vascular flow from the median nerve. During sleep, prolonged wrist flexion places the median nerve against the carpal ligament resulting in venous congestion within the nerve and nocturnal pain. Intratunnel pressure increases with prolonged wrist extension. This posturing is seen in waiters and waitresses who must carry a tray above shoulder level on an extended hand. Vibration, especially frequencies ranging from 30 to 50 Hz,[2] produces vascular damage of the small blood vessels leading to the median nerve.[12] Tenosynovitis caused by friction on the flexor tendons with repetitive hand tool use, results in excessive production of synovial fluid within the tendon sheath and within the carpal tunnel.[12,13] The median nerve sensory fibers conduct slower as ischemia occurs because of increased pressure.

Evaluation

The evaluation is composed of subjective and objective components. During the subjective evaluation, the therapist attempts to define the duration, location, and cause of the pain. Work- and activity-related factors are examined for aggravating postures. Repetitive wrist flexion and extension, ulnar deviation, and prolonged positioning of the wrist in these postures, while gripping or pinching items, can result in inflammation.[6] Sustained use of the upper extremities in one posture can also cause muscle fatigue. Working in awkward postures that require excessive reaching, twisting, or grasping and pinching aggravates the flexor tendons and the median nerve.

The objective portion of the evaluation confirms the diagnosis, identifies specific problem areas to establish a treatment program, and provides a baseline against which to compare post-treatment results. Range of motion (ROM), edema, and strength should be assessed. If active motion is limited, the patient should be carefully evaluated for signs of reduced flexor tendon gliding that result from chronic tenosynovial inflammation frequently associated with CTS. The excursion of the flexor digitorum superficialis is tested by asking the patient to flex the proximal interphalangeal (PIP) joint of one digit while holding the remaining digits in extension. In the presence of advanced compression, thenar atrophy may warrant specific manual muscle testing.

Provocative testing can include Tinel's and Phalen's signs, as illustrated in Figure 14–2. Tinel's sign is produced by tapping over the median nerve at the wrist. If the patient reports radiating electrical sensation or paresthesis, the test result is considered positive. A positive Phalen's sign is a subjective report by the patient of paresthesia or hypesthesia along the median nerve distribution within 60 seconds after the wrist is positioned in full flexion with the elbow resting on the table.[10]

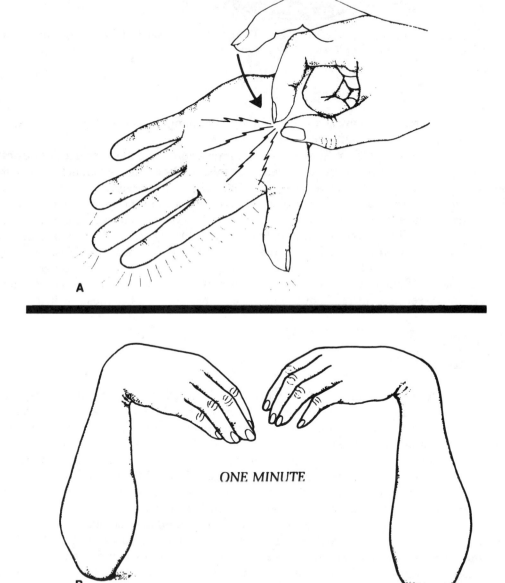

ONE MINUTE

FIGURE 14–2. *A*, Percussion over the carpal tunnel results in radiating electric shocks to the fingertips when the median nerve is compressed in the carpal tunnel. *B*, Phalen's test result is considered positive when the patient reports numbness in the thumb, index finger, and long and radial sides of the ring finger when the wrist is positioned in flexion for 1 minute.

Additional testing such as sensibility evaluation, electromyogram (EMG), and nerve conduction studies helps determine the severity of the CTS (see Chapter 4). Sensibility evaluation should include the Semmes-Weinstein monofilament test, which has been proven to correspond better with sensory nerve conduction studies than the Weber two-point test for nerve compression syndromes.[14,15] Stress testing involves a patient's performance of provocative tests (Phalen's and reverse Phalen's), repetitive squeezing of putty for 1 minute, and performance of aggravating motions on the Work Simulator, followed by testing with the Semmes-Weinstein monofilaments. The results of the stress testing are compared with the initial results obtained with Semmes-Weinstein monofilaments when the patient's hand was at rest.[15] Because the median nerve is predominantly responsible for sensation in the digits used for prehension, the Moberg pick-up test may be used to assess the patient's ability to manipulate small objects with or without vision. When vision is occluded, a patient with CTS may avoid use of the index or long finger, or both, owing to decreased sensibility.[15] Decreases in nerve conduction speed are measurable in the early stages of compression, whereas EMG findings are normal until moderate to severe neuropathy has occurred.[16]

Conservative Management

Conservative management is recommended for those patients who have only subjective sensory complaints. The presence of objective neurologic changes such as thenar weakness and atrophy indicates a more destructive lesion and requires surgical decompression.[11] Conservative treatment usually begins in the physician's office with local steroid injections, oral anti-inflammatory medication, and instruction to the patient to rest the hand. Sixty percent of the patients in one study[21] did not require further treatment after the use of local steroid injections or anti-inflammatory medication, or both. Patients who do not respond to these conservative measures are referred for further therapy.

PHASE 1: ACUTE

The focus during phase 1 is to minimize the effects of inflammation, reduce pain, and maintain normal glide of the flexor tendons in the carpal tunnel through a program of splinting, modalities, and therapeutic exercise. Splinting the wrist in a neutral position is optimal for immobilization as it minimizes pressure on the median nerve. The wearing schedule varies according to the severity of the symptoms. The splint is very helpful in relieving nocturnal pain and paresthesia that result from sleeping with the wrist in extreme flexion.[3] The median nerve is subjected to three times as much pressure during wrist flexion as when the wrist is in a neutral or slightly extended position.[12] Wearing time is slowly decreased as the inflammation and symptoms start to subside.

The problem of inflammation is also addressed using therapeutic modalities. Effective modalities for reducing inflammation may include ice, contrast baths, electrical stimulation, or phonophoresis. Once the inflammation subsides, restricted tendon excursion can be treated with heat, followed by stretching exercises of the extrinsic flexors and isolated digital flexor tendon gliding exercises to increase extensibility of the flexors and to promote normal tendon excursion (see Chapter 7).[17,18]

Tendon protection concepts as presented by Walker and Rehm[19] are reviewed with the patient. For example, the patient is instructed to avoid wrist postures that increase pressure on the median nerve. Armstrong and Chaffin[20] found that wrist flexion, ulnar deviation, and repetitive wrist flexion and extension, combined with digital gripping and pinching, are the most aggravating motions. Examples of activities that require these motions include hammering, opening valves or jar lids, gripping pliers, sawing, and turning doorknobs. Once the aggravating activities are identified, the patient is instructed to either avoid the activity or modify the way the activity is performed. For example, the usual method of picking up a bag of groceries is with wrist ulnar deviation and lateral pinch. Patients can use their forearms to cradle the bag while avoiding pinch and wrist ulnar deviation. When tools are used by the patient, their design must be assessed. If tool handles are straight, requiring wrist ulnar deviation while gripping, flexor tenosynovitis can result, causing increased pressure on the median nerve within the carpal tunnel.[6] The patient should be encouraged to use ergonomically designed tools with large, smooth handles. Some ergonomically designed tools are manufactured with a bend in their handle as seen in Figure 14–3. This type of design allows patients to use the tools with their wrist in a neutral position rather than in ulnar deviation or flexion.

As patients progress through the acute phase, the therapist must teach them to monitor their hand for signs of inflammation such as swelling or warmth. Inflammation should be treated with ice, avoidance of stressful activity, and rest. The majority of patients continue working during this acute phase; therefore, their tolerance to repetitive use of their hand can be assessed. Patients who are not working should participate in a work tolerance program to ensure that when they do return to work they will be able to perform their job duties.

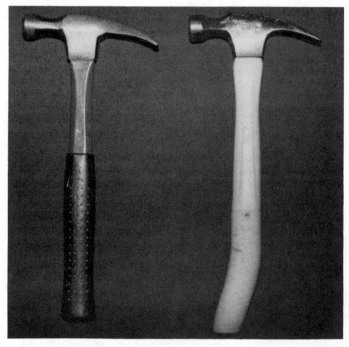

FIGURE 14–3. Ergonomic tools can minimize cumulative trauma by positioning the wrist neutrally. A bend in the handle of this hammer reduces the ulnar deviation required at the wrist during tool use.

PHASE 2: STRENGTHENING–RETURN TO WORK

Phase 2 begins with the gradual introduction of resistive exercises to increase strength. All strengthening exercises are proceeded by a warmup program of active motion to the thumb, wrist, and fingers, as well as a brief 3-minute aerobic workout. Initially, isometric exercises are used to increase strength without increasing inflammation or producing increased sensory symptoms.[21] Isometric exercises are carried out twice a day for up to 20 repetitions. The patient is instructed to make a fist and then position the wrist in a midrange (less than 30°) angle of flexion, extension, and radial and ulnar deviation. In each of these positions patients should contract their forearm muscles as much as possible. When the patient demonstrates minimal edema and full tendon excursion while completing 20 repetitions of isometric exercise, isotonic repetitive exercises are initiated.

Isotonic exercises are initiated for wrist flexion, extension, and radial and ulnar deviation. The modified Oxford technique of regressive resistive exercises is recommended to allow the patient to increase resistance without experiencing the level of fatigue reported after performing progressive resistive exercises.[22]

Endurance is gained as the patient performs job simulation.[23] If the Baltimore Therapeutic Equipment (BTE) Work Simulator is available, tools are selected that reproduce the motion performed at work. Tools that are frequently used for CTS are tool 162, which simulates use of pliers; tool 802, which simulates a wrench; and tool 901, which simulates a shovel. Assembly jobs are simulated on the Valpar Simulated Assembly Work Sample. Clerical jobs are simulated as the patient files, types, writes, folds and stuffs envelopes, and answers the telephone. Other work samples are designed for patients to simulate their specific job's physical demands of lifting, carrying, pushing, reaching, handling, and manipulating.

Standardized work samples are administered to determine if the patient's speed of coordination and endurance is adequate to ensure successful work performance at a competitive rate (see Chapter 5). Speed of coordination and endurance for mechanic work is evaluated on the Valpar Small Tools Mechanical Work Sample. Other recommended standardized tests include the other Valpar components, the box and block test, nine-hole peg test, and the Bennett hand-tool dexterity test. Before the patient can return to work, a job analysis is performed to establish the patient's job requirements and to identify ergonomic stress factors specific to CTS (see Chapter 17). The patient should be educated so that modified methods of performance can be used to decrease the ergonomic stresses in the work environment, thus minimizing the recurrence of CTS. Changes can be made by rotating the patient's job, introducing ergonomically designed tools or modifying the work site. For example, replacing the use of traditional screwdrivers with hydraulic-powered screwdrivers suspended overhead, allows workers to grip the screwdriver with their wrist in neutral rather than ulnar deviation. Pistol grips on various tools such as paintbrushes also decrease the amount of wrist motion required during performance of work activities.

Postsurgical Management

Patients who do not respond to conservative management are candidates for carpal tunnel release. The goal of surgery is to increase the volume of the carpal tunnel. The surgeon releases the transverse carpal ligament and the scar tissue is excised. An external or internal neurolysis may be performed.[11] The patient is usually referred to therapy within the first postoperative week.

PHASE 1: ACUTE

Evaluation of the patient after carpal tunnel release includes assessment of active range of motion (AROM), edema, and pain.[24] The majority of patients will experience significant relief of their symptoms after surgery. However, some patients may complain of increased postoperative pain. In these situations, the patient is educated that postoperative symptoms such as paresthesia may be a positive indication of nerve regeneration with symptoms usually subsiding within 1 to 6 months. Pain may also be present in the thenar and hypothenar eminence because of the release of the transverse carpal ligament, which can result in flattening of the palmar arch and loss of a pulley in the flexor tendon system.

Treatment priorities during this phase include rest, edema control, and tendon and nerve gliding exercises to prevent adhesion formation from restricting motion. The initial treatment may include removal of the bulky postoperative dressing and patient education regarding proper wound care. Wrist flexion should be avoided for 10 days after surgery to prevent "bowstringing" of the flexor tendons at the wrist. Edema control can usually be achieved through retrograde massage, elevation, and active exercise. Functional activities performed in elevation such as macramé can be initiated to reduce edema. If swelling persists, compression garments such as Isotoner gloves or an intermittent positive pressure pump can be applied.

According to Hunter,[25] active exercise is crucial following carpal tunnel release to limit the formation of adhesions around the median nerve within the carpal tunnel. Nerve gliding exercises, as seen in Figure 14–4, include wrist extension, finger and thumb extension, followed by supination of the forearm and extension of the elbow and wrist. A gentle passive stretch should be applied to the thumb and fingers to improve passive of motion (PROM). Tendon gliding exercises are also incorporated into the program to prevent the formation of motion-limiting adhesions between the tendons and nerves within the carpal tunnel. Frequent exercise sessions with few repetitions are recommended to discourage adhesion formation without contributing to the normal postoperative inflammatory response. If the patient complains of discomfort after exercise, or if any inflammation is noted, the number of repetitions is decreased.

Scar management begins with massage once the sutures are removed. If the scar appears thickened, Elastomer of Otoform is applied with Coban to remodel the scar. Patients who complain of hypersensitivity along the surgical incision should begin a desensitization program (See Chapter 11).[26]

PHASE 2: STRENGTHENING–RETURN TO WORK

The strengthening phase is required for those patients who have residual weakness and sensory deficits from severe compression neuropathy; patients who have continued problems with persistent edema, limitations in motion, hypersensitivity, and pain; or patients with physically strenuous jobs who must gain adequate strength to return to work. This phase of treatment begins with reevaluation of the patient. If pain, limited ROM, edema, or hypersensitivity is present, measurements are recorded and periodically reassessed to monitor progress. Although strengthening is begun as early as 4 weeks after surgery with isometric exercises, measurement of grip and pinch strength is

NERVE GLIDING PROGRAM
FOR MEDIAN NERVE DECOMPRESSION AT THE WRIST

EXERCISES TO BE DONE _____ TIMES EACH, _____ TIMES A DAY.
HOLD EACH POSITION TO A COUNT OF _____ .

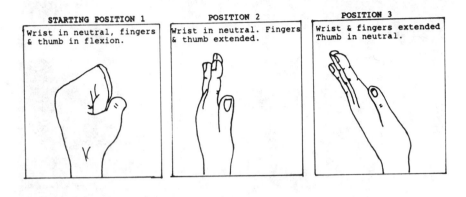

| STARTING POSITION 1 | POSITION 2 | POSITION 3 |
| Wrist in neutral, fingers & thumb in flexion. | Wrist in neutral. Fingers & thumb extended. | Wrist & fingers extended Thumb in neutral. |

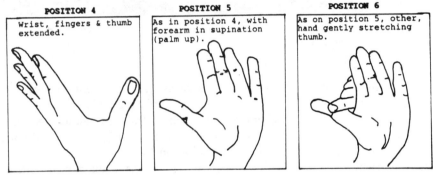

| POSITION 4 | POSITION 5 | POSITION 6 |
| Wrist, fingers & thumb extended. | As in position 4, with forearm in supination (palm up). | As on position 5, other, hand gently stretching thumb. |

FIGURE 14–4. Nerve gliding exercises. These exercises are performed in sequence to provide gliding of the median nerve.

delayed until 6 weeks after surgery if the patient complains of pain when attempting to perform the pinch and grip test. Coordination testing begins at 4 weeks following surgery and is repeated every 3 to 4 weeks. Endurance and job simulation are evaluated 8 weeks after surgery. Sensibility is not assessed until 3 months following surgery to allow sufficient time for nerve regeneration to occur.

Treatment priorities during phase 2 include recovery of full ROM of the wrist and digits, desensitization of hypersensitive skin, control of edema and pain, and recovery of adequate strength, coordination, and endurance, so that even the patient with severe neuropathy can return to a productive lifestyle.

Desensitization continues if hypersensitivity persists. If the patient develops a symptomatic neuroma, as indicated by an extremely sensitive localized area, the surgeon should be notified so that the neuroma can be monitored. Figure 14–5 illustrates how cushioning the neuroma with a Dermal Pad alleviates direct pressure and controls pain. Bicycle or work gloves may be worn to add protective padding during work.

Prolonged pain and paresthesia may persist after surgical decompression of the median nerve and may be very similar to the patient's preoperative symptoms. This

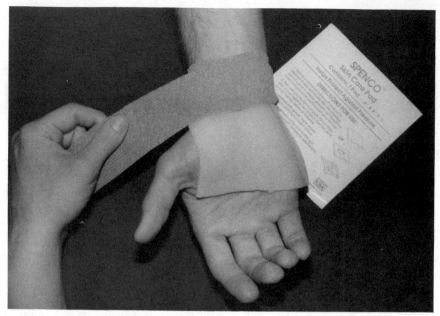

FIGURE 14–5. A dermal pad secured with Coban is used over the sensitive palmar skin to distribute pressure during activity.

continued pain may be due to the spontaneous discharge of afferent pathways without contact with a painful stimuli, which can occur not only during degeneration but also during regeneration.[11] Pain control modalities such as transcutaneous electrical nerve stimulator (TENS) units may offer relief. Phonophoresis using a hydrocortisone compound can decrease the pain related to inflammation.[8]

Vascular functioning may be impaired owing to decreased neural ability.[11] The patient may complain of color changes of the skin and cold intolerance. Contrast baths are used by patients to decrease pain and cold intolerance. During cold weather, thermal glove liners or mittens are suggested for patients with continued cold intolerance.

Patients are instructed to gradually resume normal use of their hand. Throughout this time patients learn to assess the response of their hand to activity by monitoring the presence of pain, edema, or inflammation. If necessary, aggravating activities are avoided or modified, or are performed for a limited period of time.

Based on the patient's response to treatment, the time frame for postsurgical introduction of strengthening exercise may vary from 4 to 8 weeks. At this point, management of the patient following carpal tunnel release is identical to the strengthening phase during conservative management and includes strengthening, endurance, and job simulation activities. The hand should be reevaluated on an ongoing basis and the program modified accordingly. In some patients the hand tends to swell with use; others do not experience this swelling but complain of increased pain and paresthesia. In our opinion, if swelling in the affected hand increases more than 20 percent after use, the patient must be taught to modify the time or method used for the activity. Patients who have had surgery may require a slower rate of progression in their treatment program. Patients with severe compression neuropathies may require as many as 12 weeks of therapy, while patients who respond to conservative treatment may return to productive work after only 4 to 6 weeks of therapy.

LATERAL EPICONDYLITIS

Anatomy and Etiology

Lateral epicondylitis, more commonly known as "tennis elbow," is a condition involving a lesion in the structures originating from the lateral epicondyle. The most frequently reported lesion is a tear in the common extensor tendon.[27] These tears range from microscopic to gross rupture or avulsion.[28,29] The common extensor tendon originates from the lateral epicondyle and consists of fibers from the extensor carpi radialis brevis, extensor digitorum communis, extensor digiti minimi, extensor carpi ulnaris, and superficial part of the supinator. The extensor carpi radialis brevis is the most frequently injured structure. The extensor carpi radialis longus is less commonly involved, as its origin is proximal to the lateral epicondyle.[29,30]

Lateral epicondylitis is characterized by epicondylar pain and tenderness. Forearm pain, as well as referred (radiating) pain in the ring and long fingers, may be present. Pain is often described as a constant ache, with episodes of sharp pain that cause momentary loss of grip. Pain increases with stretching of the common extensor tendon, grasping, or lifting. Localized swelling and increased skin temperature may be present and indicative of the inflammatory response to injury. Factors that may influence the onset of symptoms include age, hormonal balance (in women), as well as inadequate strength, endurance, and flexibility of the extensor muscles.[31,32]

The patient's occupational requirements can lead to this condition if repetitive forceful wrist motions and gripping are performed. Lateral epicondylitis can occur owing to eccentric muscle activity that generates forces on the wrist extensor mechanism greater than the musculotendinous unit can withstand.[21] The finger flexors act to grasp and handle objects, whereas the wrist extensors act simultaneously to stabilize the wrist. Activation of the wrist extensors is essential to power grip.[33] The demand on the extensor muscles and common extensor tendon increases when eccentric muscle activity is performed such as radial deviation with pronation. This repetitive and demanding stress can lead to overload of the common extensor tendon resulting in mechanical fatigue and microtears. As these microtears attempt to unite in the early healing stages, union may be delayed as the patient continues to use the hand during daily activities. The delay in the repair of these microtears results in chronic inflammation and the development of scar, which may become the primary source of the pain.[34] Although lateral epicondylitis is often associated with racket-type sports such as tennis or racketball, the condition can also result from other sports such as swimming, fencing, and those involving throwing.

Evaluation

A comprehensive subjective and objective evaluation identifies and differentiates lateral epicondylitis from other disorders involving the elbow. Pain is the primary complaint. Therefore, the evaluation focuses on reproduction and identification of the pain.

Lateral epicondylitis is diagnosed by reproduction of the pain and related symptoms to resistance testing, passive stretching, and palpation. Resistive muscle testing is the most provocative method of identifying lateral epicondylitis and localizing the source of pain. A positive test result reproduces the pain and weakness. Resisted muscle testing to the elbow will have a negative result, whereas application of resistance to the wrist extensors a positive one.[35] Pain may be present with resisted radial but not ulnar deviation. Resistance to the wrist flexors is also negative. All individual muscles that conjoin into the common extensor tendon should be tested to isolate the muscle(s) that are weak and painful. Resistance to the wrist extensors should be applied with the elbow both extended and flexed. Kendall[35] reported the following technique to isolate the action of the extensor carpi radialis brevis. With the patient's forearm positioned on the table, the extensor carpi radialis longus and brevis are tested by applying resistance to the dorsum of the patient's hand as the wrist is extended. The test is repeated with the patient's elbow flexed to approximately 130°. In this position, the extensor carpi radialis brevis acts alone to extend the wrist. Care should be taken to ensure the patient's fingers are kept actively flexed to eliminate involvement of the extensor digitorum communis.[35] Resistance to the supinator should not be neglected as the supinator is frequently involved and missed during evaluations. If resistive muscle testing to the individual wrist and finger extensors and supinator is negative, one should test for reproduction of pain by resisting the wrist and fingers moving into flexion. This test places more force on the wrist extensors, as eccentric contractions generate more force than isometric or concentric contractions.[21] Resistive testing by evaluation of grip strength has been reported as a means to quantify changes in pain and the patient's response to treatment.[36]

Palpation of the extensor musculature follows resistance and active stretch testing to further isolate the involvement of the individual muscles. Palpation is used also to document the presence of trigger points in the musculature. Cyriax[34] cautions that pressure of the wrist extensor musculature against the radius is normally painful and recommends palpation using a pincher-type palpation, as demonstrated in Figure 14–6. Painful palpation at the musculotendinous juncture of the extensor carpi radialis brevis may indicate a strain or tear, whereas pain with palpation of the lateral epicondyle may be due to a lesion in the subtendinous space.[37]

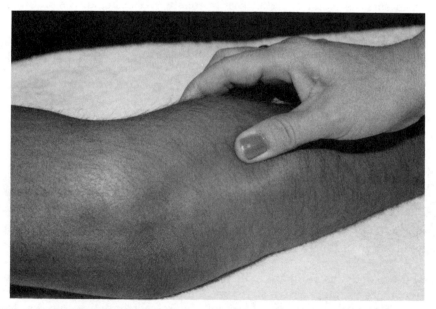

FIGURE 14–6. Pincher-type palpation is recommended by Cyriax to locate the area of strain or tear of the musculotendinous juncture of the extensor muscles.

ROM is evaluated for the elbow and wrist. PROM is usually within normal limits and eliminates any joint involvement. Limitations in active wrist extension may be present secondary to pain with contraction of the wrist extensors. Pain may also limit active wrist flexion because of the increased force occurring at the common extensor tendon with eccentric lengthening of the extensors during wrist flexion. Circumferential measurements taken at the elbow crease, as well as proximal and distal to the crease, quantify the presence of swelling and inflammation.

Associated problems, such as ulnar nerve neurapraxia, CTS, radial nerve entrapment, posterior interosseus nerve compression, intra-articular abnormalities, and joint laxity, appear independently or in combination with lateral epicondylitis. The evaluation should attempt to differentiate these conditions from lateral epicondylitis. To rule out posterior interosseus nerve compression, resistance is applied to the long finger in extension. The patient should be positioned with the wrist in neutral to eliminate recruitment of the wrist stabilizers. Pain is often reproduced with palpation of the nerve approximately 1 to 2 in distal to the lateral epicondyle in the mobile muscle mass. If these maneuvers reproduce pain, then posterior interosseus nerve compression may be present. Nerve conduction and EMG studies are then used to substantiate the presence of nerve compression.

Conservative Management

Conservative treatment focuses on pain control and decreasing inflammation. Aspirin and other nonsteroidal anti-inflammatory medications are often the first choice of treatment. In conjunction with anti-inflammatory medications, rest and elimination of aggravating activities are recommended. Local cortisone injections are also effectively used in decreasing the inflammation and pain. The number of cortisone injections given in any time frame and to one extremity is controversial. Nirschl[38] advocates that giving more than three cortisone injections is inappropriate and may lead to cellular death and potentially weakened surrounding tissue. Patients with both acute and chronic lateral epicondylitis are frequently referred to therapy for conservative treatment. Treatment consists of (1) addressing the inflammation and (2) strengthening and conditioning the involved extremity.

PHASE 1: ACUTE

The initial treatment focuses on decreasing pain and inflammation. Complete rest of the entire upper extremity musculature is avoided unless pain is extremely acute. In these cases, 1 to 3 days of rest may be necessary. Prefabricated or custom-made thermoplastic wrist splints may be used to eliminate extreme wrist flexion, reducing the stress on the common extensor tendon from eccentric contractions. A counterforce strap ("tennis elbow" strap), shown in Figure 14-7, can also be used to decrease the stress of the common extensor tendon during daily activities.[39] The counterforce strap was first described by Ilfed and popularized by Nirschl[27] and Fromisen.[29] In theory, the counterforce strap constrains full muscular expansion, thereby decreasing the muscular force at the common extensor tendon during concentric contractions.[39] Patient education during this phase is critical. Education focuses on instruction in avoidance of aggravating activities and movements that produce increased stress on the common extensor tendon.

Modalities including ice, pulsed ultrasound, interferential electrical stimulation,

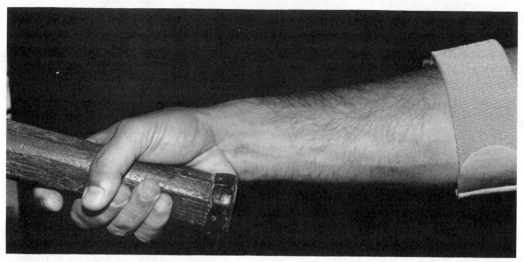

FIGURE 14–7. The counterforce brace should be worn during activities and exercises that require maximum contraction of the wrist extensors.

phonophoresis, iontophoresis, and high-voltage galvanic stimulation can be used to decrease pain and inflammation.[40–42] Nirschl[43] advocates the use of high galvanic stimulation, rather than ultrasound, in treating patients with lateral epicondylitis. He recommends four to six sessions in a 2- to 3-week period to decrease pain, inflammation, and promote healing.[43]

Following the use of modalities, transverse friction massage is applied over the common extensor tendon. Massage is helpful in stimulating circulation and mobilizing scar tissue. Ice can be used before the transverse friction massage to anesthetize the area. The treatment session concludes with gentle stretching into wrist flexion to lengthen the extensor musculature and scar tissue.

PHASE 2: STRENGTHENING–RETURN TO WORK

As the pain and inflammation become controlled, treatment priorities begin to focus on the gradual progression of strength, endurance, and conditioning. Strengthening of the entire upper extremity is critical, as weak and deconditioned muscles are more susceptible to repeated injury.[44] Active exercises are introduced to increase strength. Isolated exercises of the individual wrist extensor muscles are not necessary because the goal of the strengthening program is to promote strength of all the muscles to prevent overloading and overstretching. Strengthening the forearm flexors is beneficial in preventing muscle imbalance. According to Walmsley and colleagues,[21] eccentric exercises are recommended for the extrinsic forearm musculature to ensure that maximum strengthening occurs. Eccentric exercises (exercises that are performed as the muscle lengthens) produce greater tensile strength in the tendon than concentric exercises. Concentric exercises are added after the patient can perform eccentric exercises without excessive pain.

The patient's complaints are carefully analyzed while the extensor muscles are contracted. Stanish cautions that "pain with exercise implies that the tensile strength of the tissue is still not up to what the exercise demands and the stress on the muscle/tendon unit must be decreased,"[45] The speed and resistance of the contraction must therefore be altered. Active exercises are performed three times a day for three sets of 10 repetitions. When pain is eliminated with active exercise, resistance is added starting with a 1-lb weight. When the patient can perform pain-free wrist flexion and extension while holding a 5-lb weight, progressive resistive or regressive resistive exercises may be performed.

Most patients experience relief of pain and gradual improvement of strength within 8 weeks. For these patients, the program is progressed by increasing the resistance and speed at which the exercises are performed. Also, the Work Simulator is used to simulate job conditions. As patients practice their work activities on the Work Simulator or with equipment they use at work, the therapist teaches them to avoid postures that produce overstretching or overloading of the extensor musculature. Patients are taught to lift with the forearm in neutral. Other necessary modifications in work technique may include using the unaffected arm, change in the overall position of the forearm, and decreasing the duration and frequency of certain activities. Modifications in work equipment and tools may also be necessary. For example, increasing the girth and length of a screwdriver and hammer handle can improve the leverage, force, and torque.[6,31]

Postsurgical Management

Patients who do not respond to conservative treatment may be candidates for surgical intervention.[29] Surgery may involve repair of the common extensor tendon, lengthening of the extensor carpi radialis brevis distally, lysis of scar tissue, and inter-articular procedures involving the release of ligaments.[29]

The period of immobilization following surgery varies from 5 days to 3 weeks, depending on the surgical procedure performed. A period of immobilization following surgery is necessary to eliminate stress on the repair site and to allow for the normal postoperative inflammation to subside. Referral to therapy usually follows the period of immobilization.

PHASE 1: ACUTE

Evaluation of the patient after surgery includes assessment of the incision, AROM, edema, and pain. PROM measurements are usually deferred during the first 3 weeks to avoid stretch and stress at the surgical site. Treatment priorities during this early postoperative phase include rest, edema, and pain control, as well as active exercise. Ice, retrograde massage, and compressive stockinette are effective in controlling edema. Ice and massage are also effective for increasing circulation and decreasing pain.

AROM exercises are performed to maintain joint motion, facilitate edema reduction, and prevent adhesion formation. If joint limitations and muscle tightness exist, PROM exercises are incorporated. When performing ROM exercises, caution should be used to avoid positions that place maximum stress on the common extensor tendon. Desensitization and scar management techniques previously discussed are implemented as needed.

During the first 6 weeks after surgery, resistive exercises are avoided to prevent reinjury to the extensor musculature and common extensor tendon. Isometric exercises for the extensors can be initiated with the wrist positioned in less than 30° of flexion or extension to prevent overloading and overstretching on the extensor musculature.

PHASE 2: SCAR MATURATION

During the scar maturation phase, pain and edema continue to be assessed. ROM measurements are still documented if limitations persist. Manual muscle testing and isometric strength testing using the BTE Work Simulator or Jamar Dynamometer can be initiated at 8 weeks as the repaired structures are adequately healed. The patient's endurance and tolerance for work-related activities can be evaluated using the BTE Work Simulator and Valpar Work Samplers.

The goals of therapy and treatment during this phase are synonymous with the strengthening phase of the conservative management of lateral epicondylitis. Emphasis continues to be placed on patient education, activity, and equipment modification. A physical capacity evaluation may be necessary to determine if the patient can return to his or her previous job. On-site job evaluations with recommendations and modifications of technique and equipment can prevent recurrence of symptoms.

DE QUERVAIN'S DISEASE

Anatomy and Etiology

De Quervain's disease is a form of tenosynovitis. Tenosynovitis is inflammation of a tendon and its surrounding synovial sheath. De Quervain's disease involves inflammation of the extensor pollicis brevis (EPB) and the abductor pollicis longus (APL), as these tendons pass through the first dorsal compartment of the thumb (Fig. 14–8). The APL and EPB move in the same synovial sheath that passes in a bony groove over the radiostyloid process.[46]

De Quervain's disease is an inflammatory process. Movement of the tendons through the first dorsal compartment is facilitated by synovial fluid. When the physical demands placed on the tendons exceeds the ability of the tendons to easily glide, friction results. This friction causes inflammation to occur among the tendons, bony process, and sheath, resulting in edema and increased vascularity, further compressing the tendons within the confines of the synovial sheath. If overuse is continued, inflammation may persist causing a chronic inflammatory process characterized by continued pain and edema with decreased function.

This disease was named after the Swiss surgeon de Quervain in 1895.[49] Symptoms include pain over the radial styloid, which may radiate proximally or distally. Swelling may be noted over the first dorsal compartment. A test used in the diagnosis of this disorder is the Finkelstein's test. As seen in Figure 14–9, this test involves adducting the thumb into the palm and ulnarly deviating the wrist. A positive test result reproduces pain.

According to Mosely,[47] anatomic variations such as an aberrant APL tendon may cause this disorder. This disease has also been called "washer woman's syndrome" and has been related to activities involving repetitive thumb motions, twisting, and pinching, as illustrated in Figure 14–10. Edmonson and Crenshaw[48] report that "the cause is almost always occupational or associated with rheumatoid arthritis," and they relate the disease to repetitive types of work. The symptoms may be induced by work requiring repetitive pinching and ulnar deviation of the wrist such as assembling electronic devices or using a grocery scanner.

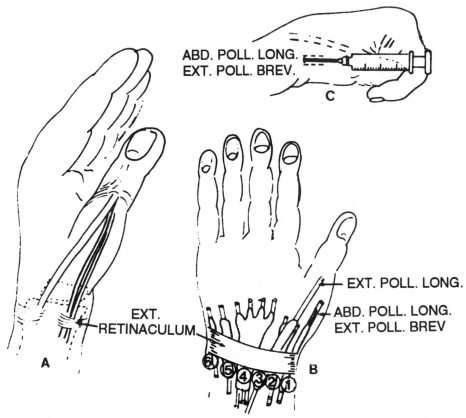

ABD. POLL. LONG.
EXT. POLL. BREV.

C

EXT. POLL. LONG.

ABD. POLL. LONG.
EXT. POLL. BREV

EXT.
RETINACULUM

A

B

FIGURE 14–8. Tenosynovitis of the extensor pollicis brevis and the abductor pollicis longus is present in the first dorsal compartment with de Quervain's disease. (From Calliet, R: Hand Pain and Impairment, ed 3. FA Davis, Philadelphia, 1982, p 120, with permission.)

Evaluation

An initial evaluation is performed to determine treatment goals and obtain baseline information to gauge progress. Pain, edema, and ROM are measured. Measurement of strength is deferred until pain decreases.

The patient's subjective report of pain is assessed with the pain analog scale and pain with palpation is recorded. Activities that cause pain are noted. The Finkelstein's test is performed.

Swelling over the first dorsal compartment is assessed visually. Edema can be measured by water displacement using the Volumeter, if there are no open wounds. Circumferential measurements at the wrist, thumb, proximal phalanx, and interphalangeal (IP) joint can be taken if a Volumeter is not available.

Goniometric measurements of thumb AROM and PROM are taken and should include flexion and extension of the thumb metacarpophalangeal (MP) and IP joints. AROM limited by pain is noted. Opposition of the thumb to the digits is measured and the web space evaluated. Wrist ROM and digital flexion are assessed. ROM measurements of the involved hand should be compared with the measurements of the contralateral side.

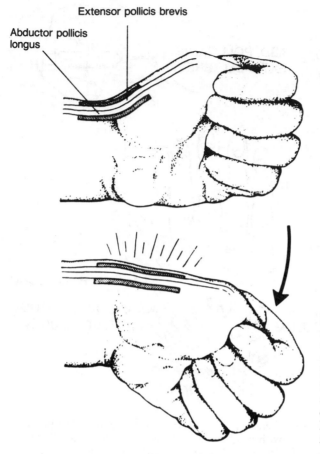

Abductor pollicis longus

Extensor pollicis brevis

FIGURE 14–9. Pain will be elicited with a Finkelstein's test when a patient with de Quervain's disease flexes the thumb into the fist and ulnarly deviates the wrist. (From The Hand: Examination and Diagnosis, American Society for Surgery of the Hand, 1983, p 76, with permission.)

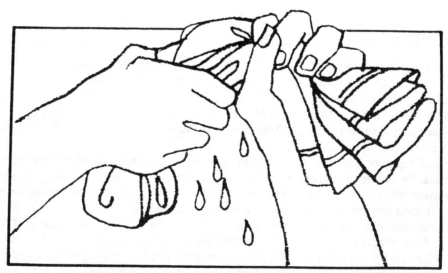

FIGURE 14–10. Gripping objects while deviating the wrists aggravates the tendons in the first dorsal compartment and contributes to the development of de Quervain's disease. (Courtesy of the Travelers Insurance Company.)

Conservative Management

PHASE 1: ACUTE

In the early stages of conservative management, the focus of therapy is to reduce pain and inflammation. Strengthening and increasing ROM cannot be addressed until these goals are achieved.

Inflammatory disorders may be managed initially by rest. With de Quervain's disease, the thumb is rested in a thumb gauntlet splint, otherwise known as a long opponens splint or long thumb spica. The splint is forearm-based to include the wrist and can support the arm volarly or, as seen in Figure 14–11, can be formed as a radial gutter splint. The wrist is placed in 15° of extension, the thumb is palmarly abducted, and the MP joint is held in 10° of flexion. This position puts the APL and EPB on slack while placing the thumb in a position of function. The patient is tested for pain with IP flexion and resisted IP extension. If these maneuvers cause pain, the IP joint is included in the splint and rested in an extended position. Immobilization is discontinued at the IP joint when the patient does not have pain with this test. Although prefabricated splints are also available, a custom-made splint is recommended for better fit.

Initially, the splint is worn both day and night and is removed only for hygiene or exercise purposes, or for the application of a modality. Three times daily the splint is removed for gentle, AROM exercises of the thumb and wrist. These exercises should avoid the extremes of wrist and thumb motion and should never produce pain. Active exercise of the unimmobilized joints should be encouraged, including tendon gliding exercises of the fingers, thumb IP joint flexion if the thumb was not included in the splint, and ROM exercises of the elbow and shoulder.

Inflammation is controlled through noninvasive techniques. Michlovitz[8] recommends the use of phonophoresis in which ultrasound is used to drive anti-inflammatory medication (such as hydrocortisone) deep into the tissues. Ice massage for 3 minutes or application of a cold pack over the inflamed tendons for 10 minutes, is performed three to four times daily.[8]

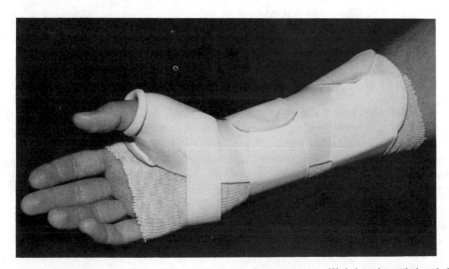

FIGURE 14–11. A radial thumb gutter splint rests the extensor pollicis brevis and the abductor pollicis longus tendons.

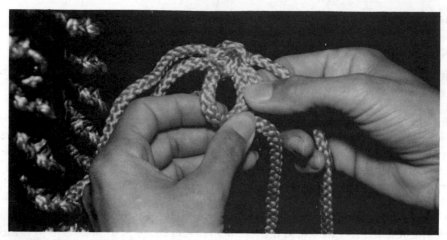

FIGURE 14–12. Knot-tying in elevation promotes prehension and reduces edema.

Progression of the patient during this acute phase depends on the patient's response to treatment. If the patient has continued pain and inflammation upon gentle active exercise, full-time immobilization is continued. If the patient can tolerate increasing levels of activity without persisting symptoms, however, the splint schedule is gradually decreased while the exercise program is progressed. Thumb ROM exercises move from general to specific, including opposition of the thumb to each digit, active thumb abduction, and thumb flexion into the palm. Light prehension activities that avoid prolonged or repetitive positioning of the thumb in the extremes of flexion and extension are initiated. Examples of such activities include making tile trivets, games involving prehension, or macramé performed in elevation, as shown in Figure 14–12. Gentle home exercises may include gathering a paper towel or newspaper into the hand or placing small foam cubes into a cup. Activities chosen at this stage should provide gentle thumb abduction and flexion with low levels of resistance.

If pain and swelling are not controlled by noninvasive means, the surgeon may inject a steroidal anti-inflammatory medication such as cortisone into the synovial sheath. The conservative management protocol is then followed.

PHASE 2: STRENGTHENING–RETURN TO WORK

The patient is in phase 2 when inflammation and pain are decreasing, and the focus can shift to hand strengthening and endurance. Strength is assessed with the Jamar Dynamometer and the pinch gauge. Pain, edema, and ROM are continually reassessed to monitor recurrence of symptoms. Coordination may be tested using standardized tests such as the nine-hole peg test, the box and block test, or the Jebson-Taylor hand function test (see Chapter 5).

Endurance may be evaluated as activity tolerance increases. The length of time that job simulation can be performed without pain is noted. Results of extended tests such as the Valpar Whole Body Work Sampler provide information about endurance. The BTE Work Simulator can be used to evaluate and provide data regarding power output that quantifies improvement.

During phase 2, if pain and swelling are resolving, the patient is completely weaned from splinting. Strengthening activities and job simulation become the focus of the patient's program with careful monitoring for recurrence of symptoms.

The program is upgraded to include strengthening exercises. Home exercises to focus on strengthening of grip and pinch are issued and may include squeezing and pinching putty. The patient is encouraged to resume use of the hand in daily activity. As pain decreases, resistance of exercises may be increased. The patient is closely monitored. If pain or edema increase, the resistance is reduced. The use of ice for 10 minutes after exercise helps control symptoms.

Various strengthening activities can be implemented during the therapy program. The goals should include strengthening of grip and pinch and increasing the patient's ability to perform job tasks. Therapeutic activities may include using clay to build ceramic pottery to strengthen pinch and promote use of the thumb. Pinching clothespins or assembling a leather link belt will also achieve pinch strengthening. Woodworking involving sustained gripping of a dowel sander can be used to increase grip strength and endurance. Job simulation is also an important part of therapy. Long sessions of repetitive activity in therapy is not recommended owing to the tendency for recurrence of symptoms.

This phase ends, it is hoped, with the patient returning to work and to pain-free daily life. However, because of the biomechanical demands placed on the thumb, recurrence of symptoms is frequent and therapy may extend beyond the 12-week schedule. The patient may require adaptations to the job site. Use of ergonomically designed tools that limit wrist ulnar deviation or job rotation to decrease time spent on repetitive pinching activities may facilitate successful return to work. The physician should be kept abreast of the patient's progress. If pain persists after conservative management, a surgical evaluation may be indicated.

Postsurgical Management

The surgical technique for relief of de Quervain's disease involves opening the first dorsal compartment and freeing the involved tendons from adhesions and compression. The wound is usually dressed for 48 hours, at which time movement is initiated and increased as tolerated.[48]

PHASE 1: ACUTE

The postsurgical evaluation begins with inspection of the wound for signs of infection including warmth, redness, and discharge. AROM is assessed. As the wound closes, skin hypersensitivity is monitored. As in conservative management, pain and edema are important considerations. When the wound is open, circumferential measures of edema must be taken rather than volumetric measures. Pain is assessed using the pain analog scale.

The goals during this stage should focus on controlling edema, maximizing ROM, and preventing adhesions as scar tissue forms during the early wound healing. To control edema, the patient is asked to elevate his or her hand as much as possible. In addition, patients are instructed to raise their hand overhead and make 10 to 20 gentle fists every hour to promote venous return. To combat serious edema, a vasopneumatic compression pump or a compression stocking may be used. Retrograde massage of the hand involving distal to proximal pressure assists in edema reduction by moving fluids toward the arm where the lymphatic system is more able to remove it.

The hand is rested in a thumb gauntlet splint, as previously described. During phase 1, the splint is worn full-time and removed for exercise periods. In phase 2, splint use will be decreased. When postsurgical edema is reduced, the splint may become too large and should be remolded. Further splinting may be necessary to correct deficits such as first web space contracture or decreased thumb flexion, if they occur.

Pain is controlled, using applications of ice. Ice can be applied over a wound that is open if the wound is dressed and a towel is placed between the wound and the ice. Use of a TENS unit will assist a patient who experiences severe pain.

Active ROM is used to facilitate tendon gliding and prevent adhesions of the APB and EPL. Active thumb carpometacarpal (CMC), MP and IP joint flexion and extension exercises are issued as well as opposition to each finger. The patient's fears of moving while sutures and open wounds are present must be dispelled by the therapist. Tendon gliding exercises should also be performed with the uninvolved digits to encourage use of the hand and prevent stiffness.

Desensitization is performed with patients who become hypersensitive to light touch on or around a scar. A very hypersensitive patient may apply textures to the areas around a wound early or desensitization may begin following wound closure. Hypersensitivity may be a problem owing to postoperative irritation of the cutaneous branch of the radial nerve.

The patient is encouraged to use the hand in gentle prehension activities during this phase. These activities may include picking up small objects such as foam cubes or gathering a paper towel into the hand.

As the wound closes, scar control techniques are used. Scar massage is performed for both desensitization and scar softening. The patient massages the scar applying firm pressure to mobilize the scar over subcutaneous tissues. Massage is performed in a circular motion three or more times daily for 10 minutes. A silastic Elastomer pad is worn at night over the scar to provide firm pressure, and worn during the day, providing the pad does not interfere with active use of the hand. The Elastomer offers positive pressure over healing scar to promote proper alignment of newly synthesized collagen.

PHASE 2: STRENGTHENING–RETURN TO WORK

The return-to-work phase for the postsurgical de Quervain's patient is the same as for the patient treated by conservative management. Job modifications may be necessary to alter hand posture or amount of repetition performed. A physical capacity evaluation may be useful to define the patient's strength and limitations (see Chapter 17).

CLINICAL DECISION MAKING—CASE STUDY

CB, a 39-year-old right hand–dominant woman, employed as a cleaning person for a railroad company, developed symptoms in her left hand including tenderness in the area of the anatomic snuffbox, pain on the radial aspect of the thumb and forearm, and difficulty lifting objects. The diagnosis of de Quervain's disease was made, cortisone was injected into the first dorsal compartment, and the patient was referred to therapy.

CONSERVATIVE MANAGEMENT

Evaluation

CB reported constant pain in the first dorsal compartment, which increased with active thumb motion. Localized swelling was present at the base of the thumb. AROM measurements were taken and are presented in Table 14–1. Grip and pinch measurements were not taken due to the acute pain the patient was experiencing.

Treatment

The goal of the acute phase of therapy is to reduce pain and inflammation. Following the cortisone injection, a thermoplastic thumb spica splint was applied, to be worn full-time for 2 weeks. Ice was applied several times daily for edema control. Gentle digit and thumb IP joint AROM exercises were performed.

By the second week, the patient could tolerate active thumb motion in the midrange without increased pain and edema. As a result, the patient was instructed to remove the splint four to five times a day and perform gentle active thumb exercises in the pain-free range, for short periods of time. Each exercise session was followed by the application of ice for edema control. As the patient improved, gentle activities such as macramé and foam cube gathering were initiated. By 6 weeks after injection, mild-resistance activities were introduced, such as ceramics and light use of the BTE Work Simulator. Throughout this time the patient was encouraged to remove the splint for increasingly longer periods of time.

After 10 weeks of conservative management, the acute pain had subsided but the patient still had significant pain with the extremes of thumb opposition and flexion. The patient complained of pain with any activity requiring tight grasp or pinch, and minimal improvement in strength was noted. Edema continued to fluctuate. Because of the persisting symptoms, the physician performed a de Quervain's release.

SURGICAL MANAGEMENT

Evaluation

At 3 days after surgery, the patient's problems were identified as pain, edema, hypersensitivity along the incision, and decreased motion.

Treatment

On the initial postoperative visit, the dressings were changed to light, dry dressings, and a thumb gauntlet splint was fabricated. The splint was worn at all times, except when exercising. Gentle, active, pain-free ROM exercises of the wrist, thumb, and fingers were performed three times a day. Because of complaints of hypersensitivity along the surgical site, a desensitization program was initiated. Once the sutures were removed, deep pressure massage was used to soften the surgical scar.

As the postoperative pain decreased, the patient gradually progressed into phase 2. The exercise program included exercises in the extremes of thumb motion

TABLE 14–1 Objective Measures—Case Study

	After Injection		10 Weeks Conservative Management		3 Days After Surgery		1 Month After Surgery		Discharge 12 Weeks After Surgery	
	R	L	R	L	R	L	R	L	R	L
Active Thumb MP Flexion	60*	30	60	30	60	20	60	30	60	35
Active Wrist Extention/Flexion	50/50	50/35	50/50	50/35	50/55	30/35	50/50	40/35	50/50	50/40
Grip (level 2) (lb)	Not assessed		70	40	Not assessed		70	30	70	55
Lateral Pinch (lb)	Not assessed		12	6	Not assessed		12	4	12	9
Tip Pinch (lb)	Not assessed		13	5	Not assessed		13	4	13	10

*All ROM measurements given in degrees.

and gentle thumb and grip resistance exercises. Ten weeks after surgery the patient was ready to begin job simulation tasks. Based on the patient interview and the employers response to the job analysis form, the demands of CB's job were identified as lifting trashcans and buckets of water, scrubbing, reaching overhead, and spraying cleaning agents. In therapy, the patient was instructed in ROM exercises to stretch and warm up her hands before performing job simulation tasks. Each of CB's job requirements was simulated in therapy, and followed by the application of ice to discourage inflammation.

At 12 weeks after surgery, the patient was able to return to work. Owing to complaints of pain with heavy lifting, a thumb gauntlet splint was worn as needed. To prevent recurrence of de Quervain's disease symptoms CB was instructed to alternate job tasks and spread out those tasks requiring extensive thumb stress.

SUMMARY

With cumulative trauma disorders, the therapist is involved in conservative management and postsurgical treatment. Edema control, splinting to rest involved structures, and pain control are initially addressed. As the patient progresses, goals turn to strengthening and preparing the patient to return to regular work and leisure activities. The patient must be carefully monitored for recurrence of symptoms. Because of the incidence of work-related cumulative trauma disorders, the therapist's role has expanded because of the need to communicate with the employer about the patient's job demands. The therapist is involved in treatment, patient education, industrial consultation, and efforts to prevent the occurrence of cumulative trauma disorders.

REFERENCES

1. National Safety Council, Chicago, IL: Telephone communication, July 1989.
2. Silverstein, BA, et al: Hand wrist cumulative trauma disorders in industry. Br J Ind Med 43:779, 1986.
3. Muffly-Elsey, D and Flinn-Wagner, S: Proposed screening tool for the detection of cumulative trauma disorders in the upper extremity. J Hand Surg 12 (5, Part 2): 931, 1987.
4. Wynn, WH: Action needed for scanner safety. United Food and Commercial Workers International Union Magazine, March, 1988.
5. Barnhart, S and Rosenstock, L: Carpal tunnel syndrome in grocery checkers. West J Med 147(1):37, 1987.
6. Armstrong, TJ, et al: Ergonomic considerations in hand and wrist tendonitis. J Hand Surg 12 (5, Part 2):830, 1987.
7. Silverstein, BA, Fine, LJ, and Armstrong, TJ: Occupational factors and carpal tunnel syndrome. Am J Ind Med 11:343, 1987.
8. Michlovitz, SL: Thermal Agents. FA Davis, Philadelphia, 1986, pp 13, 157.
9. Zachary, RB: Thenar palsy due to compression of the median nerve in the carpal tunnel. Surg Gynecol Obstet 81:215, 1945.
10. American Society for Surgery of the Hand: The hand: Diagnosis and treatment, ed 2. Churchill Livingstone, New York, 1983.
11. Sunderland, S: Nerves and Nerve Injuries. Williams & Wilkins, Baltimore, 1968, p 711.
12. Lundborg, G, et al: Median nerve compression in the carpal tunnel—functional response to experimentally induced controlled pressure. J Hand Surg 7(3):252, 1982.
13. Smith, EM, Sontegard, DA, Anderson, WH, Jr: Carpal tunnel syndrome: Contribution of flexor tendons. Arch Phys Med Rehabil 58:379, 1977.
14. Gelberman, RH, et al: Flexor tendon healing and restoration of the gliding surface. An ultrastructural study in dogs. J Bone Joint Surg 65:70, 1983.
15. Callahan, AD: Sensibility testing: State of the art. In Hunter, JM, et al (eds): Rehabilitation of the Hand, ed 2. CV Mosby, St Louis, 1984.

16. Gordon, G, Bowyr, BL, and Johnson, EW: Electrodiagnostic characteristics of acute carpal tunnel syndrome. Arch Phys Med Rehabil 68:545, 1987.
17. Wehbe, M and Hunter, JM: Flexor tendon gliding in the hand. Part II: Differential gliding. J Hand Surg 10a:575, 1985.
18. Wehbe, M: Tendon gliding exercises. Am J Occup Ther 41(3):164, 1987.
19. Walker, SE and Rehm, R: Hand therapy management for cumulative trauma disorders: Acute phase through work capacity testing. Lecture presented to the National Safety Council, March 20, 1984.
20. Armstrong, TJ and Chaffin, DB: Carpal tunnel and selected personal attributes. J Occup Med 21(7):481, 1979.
21. Walmsley, RP, et al: Eccentric wrist extensor contractions and the force velocity relationship in muscle. J Orth Sports Phys Ther, 8(6):288, 1986.
22. Zinovieff, AN: Heavy resistive exercises—the Oxford technique. Br J Phys Med 14–129, 1951.
23. Curtis, RM, Clark, GL, and Snyder, RA: The Work Simulator. In Hunter, JM, et al (eds): Rehabilitation of the Hand, ed 2. CV Mosby, St Louis, 1984.
24. Scott, J and Huskisson, E: Visual pain analogue. Pain 2:175, 1976.
25. Hunter, JM: Personal communication, September, 1988.
26. Hardy, MA, Moran, CA, and Merritt, WH: Densensitization of the traumatized hand. Va Med 109:134, 1982.
27. Nirschl, RP and Sobel, J: Conservative treatment of tennis elbow. The Physician and Sports Medicine 9(6):6, 1981.
28. Green, DP: Operative Hand Surgery. Vol I. Churchill Livingstone, 1982.
29. Fromison: Tenosynovitis and tennis elbow. In Green, DP (ed): Operative Hand Surgery. Churchill Livingstone, 1982.
30. Leach, R, and Miller, J: Lateral and medial epicondylitis of the elbow. Clin Sports Med 6:259, 1987.
31. Nirschl, R: Tennis elbow. Symposium on Sports Injuries. Orthop Clin North Am 4:787, 1972.
32. Nirschl, R: Conservative Treatment of Tennis Elbow. The Physician and Sports Medicine 9:43, 1981.
33. Travell, J and Simons, DG: Myofascial Pain and Dysfunction of the Trigger Point Manual. Baltimore, Williams & Wilkins, 1983.
34. Cyriax, J: The Elbow. In Cyriax, J (ed): Textbook of Orthopaedic Medicine, ed 8. Baillière Tindall, London, 1982, p 168.
35. Kendall, F: Lecture on manual muscle testing. Rehabilitation of the Hand Symposium, March 1988, Philadelphia.
36. Thurtle, O, Tyler, A, and Cawley, M: Grip strength as a measure of response to treatment of lateral epicondylitis (Letters to the Editor). Br J Rheumatol 23:154, 1984.
37. LaFrenier, J: Tennis elbow: Evaluation, treatment and prevention. Phys Ther 59:742, 1979.
38. Nirschl, R: Soft tissue injuries about the elbow. Clin Sports Med 5:637, 1986.
39. Nirschl, R: Muscle and tendon trauma: Tennis elbow. In Morrey, B (ed): The Elbow and Its Disorders. WB Saunders, Philadelphia, 1985, p 481.
40. Hunter, S and Poole, R: The Chronically Inflamed Tendon. Clin Sports Med 6:371, 1987.
41. Harvey, J: Tennis elbow: What's the best treatment? The Physician and Sports Medicine 18:62, 1990.
42. Binder, A, et al: Is therapeutic ultrasound effective in treating soft tissue lesions? Br Med J 290:512, 1985.
43. Nirschl, RP: Symposium on Treatment of Acute Hand Injuries. Washington Hand Symposium, Washington, DC, 1990.
44. Walker, JM: Deep transverse frictions in ligament healing. J Orthop Sports Phys Ther 6:89, 1984.
45. Curwin, S and Stanish, WD: Tendonitis: Etiology and Treatment. Collamore Press, DD Health, Lexington, MA, 1984.
46. Calliet, R: Hand Pain and Impairment. FA Davis, Philadelphia, 1981, p 119.
47. Mosley, LH: De Quervain's disease (stenosing tenosynovitis at the radial styloid) and trigger finger stenosing digital tenosynovitis. Lecture at the annual meeting of the National Hand Rehabilitation Center, Washington, DC, 1985.
48. Edmonson, A and Crenshaw, AH: Campbell's Operative Orthopaedics. Vol 1. CV Mosby, Philadelphia, 1980, p 363.
49. De Quervain, F: Korresp Bl Schweiz, Arz 25:389, 1985. In Cailliet, R: Hand Pain and Impairment. FA Davis, Philadelphia, p 119.

BIBLIOGRAPHY

Finkelstein, H: Stenosing tendovaginitis at the radial styloid process. J Bone Joint Surg 12:509, 1930.

Kirkpatrick, W: De Quervain's disease. In Hunter, JM, et al (eds): Rehabilitation of the Hand, ed 3. CV Mosby, St Louis, 1990, p 304.

McGrath, MH: Local steroid therapy in the hand. J Hand Surg 9A(6):915, 1984.

McKenzie, JMM: Conservative treatment of De Quervain's disease. Br Med J 4:659, 1972.

Medl, WT: Tendonitis, tenosynovitis, "trigger finger," and De Quervain's disease. Orthop Clin North Am 1(2):375, 1970.

Pick, RY: De Quervain's disease: A clinical triad. Clin Orthop 143:165, 1979.

Totten, P: Therapist's management of De Quervain's disease. In Hunter, JM, et al (eds): Rehabilitation of the Hand, ed 3. CV Mosby, St Louis, 1990, p 308.

CHAPTER 15

Reflex Sympathetic Dystrophy

Patricia A. Taylor Mullins, RPT, CHT

Reflex sympathetic dystrophy (RSD) is a complex of symptoms characterized by extreme pain, joint stiffness, diffuse edema, trophic skin changes, and vascular instability with discoloration. This complex of symptoms is a result of a neurochemical-controlled vasomotor phenomenon of the sympathetic nervous system. RSD is often confused with causalgia, Sudeck's atrophy, and shoulder hand syndrome. These diagnoses are not synonymous but are actually different classifications of the encompassing condition known as reflex sympathetic dystrophy.

The confusion associated with the syndrome of RSD and the various classifications reflects the difficulty in achieving proper diagnosis and treatment. For the clinician to intervene properly, he or she must understand not only the difference between the classifications but also the differences among the stages within each classification.

The objectives of this chapter are to (1) familiarize the clinician with the characteristics associated with RSD, (2) clarify the different classifications of RSD, (3) identify the three stages through which the condition (syndrome) may progress, and (4) present treatment techniques and rationale for the management of RSD throughout the three stages.

HISTORY

The earliest extensive reports of RSD were described by Silas Weir Mitchell, a neurologist, during the Civil War. He described a group of soldiers after they had sustained gunshot wounds in their extremities with subsequent partial injuries to the peripheral nerves. These patients often complained of a diffuse burning pain, which Mitchell termed "causalgia."[19]

Other writings described similar complaints of pain and disuse of the extremities without the accompanying nerve injury. One of the best known was that of Sudeck in 1900.[30] He described an injury without nerve involvement that led to an RSD appearance with accompanying bone demineralization. Sudeck called this condition "inflammatory bone atrophy."[30]

In 1916, Leriche[16] first theorized the presence of sympathetic involvement in the development of causalgia. This theory was validated by Spurling[27] in 1928. He performed a sympathectomy on a patient who developed causalgia following a gunshot wound. Total relief of pain was achieved by the procedure.

More recent writings are dominated by Omer and Thomas,[21] Lankford,[11,12] and Lankford and Thompson.[13] Though no further conditions were described than with the previous authors, Lankford established a format that delineated various characteristics of the syndrome, stages of disease, and intervention techniques. This classification formation will be used for the purpose of this chapter.

CLASSIFICATION

The characteristics of RSD are produced by an abnormal sympathetic reflex.[24] These diverse symptoms of RSD have led to a somewhat loose grouping of various clinical diagnoses such as shoulder-hand syndrome, causalgia, and Sudeck's atrophy. The difference between the different individual conditions described is important to understand. Lankford and Thompson[13] devised a distinct classification of RSD-related conditions that affords an easier understanding of the relationships of the various diagnoses (Fig. 15–1).

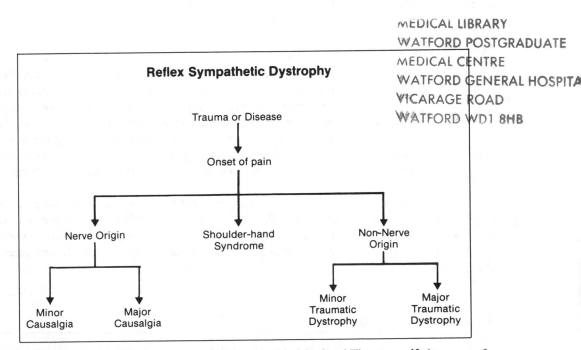

FIGURE 15–1. In a classification system devised by Lankford and Thompson,[13] the term reflex sympathetic dystrophy describes a group of vasomotor-trophic conditions. These conditions are linked by their origin from an abnormal sympathetic reflex. (From Mullins, PAT: Management of common chronic pain problems in the hand. Phys Ther 69:1050, 1989, with permission.)

Causalgia

Causalgia is the clinical type of RSD involving injury to a nerve, which is typically incomplete.[13] This classification can be divided further as a function of the degree of causalgia, depending on the size of the nerve that has been injured. The involvement of a small peripheral nerve is defined as minor causalgia, while involvement of a large peripheral nerve is referred to as major causalgia.

MINOR CAUSALGIA

Occurring in the smaller peripheral nerves, the symptoms involved with minor causalgia do not encompass the entire hand but are limited to a localized area in the hand or to a single digit. Because of the small area of involvement, the symptoms of swelling, stiffness, and pain are less severe than those seen in major causalgia. The precipitating cause is often a blow or laceration to a distal branch of a sensory nerve that leads to adhesion formation to the surrounding structures. One particularly susceptible area for an injury of this type is the dorsal superficial branch of the radial nerve. This susceptibility is due to the superficial pathway of this nerve as it lies on the dorsum of the forearm, making it prone to injury from external blows.[9] After an injury to this area, any stretching of the wrist into ulnar deviation or of the thumb into flexion causes pain over the distribution area.

What distinguishes the minor causalgia from a neuroma? A neuroma is painful only when touched; minor causalgia is painful at all times and is accompanied by other related symptoms of RSD such as edema or discoloration.[9]

MAJOR CAUSALGIA

Produced by an injury to a large peripheral nerve, major causalgia is characterized by an intense burning pain throughout the extremity.[11] This pain initially involves only the distribution of the injured nerve but may evolve to include the entire extremity.

As the pain intensifies after the injury, the patient is unable to use the hand. The hand is held protectively against the chest in a position of flexion. This posture is in contrast to other forms of RSD, which more typically display positioning in extension. The positioning can lead to flexion contractures in the joints, and these contractures are difficult to overcome.

The median nerve is the nerve most frequently involved in major causalgia of the upper extremity. Sunderland[31] found that this nerve along with the sciatic nerve in the lower extremity, has a much greater sympathetic nerve fiber population than do other peripheral nerves, which could be responsible for the increased sympathetic response to the injury.

Traumatic Dystrophy

Traumatic dystrophy, another form of RSD, can also be divided into minor and major types. Traumatic dystrophy follows generalized injury to tissue not of nerve origin such as bone or soft tissue.[11]

MINOR TRAUMATIC DYSTROPHY

An often overlooked form of RSD, minor traumatic dystrophy is probably the most common type of dystrophy seen in the clinic. The significance of minor traumatic dystrophy is often overlooked because of the fact that only a small segment of the hand is involved.

The cause of this type of dystrophy is often a minor injury, such as a sprained joint or a crushed fingertip. The pain in the digit impedes use, and the adjacent joints become stiff; in some cases, contractures result.

MAJOR TRAUMATIC DYSTROPHY

Major traumatic dystrophy, like major causalgia, has received at lot of attention because of the large proportion of the extremity involved. Major traumatic dystrophy produces the greatest amount of pain for an injury not of nerve origin.

This type of dystrophy usually follows a more severe trauma, such as a forearm fracture or crush injury to the hand. More than 50% of the cases of RSD reportedly occur after peripheral bone fractures.[25] Owing to the severity of these injuries, acute carpal tunnel syndrome, which furthers the development of RSD may develop. Lankford[12] reported that a high percentage of patients who developed RSD following Colles' fractures also displayed carpal tunnel syndrome after the initial injury.

Traumatic dystrophy may also occur after a surgical procedure such as a Dupuytren's release. As with major causalgia, the degree of pain, stiffness, and edema can lead to a total dysfunction of the hand with possible development of joint contractures in the digits and wrist. For reasons not totally understood, these same fractures or surgical procedures may occur in the majority of the population without resultant RSD.

Shoulder-Hand Syndrome

The shoulder-hand syndrome is characterized by pain that originates in the shoulder and spreads to the entire upper extremity. The cause of the initial shoulder pain may be trauma such as a rotator cuff injury, or some other factor such as adhesive capsulitis. This syndrome may also develop secondary to a disease process such as heart attack or stroke.

The pain posture of the hand in this classification is somewhat different from that described in causalgia because the fingers are held in extension. Contractures may develop in this position posturing, leading to dysfunction in the hand.

CHARACTERISTICS

There are many characteristics or symptoms of RSD displayed early in the stages of development that remain throughout the duration of the problem. Though not all of these characteristics may be present in each patient, the development of two or three of these clinical manifestations should be a key to the clinician that intervention should begin before a serious problem develops.

Reported symptoms of RSD include pain in 97% of the patients and joint stiffness in 88% of the patient population. Further symptoms include edema (69%), trophic changes (60%), and hyperesthesia (69%).[29] Other less frequent but reported symptoms include bone demineralization in the involved area and changes in skin color and temperature.

Pain

Pain is the most common and universal complaint of patients with RSD. When reported, the degree of this pain seems disproportionate to the injury. In the early stages of RSD, movement of the joints in the involved area causes pain. Later, as the RSD becomes more pronounced, patients describe the pain as constant. In a severe case of RSD, the patient may complain that even movement of air over the involved area increases the pain.

This pain is thought to be perpetuated partly through the presence of an abnormal sympathetic reflex. Afferent fibers carrying pain impulses are theorized to be the small-diameter, slow-conducting, nonmyelinated C fibers and the thinly myelinated A-delta fibers. As the patient with RSD postures the hand to prevent motion, no afferent stimulation from the large-diameter, myelinated A-alpha and beta fibers occurs from proprioceptive input due to motion. According to the Melzack and Wall[18] gate control theory of pain, such proprioceptive input could block the small-diameter afferent impulses and relieve pain. With no large afferent fiber impulses, an abnormal sympathetic reflex arc develops that continues to trigger small fiber impulses without relief, thus intensifying the pain (Fig. 15-2). Descriptions of the pain usually involve a burning sensation. Other descriptions may include throbbing, deep aching, cramping, flashing hot and cold sensations, or a complaint of an unusual increased pressure in the hand.

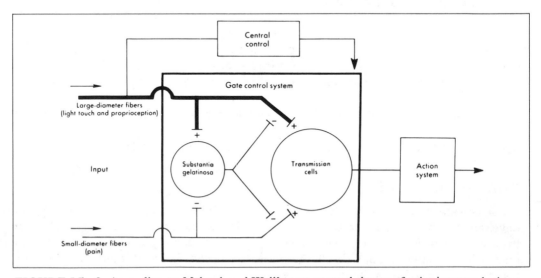

FIGURE 15-2. According to Melzack and Wall's gate-control theory of pain, increased stimulation of large-diameter fibers through motion and pressure will close the gate or block stimulation from small-diameter fibers. Absence of large-diameter fiber stimulation allows increased flow of small-diameter fiber stimulation and opens the gate for pain. (From Melzack, R and Wall, PD: Pain mechanisms: A new theory. Science 150:971, 1965, with permission.)

Stiffness

As with pain, joint stiffness results from a loss of motion that greatly exceeds the expected normal response following the injury. A crush injury to a single fingertip may lead to stiffness in all three joints of the involved digit. Even the joints of an adjacent digit may become painful to touch and resistant to motion. For example, a commonly observed problem following a Colles' fracture is generalized joint stiffness in the wrist and digits, even though the digits were free to allow motion while the patient was in a cast.

The development of limited joint motion may occur rapidly and increase with time. The resultant stiffness is further aggravated by the presence of pain. Any joint movement increases pain, leading patients to position the hand protectively in a manner to prevent motion and pain.

Edema

Another common characteristic early in RSD is extreme edema. This edema appears first as a soft fusiform swelling often relieved by retrograde massage. Later, the edema becomes hard and brawny with localization in the dorsum of the hand (Fig. 15–3).

Skin Temperature and Color Changes

When observed over a long time, the involved extremity may show temperature fluctuations from cold to hot. Early in the process the hand may have a cold, clammy feeling with a cyanotic appearance and an unusual degree of sweating, or hyperhidrosis.

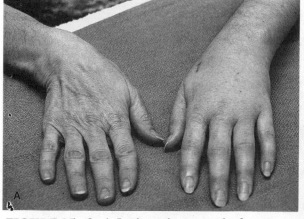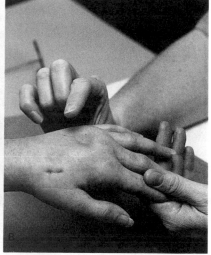

FIGURE 15–3. *A*, In the early stages of reflex sympathetic dystrophy, generalized edema is present. This edema is often localized over the dorsum of the hand in the metacarpal and PIP joint areas. *B*, The edema is usually of a pitting nature, as indicated by the indentation that remains once the pressure is removed.

Associated vasoconstriction is present at this stage. These characteristics may then change to a generalized hot feeling with redness and dry skin, indicating vasodilatation of the vessels. The increased heat of the skin may be localized over the joints, particularly the metacarpophalangeal (MP) and proximal interphalangeal (PIP) joints, with red patches often present.

Bone Demineralization

Another characteristic of RSD is seen radiographically as demineralization begins to take place in the bones of the hand. Initially represented as a localized area about the joints, over time the demineralization progresses to become more diffuse and involves the long bones of the hand. This bone demineralization is the process Sudeck[30] described as "inflammatory bone atrophy." Figure 15–4 is a radiograph demonstrating bone demineralization.

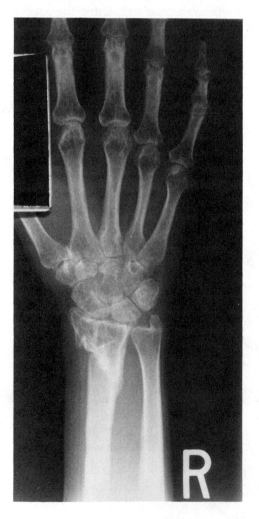

FIGURE 15–4. Radiographic changes are seen in the hand with bone demineralization. This demineralization is initially concentrated in the joint areas and carpus but later advances to involve the long bones of the hand.

Trophic Changes

Another change in appearance of the hand occurs as the skin becomes tight and shiny. This change occurs initially because of the degree of edema and continues with prolonged immobilization and the poor nutrition associated with this immobilization. Later in the disease process, the fingertips may develop a pencil-point appearance secondary to atrophy. The fingernails may grow thick and become curved. This appearance is similar to that seen in peripheral nerve injuries. Some writers have speculated that these changes are due to abnormal sympathetic activity.

STAGES

To compound the difficulty in confirming the diagnosis of RSD, there is great variance in the clinical manifestation from patient to patient, with not all characteristics present at the same time. Established patterns or stages of disease exist in RSD, with differing characteristics in each stage.[13] The disease progresses from stage 1, or the acute process of the disease state, to the more chronic stage 3 level of RSD. Not all patients will exhibit the classic characteristics or symptoms of each stage. The length of time these symptoms persist varies. For example, although one patient's symptoms may resolve in stage 1, another patient's symptoms may quickly progress to stage 2 and linger there for several months.

Stage 1

Pain is the most significant complaint in stage 1 RSD. Development of joint stiffness begins to occur from protective posturing and becomes progressively worse throughout the stage. Edema is present, particularly over the interphalangeal (IP) joints and dorsum of the hand; at this stage the edema is soft and pitting. Initially the skin is cold and clammy, it becomes dry and hot later in stage 1.

The final characteristic to develop in stage 1 is the radiographically confirmed demineralization. This change takes about 3 to 5 weeks to develop following the initial intense pain, edema, and joint stiffness. Stage 1 may last approximately 3 months.

Stage 2

In stage 2, the soft edema described in stage 1 becomes hard and brawny. This edema, unlike the soft edema, does not respond to retrograde massage and is difficult to manage. Pain continues to intensify with an associated hyperesthesia to light touch. This pain is easily aggravated with motion. Owing to the pain and the edema, joint stiffness increases. The skin is dry and hot with a generalized warmness, and the patient's skin begins to appear glossy and shiny. All of these factors lead to a disuse pattern of the hand, increasing the demineralization to a more diffuse pattern. This stage of the disease may last for approximately 3 to 9 months.

Stage 3

In the final stage, pain symptoms may peak with a gradual resolution. By this phase, the joints are extremely stiff and may display a periarticular thickening. The edema has subsided, accentuating this joint enlargement. The skin cools but remains dry and shiny. Muscle atrophy and contractures may be observed. The patient's hand may be less painful but is nonfunctional.

ETIOLOGY

Discussion of RSD stimulates the question about why some patients develop this problem while most do not. The extensive work on RSD by Lankford,[12] and Lankford and Thompson[13] indicates that three factors must be present for this condition to occur:

1. Painful lesion, either from trauma or disease
2. Diathesis or a predisposition of the individual patient to develop the problem
3. Abnormal sympathetic reflex

Painful Lesion

In patients developing RSD, a specific occurrence initiates the syndrome. This initial incident may be a trauma such as a Colles' fracture or crushed fingertip, or may be a disease process such as an arthritic flare-up or heart attack. The common factor between the initial lesions is the body's disproportionate response to the initial problem.

Diathesis

Certain patients have an inherent tendency to develop RSD; this diathasis may be physiologic or psychologic.

Patients in the physiologic diathesis group have a tendency to be hypersympathetic.[23] When questioned about their body status previous to injury, they may give a history of cold intolerance in their fingers or toes, or they may have regularly experienced sweaty palms.

Cigarette smoking may be a factor in development of RSD. In one study of a group of RSD patients, 68 percent of the group smoked regularly. The hypothesis is that cigarette smoking may be involved by enhancing sympathetic activity and vasoconstriction.[3]

Prediction of those patients who may develop RSD based on their psychologic traits is more difficult. One study[6] designed to evaluate a group of RSD patients used the Buhler-Coleman Life Goals Inventory and the Minnesota Multiphasic Personality Inventory (MMPI). The results indicated that many of these patients display a low pain threshold with a tendency to allow pain to dominate their lives. These patients were also characterized as insecure and dependent.[34] Another study,[36] using the MMPI to evaluate patients with RSD, discover that these patients scored higher on the depression, hysteria, and hypochondrical scales. Though such results are interesting, conclusions should not be drawn based on the psychologic traits that the patient with RSD is a malingerer or psychosomatic. At this preliminary stage of investigation, however, it is advised that these factors should be kept in mind when developing goals and rehabilitation programs for these patients.

Abnormal Sympathetic Reflex

The third component necessary for development of RSD is an abnormal sympathetic reflex.[24] After hand trauma that elicits a normal sympathetic reflex, afferent fibers send a pain stimulus to the posterior root ganglion into the posterior horn, and then into the lateral horn, where the stimulus reaches the sympathetic nerve cells (Fig. 15–5). The stimulus then activates the sympathetic reflex in which efferent fibers leave the anterior horn, entering the sympathetic chain at the sympathetic ganglion. At this point a synapse occurs in the postganglionic fiber and the efferent fiber leaves the ganglia and enters the peripheral nerve. Upon reaching the distal extremity, the stimulus causes vasoconstriction in the vessels. Vasoconstriction in the vessels is normal following an injury and is necessary to prevent excessive bleeding. After a few hours this vasoconstriction changes to vasodilation, a part of the reparative process that begins a normal wound healing process.[24] In an abnormal reflex, vasoconstriction continues for an abnormally long time. Ischemia resulting from this vasoconstriction causes pain. Such

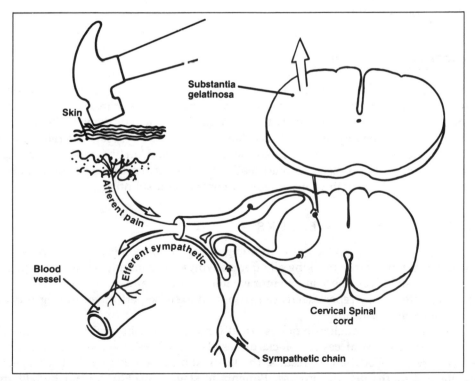

FIGURE 15–5. A normal sympathetic reflex arc resulting in vasoconstriction is initiated by painful stimulus or injury. When prolonged and uncontrolled, the abnormal reflex can lead to development of reflex sympathetic dystrophy. (From Mullins, PAT: Management of common chronic pain problems in the hand. Phys Ther 69:1050, 1989, with permission.)

pain further increases afferent fiber activity, once again initiating vasoconstriction. This cycle is the abnormal sympathetic reflex indicative of RSD.[31]

DIAGNOSIS

Diagnosis of RSD is based on the observation of the major characteristics of pain, edema, and joint stiffness. These characteristics occur in a magnitude disproportionate to the initial injury, and progressively become worse. Other symptoms may also be present such as hyperhidrosis and skin coloration changes. When these characteristics are observed, radiographic presence of demineralization will further confirm the diagnosis of RSD. Thermography has been used to detect temperature changes in the extremity associated with prolonged vasoconstriction.[32] The most definitive diagnostic tool comes when blocking the sympathetic arc actually produces some relief in the patient's clinical condition.

TREATMENT

Treatment of RSD begins with appropriate early intervention by physician and therapist.[5] No single established treatment protocol is successful for all patients, but a variety of intervention techniques are used depending on the individual clinical presentation and response to treatment.

Medical Intervention

Effective intervention in patients with RSD requires a cooperative management program between an empathetic physician and therapist. The primary goal is to eliminate the abnormal sympathetic reflex to relieve the cause of symptoms.[24] The intervention techniques commonly used by physicians to relieve the sympathetic reflex include use of stellate ganglion blocks, sympatholytic drugs, and, in the most severe cases, sympathectomy. The physician should realize the role of the therapist for comanagement of these patients with exercise, edema control, and splinting.

STELLATE GANGLION BLOCKS

Stellate ganglion blocks require an analgesic agent to be injected into the sympathetic ganglia, temporarily blocking all efferent sympathetic impulses into the extremity. After a successful block, the skin will immediately warm up and return to a more normal color. The patient may report decreased pain, and exercise performed during this time will be much less painful.

A single stellate ganglion block is usually not effective in total relief of the RSD pattern. Usually 4 to 6 successive blocks are used over a 3-week period before complete relief is observed. For the best results, the block should be initiated during stage 1 or early stage 2 of the disease process. Patients in stage 3 usually do not benefit from sympathetic ganglion blocks.

The administration of a stellate ganglion block is often difficult and requires a thorough understanding of the regional anatomy and possible drug response to the injection. The injection is most often performed by an anesthesiologist in a facility where equipment necessary to treat possible anaphylactic shock reaction is available.

The injection is performed from an anterior approach into the stellate ganglion which lies anterior to the seventh cervical lateral mass. The medication consists of a solution of either 1% Xylocaine or 0.5% Marcaine.[20] With proper injection of the agent, the patient will develop a Horner's sign with drooping of the eyelid, pupil constriction, and warming of the ipsilateral side of the face. The first signs of the block may be apparent within 5 to 10 minutes of the injection.

The associated interrupted function of the sympathetic nerve fibers will last approximately 2 hours with the Xylocaine and 10 to 18 hours with the Marcaine, but there may be an interruption of the hyperactivity of the sympathetic reflex for several days. Further blocks are held until return of this hyperactivity is noted with its associated symptoms.

SYMPATHOLYTIC DRUGS

An alternative to the use of a stellate ganglion block would be the use of oral medication to inhibit the sympathetic function. Most of these medications are alpha-adrenergic blocking agents and have the effect of decreasing the vasoconstriction of the vessels in the extremity. These medications may also produce orthostatic hypotension and therefore should be used with caution.

Dibenzyline[8,10] is the most commonly used and the most effective of these agents. Other, less frequently used, agents include Regitine and Priscoline. These medications are all effective alpha-adrenergic blockers, but the Regitine and Priscoline cause side effects not seen in Dibenzyline use.

Another sympatholytic agent used is reserpine, which acts through a catecholamine or norepinephrine depleting action on the vessel wall. Given by intra-arterial or intravenous injection, reserpine is more difficult to administer than oral medication because its administration requires medical assistance with each dose.[21] Oral administration of this medication is possible but requires such a high dosage to be effective that systemic side effects are observed.

Most of the clinical advances being made in the care of the patient with RSD are occurring in the area of drug intervention. The author encourages review of the most current medical literature in this everchanging subject.

SYMPATHECTOMY

In severe cases of RSD or in cases of late intervention, stellate ganglion blocks may not be successful. In these cases it may be necessary to perform a surgical sympathectomy before relief of the abnormal sympathetic reflex is achieved.

After a simple sympathectomy, the greatest change is the drastic decrease in pain.[35] Improvement in circulation results in less edema and better skin color.[17] The decreased pain and edema allow a more productive exercise program to increase range of motion (ROM).

A surgical sympathectomy may leave the patient with a permanent Horner's syndrome. If care is taken to remove only the upper thoracic ganglia, Horner's syndrome is seldom seen.

Therapeutic Intervention

Hand rehabilitation is essential in treating RSD. The presentation of a severely involved RSD patient can be overwhelming with the many clinical problems manifested. The therapy program must be vigorous enough to be beneficial without increasing pain and perpetuating the problem. Therapists must be patient and evaluate the results of each session to determine if the program should be adjusted.

EVALUATION

In RSD, initial evaluation requires observation of many aspects of the patient. The patient with RSD should be questioned as to the degree of pain and whether motion increases the pain. The hand is palpated to determine skin temperature and the quality of the edema—whether it is soft and pitting or hard and brawny. The therapist should record passive and active ROM measurements and determine whether limitations are due to joint tightness or lack of tendon excursion.

Information received from the evaluation helps set priorities in treatment goals. To provide an effective rehabilitation program, periodic evaluations should be performed to ascertain the response of the patient to treatment. If pain limits the exercise program, then the primary initial goal is to control the pain. When pain is under control, the program should be adjusted to concentrate on gaining ROM and controlling edema.

The rest of the chapter discusses the use of exercise, modalities, and splinting techniques commonly used to manage RSD.

EXERCISE PROGRAM

In the early stages of RSD all exercises should be gentle and active. Exercise is needed to overcome the rapidly increasing stiffness but a too-vigorous exercise program may actually increase the pain, causing the joints to become more reactive and stiff. The best program is to support and slowly exercise each joint actively for a short time and then to teach the patient the importance of following such a program every hour at home. Brief exercise programs activate large afferent fiber stimulation, which decreases pain impulses.[18] Brief exercise also causes less tissue reaction than do vigorous, long exercise programs. In addition to the exercises of isolated joint motion, the program should include hook fisting and full fisting to achieve differential tendon gliding.

As pain begins to decrease, gentle passive range of motion (PROM) and joint mobilization can be initiated. An increase in pain or edema alerts the therapist that PROM was too forceful and may need to be temporarily discontinued. After a sympathetic block, pain reduction may be sufficient to let the therapist perform some passive joint mobilization without causing pain. During this time, care should be taken to avoid stressing the joints and gaining large increases in passive motion.

While monitoring progress in the joints of the hand, evaluation of stiffness in the adjacent joints, such as the shoulder and elbow, should not be overlooked. The shoulder in particular may quickly become painful and stiff during the RSD process because of protective positioning and reluctance on the part of the patient to move the extremity. An active exercise program of the uninvolved joints should be developed to prevent stiffness. As a patient progresses through stage 3, the pain begins to "burn out," or decrease. This is a time when more vigorous passive motion can be instituted. Unfortunately, at this stage the joints are often so limited that little response to exercise or splinting is seen. If no objective improvement in joint motion or function is seen for several weeks, the surgeon may consider surgical intervention to gain motion, such as performing capsulotomies at the MP or IP joints.

MASSAGE

Retrograde massage is a useful tool in early management. In stage 1, the edema is soft and pitting and responds well to massage.[28] Massage should be performed before exercise to aid in decreasing the bulk of the fingers. Retrograde massage will alleviate some of the tight feeling and thereby encourage further active exercise. Performing massage after exercise may help to decrease the reactive edema sometimes seen after exercise.

In stage 2, as the edema becomes more brawny, retrograde massage will have little effect. During this stage the brawny edema can be softened by applying heat before exercise.

THERAPEUTIC MODALITIES

Thermal Modalities

Many therapists are reluctant to use heat with RSD as they fear it will cause increased edema. The use of vigorous heat should be avoided in stage 1 because of the presence of acute edema. Heat can produce a mild inflammatory response, if applied in a vigorous fashion, leading to release of histamine. This release of histamine and bradykinin acts on vessels to cause vasodilation, allowing fluid filtration into the extra-vascular space, which can cause a mild edema.[18a] However, heat application has many positive effects such as increased tissue extensibility, decreased joint stiffness, and increased blood flow.[14] The apprehension over causing edema can be overcome by applying heat with the limb held in an elevated position, using gravity to assist in venous and lymphatic flow. Evaluation of edema before and after heat will aid in determining the appropriateness of the heat application. In stage 3, heat application will not cause more edema and should be used vigorously to increase tissue extensibility. Different forms of heat are available, each with different qualities.

Hot Packs. Application of moist heat or hot packs before exercise is effective in decreasing pain and increasing tissue extensibility with exercise.[14] Hot packs are the easiest form of heat to apply to the limb held in an elevated fashion. If joint stiffness is limited to the hand, this procedure can be performed while seated with the hand propped on a foam wedge or pillow to ensure elevation. If the shoulder also needs heat, it is best to have the patient supine, allowing elevation of the entire extremity.

Whirlpool. Whirlpool is often used in therapy with the idea that active exercises can be performed while the hand is underwater. However, whirlpool is not the preferred choice for heat application with RSD. Studies[26,33] show that the dependent position of the extremity actually increases edema. Because increased edema is one of the primary symptoms in the development of RSD, whirlpool should be avoided. The only indication for whirlpool use would be in the presence of an open wound where the whirlpool is needed for debridement. Whirlpool should then be followed with elevation, massage, and exercise to overcome possible edema formation.

Paraffin. In the later stages of RSD, paraffin use is effective in conjunction with passive stretch to increase joint mobility. This stretch can be obtained by application of

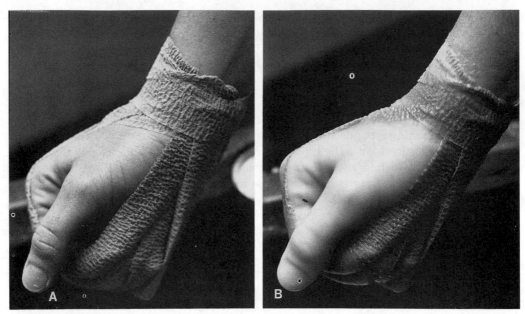

FIGURE 15–6. Application of Coban to pull the fingers into passive flexion (*A*), is followed by dipping the hand into paraffin (*B*). This is an effective means of applying stretch while tissue is being heated.

Coban* pulling the fingers into a flexed position, followed by dipping into the paraffin (Fig. 15–6). The patient may not tolerate the use of paraffin during early stages of RSD because the temperature of the paraffin is greater than that of hot packs, which may cause discomfort in the hypersensitive hand.

   Ultrasound. Ultrasound can be effective when the tissues to be heated before exercise cannot be reached by the more superficial forms of heat such as hot packs.[14] Ultrasound over individual finger joints can aid in increasing extensibility of the joint structures, thereby allowing increased ROM. If limited flexor tendon glide prevents good motion, use of ultrasound can lead to increasing extensibility of motion-limiting adhesions at a deeper level than other forms of heat.[15]

   Fluidotherapy. Fluidotherapy,† a form of dry heat, circulates a dry medium or particles about the hand to cause increases in tissue temperature.[4] The texture stimulation from the particle bombardment to the hand can be effective in desensitization. Fluidotherapy cannot be performed in an elevated position. If Fluidotherapy is to be used for desensitization when edema is a concern, a low temperature setting is recommended.

Electrical Modalities

   The use of various electrical modalities has been advocated to help control RSD. Goals include decreasing pain, decreasing edema, and increasing muscle strength. Each

---

*3M Medical Surgical Division, St. Paul, MN 55144-1000.
†Henley International, 104 Industrial Blvd., Sugarland, TX 77478.

form of stimulation has its merits, but evaluation of individual patient problems is necessary to ensure judicious use.

Transcutaneous Electrical Nerve Stimulators. The use of transcutaneous electrical nerve stimulators (TENS) to decrease pain has been a useful adjunct in the rehabilitation process.[2,18] The associated decrease in pain facilitates exercise and increases functional use of the hand. TENS should be applied in the early stages of RSD when pain is greatest. While the patient is undergoing a series of stellate ganglion blocks, the TENS may be used between injections to lengthen the time of decreased pain.

TENS may bring only partial relief of pain to this group of patients. This fact should be presented to the individual patient to avoid unrealistic expectations and disappointments. The patient should turn the unit off for increasing periods of time to avoid dependence on the unit. Further discussion of the use of TENS appears in Chapter 8.

High-Voltage Galvanic Stimulation. High-voltage galvanic stimulation (HVGS) used with parameters of a low-pulse rate stimulation can activate a muscle-pump action in the extremity to aid both in venous return and decreasing edema.[36] The intensity of stimulation should be sufficient to create a muscle contraction, while also affording comfort to the patient. In my experience, stimulation is tolerated well by this patient group, and the facilitation of the muscle contraction seems to encourage the patient's active exercise program in the early stages. Volumetric measurements taken before and after stimulation will assist in the decision regarding its effectiveness.

Functional Electrical Stimulation. Muscles immobilized for long periods of time owing to painful posturing or cast immobilization may benefit from facilitation achieved with functional electrical stimulation units. The alternating current stimulation can be used in any stage of the disease. For example, stimulation of the wrist extensors after removal of the cast in a Colles' fracture will elicit wrist extension independent of finger extension.

Patients with RSD have a difficult time tolerating a stimulus sufficient to elicit a strong contraction of the extrinsic finger flexors. The proximity of the motor points in these muscles to the sensory fibers of the median nerve may aggravate the hypersensitivity, causing increased pain.

STRESS LOADING

One form of exercise that has gained attention in treatment of RSD is stress loading.[7] This technique involves active exercises that require stressful use of the upper extremity without forcing joint motion. The success of this exercise is based on the application of pressure or resistance to the hand, which increases the large fiber afferent impulses which, in turn, helps relieve pain.[18]

Stress-loading programs described by Carlson and Watson[7] involve the patient using a scrub brush for resistive application of pressure (Fig. 15-7). To be the most beneficial, stress loading should be initiated in stage 1 or 2 of RSD when pain is greatest.

CONTINUOUS PASSIVE MOTION DEVICES

The use of continuous passive motion (CPM) devices has gained popularity recently. The theory behind the effectiveness of CPM is based largely on studies by Akeson and associates,[1] in which increased tissue nutrition is seen with passive motion compared with immobilization. CPM has been advocated in various conditions, including RSD. Used periodically during the day or at night, the device passively moves the

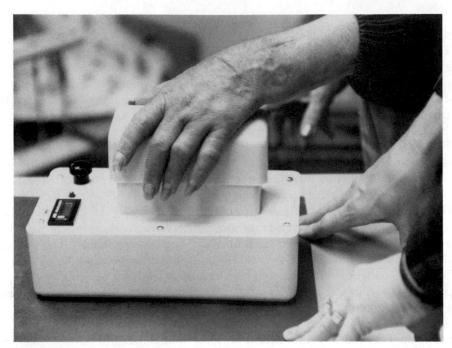

FIGURE 15–7. Some studies report decrease of pain after applying pressure stimulation to the extremity during exercise programs.[7] The figure depicts use of a Dystrophile (Joint-Jack, 108 Britt Road, East Hartford, CT 06118) to achieve this goal.

finger joints through their ROM (Fig. 15–8). The goal of using CPM is not to passively force the joints into greater motion but rather to move the joints through the comfort range. Reports from clinicians of decreased edema and pain warrant the use of CPM devices even though research studies have not been performed to support the theory.

CPM devices are not meant to replace active motion but to serve as an addition to the more conventional rehabilitation program. Continuation of active range of motion (AROM) programs is extremely important to maintain tendon gliding.

SPLINTING

Splinting is important in the rehabilitation of RSD. In the initial painful stages of RSD, splinting can be effective because it rests the hand. The resting splint should position the wrist in approximately 10° to 20° of extension, the MP joints in 60° to 70° of flexion, and the IP joints in extension. The patient should understand that the splint is not to be worn at all times, as this discourages active motion and use of the hand. Using the splint at night or for periodic day use may increase patient comfort, thus allowing sleep.

As described earlier in the text, the fingers can assume either an extended or a flexed posture as a result of the pain from RSD. Long-term posturing in these positions, coupled with chronic edema, can lead to joint contractures. These contractures may present as MP joint extension contractures, PIP flexion contractures, or PIP extension contractures. Quite often, the PIP joints may be limited in both flexion and extension.

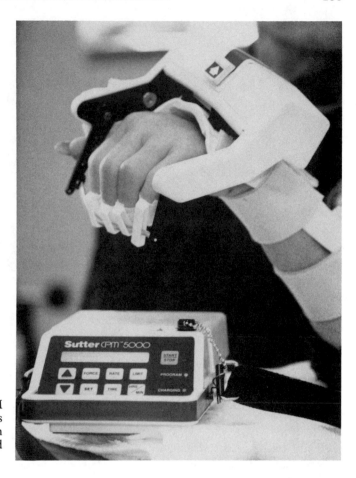

FIGURE 15-8. Use of CPM devices for intermittent periods during the day to maintain joint mobility has had reported clinical success.

Individual evaluation of each patient is necessary to determine the necessary splinting. Dynamic splinting can be used effectively in later stages of RSD to manage the developing contractures, but care must be taken to avoid excessive dynamic force which may cause an exacerbation in the pain cycle. Dynamic splints should be worn briefly, 20 to 30 minutes at a time, several times a day. This will help prevent reactive pain and edema.

Serial static splinting can be used on individual PIP joints to increase extension. The splints are applied with the joint in maximum extension and worn for 6 to 8 hours at a time. On each therapy visit, the splints are examined and adjusted as PIP extension increases. Serial casting to individual PIP joints may also be used, but these casts are typically worn at all times which does not allow for daily exercise programs.

A splinting program using a combination of different splints to achieve different goals is the most effective. In those patients who lack MP and PIP joint flexion, periodic use of dynamic flexion splinting during the day can be initiated while using static serial splinting at night to increase PIP extension (Fig. 15-9).

Patients should not be overwhelmed by the use of several different splints. Although there may be many joints that could benefit from splinting, no more than two splints should be provided at a time. As an improvement is observed in one area, a new splint can be fabricated for another area. By limiting the splinting program the patient

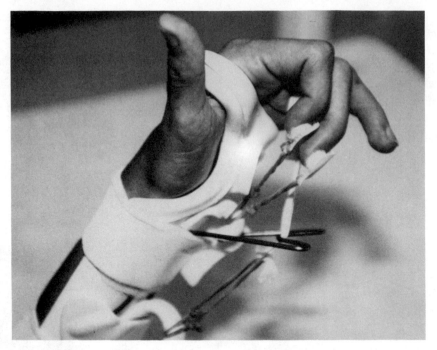

FIGURE 15–9. One complication of long-term reflex sympathetic dystrophy is joint contractures. Each digit must be evaluated and splinted based on individual deficits.

will not become frustrated with the daily splint schedule, and this may cause more compliance with splint usage.

FUNCTIONAL ACTIVITIES

Use of functional activities can be very beneficial with RSD patients. As a therapist works on an exercise program with these patients, it may be difficult for patients to relate such a program to the ability to use the hand in functional activities at home. Initiation of craft activities in the clinic will help patients develop confidence in the functional ability of their hand. The therapist may find it useful to initiate these programs under clinical supervision rather than give the patient tasks to be performed at home. When functional activities are performed in the clinic, the therapist is present to reinforce the activity, increasing the patient's confidence. These activities can begin in stage 1 and 2 with simple pegboard activities and progress to more difficult activities, such as leatherwork, in later stages. Each accomplishment will encourage patients to view their hand as a functional part of their body and will bring a realization that their hand is capable of returning to a more normal state.

STRENGTHENING

As with any longstanding disability, disuse leads to weakness in the involved extremity. In the final stages of rehabilitation, edema may be absent and joint stiffness greatly improved, yet continued weakness may prevent functional use of the hand. To gain further use of the hand, the therapist should begin a strength and endurance program.

The aforementioned functional activities may be capable of maintaining some level of endurance for the extremity. Endurance can be increased by lengthening the periods of time spent in craft projects. Although functional activities may improve dexterity and endurance, they do not adequately increase strength. To increase strength, it will also be necessary to initiate a direct strengthening program.

Inexpensive exercise equipment that can be used at home includes Theraputty or the rubberband-resisted Hand Helper. These are compact and easy for patients to use independently but do not address all muscle groups of the upper extremity. Use of exercise equipment such as the BTE Work Simulator or Cybex can then provide a dynamic resistive program that can resist all muscle groups.

The BTE Work Simulator can be initiated with low resistance and can be increased in both resistance and time of use as the patient improves. Multiple tool end devices allow a multitude of exercise regimens (Fig. 15–10). As the patient works, the equipment will display information relating to the amount of force being applied and the distance that the exercise arm has been moved. The display screen serves as a motivating device for the patient allowing them to see objective feedback on their improvement.

If strengthening equipment is not available or if the patient is unable to return to the clinic on a regular basis, a home program of exercises becomes the primary treatment tool. A combination of Theraputty or a Hand Helper in addition to Theraband and cuff weights can be used as an independent home program. Exercises should be incorporated for the entire upper extremity.

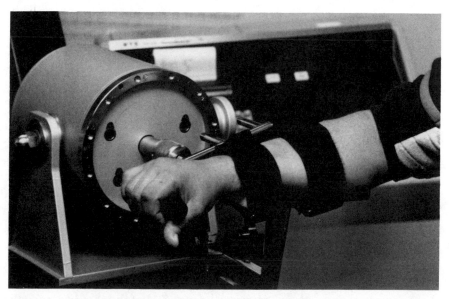

FIGURE 15–10. Use of BTE with its various tools offers a variety of resistive exercises.

CLINICAL DECISION MAKING—CASE STUDY

GD is a 34-year-old right hand–dominant man who was employed as a painter. While at work he fell from a ladder, landing on his extended wrist, which resulted in an open Colles' fracture to the right forearm.

SURGICAL REPORT

To achieve maximum alignment and stabilization, an external fixator was applied on the day of injury to immobilize the fracture. Three days after the stabilization, decompression of the median nerve was necessary secondary to the development of an acute carpal tunnel syndrome.

THERAPEUTIC MANAGEMENT
Stage 1 RSD: 1 to 3 Months

The patient was referred to hand therapy 4 weeks after injury, when the physician noted an undue amount of pain and edema in the involved hand.

Initial Evaluation

Upon evaluation, the patient exhibited soft fusiform edema throughout the hand. Circumferential measurements were taken of the MP and IP joints as the fixator prevented volumetric measurements. ROM in the hand was extremely limited with pain elicited on movement of the joints. The proximal elbow and shoulder joints revealed no limitations or pain with motion. General appearance of the skin was reddened and shiny, with localized increased redness over the MP and IP joints. The initial AROM measurements were as follows:

AROM	MP	PIP	DIP
Thumb	10/20	15	
Index	30/45	20/55	20
Middle	35/50	15/60	20
Ring	30/60	15/55	25
Little	20/35	20/60	30

Treatment Goals

The initial therapy program for the patient included goals of edema control, increased joint mobility, and pain relief.

Edema Control. Retrograde massage was performed with the patient and was included in the home program. The edema was responsive to this form of massage as indicated by a decrease in circumferential measurements. The patient also reported decrease in pain after massage.

Range of Motion. Gentle AROM was performed with stabilization of the individual fingers to minimize pain during the exercise. The patient was given a written home program of exercises and encouraged to perform the exercises for short periods of time, several times each day. ROM of the shoulder and elbow was within normal limits and AROM exercises were initiated to maintain the motion.

A resting splint was applied to hold the hand in a protected position when not exercising. Adjustments were made as needed to ensure fit around the fixating device.

Pain Control. Application of a TENS unit, using the conventional mode of treatment, proved only moderately successful. Electrode placement was attempted both proximally at the shoulder and distally at the hand. The position of the fixator made the application of the electrodes difficult as the rods were located in the desired electrode placement area.

Some relief of pain was seen as edema decreased and joint motion increased. The high level of pain prevented the patient from complying with all aspects of therapy program. Because of limited success from TENS, the referring physician began to consider the patient a candidate for a series of stellate ganglion blocks for pain control.

Sensibility Evaluation. Because of the necessary decompression of the median nerve, periodic evaluations were performed to evaluate the level of sensation. The tools used in these evaluations were the Semmes-Weinstein monofilaments to test pressure threshold and calipers to test two-point discrimination of the fingertips.

Desensitization. Hypersensitivity was present in all fingertips, particularly those in the median nerve distribution. As the fixator prevented use of Fluidotherapy for desensitization, the patient was instructed in application of various textures and objects to the fingertips periodically during the day to desensitize the fingers.

Functional Activities. The patient was started on light functional activities early in the rehabilitation process. The position of the wrist immobilization limited some activities, but pegboard and beading activities were possible with adaptive positioning of the projects.

Stage 2 RSD: 3 Months

Reevaluation

Before total removal of immobilization for the fracture, the patient was advanced from an external fixator to cast immobilization. At the time of reevaluation there was no form of immobilization and patient was free to move all joints of the hand and forearm. Radiographic evaluation by the physician revealed a generalized demineralization throughout the hand.

The edema had changed to a brawny, hard edema. Pain continued with hyperesthesia to light touch, and pain was elicited with joint motion. The skin was red, dry, and hot to touch.

Sensibility evaluation using the Semmes-Weinstein monofilaments continued to show a gradual return of sensation in the median nerve distribution.

Because of the degree of pain and stiffness, the physician chose to intervene with a series of stellate ganglion blocks. The patient was hospitalized, allowing ease of postinjection therapy. After a series of three injections in 1 week, the pain was greatly reduced, allowing a more vigorous exercise program. Discoloration was greatly improved, with less redness and warmth.

AROM was improved after stellate ganglion blocks:

AROM	MP	PIP	DIP
Thumb	5/30	0/25	20/60
Index	10/65	0/20	5/60
Middle	5/60	10/70	0/20
Ring	10/65	10/70	0/30
Little	10/55	10/65	0/35
Wrist			
Extension/Flexion	−5/40		
Radioulnar deviation	5/10		
Forearm			
Supination/Pronation	0/45		

Reestablishing Treatment Goals

Goals at this time were to maintain the improvement seen after injection. The decreased pain allowed more vigorous exercise to gain ROM.

Range of Motion. The patient was seen immediately following stellate ganglion injections for AROM and gentle PROM. Shoulder ROM remained pain-free without limitations. To maintain the increased motion in the digits, the patient was fitted with a CPM device to be worn at night. The parameters of the machine were set to the maximum ROM tolerated without pain. During the day, the machine was removed and the patient was encouraged to use the hand in functional activities.

Edema Control. As GD began using the hand in a functional manner, edema began to decrease. To further aid in edema control, an elasticized (Isotoner) glove was worn for compression. The glove was worn periodically during the day as fluctuations in edema were noted.

Pain Control. With the increased use in motion of the extremity, pain was greatly decreased in the hand. Some hyperesthesia was present around the incision site of the surgical carpal tunnel release. The patient was begun on a localized program of desensitization using scar massage and various modes of texture stimulation to help relieve hypersensitivity.

Stage 3 RSD: 4 to 5 Months

Reevaluation

All signs of acute RSD are resolved with decrease in pain, discoloration, and edema. Upon evaluation, the patient continued to display some ROM limitations:

AROM	MP	PIP	DIP
Thumb	0/35	0/40	0/60
Index	0/60	0/100	0/40
Middle	0/70	0/100	0/40
Ring	0/85	5/110	0/50
Little	0/80	0/95	0/55
Wrist			
Extension/Flexion	15/60		
Radioulnar deviation	8/18		
Forearm			
Supination/Pronation	20/65		

Reestablishing Treatment Goals

With resolution of pain, more vigorous ROM exercises and strengthening were incorporated into the program to improve functional capabilities.

Range of Motion. Stretch techniques were used in conjunction with heat to increase the ROM progress. Coban was applied, pulling the digits into flexion; the hand was then dipped into paraffin.

Dynamic splinting was begun to increase mass flexion of all joints. Though individual joint motion was good, when mass fisting was performed, the individual joint flexion decreased. Patient was fitted with a volar splint with dynamic pull on the fingertips into the palm to increase mass flexion. Splints were used periodically during the day with continuation of functional activities.

Strengthening. Resistive activities were begun on a gradual basis with use of Theraputty. As the patient tolerated it, a more vigorous program for the entire upper extremity was initiated using the BTE Work Simulator, with gradual increase in both resistance and endurance levels of the machine.

Discharge Status

At discharge, between 4 and 5 months after injury, the patient exhibited full ROM of the involved digits. Some loss in wrist dorsiflexion and forearm supination remained but continued to slowly improve. Grip and pinch measurements were approximately 30% less on the affected side than in the uninvolved extremity.

The patient was placed on a home program of ROM exercise to maintain gains made in the digits and to increase the motion in the wrist and forearm. Strengthening continued as the patient returned to more normal functional activities.

SUMMARY

Reflex sympathetic dystrophy describes a group of vasomotor conditions including causalgia, shoulder-hand syndrome, and Sudeck's atrophy. This complex of conditions exhibits common clinical characteristics of pain, joint stiffness, edema, and vasomotor instability, with pain being the predominant feature. These characteristics develop following injury or disease and are more severe than would ordinarily be expected.

Five types of RSD are classified by Lankford:[11,12] They are as follows:

1. Minor causalgia
2. Major causalgia
3. Minor traumatic dystrophy
4. Major traumatic dystrophy
5. Shoulder-hand syndrome

For RSD to occur, there must first be an initial painful lesion accompanied with an abnormal sympathetic reflex. When these conditions are present in a patient who also has a predisposing diathesis or susceptibility, RSD is likely to develop. To control RSD, the sympathetic reflex must be interrupted through stellate ganglion blocks, sympatholytic drugs, or, in severe cases, sympathectomy.

Therapy is important to use in conjunction with medical intervention. Evaluation of individual patient problems can lead to establishment of modalities and exercise programs to control pain, increase joint mobility, and decrease edema. Care should be taken to avoid overly vigorous programs that increase pain and edema. Frequent evaluation of progress should be performed to allow appropriate adjustment of the rehabilitation program. With a cohesive, comprehensive approach from both the therapist and physician, this difficult problem can be managed.

REFERENCES

1. Akeson, WH, et al: Effects of immobilization on joints. Clin Orthop 219:28, 1987.
2. Ali, J, Yaffe, CS, and Serett, C: The effect of transcutaneous electrical nerve stimulation on postoperative pain and pulmonary function. Surgery 89:507, 1981.
3. An, HS, Hawthorne, KB, and Jackson, WT: Reflex sympathetic dystrophy and cigarette smoking. J Hand Surg 13(3):458, 1988.
4. Borrell, RM, et al: Fluidotherapy: Evaluation of a new heat modality. Arch Phys Med Rehabil 58:69, 1977.
5. Bossi, L, et al: Algodystrophy: Treatment. Func Neurol 4(2):157, 1989.
6. Buhler, C and Coleman, WE: Life goals inventory manual. University of Southern California School of Medicine, Los Angeles, 1965.
7. Carlson, L and Watson, HK: Treatment of ref sym dys using the stress-loading program. J Hand Ther 4:149, 1988.
8. DeSaussure, RL: Causalgia. Clin Neurosurg 25:626, 1978.
9. Eaton, R: Painful neuromas. In Omer, GE, Jr and Spinner, M (eds): Management of Peripheral Nerve Problems. WB Saunders, Philadelphia, 1980.
10. Fowler, FD and Moser, M: Use of hexomethonium and dibenzyline in diagnosis and treatment of causalgia. JAMA 161:1051, 1956.
11. Lankford, LL: Reflex sympathic dystrophy. In Hunter, JM, et al: Rehabilitation of the Hand, ed 3. CV Mosby, St Louis, 1990.
12. Lankford, LL: Reflex sympathetic dystrophy. In Omer, GE, Jr and Spinner, M (eds): Management of Peripheral Nerve Problems. WB Saunders, Philadelphia, 1980.
13. Lankford, LL and Thompson, JE: Reflex sympathetic dystrophy, upper and lower extremity: Diagnosis and management. In American Academy of Orthopaedic Surgeons: Instructional course lectures. Vol 26. CV Mosby, St Louis, 1977.
14. Lehman, JF: Therapeutic Heat and Cold, ed 3. Williams & Wilkins, Baltimore, 1982.
15. Lehman, JF, et al: Effect of therapeutic temperatures on tendon extensibility. Arch Phys Med Rehabil 51:481, 1970.
16. Leriche, R: The Surgery of Pain. Ballière, Tindall and Cox, London, 1939.
17. McGrath, MA and Penny, R: The mechanisms of Raynaud's phenomenon, Part I. Med J Aust 2:238, 1974.
18. Melzack, R and Wall, PD: Pain mechanisms: A new theory. Science 150:971, 1965.
18a. Michlovitz, SL (ed): Thermal Agents in Rehabilitation, ed 2. FA Davis, Philadelphia, 1991.
19. Mitchell, SW, Morehouse, GR, and Keen, WW: Gunshot Wounds and Other Injuries of Nerves. JB Lippincott, Philadelphia, 1864.
20. Moore, DC: Regional Block. Charles C Thomas, Springfield, IL, 1967.
21. Omer, GE, Jr and Thomas, SR: The management of chronic pain syndromes in the upper extremity. Clin Orthop 104:37, 1974.
22. Porter, JM, et al: Effects of intra-arterial injection of reserpine on vascular wall catecholamine content. Surg Forum 22:183, 1972.
23. Owens, JC: Causalgia. Am Surg 23:636, 1957.
24. Procacci, P and Maresca, M: Reflex sympathetic dystrophies and algodystrophies: Historical and pathogenic considerations. Pain 31:137, 1987.
25. Rowlingson, SC: The sympathetic dystrophies. Int Anesthesiol Clin 21(4):117, 1983.
26. Schultz, KS: The effect of active exercise on edema. J Hand Surg 8(5):625, 1983.
27. Spurling, RG: Causalgia of the upper extremity: Treatment by dorsal sympathetic ganglionectomy. Arch Neurol Psychiatry 23:784, 1930.
28. Stillwell, GK: Psychiatric management of postmastectomy lymphedema. Med Clin North Am 46:1051, 1962.
29. Subbaro, J and Stillwell, GK: Reflex sympathetic dystrophy syndrome of the upper extremity: Analysis of total outcome of management of 125 cases. Arch Phys Med Rehabil 62:549, 1981.

30. Sudeck, PHM: Ueber die acute entzundliche Knockenatrophie. Arch Klin Chir 62:147, 1900.
31. Sunderland, S: Pain mechanisms in causalgia. J Neurol Neurosurg Psychiatry 39:471, 1976.
32. Uricchio, JV: Thermography and the evaluation of causalgia in medical thermography. In Abernathy, A and Uematsu, S (eds): Medical Thermology. American Academy of Thermology, Washington, DC, 1986.
33. Walsh, M: Hydrotherapy: The use of water as a therapeutic agent. In Michlovitz, SL (ed): Thermal Agents in Rehabilitation. ed 2. FA Davis, Philadelphia, 1991.
34. Waylett-Rendall, J: Therapist's management of reflex sympathetic dystrophy. In Hunter, JM, et al: Rehabilitation of the Hand, ed 3. CV Mosby, St Louis, 1990.
35. White, JC: Sympathectomy for relief of pain. In Bonica, JJ (ed): Advances in Neurology. International Symposium in Pain, Vol 4. Raven Press, New York, 1974.
36. Williams, R, and Carey, L: Studies in the production of standard venous thrombosis. Ann Surg 149:381, 1959.
37. Zucchini, M, Alberti, G, and Moretti, MP: Algodystrophy and related psychological features. Func Neurol 4(2):153, 1989.

CHAPTER 16

Traumatic Injuries of the Hand: Crush Injuries and Amputations

James W. King, MA, OTR, CHT

Traumatic hand injuries are often seen in hand rehabilitation programs. Trauma to body parts occurs frequently in mechanized industry in which people interact with machines, at home, and in recreation and sports activities. These injured workers, "weekend carpenters," and sports enthusiasts will require the services of hand surgeons and hand rehabilitation specialists to enable them to return to vocational and daily living activities. Two types of trauma to the hand, crush injuries and amputations, are the subject of this chapter.

The objectives of this chapter are to:

1. Review the etiology and therapeutic management of crush injuries to the hand
2. Present the therapeutic management of finger and partial hand amputations
3. Present guidelines for classifying an individual's level of hand function after finger or partial hand amputation
4. Discuss the preparation for return to work of individuals who have suffered hand crush injuries or amputations, or both
5. Discuss considerations of impairment and disability after crush injury or amputation.

The chapter concludes with a clinical case study that reviews the treatment of a patient with a severe crush injury.

THE RELATIONSHIP OF WOUND HEALING TO TRAUMA

Therapists must understand the healing response of injured tissue before they can effectively rehabilitate the hand. The quantity of scar deposited is directly proportional to the amount of tissue injury. Epithelialization can begin in as few as 48 hours in a clean, sharply incised (so-called tidy) wound.[1] However, many traumatic hand injuries have wounds that are not only difficult or impossible to close but also infiltrated with debris and bacteria. The presence of excessive trauma and foreign matter in the untidy wound may increase the length of time in which the acute inflammatory phase of healing persists. Fractures and lacerations of tendons, ligaments, skin, and nerves may occur simultaneously, adding complexity to the patient's care. Prolonged pain, edema, and the patient's subsequent inability or unwillingness to move the injured part all present challenging treatment implications for the therapist.

Collagen synthesis (and ultimately scar formation) is both friend and foe of the hand therapist and will affect the results of surgical and therapeutic management. The nature of scar is to contract and adhere. The body forms scar to heal the damaged tissue of the hand and restore its integrity. Severe wounds, however, often result in excessive scar tissue that is randomly deposited by the healing process. This excessive scar formation, has the effect of adhering and contracting the various fixed and mobile units of the hand.

An understanding of the wound healing process forms the basis for intervention strategies designed by the therapist. Rehabilitation of severe traumatic injuries should emphasize prevention of complications from the inflammatory response to the injury and application of appropriate scar management techniques. As the patient's hand progresses through the three phases of healing, the therapist chooses from a wide selection of exercise, activities, physical agents, and splints to affect the collagen formation process. The ultimate goal of surgery and rehabilitation is to restore a functional, more cosmetically acceptable hand to the patient.

CRUSH INJURIES

Crush injuries to the hand are often complex, requiring a multitude of skills by the treating therapist. A crushed hand can result in fractures, lacerations of major hand structures, and closed soft tissue trauma ranging from minimal to severe. Some crush injuries have little or no skin breakage and, upon examination, the major structures of the hand have maintained their integrity.

Although fractures and lacerations receive much attention, the internal wound — the closed, soft tissue damage present to some degree in all crush injuries — may provide the most substantial obstacle to patient progress. Brown[2] describes the sequelae following crush injury as, "Great pressures applied to the hand shear, compress, and twist tissues . . . causing hemorrhage and the escape of intra- and extracellular fluids into potential spaces and tissue planes. The net result is the formation of hematoma and progressive edema that, in turn, leads to the precipitation of proteins, fibrosis, and stiffness."

Another unique and difficult management concept for the crushed hand is that multiple injuries often occur simultaneously. Describing the multiple system trauma that exists in a crush injury, Wynn Parry[3] stated, ". . . what makes these [crush] injuries so much more disabling than each of these lesions on its own is the outpouring of reactive

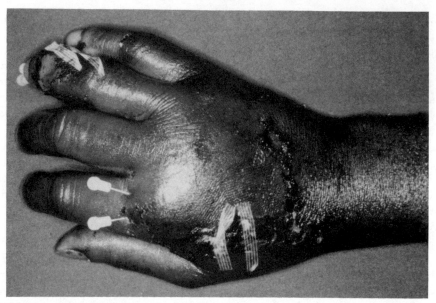

FIGURE 16–1. This crushed hand represents the ultimate challenge for therapists working with these injuries: a combination of open and closed wounds, fractures, and significant soft tissue damage all occurring simultaneously.

fluid in the soft tissues. This organizes and causes severe fibrosis leading to a 'frozen hand'."

Multiple system damage in the presence of severe soft tissue injury is the ultimate challenge for the therapist. A patient may have large areas of skin loss, and tendon or nerve lacerations in one portion of the hand, while sustaining fractures in other areas (Fig. 16–1). Moreover, with the crushed hand, the therapist must also deal with tissues that are in different phases of wound healing at the same time. In such instances, the therapist must use a thorough knowledge of tissue healing to mobilize (and immobilize) the hand appropriately.

Therapeutic Management

INFLAMMATORY/FIBROPLASIA PHASES

The initial response of the acutely injured hand is inflammation, characterized by pain and edema. The therapist's first consideration in the management of an acute crush injury to the hand is to prevent complications from excessive edema. Excessive edema can lead to tissue ischemia and subsequent fibrosis and stiffness. The goals of therapy are to minimize pain and reduce edema; to provide wound care; and, through splinting, activity, and exercise, to rest and mobilize healing tissues appropriately. To what degree the therapist will use these techniques to manage the symptoms depends primarily on the presence of fractures or other surgically repaired structures.

If fractures are surgically stabilized, open wounds and the symptoms of acute inflammation in the crushed hand can be treated more aggressively. Treatment permitted by surgical stabilization includes using whirlpool to help cleanse untidy wounds,

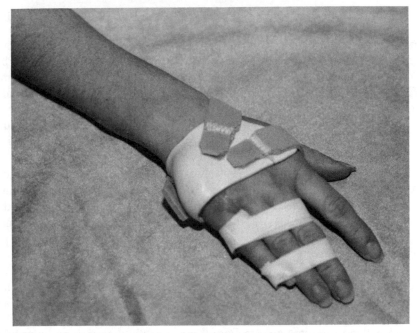

FIGURE 16-2. This splint allows for the appropriate immobilization of metacarpal fractures that have been pinned and mobilization of the adjacent fingers.

decongestive retrograde massage, and active range of motion (AROM) with the fracture area manually supported.

The possibility of fracture displacement limits the use of aggressive techniques by the therapist in the presence of an unstable fracture. Yet the nature of crush injuries, with their potential for resulting stiffness, requires an approach that often combines mobility with stability. This notion is exemplified by the crush injury resulting in a nondisplaced fracture of a single metacarpal. By appropriately immobilizing the fracture in a splint, the patient can mobilize the affected and adjacent fingers and prevent rotation by taping them together (Fig. 16-2).

Edema Control

The edematous response varies depending on the extent of the injury. The inflammatory phase of healing, is usually characterized by pitting edema—so-called because impressions in the edematous area from external forces will remain visible for some time after the force is removed. Edema may be minimal with the hand appearing puffy, or massive with the hand achieving immense size. The *amount* of edema filling the interstitial spaces is of greatest concern. In cases when edema seriously compromises vascular and neurologic function, surgical decompression may be required.[4]

Effects of Edema. The hand often assumes characteristic postures in the presence of excessive edema. Uncontrolled, edema may lead to intrinsic muscle ischemia with contracture and fibrosis of the intrinsic musculature. Excessive edema results in an intrinsic-plus posture, characterized by a flexion contracture of the metacarpophalangeal (MP) joints. More commonly, though, the hand assumes the intrinsic-minus posture. This position includes MP joint extension, interphalangeal (IP) joint flexion, and adduction of the first web space. The therapist must properly evaluate the hand to determine which hand structures are contributing to the contracture.

The posture assumed by the hand in the presence of edema also masks conditions that become more evident as the acute edema subsides. The therapist may often become aware of conditions such as tendon rupture or neuropraxia as more acute symptoms subside. For example, in blunt trauma over the dorsum of the proximal interphalangeal (PIP) joint, in the absence of a fracture, injury to the central slip of the extensor tendon should be considered. This injury is masked by the position that the finger assumes in the presence of significant amounts of edema. Often the therapist recognizes the central slip injury as edema diminishes and inability to extend the PIP joint persists (Fig. 16–3).

Treatment of Edema. When the crush injury requires immobilization, due to the presence of surgically repaired structures or structures with questionable stability, the most effective method of edema reduction is elevation. Elevation can be achieved with a sling, manually, or through support of the extremity with an external device such as an arm elevation pillow (Fig. 16–4). Appropriate compression dressings also help prevent edema and minimize bleeding[5] (Fig. 16–5).

Even when structures of the hand are stable, elevation is still the best method of reducing edema.[6] Other methods such as an intermittent air compression unit, compression garments, manual retrograde massage (Fig. 16–6), and early AROM are also available to the therapist to help reduce edema when the condition of the hand allows.

The therapist can fabricate splints from thermoplastic materials to immobilize the hand appropriately following crush injuries. Splinting helps to rest injured tissue, decreasing inflammation and, subsequently, edema and pain.[7] When not otherwise

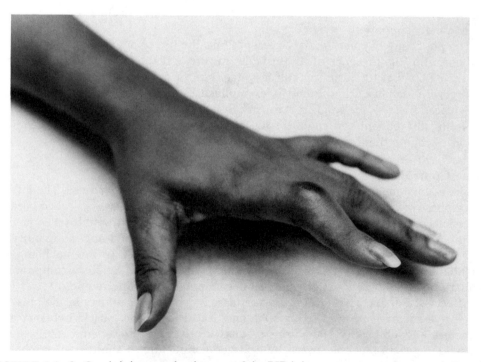

FIGURE 16–3. Crush injury to the dorsum of the PIP joint may rupture the central slip with secondary development of a boutonnière deformity.

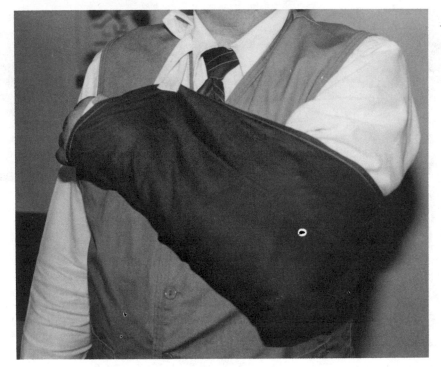

FIGURE 16–4. When using a sling to support and elevate a crushed hand, the hand should be positioned above the elbow.

indicated by protocols for specific injuries, the "safe position" splint should be used.[8] This position maintains tissue length through MP joint flexion, IP joint extension, and abduction and extension of the first web space (Fig. 16–7). Using circumferential splints on an edematous extremity requires caution to avoid a buildup of pressure within the splint, resulting in neuromuscular damage. The therapist must warn the patient of this danger and instruct him or her to monitor the splinted hand for signs of neuromuscular compromise, including increasing pain, numbness, and discoloration.

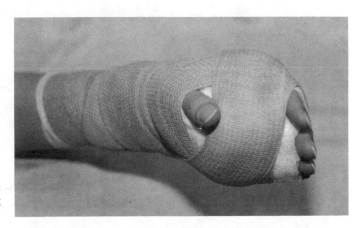

FIGURE 16–5. Appropriate bandage to minimize bleeding and edema.

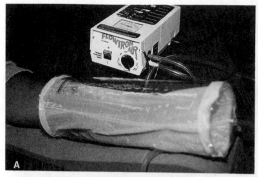
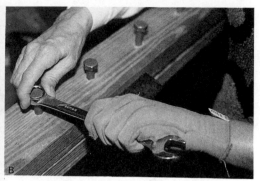
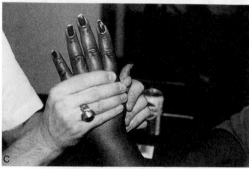

FIGURE 16–6. With relative stability of injured and/or repaired tissue, other means to reduce edema include A, intermittent air compression unit, B, compression garments; and C, manual retrograde massage.

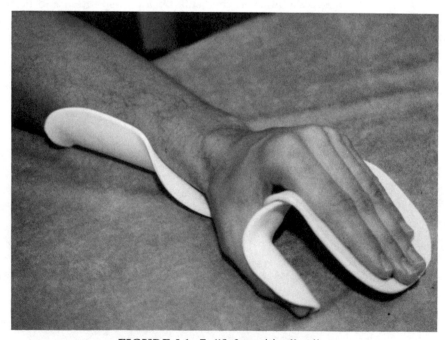

FIGURE 16–7. "Safe position" splint.

Pain Management

Management of pain during the acute phase of injury may be the key to patient compliance. Therapists have several therapeutic agents that, along with patient education and medication prescribed by the physician, can minimize this problem. Few patients have pain that is incapacitating after crush injuries. The patient who presents with an edematous hand and describes severe pain that inhibits sleep and daily life tasks must be a concern to the therapist. This patient has the greatest risk of developing significant hand stiffness in later stages of healing.

During the first two healing phases, the use of transcutaneous electrical nerve stimulation (TENS), elevation, ice, and appropriate prescribed medications will help decrease pain and improve compliance with early mobilization treatment programs. TENS is effective for relieving pain and can be used in the presence of open wounds and hand splints by placing the electrodes proximally over nerve routes, dermatomal patterns, or proximal trigger points. Ice and elevation are also techniques that can be used to help decrease pain when not contraindicated by vascular compromise. Edema, pain, and other signs of inflammation are normal early in the course of treatment following a crush injury; however, the persistence of these symptoms should alert the therapist to the possibility of the development of reflex sympathetic dystrophy (RSD).

Wound Care and Scar Management

Management of open wounds from a crush injury may be complicated by the presence of fractures or newly repaired structures. If the fractures are reduced and fixated, wound care can proceed with sterile soaks or washes. Whirlpool with very slight agitation is also acceptable. Manual debridement of necrotic tissue assists the macrophage cells in cleaning the wound of necrotic tissue, bacteria, and debris.

Collagen synthesis begins as the inflammatory phase decreases and reaches a peak at 3 to 4 weeks postinjury in the fibroplasia phase. Collagen formation continues for up to 1 year in the scar maturation phase. While the adhering and contractile nature of external scar is visible, the developing internal scar is just as likely to limit the final functional outcome. For example, if a skin laceration crosses joint surfaces, the contractile nature of the myofibroblasts and randomly deposited collagen fibers in the wound will ultimately adhere and contract the joint if not appropriately treated. Similarly, the nature of the internal scar may produce adhesions of muscle-tendon units within the hand, inhibiting their gliding ability and producing the characteristic fibrotic, hard feel of the hand as the healing phases proceed.

Management of healing tissue in the fibroplasia phase should include pressure through manual massage, vibration, compression garments, and splinting. Pressure is one method of applying stress to help the collagen fibers in the newly forming scar become organized and thus less adherent to surrounding healing or intact tissues.[9] Experienced therapists use their hands to massage, recognizing the value of feeling the tissue and applying pressure to the hardened, edematous areas.

Application of pressure using compression garments such as gloves or digital sleeves minimizes hypertrophic scarring and edema. The application of mechanical vibration is an additional method to soften the forming scar.

During the inflammatory phase of healing, static splinting is best employed to maintain ROM.[10] The patient's hand can be immobilized in the safe position of MP joint flexion, IP joint extension, and abduction and extension of the first web. If the patient develops contractures during the fibroplasia phase of healing, dynamic splints are more appropriate than static splints to place low-load, progressive stress to the healing tissues.

Use of dynamic splinting lets the tissues heal in an elongated position that will lead to a better functional outcome.[11] Common problems that can be splinted with dynamic splints are PIP joint flexion contractures, MP joint extension contractures, and adduction contractures of the first (thumb) web space. The splints will need to be adjusted regularly to allow for decreasing edema and improving ROM.

Exercise and Activity

Incorporating therapeutic exercise in the program can reduce edema, maintain joint mobility, and promote tendon gliding. During the inflammatory phase, the use of exercise must be carefully balanced with the need for rest. Too much activity will only aggravate the inflammatory response. The appropriate program would incorporate gentle AROM in an elevated position three to four times per day. For the patient who has severe pain or edema, complete immobilization in a functional position for up to 72 hours may be indicated to rest traumatized tissue.

As the pain and edema of the inflammatory phase start to subside, more aggressive exercise is appropriate, even if open wounds persist. In developing a program, the therapist must first have a detailed understanding of which joints or structures require immobilization or protected motion, and which will tolerate full motion. For example, a patient with a first metacarpal fracture can use a properly fitted, forearm-based thumb spica orthosis to immobilize the fracture and its adjacent joints. To prevent adhesion and contracture of the soft tissues adjacent to the fracture, the splint should be fabricated to allow for flexion and extension of the IP joint of the thumb (Fig. 16–8).

AROM and gentle passive range of motion (PROM) exercises, as well as joint

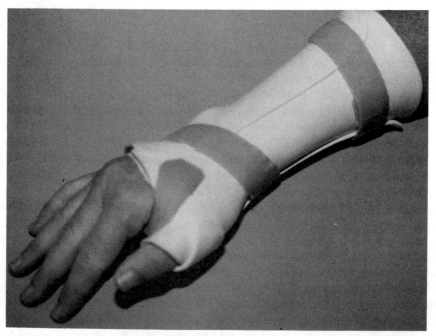

FIGURE 16–8. Splint for a first metacarpal fracture allows for mobilization of joints adjacent to the site of fracture, which maintains gliding structures and allows the patient some functional use of the hand.

mobilization techniques, are introduced to maintain mobility of all nonimmobilized joints. Continuous passive motion (CPM) machines are an effective modality to maintain joint motion during the scar formation phase but should be used with active exercise as well. When significant amounts of edema have been present, intrinsic stretching exercises should be initiated before intrinsic tightness becomes a problem. Exercises that promote tendon gliding are essential even in the absence of direct trauma to the tendon. During the scar formation phase, the exercises and activities can be preceded by heat modalities that increase tissue elasticity, relieve pain, and increase circulation.

Exercise and activities to improve strength should be initiated once all injured structures are strong enough to withstand resistance. Improving strength is particularly important as the patient's hand progresses from the fibroplasia phase into the scar maturation phase and experiences increased internal resistance to motion. A common problem when initiating strengthening exercises and resistive activities with the crushed hand is the reappearance of inflammation. When therapeutic activity exceeds the tissue's strength and tolerance to stress, the weaker tissues may become reinjured and edema will result. Strengthening exercises should be progressed very gradually, with the therapist monitoring the patient's response to exercise through volumetric measurements and patient complaints of pain. The therapist should prevent deconditioning of unaffected portions of the extremity through a program designed to maintain or increase strength and endurance. A general fitness program such as walking each day will also minimize the effects of prolonged inactivity.

SCAR MATURATION PHASE

When a patient's hand reaches the third phase of healing, the preceding events have usually established a pattern of hand function or dysfunction. Unresolved problems, such as joint contractures and tendon adhesions, become more resistant to motion, reflecting the increasing tensile strength of the maturing scar. The goals of therapy during this phase of healing are to (1) continue ROM, strengthening, and functional activity programs to achieve as much function as possible; (2) treat chronic pain and edema; and (3) facilitate return to independent vocational and daily living activities.

Despite optimum treatment, fingers and hands can become stiff. Each injury has its own potential for improvement, which is dependent on the patient's age, the severity of the soft tissue injury, and the need for immobilization of injured bones and tendons. Surgical intervention may improve the potential but a limited potential may still exist. The goal of therapy is to reach this potential. Chronic conditions such as edema and pain, joint and tendon adhesions, late-stage RSD, and scar contracture all lend themselves to development of a stiff hand or finger.

The severely crushed hand may literally have had most of its structures injured. In addition, the presence of an untidy and possibly infected wound can prolong the inflammatory phase of healing, thus increasing the scar tissue response. When excessive amounts of scar tissue have been deposited, the chance of significant stiffness and relative inability to perform normal prehensile and grasp patterns increases. The ability of the patient to achieve maximum potential depends on the quality of the therapeutic intervention and the patient's willingness and ability to follow through with the prescribed program.

Edema Control

The edema that was liquidlike in the inflammatory phase and pitting during healing in the fibroplasia phase becomes brawny and thick in the scar maturation phase. This brawny edema is less amenable to passive techniques such as elevation alone. The therapist must use methods to increase tissue hydrostatic pressure, which creates a pressure gradient and forces the fluid across the capillary and lymphatic membranes back into the vessels. This pressure gradient can be achieved with compression gloves, the application of self-adherent wrap circumferentially to the hand, and firm retrograde massage. The use of an inflatable air compression pump for chronic edema usually requires lengthy treatment sessions if the modality is to be effective enough to justify its use. The patient can rent or buy a unit for home use. Because the lengthy treatment sessions require prolonged immobilization, the benefit must be justified to balance the increased stiffness that may occur.

Performing AROM exercises and functional activities with the affected limb elevated helps reduce chronic edema and stiffness. Grasp and release activities such as squeezing Therapy Putty and using hand "pipe trees" improve circulation and strength (Fig. 16–9). The use of grasp and release activities promotes circulation, mobility, and strength.

Pain Management

Chronic pain is a significant problem from both etiologic and treatment perspectives of scar maturation. The perceptive therapist can often anticipate the sequelae of events that may lead to shoulder-hand syndrome.[12] The patient with chronic hand pain often avoids using the extremity, which leads to shoulder and other proximal joint stiffness. Stiffness of the joints can increase pain with motion, thus encouraging the

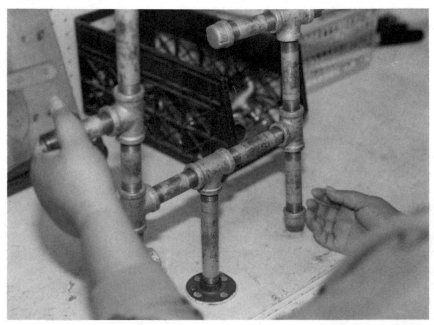

FIGURE 16–9. Using hand "Pipe Trees" improves circulation and strength to help decrease edema and increase functional use.

patient to hold the shoulder in a protected position of adduction and internal rotation. With the shoulder so positioned, the hand is held in a dependent manner leading to increased edema, more hand pain, and, ultimately, dysfunction. This pattern of behavior during the scar maturation phase is both a symptom and an etiologic factor in the development of the stiff hand.

Treatment of the painfully stiff hand or finger requires a different approach by the therapist during the maturation phase than during earlier phases. As before, TENS and medication may help; in this stage of healing, however, pain relief alone will not increase motion, because the basis for dysfunction is tendon adhesion and joint contracture. If the patient's pain can be attributed to sympathetic nervous system activity, even more caution should be taken to avoid painful stretching exercises.

Scar Management

Management of chronic scar contracture can include pressure, splinting, and active and gentle passive exercise. As before, the use of CPM machines, joint mobilization, and heat modalities may be effective in mobilizing adherent tissue but should be used in moderation. CPM is effective primarily in the early phases of healing when scar tissue is forming.[13] The cost of implementing CPM can be justified when the patient cannot or will not actively move, as is often the case in those with a chronically stiff hand. Using CPM in the pain-free ROM allows for the benefits of motion—improved gliding, nutrition of tissue, and scar lengthening—without increasing the patient's pain or apprehension. Likewise, joint mobilization techniques to increase the accessory and physiologic joint motions can be performed in pain-free ranges.[14] Paraffin treatments with the hand elevated and the fingers wrapped in a flexed position with self-adherent wrap (Fig. 16–10) is an effective method of applying heat and stretch to restore finger flexion. Use of ultrasound before exercise improves tissue elasticity before and during gentle PROM and other exercise programs. Again, the key to treatment in this stage of healing is motion without pain.

During the scar maturation phase, the type of splinting used should be serial progressive and static progressive splints (Fig. 16–11 A,B). These types of splints have

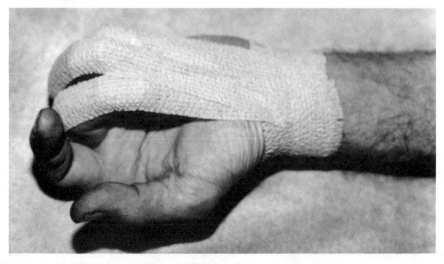

FIGURE 16–10. The fingers can be flexed using self-adherent wrap to produce a gentle dynamic force during rest or application of heat.

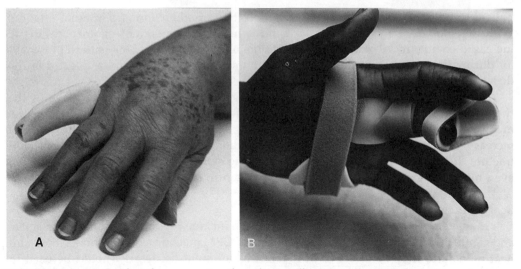

FIGURE 16–11. During the scar maturation phase, splints that allow comfortable use for long periods of time are recommended, such as these for PIP flexion contractures. *A*, Serial cylindric splint. *B*, static progressive splint.

the advantage of placing stress on the tissue that is tolerable or adjustable for the patient, thus increasing compliance and wearing time. This is imperative in the final stage of healing, because the collagen formation and reabsorption process is slow and takes longer to affect with external stress.

If the conservative management techniques are unsuccessful in providing optimum results, the treatment team (including the patient) may opt for further surgical intervention. Examples of secondary surgeries performed when the outcome from a crush injury was less than optimal are joint capsulectomy, tenolysis, and web space releases. The goal of postoperative therapy is to maintain the motion gained with surgery. Therapeutic management following secondary surgeries is particularly challenging because of the tendency for deformities to recur.

Exercise and Activity

Activity and exercise programs during the final phase of healing should center on strengthening and functional activities. Such activities include work simulation for the patient who has the potential to return to work and adaptation of daily living activities for the patient who will have significant residual hand impairment. Even this late after injury, tissues in various stages of wound healing within the same hand will have different levels of tolerance to resistance.

One way to determine the appropriate exercise program is to view tissues in earlier stages of healing as the weak link and to use only therapeutic activities that do not exceed the strength of these weaker tissues. Increased edema and pain following exercise is a sign that the exercise dose has been excessive and should be reduced. Static or isometric assessments during this phase of healing can help determine the level of resistance at which to proceed. Different exercise strategies for increasing both strength and endurance have been advocated.[15,16]

SUMMARY

In summary, the management of crush injuries is complex, requiring the therapist to consider carefully the healing phase of injured structures, as well as the presence of a significant internal scar. With knowledge of the healing process, decisions to mobilize and/or immobilize injured skin, nerves, tendons, and bones can be made. Effective treatment (e.g., decreasing edema and pain; providing wound care and scar management; and using splints, exercise, and activity at appropriate times) can help patients achieve their functional potential.

FINGER AND PARTIAL HAND AMPUTATIONS

Unlike crush injuries, where the chance to regain functional ability of the injured part exists, amputation of a finger or amputation that extends into the hand has an immediate physical and psychologic impact on the patient.

Many injuries result in amputations. Severe crush injuries with significant bony and soft tissue damage can result in such vascular compromise that amputation is necessary (Fig. 16–12). Even when viability of the finger is likely, a severe injury leaves the possibility of significant stiffness, secondary hypersensitivity, pain, cold intolerance, and a lengthy rehabilitation period. These complications may influence certain patients to choose amputation as an option. In cases when amputation of a finger or hand occurs traumatically, the surgeon and patient must decide whether to revise the amputation or attempt reattachment.

These and other treatment decisions are made after considering several factors including age and occupation of the patient, viability of the residual tissues, and status of the amputated part. When reattachment is impossible, the surgeon must consider the type of skin coverage for the finger.

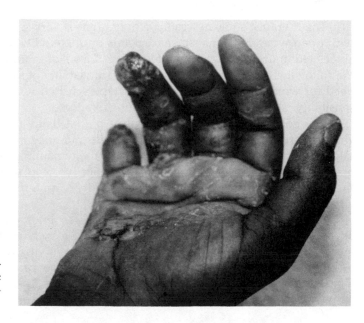

FIGURE 16–12. A mutilating injury can cause multiple finger injuries including amputations.

Skin Coverage

Fingertip amputations that are allowed to heal on their own[17] have the advantage of better sensibility after healing and improved cosmesis. Only small defects can be treated in this manner, and this method is not acceptable if bone is exposed. The therapist manages this type of injury by dressing the wound with a nonadherent gauze, providing a protective splint, and teaching the patient maintenance ROM exercise. Most traumatic amputations, though, require revision with one of several surgical methods for skin coverage. The type of coverage chosen will have implications for the treating therapist.

Skin coverage can take the form of full- or split-thickness skin grafts. Full-thickness grafts have the advantages of being (1) more durable, (2) more likely to develop functional sensibility, and (3) better able to cover bony prominences.[18] Pedicle (island) flaps[19] with intact neurovascular supplies or a variety of intrinsic grafts from the hand may give the patient a more functional and cosmetic result.

Skin grafting with local flaps that have neurovascular supplies intact maintains immune mechanisms and decreases the chance of infection. The volar and lateral v-y (Fig. 16–13, A, B) advancements, although not always indicated, have the advantage over the Moberg slide (Fig. 16–13, C) of not requiring immobilization of the finger in a flexed position, thus minimizing the chance of contracture. With the cross-finger flap (Fig. 16–13, D) and flaps from the palm, suturing of the amputated site occurs in a position of flexion for up to 3 weeks. The methods (Fig. 16–13 C, D) have the disadvantage of requiring two surgeries and significant risk of digital stiffness because of the initial flexed posture of the finger.

Therapeutic Management

The therapist's role in treating amputations is very similar to that for crush injuries with open wounds. Management depends on the quality and degree of skin coverage, associated injuries, presence of infection, and level of injury. Therapists should evaluate the following to establish the treatment plan: viability of skin coverage to determine the need for wound care, edema, pain and hypersensitivity, ROM, and, as healing allows, sensibility, strength, endurance, and functional use.

The goals for therapy after digital or partial hand amputation should emphasize wound care and edema management while minimizing pain, hypersensitivity, cold intolerance and regaining optimum ROM of the remaining joints. Every effort should be made to provide the patient with as cosmetically acceptable a hand as possible. Early therapeutic intervention increases the possibility of an improved functional and cosmetically acceptable outcome.

Another important aspect of the therapist's intervention is the emotional and psychologic adjustment of the patient to loss of a body part. This psychologic adjustment is generally minimal in fingertip injuries involving one finger but may increase proportionally with full finger, multiple finger, and partial hand amputations. Psychologic counseling may be necessary if the patient has difficulty adjusting to the amputation.

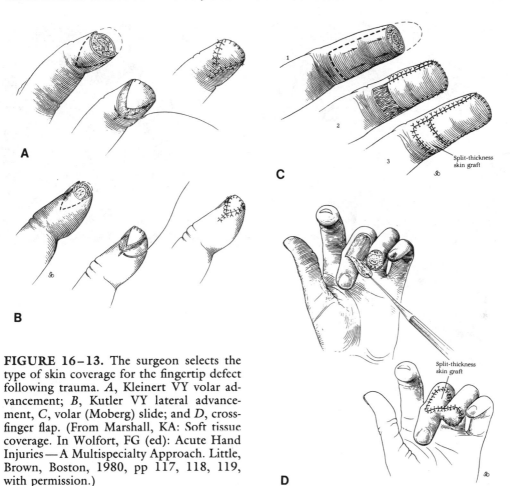

FIGURE 16–13. The surgeon selects the type of skin coverage for the fingertip defect following trauma. *A*, Kleinert VY volar advancement; *B*, Kutler VY lateral advancement, *C*, volar (Moberg) slide; and *D*, cross-finger flap. (From Marshall, KA: Soft tissue coverage. In Wolfort, FG (ed): Acute Hand Injuries — A Multispecialty Approach. Little, Brown, Boston, 1980, pp 117, 118, 119, with permission.)

WOUND CARE AND SCAR MANAGEMENT

When adequate and viable skin coverage has been achieved over an amputated finger, the inflammatory phase may be brief with progression to collagen synthesis and wound healing occurring rather quickly. Successful skin grafting relies on absolute immobilization of the graft in the recipient bed. In less tidy injuries, the therapist's role for wound care requires particular attention to careful debridement and early bandaging. Edema should be managed using appropriate methods for each phase of healing, such as those described earlier in this chapter.

In addition to edema control, the final appearance and function of the finger can be improved by wrapping the residual digits with self-adherent wrap and gauze initially, followed later with compressive garments for the fingertips (Fig. 16–14). The constant pressure from this procedure also seems to minimize the hypersensitivity and pain often seen in fingertip amputations.

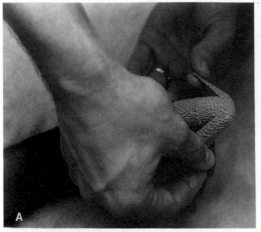
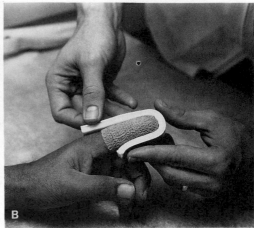
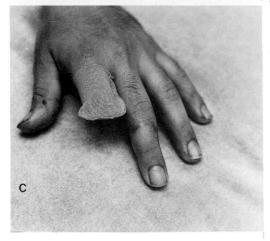

FIGURE 16–14. Wrapping the finger amputation to improve shape of the residual finger and decrease hypersensitivity. *A*, Self-adherent wrap is placed on the finger vertically, then circumferentially, followed by a horizontal wrap over the top. *B*, A protective splint can be used. *C*, After healing, compressive garments will continue to shape the finger.

PAIN AND HYPERSENSITIVITY

The patient can begin with desensitization procedures after removal of the postoperative dressing by tapping the fingers gently. This proprioceptive input also helps with resolution of phantom limb sensations the patient may be experiencing. Aggressive desensitization activities should not begin until the third postoperative week as the wound will not withstand aggressive rubbing or other desensitization activities. If blisters occur initially, one should wait longer. Once the wound is strong enough, more aggressive activities can be started such as rubbing different textures (Fig. 16–15 *A*, *B*), feeling vibration, and using the fingers for light activities.

Normal postoperative pain should diminish during the first 2 to 3 weeks. Occasionally a digital nerve neuroma may develop. A neuroma is a single, often palpable, area of hypersensitivity in the anatomic distribution of the ulnar or radial digital nerve. If desensitization activities in the area of the neuroma aggravate the pain, pressure should be applied with self-adherent wrap and silicon Elastomer, as seen in Figure 16–16A. TENS application on the fingertip or proximally in the appropriate nerve distribution is also helpful (Fig. 16–16B). Eventually, surgical resection of the neuroma may be necessary to achieve a successful outcome.[20]

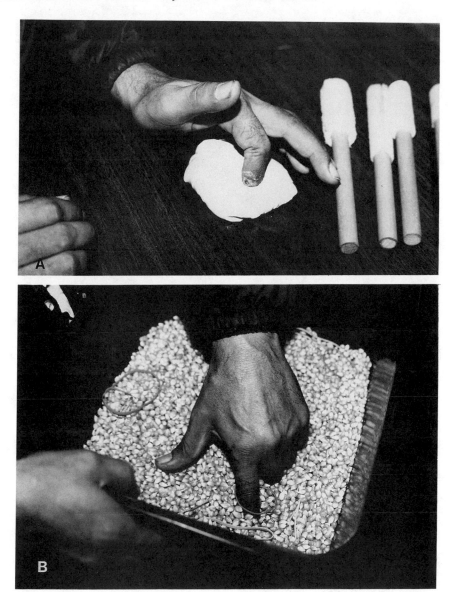

FIGURE 16-15. Desensitization activities. *A*, Tapping and texture sticks. *B*, Rubbing the finger in popcorn.

RANGE OF MOTION EXERCISE

ROM exercise for the residual joints should be started as soon as possible after surgery. The initiation of motion is particularly important for the proximal joints to prevent limitations in motion owing to disuse syndromes. A specific example of a disuse syndrome is called extensor habitus. This syndrome occurs when the patient holds the injured finger in an extended position and does not use it in hand function or daily activities. The phenomenon is often seen after the index finger is injured, because that digit is easily left out of grasp and prehension patterns. Extensor habitus is usually a

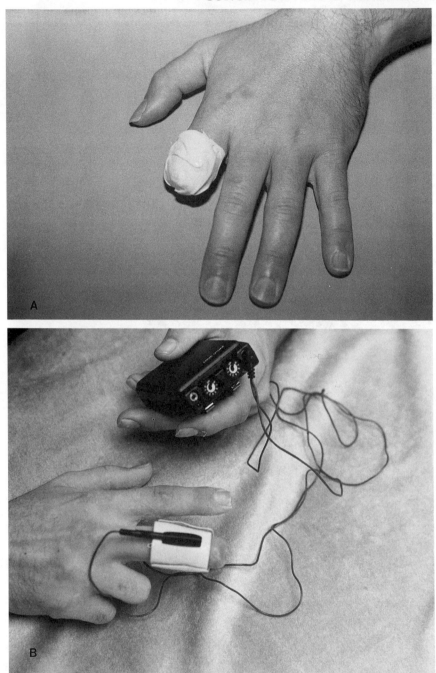

FIGURE 16–16. *A*, Application of silicone elastomer for the residual finger that can be held on with self-adherent wrap. *B*, TENS electrode placement for digital hypersensitivity or neuroma.

manifestation of an underlying pain, hypersensitivity, or joint motion problem. In addition to treating the causal factors, taping the injured digit to the adjacent finger(s) will encourage its use.

The goal is optimum, nonpainful ROM of the residual joints of the amputated finger(s). Assuming no injury to the residual joints, if the level of amputation is at the

PIP joint or more proximal, up to 70° of flexion of the MP joint can be expected. Limited MP joint flexion has an anatomic and biomechanical rationale. When the amputation of the finger occurs closer to the MP joint, the mechanical advantage of the extrinsic flexor in assisting this motion is lost. The lumbrical muscle originates on the flexor digitorum profundus tendon and flexes the MP joint. This function is assisted by the extrinsic flexors. If the amputation occurs distal to the PIP joint, this relationship usually remains intact and normal motion can be expected at the MP joint.

Functional Results by Level of Amputation

In general, a patient's ability to use an injured hand after finger or partial hand amputation for functional activities has three considerations: the finger(s) or part of the hand affected, the level of the amputation, and the presence of complications. Complications usually take the form of pain, hypersensitivity, or insensibility.

The countless uses of the thumb in prehension and grasp patterns, stabilizing objects, and sensory functions all contribute to significant disability from loss of any length of the thumb. Amputation at the IP joint of the thumb in the absence of complications leaves a functional post for performing most activities. Activities will be limited to the less refined grasp and pinch patterns because of the loss of fine manipulative ability that the normal thumb tip and normal sensibility allow (Fig. 16–17). With an amputation proximal to the IP joint, thumb function becomes limited to stabilizing objects for opposition and lateral pinch. In the absence of a prosthesis, complete loss of the thumb limits hand function to grasp and release, and prehension by abducting and adducting the fingers.

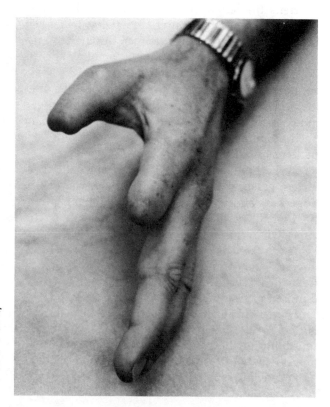

FIGURE 16–17. Loss of the tip of the thumb still allows for modified prehension but the shape of the residual thumb is not conducive to fine prehension, and the residual thumb lacks discriminative sensibility.

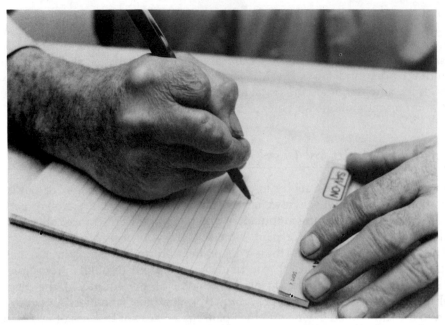

FIGURE 16–18. Loss of length in radial fingers requires shifting to the longer fingers for functional activities.

The index and middle fingers are usually used for prehension patterns, whereas the ring and small fingers are more effective for grasp. When a patient's amputation shortens the length of the index or middle finger, or both, changing of prehension patterns is required during functional activities. The patient often switches to using the thumb and either the next longer amputated finger or uninvolved finger (Fig. 16–18).

In the presence of an amputation of a finger proximal to the PIP joint, patients who do not need the full breadth of their hand for heavy manual labor may choose to have a surgical ray resection. In this operation, the residual finger and distal portion of the metacarpal are excised, which widens the first web space significantly in the case of an index finger injury, or closes the gap left in the hand when one of the middle fingers has been amputated (Fig. 16–19). These surgeries often allow the patient to have better prehension and improved cosmesis.

Whereas disruption of prehension patterns occurs when the radial digits are affected, grasp, particularly for large objects, will be more difficult when the ulnar two fingers are affected. Loss of length in the ulnar fingers will affect the patient's attempt to hold small, particularly cylindrical, objects or to use the ulnar fingers for a cupping effect when holding multiple objects in the hand. This loss of function is particularly evident when the ulnar side of the palm is amputated obliquely in addition to the fingers. When amputations of all the fingers occur at a level where they become useless, the patient will require a prosthesis or will have only adduction prehension between the thumb and residual hand.

Functional and cosmetic prostheses can improve hand function and the psychologic outlook of the patient (Fig. 16–20).[21] Obviously, prostheses do not replace the critical sensibility of the hand. Use of a prosthesis usually requires patients to observe their hand activity, which slows dexterity and decreases effectiveness. Prostheses facilitate hand function most effectively when the patient has lost the thumb proximal to the IP

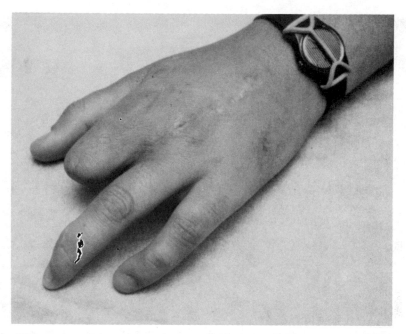

FIGURE 16–19. Cosmetic results are improved with middle ray resection following amputation of the middle finger.

joint (Fig. 16–21*A*) or has lost one or more fingers on the ulnar side of the hand proximal to the PIP joint (Fig. 16–21*B*). Most functional prostheses improve opposition of the hand and also function as a hook for carrying objects in the injured hand.

PREPARATION OF THE TRAUMA PATIENT FOR RETURN TO WORK

Because many traumatic injuries occur in the workplace, their disabling effects may necessitate changes in jobs or adaptations of the workplace. This consideration should be initiated early in the patient's treatment. Functional activities, such as the use of hand tools and craft techniques can improve outcome by increasing the patient's ability to compensate following trauma. Use of computerized work simulators (Fig. 16–22) and other functional activities are important for evaluating the strength of the hand, increasing tolerance to touching tools for hypersensitive fingers and allowing patients to adapt the manner in which they use the hand for performing certain activities.

Examples of modifications of tools for the impaired hand include adjusting handle size, extending triggers, and minimizing exposure to temperature and vibration. Depending on the injury, the tool handle size may be too large or too small.[22] If the amputation leaves the fingers very short, most hand tools will be too large. Changing tools or hand dominance may be necessary. If limitation of motion or weakness is the problem, the tool can be adapted by increasing its size. When the amputation affects the index finger and the usual occupation requires the use of power tools with triggers, adjacent fingers or the other hand may be used. When it is impractical or impossible to use adjacent fingers, an adaptation for the tool can be implemented.

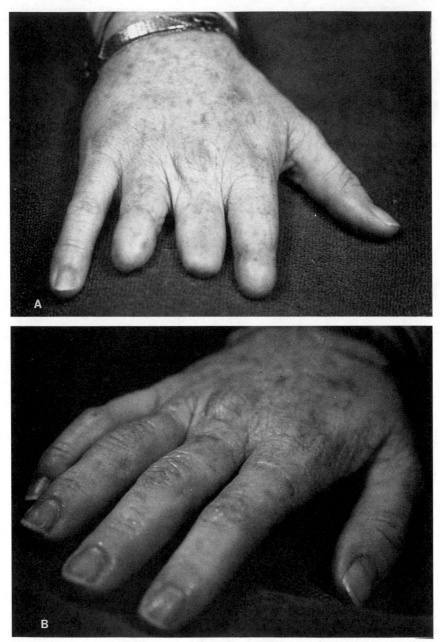

FIGURE 16–20. *A* and *B*, Cosmetic prosthesis for partial hand amputation. (Special credit to Life-Like Laboratory, Dallas, TX; Horst Buckner, MDT, CDT. Used with permission.)

Traumatized hands are often intolerant of extreme temperatures and vibration. The use of neoprene gloves or sleeves (for temperature extremes) and shock-absorbing gloves (for vibration) will increase tolerance to these conditions. Sometimes, adaptation for cold intolerance or hypersensitivity may be as simple as wrapping tape around a tool's handle.

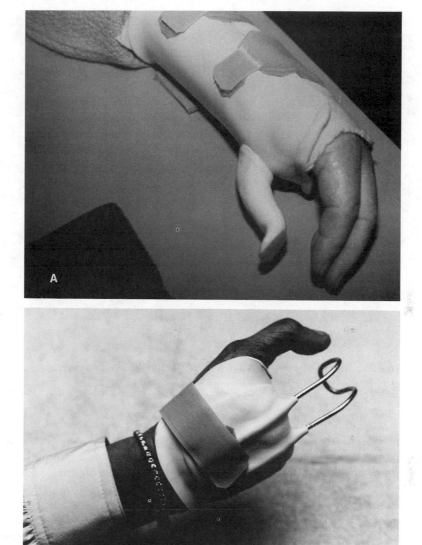

FIGURE 16–21. *A*, Temporary thumb prosthesis. *B*, Partial hand prosthesis for loss of the ulnar side of the hand.

IMPAIRMENT AND DISABILITY CONSIDERATIONS

At the conclusion of the surgical and therapeutic treatment of a crush injury or amputation, the therapist or physician may be asked to provide information regarding the patient's level of impairment or disability. The therapist may be consulted, for instance, as to the type of work the patient can safely do or as to whether the patient can safely return to work at all. In some (but not all) states, the guidelines for rating the level of impairment are set by law or regulatory agencies. Several concerned groups[23] and individuals[24] have published such guidelines as well (Fig. 16–23). One of the best

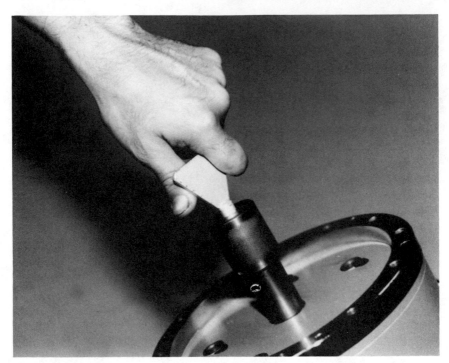

FIGURE 16–22. Use of computerized work simulator allows for practicing activities and desensitizes the finger for normal activities.

methods of determining safe work levels or the level of compensable impairment, or both, is the physical capacity evaluation (see Chapter 17). A well-designed physical capacity test enables the physician or therapist to measure ROM, strength, sensibility, dexterity, level of effort, lifting ability, and other functional abilities and physiologic responses.

The physician or therapist develops an impairment rating based on loss of function and the anatomic part affected. Thumb amputations are the most significantly impairing digital amputation, whereas complete arthrodesis and sensory loss in a finger is the equivalent of amputation. Disability can be defined as the social consequence of impairment and is usually a legal determination based on the injured worker's future loss of wage earning capacity and ability to perform his or her previous job because of the injury.

Because of the financial incentives in litigation and worker's compensation cases based on the results of testing, therapists must include portions of their functional capacity evaluations that assess whether an acceptable effort has been given by the patient.[25] These tests should be fair to the patient but must be designed to demonstrate clearly the patient's level of effort. Pain must be measured by how it affects function rather than by the patient's subjective report.

CLINICAL DECISION MAKING—CASE STUDY

This clinical case analysis is presented as the typical crush injury—complicated, untidy, and involving multiple systems of the hand.

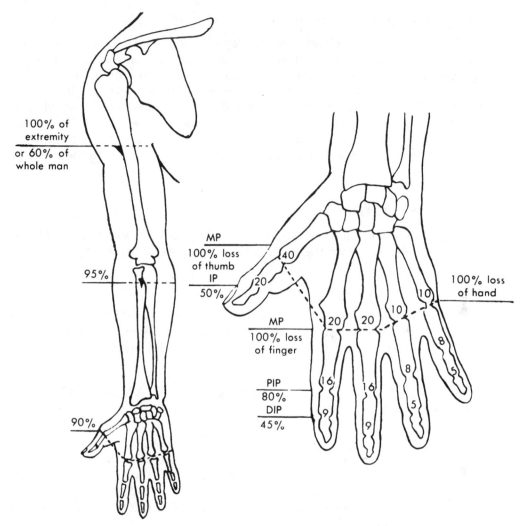

FIGURE 16–23. Amputation impairment guide. (From Swanson, AB, Goran-Hagert, C, and deGroot Swanson, G: Evaluation of impairment of hand function. In Hunter, JM, et al (eds): Rehabilitation of the Hand, ed 2. CV Mosby, St Louis, 1984, p 112, with permission.)

HISTORY

WH, a 59-year-old man, sustained multiple lacerations, abrasions, and fractures of the fingers to his right dominant hand when the backhoe he was operating overturned. The injuries included (1) index finger—distal phalanx fracture; (2) middle finger—comminuted fractures of the middle and distal phalanges, dislocation of the PIP joint, and laceration of the extensor tendon in zone 3; and (3) ring finger—open, comminuted intra-articular fracture of the distal phalanx and distal interphalangeal (DIP) joint. In addition, he had multiple soft tissue injuries with degloving-type skin loss over the dorsum of the hand.

Surgical Report

The surgery was performed on the day of injury. Under general anesthesia, the patient underwent debridement and irrigation of the open wounds, removal of the nails of the long and ring fingers, and open reduction with Kirschner's wire fixation of the middle and ring finger fractures following repair of the extensor tendon. The surgeon determined that the dorsal skin loss would probably heal without grafting. Loose closure of untidy wounds was performed. The patient tolerated the surgical procedures well, and his hand was placed in a bulky, postoperative dressing with immobilization of the entire hand with the exception of the thumb.

Past Medical History

The patient had a longstanding history of hypertension and diabetes. He was taking oral medication for these conditions at the time of his injury.

Vocational History

WH's job involved handling of tools, particularly a shovel and pick, operation of levers, and maintaining his tractor with small hand tools and occasionally larger tools such as a tire tool and jack. He was required to lift up to 75 lb.

THERAPEUTIC MANAGEMENT: INFLAMMATORY/ FIBROPLASIA PHASE

Evaluation

Initial evaluation occurred 1 week after surgery. Observations made at that time included moderate edema with external pins exiting the distal end of the long and ring fingers. The surgical-traumatic wounds were still open. ROM for proximal portion of the extremity was within normal limits. AROM for the wrist and hand was as follows:

Wrist extension/flexion			35/35°
Radioulnar deviation			12/12°

Digits	MP	PIP	DIP
Thumb	0/50	0/30	
Index	0/60	30/60	NT
Middle	0/60	NT	NT
Ring	0/45	30/60	NT
Small	0/60	30/60	0/10

PROM was not assessed owing to the length of time since the injury. Sensibility evaluation of the patient's hand showed no specific nerve involvement but did demonstrate slightly decreased static two-point discrimination of 7 mm in the tips of all fingers. Because of the roughness of the skin and open wounds, moving two-point discrimination was not assessed. The patient had limited ability to use his right hand, including restricted lateral pinch between the thumb and proximal phalanx of the index finger. The patient was using his nondominant left hand for most daily living activities.

Treatment

1 Week After Surgery

Because of his diabetes, a slower healing rate and the possibility of infection were anticipated. WH was taking prescribed oral antibiotics. His skin, which was thick and heavy before the injury, was sloughing, and there was necrotic tissue in the wounds. Edema was the most significant complication factor at the initial evaluation. The treatment program was developed as follows:

1. How might the edema be decreased? Edema management occurred initially through elevation, retrograde massage, and AROM of the unaffected fingers and wrist. An arm elevation pillow was used at night and a sling that held the hand above the elbow was used during the day.
2. What type of splinting program would be most appropriate. Splints for the fingers included volar, static splints for the index, middle, and ring fingers extending beyond the pins to protect them from becoming caught in clothing or hit during active use. These splints were fabricated of ¹⁄₁₆-in thermoplastic, which was selected because of the lightweight and conforming nature of the material. Individual finger splints were chosen during the day to give support and protection while allowing the uninjured joints to remain mobilized. At night, the finger splints were removed and the patient used a resting hand splint made of ¹⁄₈-in thermoplastic material. This resting splint held the wrist in 30° of extension to promote venous drainage. The MP joints were placed in 45° of flexion while the nonsurgically fixated PIP joints were maintained in as much extension as possible. The thumb web space was maintained in its most open position for abduction and opposition.
3. How could wound healing be facilitated? Sterile whirlpool was used with gentle agitation followed by debridement and redressing of the wounds using nonadherent gauze and wrapping with self-adherent wrap to help diminish edema and facilitate closure of the wounds. WH's hand required extensive whirlpool treatments to help debride necrotic tissue, improve circulation of the hand, soften tissue for manual debridement, and allow for application of disinfectant to decrease the bacterial count of his wound. Although the wound continued to heal, cultures revealed a persistent gram-positive *Staphylococcus* infection. The presence of infection implied that the acute inflammatory phase of healing would be prolonged. Manual debridement was also performed. Initially, a bulky dressing with three layers was applied—nonadherent gauze on the wound as the intimate layer; loose, fluffy gauze to absorb drainage as an intermediate layer; and roll gauze and stretch wrap as a protective outer layer.
4. How could ROM be maintained and improved? The joints that were not pinned were mobilized with gentle AROM and PROM as well as light functional activities. Maintenance ROM activities were initiated for the proximal joints of the wrist, elbow, and shoulder.
5. What type of home program should be initiated? A home program was developed to facilitate care between therapy sessions. Edema reduction techniques, ROM of the less affected joints of the hand, and strengthening of the wrist

musculature were emphasized. The patient was encouraged to use compensatory techniques to allow for independence in activities of daily living.

4 Weeks After Surgery

One month after surgery the pins were removed. Wound closure was almost complete, AROM of the wrist and thumb was normal, and edema was decreased. The ROM of the fingers and hand improved as well. What appropriate treatment strategies should be used at this time?

1. Edema reduction techniques, such as wrapping with compressive wrap, elevation, massage, and active exercise in an elevated position should be continued.
2. Sterile whirlpool should be discontinued in favor of hot packs with elevation. The use of moist heat to increase circulation to the area would improve phagocytosis, infiltration of leukocytes and antibodies, and flushing of waste products from the wound. In addition, the moist heat from the hot pack would soften the dry, peeling skin and provide heat to increase the tissue elasticity.
3. Day splints should be continued for an additional 2 weeks for the middle and ring finger to protect the healing fractures and extensor tendon.
4. After removal of the pins, gentle blocking exercises should be started on the long and ring finger PIP and DIP joints. PROM and AROM exercises should be continued on all other joints.

THERAPEUTIC MANAGEMENT: SCAR MATURATION PHASE

Evaluation

Two months after injury, edema continued to decrease while hand function increased. Digital ROM was as follows:

Digits	MP	PIP	DIP
Index	0/70	10/80	0/25
Middle	0/80	25/65	0/20
Ring	0/80	20/75	0/20
Small	0/80	10/80	0/40

The patient's initial grip strength was taken using standardized assessment techniques and was found to be 25 lb on the right hand compared with 80 lb on the left. WH was independent in self-care skills.

Treatment

Two Months After Surgery

Two months after surgery the patient was in the scar maturation phase of wound healing characterized by hardening of the residual edema and increasing resistance to joint motion. With the resolution of the inflammatory stage, the patient was ready for a more aggressive therapy program that addressed the problems of limited motion and weakness. How should the therapy program be modified in the scar maturation phase of wound healing?

1. Edema reduction techniques should be continued emphasizing heat, deep pressure massage, and compression gloves.
2. Restoration of joint ROM should be aggressively pursued. Joint mobilization should be used and AROM and PROM exercises, particularly for PIP extension and DIP flexion, encouraged. Dynamic splinting progressing to static progressive splinting or serial cylindrical splinting should be initiated as the fractures had healed sufficiently to use these more aggressive devices. The relative equality in immobility of the PIP and DIP joints allowed for use of a flexion mitt for the middle and ring fingers. A forearm-based hand splint with MP block and low-profile PIP extension assist was fabricated to increase PIP joint extension.

Three Months After Surgery

At 3 months after surgery, WH continued strengthening through functional activities and use of the Work Simulator. His grip strength had improved to 40 lb and he was able to use the hand for light to moderate activities at home. His pain had decreased significantly and edema was no longer present. Except for occasional use, the extension splint and flexion mit were discontinued. WH continued in therapy two to three times weekly with emphasis on improving work tolerance with activities such as lifting, using hand tools, general conditioning, and other tasks performed at work.

FINAL EVALUATION

Four months after surgery, a physical capacity evaluation was ordered by his physician to provide information for determining an impairment rating and functional level. WH's performance on the evaluation, as measured by validity factors, represented maximum voluntary effort. Evaluation showed no edema, either at rest or with activity. The following objective measurements were recorded:

TAM right vs left	670° vs 940° = 71%
Grip strength	70 lb
Pincer prehension	12 lb
Tripod prehension	13 lb
Lateral prehension	15 lb
Two-handed lifting	
Floor to waist	70 lb
Waist to shoulder	44 lb
Shoulder to overhead	24 lb
One-handed lifting	
Floor level (right hand)	52 lb
Pushing	30 lb
Pulling	50 lb

The patient had some residual stiffness of the fingers, but considering the severity of his injury, early infection, and premorbid state of the patient, the outcome was acceptable. Sensibility of the injured hand was essentially equal to the uninvolved hand. WH had decreased dexterity as noted by Purdue pegboard testing. His right hand was below the first percentile, whereas the left was in the 15th percentile when compared with male maintenance and service workers' results.

From this information, his physician's evaluation indicated a permanent impairment of 40% of the hand, based on loss of strength, motion, and dexterity. He was able to return to the same company with lifting restrictions, as previously noted. Upon return to work he was primarily performing equipment maintenance and heavy machinery operations.

SUMMARY

This chapter has reviewed two sequelae of serious trauma to the hand—crush injuries and amputations. The number and magnitude of problems seen in this patient population require a goal-oriented, problem-solving approach by the treating therapist. The therapist's role is maximized through early referral, intervention, and prevention of problems by aggressively treating the patient within the presenting stages of wound healing. Through careful evaluation and treatment, the optimum potential recovery for each of these injuries can be attained.

REFERENCES

1. Kelly, JM and Madden, JW: Hand surgery and wound healing. In Wolfort, FG (ed): Acute Hand Injuries—A Multispecialty Approach. Little, Brown, Boston, 1980, p 48.
2. Brown, PW: Open injuries of the hand. In Green, DP (ed): Operative Hand Surgery, ed 2. Churchill Livingstone, New York, 1988, p 1637.
3. Wynn Parry, CB: Rehabilitation of the Hand, ed 3. Butterworths, London, p 210.
4. Tsuge, K: Comprehensive Atlas of Hand Surgery. Year Book Medical Publishers, Chicago, p 253.
5. Chase, RA and Hentz, VR: The philosophy of hand salvage and repair. In Wolfort, FG (ed): Acute Hand Injuries—A Multispecialty Approach. Little, Brown, Boston, 1980, p 12.
6. Miles, W: Soft tissue trauma. Hand Clin 2(1):33, 1986.
7. Cailliet, R: Hand Pain and Impairment, ed 3. FA Davis, Philadelphia, 1982, p 216.
8. Fess, EE, Gettle, KS, and Strickland, JW: Hand Splinting Principles and Methods. CV Mosby, St Louis, 1981, p 221.
9. Madden, JW: Wound healing: The biological basis of hand surgery. In Hunter, JM, et al (eds): Rehabilitation of the Hand, ed 2. CV Mosby, St Louis, 1984, p 142.
10. Fess, EE, Gettle, KS, and Strickland, JW: Hand Splinting Principles and Methods. CV Mosby, St Louis, 1981, p 185.
11. Braun, RM and McGough, C: Immobilization, mobilization, and rehabilitation of the injured hand. In Sandzen, SC (ed): The Hand and Wrist. Williams & Wilkins, Baltimore, 1985, p 330.
12. Lankford, LL and Thompson, JE: Reflex sympathetic dystrophy, upper and lower extremity: Diagnosis and management. In American Academy of Orthopaedic Surgeons: Instructional Course Lectures, Vol 26. CV Mosby, St Louis, 1977, p 163.
13. Salter, RB, et al: The effects of continuous passive motion on healing of full thickness defects in articular cartilage. J Bone Surg 62A:1232, 1980.
14. Mennell, JM: Joint Pain: Diagnosis and Treatment Using Manipulative Techniques. Little, Brown, Boston, p 40.
15. Baxter, PL and Freid, SL: The work tolerance program of the Hand Rehabilitation Center in Philadelphia. In Hunter, JM, et al (eds): Rehabilitation of the Hand, ed 2. CV Mosby, St. Louis, 1984, p 895.
16. Blackmore, SM, et al: A comparison study of three methods to determine exercise resistance and duration for the BTE Work Simulator. J Hand Ther 1:165, 1988.
17. Grad, JB and Beasley, RW: Fingertip reconstruction. Hand Clin 1(4):670, 1985.
18. Grad, JB and Beasley, RW: Fingertip reconstruction. Hand Clin 1(4):670, 1985.
19. Markley, JM: Island flaps of the hand. Hand Clin 1(4):689, 1985.
20. Herndon, JH: Neuromas. In Green, DP (ed): Operative Hand Surgery. Churchill Livingstone, New York, 1988, p 1408.
21. Godfrey, SB: Workers with prostheses. J Hand Ther 3:101, 1990.

22. Johnson, SL: Ergonomic design of hand-held tools to prevent trauma to the hand and upper extremity. J Hand Ther 3:86, 1990.
23. Engelberg, AL (ed): American Medical Association Guides to the Evaluation of Permanent Impairment, ed 3. American Medical Association, Chicago, 1988, p 14.
24. Swanson, AB, Goran-Hagert, C, and Swanson, G: Evaluation of impairment of hand function. In Hunter, JM, et al (eds): Rehabilitation of the Hand, ed 2. CV Mosby, St Louis, 1984, p 101.
25. King, JW and Berryhill, BH: A method of determining the probability of maximum effort during upper extremity functional testing. WORK 1:65–76, 1991.

BIBLIOGRAPHY

American Society for Surgery of the Hand: The Hand—Examination and Diagnosis. American Society for Surgery of the Hand, Aurora, CO, 1978.

Baxter, PL and Ballard, MS: Evaluation of the hand by functional tests. In Hunter, JM, et al (eds): Rehabilitation of the Hand, ed 2. CV Mosby, St Louis, 1984, p. 91.

Beasley, RW: Management of upper limb amputations. Orthop Clin of North Am 12(4):767, 1981.

Boyes, JH: A philosophy of care of the injured hand. Bull Am Coll Surg 50:341, 1965.

Bright, D and Wright, S: Post-operative management in replantation. In American Academy of Orthopaedic Surgeons: Symposium on Microsurgery: Practical Use in Orthopaedics. CV Mosby, St Louis, 1979.

Bunnell, S: Ischemic contracture, local, in the hand. J Bone Joint Surg 35A:88, 1953.

Cochran, TC: Fingertip injuries. In Wolfort, FG (ed): Acute Hand Injuries—A Multispecialty Approach. Little, Brown, Boston, 1980, p 227.

Entin, MA: Crushing and avulsing injuries of the hand. Surg Clin North Am 44:1009, 1964.

Frazier, SH and Kolb CC: Psychiatric aspects of pain and the phantom limb. Orthop Clin North Am 1:481, 1970.

Hardy, MA and Moran, CA: Desensitization of the traumatized hand. Va Med 109:134, 1982.

Littler, JW: Mobilization of the stiffened proximal interphalangeal joint. J Bone Joint Surg 46A:917, 1964.

Littler, JW: On making a thumb: One hundred years of surgical effort. J Hand Surg 1:135, 1976.

Linscheid, RL and Dobyns, JH: Common and uncommon infections of the hand. Orthop Clin North Am 6:1063, 1975.

Marshall, KA: Soft tissue coverage. In Wolfort, FG (ed): Acute Hand Injuries—A Multispecialty Approach. Little, Brown, Boston, 1980, p 116.

Neider, H, et al: Reduction of skin bacterial load with use of the therapeutic whirlpool. Phys Ther 55(5):482, 1975.

Nemeth, GE: Phalangeal fractures treated by open reduction and Kirschner wire fixation. Ind Med Surg 23:148, 1954.

Peacock, EE, Jr: Dynamic splinting for the prevention and correction of hand deformities. J Bone Joint Surg 34A:789, 1952.

Peacock, EE, Jr: Some biochemical and biophysical aspects of joint stiffness: Role of collagen synthesis as opposed to ultra-molecular binding. Ann Surg 164:1, 1966.

Pratt, DR: Joints of the hand and fingers—their stiffness, splinting and surgery. Cal Med 66:22, 1947.

Sturnam, MJ and Duran, RJ: Late results of fingertip injuries. J Bone Joint Surg 45A:289, 1963.

Swanson, AB: Restoration of hand function by the use of partial prosthesis. J Bone Joint Surg 45A:276, 1963.

Tajima, T: Treatment of open crushing type of industrial injuries of the hand and forearm: Degloving, open circumferential, heat press, and nail bed injuries. J Trauma 14:995, 1974.

Weeks, PM and Wray, RC: Management of the stiff hand. In Management of Acute Hand Injuries, ed 1. CV Mosby, St Louis, 1973, p 255.

CHAPTER **17**

Returning the Hand-Injured Patient to Work

Susan M. Blackmore, MS, OTR, CHT
Laura Bruening-Reilly, OTR/L

Rehabilitation following hand injuries is not considered completed until the patient can participate in work and leisure activities. As a result, therapy programs that facilitate the performance of work and leisure activities have become an important component of the rehabilitation process.

There has been renewed interest in work therapy programming over the past 10 years, although prevocational therapy began in the 1920s with the enactment of the Vocational Rehabilitation Act.[1-3] Table 17-1 presents a timeline of the major events that lead to the development of return to work programs. Over the years, numerous terms have been used to describe work-related programming including work hardening, return to work programs, work conditions, work capacity testing, work tolerance training, and work therapy. For consistency, the term "work therapy" will be used in this text.

A comprehensive work therapy program includes many phases. Initially a job analysis is performed to identify the patient's job requirements. Next, a rehabilitation program is designed to help the patient develop the strength, endurance, and coordination necessary to perform his or her job. A work capacity evaluation is used to assess the patient's physical capabilities and limitations with regard to work. If the patient is unable to return to work after participating in a rehabilitation program, then modification of the work environment, tasks, or tools is explored. A successful return to work program involves the coordinated efforts of the patient, therapist, physician, employer, rehabilitation specialist, insurance company, and attorney.

The objectives of this chapter are to (1) describe the performance of a job analysis; (2) describe the four components of a work therapy program including flexibility, strength, endurance, and job simulation; (3) describe the testing procedures used in a work capacity evaluation (WCE); (4) outline possible job alternatives based on the patient's physical limitations; and (5) present a case study that demonstrates how the

504

TABLE 17-1 Timeline

1900s	Returning soldiers from World War I	Concerned about return to work for these
1910	Victims of polio epidemic	individuals; used crafts in rehabilitation
1916	Industrial and auto accident victims	process
1920	Vocational Rehabilitation Act	

1920   Federal government matches state funds for the disabled. The rehabilitation of disabled individuals includes the goal of returning these individuals to work.

Community-based workshops were developed by Barton to return individuals to work.

Dinton focused on developing work habits for psychiatric patients with work programs that last all day.

Kidner worked with industrial injuries. He provided activity as a component of therapy to return individuals to work.

1930   Therapists incorporated activities as a part of their treatment plans such as bookbinding, printing, and cement work.

1934   Social Security Act provided that physically disabled individuals needed vocational rehabilitation for return to work. Job modifications needed to be considered.

1938   Canadian Workmen's Compensation Board formed a workshop to decrease compensation costs. The workshop had injured workers complete occupation-related tasks.

1943   Vocational Rehabilitation Act Amendment of 1943, provided that disabled individuals who have never worked be given vocational training.

1950s   Therapists focused on developing work habits and work hardening program. The Testing Orientation and Work Evaluation in Rehabilitation (TOWER) system was developed.

1960s   The Stout Vocational Rehabilitation Institute was developed to be a database for information about work programs.

1970s   Rehabilitation Act of 1973 and Rehabilitation Act of 1975; both acts stated that therapy for children to be provided for and paid for by the school systems.

More work hardening programs developed with the focus on the individual's physical demands.

1980s   Therapists began to look at injury prevention as a component of their programs. More therapists began to consult with private industry.

---

job analysis, work therapy program, and WCE contribute to returning the patient to work.

JOB ANALYSIS

The first phase of preparing the hand-injured patient for returning to work is to obtain a thorough job analysis by cross-referencing four sources. The sources described here include a patient interview, employer contact, the *Dictionary of Occupational Titles*,[4] and the therapist visiting the job site.

Patient Interview

The structured patient interview allows the therapist to identify the patient's perception of the injury and job requirements, as well as plans for the future. The patient's description of the type of physical demands involved in the particular job and the frequency with which the demands are performed are also documented on a specially designed form (Fig. 17-1). Tables 17-2 and 17-3 explain the meaning of the ratings

THE NEW YORK HOSPITAL DEPARTMENT OF REHABILITATION MEDICINE
JOB ANALYSIS

Employee: _____ Date: _____
Occupation: _____
Subjective Description: _____
DOT Title: _____ DOT Number: _____
Level of Work: (circle): Sedentary (Max 10lb) Light (Max 20lb) Medium (Max 50lb)
Heavy (Max 100lb) Very Heavy (Max over 100lb)
Comments: _____

Frequency				Physical Demand
Never	Occ.	Freq.	Const.	
1.				1. Finger-Objects: _____
2.				2. Handle-Objects: _____
3.				3. Reach-Objects, Range: _____
4.				4. Push/Pull-Objects, Tools: _____
5a.				5a. Lift (bilateral)-Objects, Range: _____
5b.				5b. Lift (unilateral)-Objects, Distance: _____
6.				6. Carry-Objects, Distance: _____
7.				7. Feel: _____
8.				8. Climb: _____
9.				9. Balance: _____
10.				10. Stoop: _____
11.				11. Kneel: _____
12.				12. Crouch: _____
13.				13. Crawl: _____
14.				14. Stand: _____
15.				15. Sit: _____
16.				16. Walk: _____
17.				17. Repetitive Motions: _____
18.				18. Torque: Objects, Tools: _____
19.				19. Body Twist: _____
20.				20. Write: _____
21.				21. Tools-Type:. _____
22.				22. Machines: _____
23.				23. Drive: _____

Is light duty work available: Yes_____ No_____ Unsure_____ Describe: _____

Is Minor job modification feasible? Yes_____ No_____ Unsure_____

Is the job unionized? Yes_____ No_____

Plan of action: _____
_____

FIGURE 17–1. The patient and employer describe the type and frequency of physical demands made by his or her job on the job analysis form.

TABLE 17–2 Physical Demands[4,5]

Lifting: The ability to raise an object from floor level to waist level and overhead
Carrying: The ability to move an object by holding it in both arms or by one hand
Pushing: The ability to move an object away from the body using the upper extremities
Pulling: The ability to move an object toward the body using the upper extremities
Reaching: The ability to move the upper extremities forward, overhead, behind, or downward from the body
Fingering: Using the manipulation skills (i.e., fingertips)
Handling: The ability to manipulate with the hand
Walking: Moving on foot
Standing: The ability to bear weight on one or both feet while standing in one location
Kneeling: To assume position on knees
Stooping: To assume position with knees bent but not touching the floor
Crawling: Using hands and knees to move
Climbing: The ability to go up and down stairs and ladders
Feeling: Perceiving size, shapes, and texture of an object through sensory receptors in the fingers

used in the form. The interview is used to build rapport with the patient and discover his or her perceived limitations due to the injury. The patient's future goals are discussed to identify whether the patient wants to return to former work.

Employer Contact

After completion of the patient interview, the same job analysis form is sent to the employer to gain the same information about the job requirements as obtained from the patient. A comparison can be made between the job descriptions completed by the patient and those of the employer to identify perceived and actual work requirements. It is not uncommon for a patient to add tasks to the required job demands to help co-workers or to speed a production process. Sending the analysis form to the employer during the early phase of a patient's treatment program serves to establish communication between the therapist and the employer. Also, the feasibility of alternative return-to-work issues can be examined.

Dictionary of Occupational Titles

The third source for completion of the job analysis is through the *Dictionary of Occupational Titles (DOT)* and selected characteristics of occupations as defined in the *DOT*.[4] The United States Department of Labor publishes these texts to provide a

TABLE 17–3 Frequency Rating for Physical Demands Per 8-Hour Day[5]

NA	Not present
Rarely	Less than 58 min/day
Occasionally	Between 59 min and 2½ hours/day
Frequently	Between 2½ hours and 5 hours/day
Continuously	Greater than 5 hours/day

description of jobs as well as to list the critical physical demands involved in each job. The job description paragraph in the *DOT* is read to the patient to assess the accuracy of the listed job compared with the patient's actual job.

On-Site Visit

The final way to obtain a job analysis[5] is for the therapist to visit the job site to perform an activity analysis for the components of the patient's job. The on-site visit is most often performed as the patient progresses in strengthening activities and when job simulation tasks need to be incorporated into the therapy program.

The on-site visit job analysis is performed by breaking the job into task performance segments, then analyzing each task according to the physical demand and the frequency with which the demands are performed. The job tasks can be described from the following perspectives: biomechanical, resistance level of the activity, extremes of motion, temperature, vibration, repetitions of motion required to complete the task, and repetitions of the completed task per day. Tools or equipment that help the therapist perform the job analysis include a camera, stopwatch, measuring tape, and push-pull gauge.

A visit to the job site can give the therapist a clear concept of the job requirements, as well as a perspective on the psychosocial and cultural aspects of the workplace. The work environment is often a critical component that can affect the patient's readiness in return to work.

WORK THERAPY PROGRAM

Once the job requirements of the patient are defined, a work therapy program is designed for conditioning the patient prior to working. Patients who participate in a work therapy program usually require reconditioning before returning to their jobs. Reconditioning can involve strengthening, endurance training, technique training to decrease potential stresses placed on the upper extremities, or coordinating training. Reconditioning for many patients may include strengthening, but for the work therapy patient job activities are useful in the treatment program.

The program begins with an initial evaluation of the patient's upper extremity function[6] to establish baseline measurements, to assist with the determination of the entry level into the work therapy program, and to identify any problem areas.

This evaluation includes the measurement of range of motion (ROM), grip strength, pinch strength, coordination, sensibility, edema, and muscle function (see Chapters 3, 4, and 5).

In addition to standard measurements of upper extremity function, the patient is evaluated for the ability to manage both the weight and duration of resistive exercises[7] (Table 17–4). If a patient's therapy program is restricted to active motion without resistance, then the patient begins the work therapy program at level 1 for the purposes of edema control and beginning active hand movement. Patients are advanced in 1-lb increments when resistive exercises are allowed.

Level 2 programming begins when resistive activities and exercises are allowed. The patient participates in a level 3 program to begin upper extremity conditioning and strengthening. Levels 4 and 5 incorporate job simulation. The patient may begin at any

TABLE 17–4 Work Therapy Program Level and Activities

Program Level	Activities
Level 1: 0–1 lb	Prehension activities and edema control
Level 2: 1–3 lb	Focusing on active motion
Level 3: 3–30 lb	Work hardening and
Level 4: 30–60 lb	Job simulation
Level 5: 60–100 lb	Heavy job simulation, if necessary

level of the program depending on precautions and the patient's limitations. Reevaluations are done monthly, or more frequently if needed, with the hand evaluations listed earlier.

After the completion of the upper extremity functional evaluation, the patient is ready to begin the work therapy program. Patients can participate in a work therapy program when active range of motion (AROM) is allowed. Often acute injury management and the work therapy program overlap. Early involvement in work therapy is desirable to limit the possible loss of function due to immobilization and lack of performance of daily tasks. A patient is often involved in work therapy before being strong enough to perform work tasks.

The work therapy program is based on four component areas: flexibility, strength, endurance, and job simulation. Patients usually begin with flexibility and strengthening activities and progress to endurance training and job simulation.

Flexibility

Flexibility is defined as the "ability for the patient's musculoskeletal system to relax against passive resistance."[8] The patient who is not working usually experiences a decrease in activity level and might even guard the injured hand by not moving the shoulder, resulting in decreased flexibility in areas other than the injured hand. Flexibility is emphasized to prevent proximal ROM limitations.

Performance of work and leisure tasks requires composite movements of the upper extremity. Composite movements, such as reaching overhead to place a stack of paper on a shelf, requires elongation of the finger flexors. If the end range of musculoskeletal length cannot be obtained, then the patient may have to alter patterns of movement to perform tasks. For example, when stacking paper on a high shelf, the patient may need a step ladder to reach the shelf.

The flexibility component of the therapy program includes warmup exercises and aerobic activity, followed by maximal elongation of the musculoskeletal system. Warmup activities include circumduction of the shoulder, wrist and thumb and full ROM exercises for the elbow and fingers to move the joints through their available ROM. Aerobic activity can be as simple as marching in place. Equipment for aerobic activity can include the upper body ergometer or the Baltimore Therapeutic Equipment (BTE) Work Simulator, rowing machine, bike, or treadmill. Patients must have medical clearance before performing aerobic exercise. The light work performed by large muscle groups enhances the delivery of oxygen to the muscles, to prevent postexercise soreness.[8]

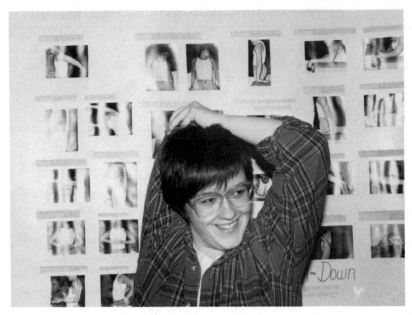

FIGURE 17–2. Upper extremity stretching to improve composite range of motion.

After warmups and aerobic exercise, the patient performs gentle prolonged (30-second) stretches to the areas with limited ROM to enhance composite ROM (e.g., simultaneous wrist and digit extension). Upper trunk stretching (Fig. 17–2) is also included if there are no contraindications such as back or neck problems.

Strength

As the patient gains flexibility, the strengthening component of the work therapy program is initiated. Strength is defined as the "maximal force exerted by a muscle."[8] Patients perform activities and exercises to enhance isometric, concentric, and eccentric muscle contractions because all three types of contractions are used in work task performance. The strengthening program is individually designed for each patient depending on diagnosis, limitations, and job requirements. Patients usually begin with isometric conditioning and advance to isotonic exercises because the patient must be able to hold an item before attempting to move the item (Fig. 17–3). One exception to this program applies to patients who have a diagnosis of cumulative trauma. Often their strengthening program is limited to isometric exercises and they are taught alternative techniques for job performance requiring repetitive motion.

Some of the equipment and activities used most frequently for strengthening are seen in Figure 17–4, including regressive resistive exercises for forearm musculature,[9-11] Theraputty, Theraband, resistive gripping devices, the BTE Work Simulator, woodworking, clay molding on the potter's wheel, wall pulleys, weight well, and the Bioflex Wrist Exerciser (Fig. 17–4). The patient not only strengthens musculature weakened by the injury but also reconditions muscles that he or she uses for work activities.

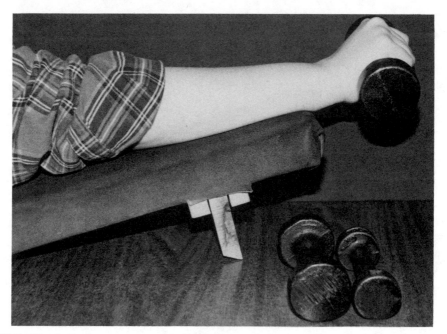

FIGURE 17–3. Patients progress to isotonic exercises after they satisfactorily complete the isometric program.

Endurance

As the patient gains strength to perform work tasks, endurance training is emphasized. Endurance is defined as "the ability to continue a specific task."[9] General endurance conditioning begins early in the program with aerobic exercise. Endurance training for job-specific tasks begins when the patient has the motion, coordination, and strength to complete one repetition of the task. Time or repetition of work activities are increased at every other visit; this schedule maximizes successful performance of work tasks. We believe that patients who tolerate one-half day of job simulation can perform a full day of work.

Job Simulation

Job tasks are introduced into the work therapy program as the patient achieves soft tissue mobility, maximum joint motion, tendon excursion, coordination, and strength. Information from the job analysis provides the therapist with the specific physical demands[4,5] and the tools used on the job. The modality of treatment is advanced to include work tasks. Patients are often asked to bring work supplies to therapy to accurately simulate work tasks.

When setting up a work area, the prominent area industries should be identified and materials and activities commonly used in jobs in those industries should be incorporated. Work stations can be designed to simulate several components of one job. Each work station includes the necessary equipment and supplies (Fig. 17–5), patient

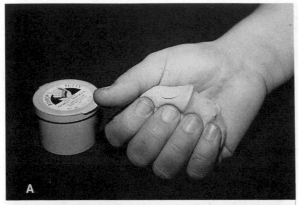
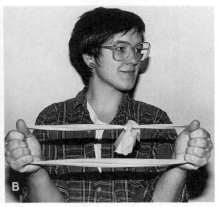
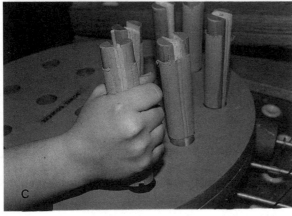

FIGURE 17–4. Exercise equipment used to increase strength includes *A*, putty; *B*, theraband; *C*, dowel squeeze;

instructions (Table 17–5), and, for each type of job, a form for monitoring patient progress (Fig. 17–6). After initial instruction in each task in the job simulation, each patient works independently with distant supervision from the therapist.

In addition to work tasks, the BTE Work Simulator is a space-efficient piece of equipment used to simulate many job tasks. This equipment allows the therapist to grade resistance, duration, and the amount of movement the patient performs (Fig. 17–7). Creativity and adaptability are needed when designing a job simulation program. Each program will be different according to the patient's limitations and job requirements.

WORK CAPACITY EVALUATION

A WCE, also known as a physical capacity or functional capacity evaluation, assesses a patient's physical capabilities and limitations with regard to work. By outlining the patient's strengths and weaknesses, the WCE is completed to determine if the patient is capable of performing his or her job requirements. The information obtained from the evaluation assesses the individual's ability to return to work safely[5,13] and provides useful information when considering alternative job placements. The WCE has five components: medical and work history, hand function, standardized testing, physical demands of work, and effort consistency.[12]

Various methods are used to complete a WCE. The assessment can be completed in 3 hours or can be broken into several components over several days. Even though not

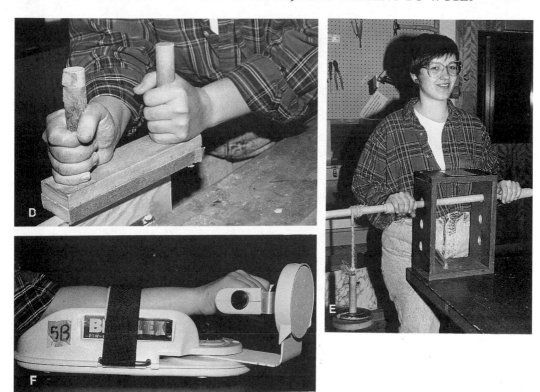

FIGURE 17–4. *D*, hand sanding; *E*, weight well; *F*, Bioflex wrist and forearm exercise.

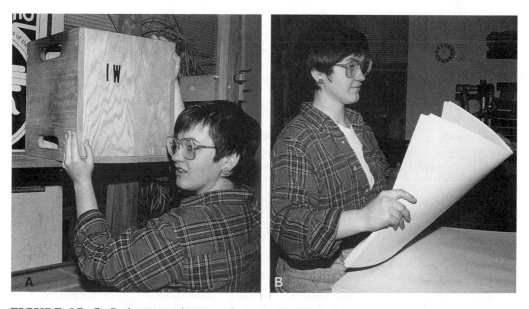

FIGURE 17–5. Patients are instructed to complete activities that simulate their jobs. *A*, Overhead lifting; *B*, manipulating paper.

TABLE 17–5 Work Station: Nurse's Aide and
Laboratory Technologist

Instructions for the patient:

1. Ride the bike or walk; the time is listed on your therapy card.
2. Wheelchair: You must ask one of the staff to obtain the wheelchair for you. Place the designated amount of sandbag weight in the chair. Push the chair around the tables for the time listed on your card.
3. Making a bed: Check with your therapist on the availability of a room where you can practice this task. Use the sheet and pillowcase provided to complete the task.
4. Stacking trays and/or jars: Either in a seated or standing position in front of the lifting frame, move the trays/jars from waist height to overhead and return to waist height. Move repetitively for 5 minutes (or the time designated on your therapy card) using both hands.
5. Carrying trays/jars: Place the designated amount of sandbag weights on the tray or around the jars. Using both hands, carry the objects around the tables for the time designated on your therapy card.
6. Thumbciser: Use the Thumbciser for 20 repetitions. Perform the motion very slowly. Add rubberbands when you can tolerate additional resistance. Repetitions may be advanced by your therapist as you gain strength and endurance.
7. Ear syringe: Use the ear syringe to transfer water from one jar to another. Continue this for 3 to 5 minutes or as designated on your therapy card.
8. Rubberbands and paper: Use the rubberbands provided to secure paper around the jars. Practice placing the paper on and removing it for the time listed on your therapy card.
9. Tongue depressor: Use the tongue depressor to stir the liquid in the jar for 50 repetitions or for the amount of repetitions listed on your card.
10. Minnesota Range of Manipulation Test: Place the board on a tabletop and practice placing or turning the red disks as instructed by your therapist.
11. Valpar Simulated Assembly: Your therapist will instruct you on the operation of this piece of equipment. Complete the assemblies for the time designated on your therapy card.
12. Valpar Whole Body Test: Stand in front of the frame and remove the bolted nuts from the bolts and place the nuts in the container on the middle of the frame. Move the colored shapes from one panel to the next. Return the bolted nuts to the board to hold the shapes in place. Repeat this to return the shapes back to panel one.
13. HI-Q: This activity will be explained by your therapist. You will use the tweezers to remove and replace the hex nuts from the pegboard.
14. Work Simulator: Your therapist will instruct and monitor you with this piece of equipment.

always feasible, spreading the test over several days offers many advantages. If the evaluation is completed in 1 day, the therapist cannot assess swelling, discomfort, or pain that may occur later. Completing a WCE over several days allows for retesting in specific areas. For example, edema may not be significant immediately after the WCE but may occur the morning after repetitious job performance. The physical demands section of the WCE can be broken down so that one component is repeated for 2 to 3 hours. Repeating the performance of job tasks is used for patients with limitations resulting from cumulative trauma. Then the component that causes the most inflammation can be identified.

Medical and Work History

A medical history is obtained by reviewing the medical chart. The mechanism of injury, medical treatment, surgical intervention, and therapy program can provide an accurate picture of the patient's course of rehabilitation. A patient interview will disclose the injury's impact on the patient's level of functioning.

WORK STATION
NURSE'S AIDE AND LABORATORY TECHNICIAN

TASK/MEASUREMENT	DATE									
BIKE OR WALK/ Time										
WHEELCHAIR/ Time, Wt										
BED/ Reps										
STACK TRAYS/ HT, Wt, Reps										
CARRY TRAYS/ Wt., Reps										
THUMBCISER/ Reps										
EAR SYRINGE/ Reps										
PAPER AND R.B./ Reps or Time										
STIRRING/ Reps or Time										
MRMT/ Time, Reps, Ht.										
SIM ASSEM/ Time										
WHOLE BODY/ Time/Transfers										
HI-Q/ Time										
BTE WS/ Force										

FIGURE 17–6. The work station consists of job components that are independently performed by the patient and supervised by a therapist while attending therapy.

A work history is obtained through an interview with the patient. Previous work experience is discussed. The patient may have transferable skills from a previous employment that may be beneficial for alternative placement. Obtaining information regarding present job descriptions was discussed in the job analysis section of this chapter.[12]

Hand Function

The assessment of hand function consists of measuring strength, ROM, sensibility, edema, and coordination (see Chapter 3).

Strength measurements are taken for grip and pinch. Grip measurements are taken on the five levels of the Jamar Dynamometer.[14] The percentage differences between hands should be recorded because it places the grip and pinch strength measurements of the injured hand in a more meaningful context.

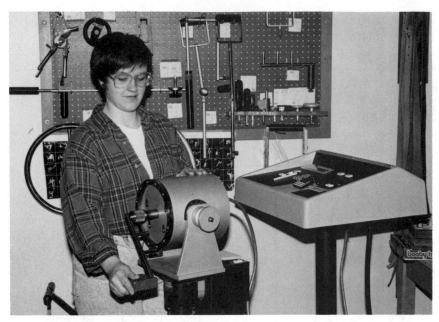

FIGURE 17–7. The work simulator is used for increasing strength and endurance, as well as job simulation. This person is simulating a movement completed frequently as a paper cutter.

The evaluation assesses function deficits, so AROM is measured more often than PROM. ROM is measured for all joint motions of the hand, wrist, elbow, and shoulder. Any deficits are compared with measurements from the noninjured extremity.[6]

The third section of hand evaluation focuses on sensation. Sensation is needed for full hand function.[15,16] In the work environment, employees are exposed to extremes of temperature, moving machinery, tools, and sharp objects. The Moberg pickup test[17] identifies compensation techniques in fine prehension if the median nerve is impaired. Sensibility loss varies in severity and the Semmes-Weinstein monofilament test grades any loss in four categories ranging from light touch to deep pressure. Recommendations for return to work may be influenced by the degree of sensibility in the patient's hand.[16]

The measuring of edema is completed at least twice during the evaluation using a Volumeter.[18] A baseline measurement is taken of both hands before the assessment is begun. Another measurement is taken at the end of the WCE to determine if the patient's hand edema has increased. If the patient has overworked and did not tolerate the evaluation well, the hand may swell. Edema measurements can be taken many times throughout the assessment to determine if one activity causes more edema than others. This technique can be beneficial in identifying a repetitive motion that is causing inflammation.

Coordination is evaluated through standardized tests (see Chapter 3). Both gross and fine coordination are assessed as applicable to job requirements.

Standardized Tests

The importance of incorporating standardized tests in a WCE cannot be overestimated.[13] The results from these tests validate conclusions and recommendations. Many therapists have found that standardized testing increases the validity of the WCE, especially in litigation circumstances.

Each WCE is different depending on the purpose of the evaluation. If the test is administered to determine whether the patient can return to former work, then the test focuses on skills needed for the specific job. For example, in testing a patient who works on a conveyor line putting machine parts in a box, information about speed and endurance may be most beneficial. The Valpar simulated assembly work sample is useful for testing speed and endurance for the upper extremity.

If the work capacity evaluation is being administered to determine a work level,[12] the goal is to obtain information about upper extremity function. The Jebsen-Taylor hand function assessment[19] and the Valpar upper extremity work sample would be appropriate, because these assessments focus on handling and manipulation but may not be job specific.

Many standardized tests are available to the therapist. Availability of a variety of tests emphasizing the work population treated most frequently by the clinic is optimal. The following tests are particularly useful in performing WCEs, because they are easy to administer, apply to a large population, and provide good insight into the patient's ability to perform certain jobs.

The Jebsen-Taylor hand function assessment[19] evaluates unilateral grasp and prehension patterns. Although this test cannot be purchased commercially, it can be assembled inexpensively by the therapist. The Jebsen-Taylor hand function test is fast and easy to administer

The nine-hole peg test[20] evaluates unilateral fine manipulation. Fingertip prehension of ¼-in pegs is required. This test is also fast and easy to administer.

The Purdue pegboard test[12] consists of four subtests. This test provides information on fine coordination and speed of manipulation, necessary for many assembly-type jobs. For patients with jobs that require precise fine manipulation, such as jewelers or electronic assemblers, these tests can provide important information about the ability to return to work.

The *Valpar work sample assessment tools*[12] are a group of tests that come with scores from a working population. By comparing the patient's scores with those of a normal working population, the therapist can determine how the patient will function in the work force.

The Minnesota rate of manipulation test[12] consists of four subtests, which assess unilateral and bilateral coordination. Each subtest has four trials that allow for the assessment of endurance. They also test an individual's ability to reach forward while sitting.

Physical Demands

Additional information about the patient's work performance can be gained through observing task performance. Patients demonstrate their ability to complete the physical demands that are commonly seen in a workplace. The test can involve finding maximum abilities and limitations for the physical demands of work (see Table 17–2). Individual job tasks can be added so that the evaluation can be more job specific.

Physical demand testing requires the use of boxes, crates, wall pulleys, buckets, weighted cans, stairs, ladders, shelves at various heights, and objects for fine and gross manipulation to simulate the tasks listed in Table 17–2. The patient's performance of work tasks is examined for speed, accuracy, tool use, coordination and endurance. The patient's tolerance for sustained positions, temperature, vibration, repetitive motions, and amounts of resistance is documented. The patient's body mechanics, compensatory movements, and hand use with vision occluded are observed.[5]

During work simulation, modifications may be made for tools, work stations, and techniques of tool use. If the modifications enable the patient to safely perform work tasks during the WCE, then these modifications are suggested to the employer.

Effort Consistency

During a WCE, determining if the patient is working to maximum ability is often difficult. Patients are instructed to work within pain limits and to lift and carry only the weight that can be lifted safely. In some cases, when patients are not trying their hardest, the results will not provide a true picture of their functional ability. Throughout the evaluation, there are methods to ensure that the patients' performance is consistent and that they are performing to their maximum capacity. The following tests are designed to assess the patient's maximal effort performance.

A patient's lifting ability is assessed initially with a wooden box that weighs approximately 18 lb. The weight of the box plus the amount of weight placed in the box is never mentioned to the patient. The therapist simply asks the patient to lift the box with weights to determine a maximum lifting ability. For example, a patient may be able to lift 60 lb in the wooden box. The patient is then asked to lift to his or her maximum with a plastic crate that may weigh 1 lb. In order to show consistency in his lifting ability, the patient should lift approximately 60 lb plus the 18-lb weight of the wooden box.

Stokes[14] documented that grip strength should follow a bell-shaped curve for the five levels of the Dynamometer when the individual is working to his or her maximum potential. In other words, strength measurements should be highest on levels 2 and 3 of the Dynamometer.

Bechtol[21] in 1955 reports that effort consistency can be calculated by determining the coefficient of variance between three trials of grip measurements on the Jamar Dynamometer. This research showed that the coefficient of variance should not exceed 10% for adults.

Effort consistency can be determined with the Work Simulator as reported by studies by Berlin and Vermette.[22] The tool that simulates gross gripping (tool 162) or wrist extension and flexion (tool 701) is used to calculate the coefficient of variance. This study reports that the coefficient of variance should not exceed 12% for men and 15% for women.

Report of Findings

A written report is completed to summarize all the findings during the WCE. If the patient can perform work demands independently and without symptoms or significant discomfort, then a return to regular duty is recommended. The patient can then work the regular hours and safely complete the job. Sometimes employees can safely complete job tasks but do not have the endurance capacity to work a full day. In this situation, these patients can start to work at a part-time level for 1 or 2 weeks and then increase to full-time work.

The need for light or modified duty depends on the patient's physical abilities. An example of job modifications could be limiting a patient's lifting to 20 lb but resuming the regular duties of machine operation.

Patients who do not meet the physical demands of the job may be given a different job (e.g., a waitress who is given the job of hostess). Before modified duty is recommended, the options should be discussed with the employer to determine feasibility.

CLINICAL DECISION MAKING—CASE STUDY

HISTORY

BK, a 27-year-old right hand–dominant paper cutter, sustained a crush injury to his left hand, resulting in the following:

1. Index finger—fracture of middle phalanx
2. Long finger—Fracture subluxation of the proximal interphalangeal (PIP) joint and open dislocation of the distal interphalangeal (DIP) joint
3. Middle finger—Fracture of the middle phalanx

The DIP joint of the long finger was pinned, closed reduction of the other fractures was accomplished, and the hand was casted. At 3 weeks after injury, the cast was removed and therapy initiated. A protective splint was fabricated and active motion was started on the nonimmobilized joints. At 5 weeks, the pin was removed and AROM was initiated for the long finger DIP joint. At 9 weeks BK started on a work therapy program, with generalized limitations including decreased upper extremity endurance, hypersensitivity of the tip of the long finger, and decreased ROM of the long and ring fingers.

JOB ANALYSIS

Patient Interview

BK was employed as a paper cutter, and described his job as lifting up to 100 lb and performing frequently to constantly the following activities: lifting, carrying, pulling, pushing, reaching, and manipulating. He stated that he used ratchets and a logging block and that light duty work was not available.

Employer Contact

BK's employer stated that the job can be completed by lifting 20 lb of paper at a time, but the paper-cutting machine must then be loaded more frequently. BK's employer also stated that light duty work could be arranged.

Dictionary of Occupational Titles

For BK's job as a paper cutter, the *DOT* states the following: "Light work with physical demands of lifting 20 pounds maximum, with frequent lifting and/or carrying of objects weighing up to 10 pounds. Individual tends power shear that cuts sheets of material such as paper, press board, foil, cardboard, cork or plathing material to specific dimensions for items such as cartons, wrappers, labels, business forms, or gaskets; adjusts guides on machine to regulate width of cut using ruler or by following calibrated scale on machine bed. Positions and aligns sheets against guides and presses lever to clamp sheets to bed of machine. Adjusts guides and repositions material to trim or square edges to specifications. Maintains shear blade, using hand tools. May be designated according to type of material cut as cardboard cutter; cutter, plastic sheets; paper cutter. May cut material manually, using hand powered shear and be designated paper cutter, hand."[4]

On-Site Visit

An on-site visit was not performed because the job requirements were clearly identified through the patient interview, employer contact, and the *Dictionary of Occupational Titles.*

WORK THERAPY PROGRAM

The work therapy program began on level 3 with isometric forearm strengthening, desensitization, coordination skills, activities of daily living (ADLs) review, and sustained gripping activities. Level 3 was chosen because the fractures were well healed and the patient could tolerate light resistance to increase his ROM. As BK progressed, he completed 15 minutes of hand sanding. Large-lever arm tools on the BTE Work Simulator (e.g., tools 801, 444, and 131) were used for proximal musculature strengthening. All hand tools and weights were built up to accommodate BK's decreased finger flexion because there must be finger contact with tool surface to facilitate flexor tendon excursion. Edema was monitored at each visit to determine if BK was working within his tolerance. Increased edema would indicate overworking or too much resistance with his program.

Within 1 week, BK's program was updated by increasing repetitions while maintaining a low resistance level. Gradually the resistance was increased and additional repetitions were added. Wall pulley exercises for biceps and triceps strengthening were added to his program for continued proximal strengthening owing to the great amount of overhead lifting BK needs to perform at work. The weight well was included to facilitate the hand's functional strength position of wrist extension with finger flexion. BTE tool 161 was added to increase grip strength 2 weeks into his work therapy program. Isometric exercises were changed to isotonic regressive resistive exercises after 1 month of work therapy (13 weeks after surgery). In our clinical experience, when the patient can tolerate 5 lb of isometric strengthening, isotonic strengthening can be initiated. When beginning the regressive resistive exercise program, BK started using 3-lb, 2-lb, and 1-lb weights to increase forearm muscle strength.

At 17 weeks after surgery, BK was performing a level 4 program, including isotonic exercises of 7 lb, 5 lb, and 3 lb for his forearm musculature. Additionally, BTE tool 704 was added to simulate grasping paper. Lifting from ground to waist level to overhead was integrated into his program to begin job simulation (Fig. 17–7) BK's employer provided two cases of paper to assist in job simulation.

WORK CAPACITY EVALUATION

Hand Function

After 5 months in a work therapy program, BK's measurements of grip strength on level 3 of the Jamar Dynamometer were 60 lb for the right hand and 15 lb for the left hand. AROM was within normal limits in all joints, except for the following:

		Extension/Flexion
Digit 2	PIP	25/70
	DIP	30/40
Digit 3	PIP	0/85
	DIP	0/35

Standardized Tests

When tested on the Valpar whole body ROM work sample, BK performed in the 85th percentile, which is an acceptable result for his job requirements. This test was chosen because it required BK to reach in all planes of shoulder motion and assessed bilateral manipulation with sustained overhead reaching. BK was also tested on the Jebsen-Taylor hand function test, scoring within normal limits on six of the seven subtests. Because of the limitations in motion in his index and middle fingers BK had difficulty with the subtest that required manipulating small objects.

Physical Demands

For the physical demands of carrying, pushing, and pulling, BK was able to manage the amount of weight necessary for his job requirements. BK was able to maximally lift 40 lb, but could only repetitively lift 20 lb for 30 minutes before his hand cramped. Endurance for standing was 2 hours and repetitive tool handling was tolerated for 20 minutes.

Report of Findings

Recommendations were made for BK to return to modified duty, requiring lifting for 30 minutes, followed by rest or performance of an alternative job task. BK worked half days for 2 weeks, followed by a return to full-time, unrestricted work.

SUMMARY

The final component of the hand rehabilitation process is the work therapy program. Once the patient's job requirements are identified, a therapy program is designed to improve his or her flexibility, strength, endurance, and coordination for job tasks. The WCE is completed at the end of the therapy program to determine the patient's ability to return to work. Ideally, the goal of the work therapy program is to return patients to their previous occupation. When this is not possible, job modifications are considered. The success of any hand therapy program should be gauged not only by gains in strength and ROM measurements but also by the patient's ability to return to work.

REFERENCES

1. Jacobs, K: Occupational Therapy: Work Related Programs and Assessments. Little, Brown, Boston, 1985.
2. Harvey-Kvefting, L: The Concept of Work in Occupational Therapy: A Historical Review. Am J Occup Ther 39:301, 1985.
3. Matheson, LM, et al: Work hardening: Occupational therapy in industrial rehabilitation. Am J Occup Ther 39:314, 1985.
4. US Department of Labor: Dictionary of Occupational Titles and Selected Characteristics of Occupations, ed 4. US Government Printing Office, Washington, DC, 1977.
5. Schultz-Johnson, K: Work-Oriented Evaluation of the Hand and Upper Extremity, ASHT Certification Review Course, Baltimore, Nov 11–12, 1989.
6. Aulicino, PL and Depuy, TE: Clinical examination of the hand. In Hunter, JM, et al. (eds): Rehabilitation of the Hand, ed 2. CV Mosby, St Louis, 1984.
7. Ballard, M, et al: Work therapy and return to work. Hand Clin 2(1):247, 1986.
8. Delateur, B: Exercise for strength and endurance. In Basmajian, JV (ed): Therapeutic Exercise, ed 4. Williams & Williams, Baltimore, 1984.
9. Trombly, C and Scott, A: Occupational Therapy for Physical Dysfunction. Williams & Wilkins, Baltimore, 1977.
10. Zinovieff, AM: Heavy resistive exercises—The Oxford technique. Br J Phys Med 14:129, 1951.
11. Baxter, P, Bruening, L, and Blackmore, S: Work Tolerance Program of the Hand Rehabilitation Center in Philadelphia. In Hunter, JM, Schneider, LH, Mackin, EK, and Callahan, AP (eds): Rehabilitation of the Hand, ed 3. CV Mosby, St Louis, 1990.
12. Baxter, P, Bruening, L, and Blackmore, S: Physical capacity evaluation. In Hunter, JM, et al (eds): Rehabilitation of the Hand, ed 3. CV Mosby, St Louis, 1990.
13. Schultz-Johnson, K: Functional Capacity Evaluation of the Hand and Upper Extremity. Presentation at Functional Evaluation Course, Boston, 1987.
14. Stokes, H: The Seriously Uninjured Hand—Weakness of Grip. J Occup Med 25(9):683, 1983.
15. Moberg, E: Criticism and study methods of examining sensibility in the hand. Neurology 12:8, 1962.
16. Callahan, AP: Sensibility Testing: Clinical Methods. In Hunter, JM. (eds): Rehabilitation of the Hand, ed 2. CV Mosby, St Louis, 1984.
17. Moberg, E: Objective methods for determining the functional value of sensibility in the hand. J Bone Joint Surg 408:454, 1958.
18. Hunter, JM and Mackin, EK: Edema and bandaging. In Hunter, JM (eds): Rehabilitation of the Hand, ed 2. CV Mosby, St Louis, 1984, p 407.
19. Jebsen, R and Taylor, N: An objective and standardized test of hand function. Arch Phys Med Rehab 50:311, 1969.
20. Mathiowetz, V, et al: Adult norms for the nine hole peg test of finger dexterity. J Occup Ther Res 5(1):25, 1984.
21. Bechtol, C: Grip tests. J Bone Joint Surg 34A(4):820, 1954.
22. Berlin, S and Vermette, J: An exploratory study of work simulator norms for grip and wrist flexion. Vocational Evaluation and Work Adjustment Bulletin, p 61, Summer 1985.

BIBLIOGRAPHY

Carlton, RS: The effects of body mechanics instruction on work performance. Am J Occup Ther 41:16, 1987.

Hoppenfeld, S: Physical Evaluation of the Spine and Extremities. Appleton-Century-Crofts, New York, 1976.

King, JW and Berryhill, BH: A comparison of two static grip testing methods and their clinical applications: A preliminary study. J Hand Ther 1(56):204, 1988.

Matheson, L: Symptom magnification syndrome. In Isenhage, SJ (ed): Work Injury: Management and Prevention. Rockville, MD, 1988.

Matheson, L and Ogden, L: How do you know that he tried his best? The Reliability Crisis in Industrial Rehabilitation. Ind Rehabil Q 1(1):1, 1988.

Schmidt, RT and Toews, JV: Grip Strength as Measured by the Jamar Dynamometer. Arch Phys Med Rehabil 3:321, 1989.

Schultz, KS: The Schultz structured interview for assessing upper extremity pain. Occup Ther Health Care 1(3):69, 1984.

Swanson, AB, Hagert, CA, and Swanson, CT: Evaluation of impairment of hand function. J Hand Surg 8(5)(Part 2):709, 1983.

Hand Volume Measurement

METHOD

The method recommended by the manufacturer should be followed for all trials.

1. The Hand Volumeter* is filled with tepid water until the water overflows into the beaker. The beaker is then emptied.
2. The patient is instructed to immerse the hand slowly in the Volumeter until the fingers firmly straddle the rod. Water then overflows into the beaker. (Normal positioning is with the thumb toward the overflow spout, the ring and middle fingers straddling the rod, and the forearm in pronation. When the condition of the patient's hand requires a variation of this position, make a notation in the record. The patient should assume the same position with subsequent measurements.)
3. The water is poured from the beaker into a graduated cylinder and the volume displaced by the hand is then recorded. (Note that each division is 5 ml—the PMP cylinder has no meniscus to interfere with reading.)
4. If more than 500 ml is displaced, the cylinder should be filled twice and both volumes of displaced water added.
5. To understand the accuracy and reproducibility of measurement, the therapist should make several trials in succession with his or her own hand. Small differences of hand position and firmness of pressing on the rod will result in variations of about 5 ml, plus or minus, or about 1%. There need be no concern about dripping because the loss of many drops will not affect accuracy; 15 drops equal only 1 ml.

---

*Volumeters Unlimited, Idyllwild, CA.

APPENDIX B

Measurement of Joint Motion for the Forearm, Wrist, Digits, and Thumb

An accurate range of motion (ROM) evaluation is critical in the total evaluation of the hand patient. The purpose of ROM measurements is to:

1. Determine the presence of limitations
2. Determine treatment techniques
3. Assess the success of treatment
4. Assess patient motivation

The objectives of this appendix are to (1) review definitions of terms relating to ROM, (2) discuss general considerations when evaluation ROM, and (3) present proper technique for the evaluation of ROM of the forearm, wrist, digits, and thumb.

DEFINITION OF TERMS

The following definitions were taken from Norkin and White's[1] text, *Measurement of Joint Motion: A Guide to Goniometry.*

Goniometry—This term is derived from two Greek words, "gonia," meaning angle, and "metron," meaning measure. Goniometric measurements can be used to determine a particular joint position and the total amount of motion available at a joint. Measurements are obtained by placing the parts of the measuring device along the proximal and distal bones adjacent to the joint under consideration.

Goniometer—Measuring device used to measure ROM; the arms of the goniometer are designated as the stationary and moving arms. The stationary arm is a structural part of the body of the goniometer and cannot be moved independently from the body, whereas the moving arm is attached to the fulcrum in the center of the body by a screw-type device that permits the arm to move freely on the body.

525

Range of motion (ROM)—The amount of motion that is available at a specific joint.

Active range of motion (AROM)—The amount of joint motion that is attained by a subject during the performance of unassisted voluntary joint motion.

Passive range of motion (PROM)—The amount of motion attained by an examiner without any assistance from a subject during the performance of a joint motion.

"End feel"—The feeling that is experienced by an examiner as a resistance to further motion at the end of PROM.

GENERAL CONSIDERATIONS

Consistent measurements by one tester is important. Consistency in time of day or time during the treatment session in which ROM is evaluated is encouraged. Although it is always not feasible to measure ROM at the same time of the day owing to changes in patient appointments and the therapist's schedule, it is usually feasible to evaluate ROM in the same treatment order. For example, if a patient's ROM was evaluated after Fluidotherapy treatment and AROM and PROM exercises, be consistent and always reevaluate ROM after these treatments. The time of day in which ROM was evaluated should be documented on the ROM evaluation form.

The type of goniometer should be appropriate in size for the joint being measured. Figure B–1 illustrates the various types of goniometers used in evaluation of the forearm, wrist, digits, and thumb. Be consistent by always using the same goniometer when taking serial joint measurements.

Factors that may affect the placement of the goniometer include edema, wounds, scars, dressings, and deformities. When placement is altered, the altered placement should be noted on the evaluation form. For example, the note on the ROM form may read as follows: "Dorsal placement of the goniometer was not feasible when measuring

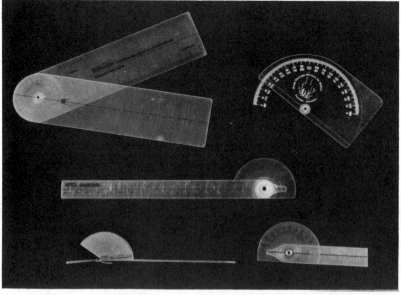

FIGURE B–1. Several kinds of goniometers are appropriate for ROM measurement of the forearm, wrist, digits, and thumb.

MP joint flexion of digits 2 and 3 owing to the presence of severe edema; therefore, a lateral placement was used."

When a lateral placement is being used, the goniometer needs to be placed so the arms are parallel to the long axis of the adjacent bones forming the joint. The fulcrum of the goniometer should be as close to the axis of motion as possible.

When a dorsal placement is being used, the fulcrum of the goniometer should be centered dorsally over the joint with the arms lying along the long axis of the bones.

When evaluating ROM of the fingers, the wrist should be positioned in neutral to eliminate the tenodesis effect of the long extensors and flexors of the digits. The forearm should be positioned in neutral when measuring the wrists to eliminate the effect of forearm positioning on the wrist.

ROM of the uninvolved side should be evaluated as a basis for comparison. ROM measurements can also be compared with norms established by the American Medical Association (AMA), *Guides to the Evaluation of Permanent Impairment*.[2]

TECHNIQUE

The normal degree of range of motion for each of the following joint positions is taken from the AMA *Guides to the Evaluation of Permanent Impairment*.[2] Table B–1 compares several sources on average range of motion measurements of the forearm, wrist, digits, and thumb. Based on a review of the literature, ROM measurement techniques were found to be variable.[1,3–8] The following placements are based on the AMA *Guides to the Evaluation of Permanent Impairment*[2] and *Measurement of Joint Motion, Guide to Goniometry*,[1] as well those placements that are commonly used in clinical practice. When more than one placement is cited for the goniometer alignment, the placement recommended by the AMA is identified for the reader.

Forearm Radioulnar Joint

PRONATION

Normal Range 0°–80°
Position: Position the elbow at 90° with the arm close to body to prevent substitution from the shoulder. The forearm should be in midposition with the palm vertical in relation to the floor.
Goniometer alignment (Fig. B–2)

1. Center the fulcrum of the goniometer lateral to the ulnar styloid process.
2. Align the stationary arm parallel to the anterior midline of the humerus.
3. Align the moving arm across the dorsal aspect of the forearm just proximal to the styloid processes of the radius and ulna.

SUPINATION

Normal range 0°–80°
Position: Position is the same as for pronation.
Goniometer alignment (Fig. B–3)

TABLE B-1 Average Ranges of Motion for the Forearm, Wrist, Digits, and Thumb

Joint	Motion	Amer Acad Ortho Surg[9]	Kendall McCreary[10]	Hoppenfeld[11]	Kapandji[12]	AMA Guides to Evaluation of Permanent Impairment[2]
Forearm						
	Pronation	0-80	0-90	0-90	0-85	0-80
	Supination	0-80	0-90	0-90	0-90	0-80
Wrist						
	Extension	0-70	0-70	0-70	0-85	0-60
	Flexion	0-80	0-80	0-80	0-85	0-60
	Radial Deviation	0-20	0-20	0-20	0-15	0-20
	Ulnar Deviation	0-30	0-35	0-30		0-30
Thumb CMC						
	Abduction	0-70	0-80	0-70	0-50	0-50
	Flexion	0-15	0-45			
	Extension	0-20	0			
	Opposition	Tip of thumb to base or tip of fifth digit	Pad of thumb to pad of fifth digit	Tip of thumb to tip of fingers		0-8 cm
MCP						
	Flexion	0-50	0-60	0-50	0-80	0-60
IP						
	Flexion	0-80	0-80	0-90	0-80	0-80
Digit 2-5 MCP						
	Flexion	0-90	0-90	0-90		0-90
	Extension	0-45		0-45		
	Abduction			0-20		
PIP						
	Flexion			0-100		0-100
DIP	Flexion			0-90		0-70
	Extension			0-10		

Adapted from Norkin, CC and White, DJ: Measurement of Joint Motion: A Guide to Goniometry. FA Davis, Philadelphia, 1987, p. 138.

1. Center the fulcrum of the goniometer medial to the ulnar styloid process.
2. Align the stationary arm parallel to the anterior midline of the humerus.
3. Place the moving arm across the volar aspect of the forearm, just proximal to the styloid processes.

WRIST FLEXION

Normal range 0°-60°
Position: The elbow is flexed and the forearm is positioned in neutral pronation/supination and the wrist positioned in neutral flexion/extension and radioulnar deviation. The fingers should be relaxed avoiding active finger flexion.

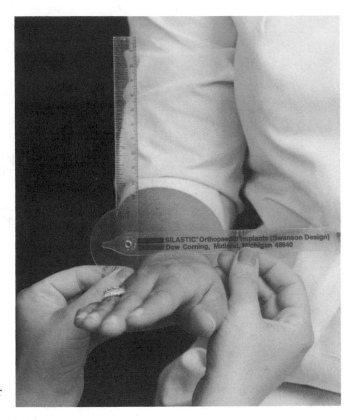

FIGURE B–2. Radioulnar pronation.

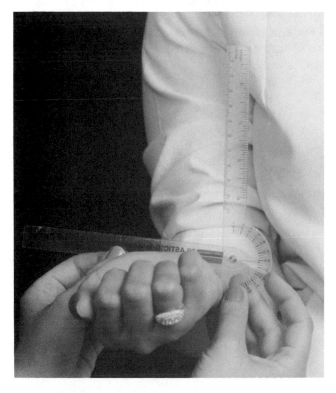

FIGURE B–3. Radioulnar supination.

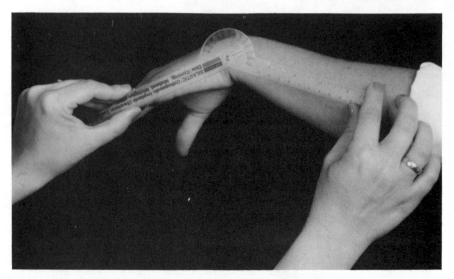

FIGURE B–4. Wrist flexion, ulnar placement.

Ulnar Placement

Goniometer alignment (Fig. B–4)

1. Center the fulcrum of the goniometer over the ulnar aspect of the wrist close to the triquetrum.
2. Align the stationary arm with the midline of the ulna using the olecranon process for reference.
3. Align the moving arm with the midline of the fifth metacarpal.
4. This placement is often not recommended secondary to the mobility of the carpometacarpal joints of the fourth and fifth metacarpals.

Radial Placement

Goniometer alignment (Fig. B–5)

1. Center the fulcrum of the goniometer over the radial aspect of the wrist approximately at the level of the radial styloid.
2. Align the stationary arm with the radius.
3. Align the moving arm with the second metacarpal.

Dorsal Placement

Goniometer alignment (Fig. B–6)

1. Center the fulcrum of the goniometer over the dorsal aspect of the wrist using the capitate as a reference.
2. Align the stationary arm with the dorsal midline of the forearm using the lateral epicondyle of the humerus for a reference.
3. Align the moving arm with the dorsal midline of the third metacarpal.

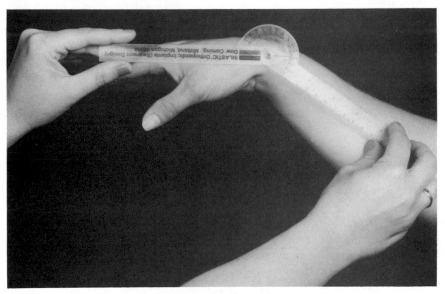

FIGURE B–5. Wrist flexion, radial placement.

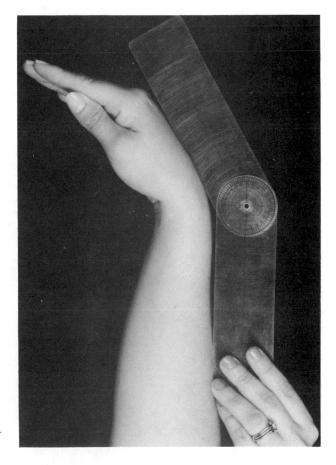

FIGURE B–6. Wrist flexion, dorsal placement.

4. This placement is often not recommended in the presence of dorsal edema.
5. This placement is the recommended placement by the AMA *Guides to the Evaluation of Permanent Impairment*.[2]

WRIST DORSIFLEXION (EXTENSION)

Normal range 0°–60°
Position: Same position as for wrist flexion.

Ulnar Placement

Goniometer alignment (Fig. B–7)

1. Center the fulcrum of the goniometer over the lateral aspect of the wrist between the triquetrum and ulnar styloid.
2. Align the stationary arm with the lateral midline of the ulna, using the olecranon process for reference.
3. Align the mobile arm with the lateral midline of the fifth metacarpal.
4. This placement is often not recommended secondary to the mobility of the carpometacarpal joint of the fourth and fifth metacarpals.

Radial Placement

Goniometer alignment (Fig. B–8)

1. Center the fulcrum of the goniometer over the radial lateral aspect of the wrist approximately at the level of the radial styloid.

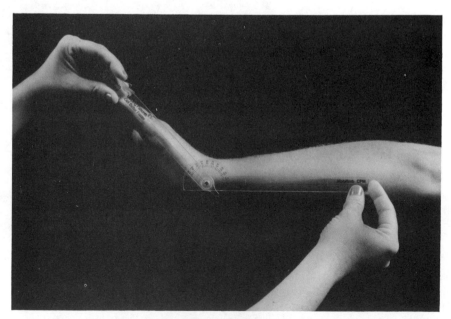

FIGURE B–7. Wrist dorsiflexion, ulnar placement.

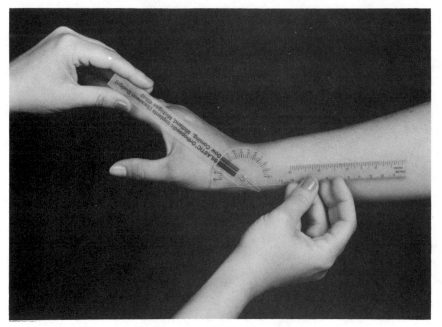

FIGURE B–8. Wrist dorsiflexion, radial placement.

2. Align the stationary arm with the radius.
3. Align the moving arm with the second metacarpal.

Volar Placement

Goniometer alignment (Fig. B–9)

1. Center the fulcrum of the goniometer over the wrist joint at the level of the capitate.
2. Align the stationary arm with the volar midline of the forearm.
3. Align the moving arm with the volar midline of the third metacarpal.
4. Volar placement is often not recommended secondary to the difficulty aligning the goniometer along the contours of the palm.
5. This is the recommended placement in the AMA *Guidelines to the Evaluation of Permanent Impairment.*[2]

WRIST RADIAL DEVIATION

Normal range 0°–20°
Position: The forearm is positioned in pronation with the wrist in neutral flexion/extension and radioulnar deviation.
Goniometer alignment (Fig. B–10)

1. Center the fulcrum of the goniometer over the middle of the dorsal aspect of the wrist in line with the capitate.
2. Align the stationary arm with the dorsal midline of the forearm using the lateral epicondyle of the humerus for a reference.
3. Align the moving arm with the dorsal midline of the third metacarpal.

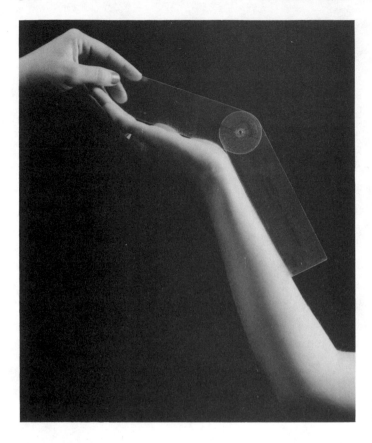

FIGURE B–9. Wrist dorsiflexion, volar placement.

WRIST ULNAR DEVIATION

Normal range 0°–30°
Position: Same as for radial deviation.
Goniometer alignment (Fig. B–11)

1. Center the fulcrum of the goniometer over the middle of the dorsal aspect of the wrist in line with the capitate.
2. Align the stationary arm with the dorsal midline of the forearm, using the lateral epicondyle of the humerus for reference.
3. Align the moving arm with the dorsal midline of the third metacarpal.

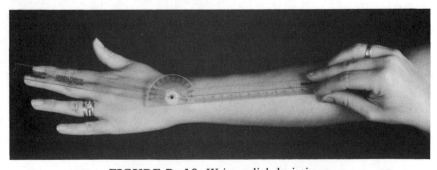

FIGURE B–10. Wrist radial deviation.

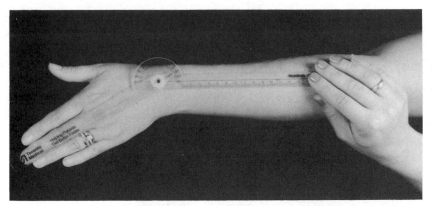

FIGURE B–11. Wrist ulnar deviation.

FINGERS

Metacarpophalangeal (MCP) Joints

Position: Position the forearm in neutral pronation/supination and neutral wrist flexion/extension and radioulnar deviation.

MCP FLEXION

Normal range of flexion 0°–90°

Dorsal Placement

Goniometer alignment (Fig. B–12)

1. Center the fulcrum of the goniometer over the dorsal aspect of MCP joint.
2. Align the stationary arm over the dorsal midline of the metacarpal.
3. Align the moving arm over the dorsal midline of the proximal phalanx.
4. Dorsal placement is recommended for consistency in measurement.
5. This placement is recommended by the AMA *Guidelines for Evaluation of Permanent Impairment.*[2]

Lateral Placement

Goniometer alignment

1. Center the fulcrum of the goniometer lateral to the MCP joint.
2. Align the stationary arm lateral to the midline of the metacarpal.
3. Align the moving arm on lateral midline of the proximal phalanx.
4. Lateral placement is recommended in the presence of edema, an open wound, or a deformed metacarpal head.
5. Lateral measurement of the middle and long fingers is difficult.

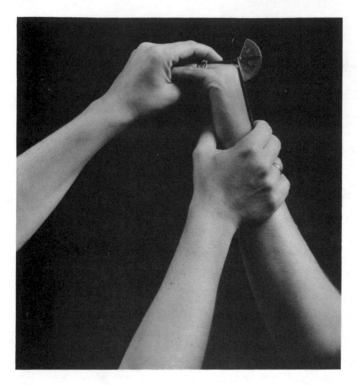

FIGURE B–12. MCP flexion, dorsal placement.

MCP EXTENSION

Normal range of extension 0°
Goniometer alignment

1. Center the fulcrum of the goniometer over the dorsal aspect of the MCP joint.
2. Align the stationary arm over the dorsal midline of the metacarpal.
3. Align the moving arm over the dorsal midline of the proximal phalanx.

MCP HYPEREXTENSION

Normal ROM is established by evaluating the uninvolved hand.
Goniometer alignment (Fig. B–13)

1. Center the fulcrum of the goniometer on the volar aspect at the metacarpophalangeal (MCP) joint.
2. Align the stationary arm on the volar aspect over the midline of the metacarpal.
3. Align the moving arm on the volar aspect over the midline of proximal phalanx.

MCP hyperextension can also be measured dorsally; the goniometer placement is the same except on the dorsal aspect.

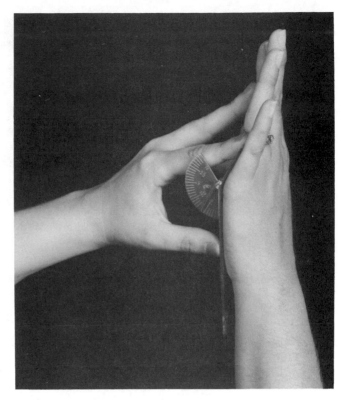

FIGURE B–13. MCP hyper-extension.

MCP ABDUCTION (RADIAL DEVIATION)

Position: The forearm is fully pronated; the wrist is positioned in neutral flexion/extension and radioulnar deviation. The MCP joint in 0° of extension. The forearm and hand are supported on a flat surface.

Goniometer alignment (Fig. B–14)

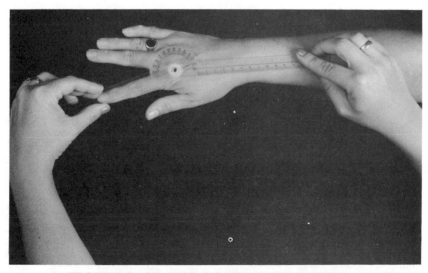

FIGURE B–14. MCP abduction (radial deviation).

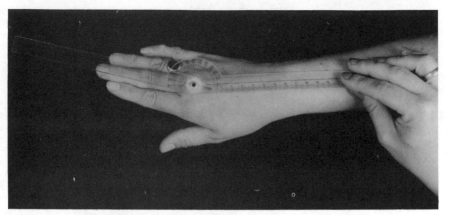

FIGURE B–15. MCP adduction (ulnar deviation).

1. Center the fulcrum of the goniometer over the dorsal aspect of the MCP joint.
2. Align the stationary arm over the dorsal midline of the metacarpal.
3. Align the moving arm over the dorsal midline of the proximal phalanx.

MCP ADDUCTION (ULNAR DEVIATION)

Position: Same as for MCP abduction.
Goniometer alignment (Fig. B–15)
Same as for MCP abduction.

Proximal Interphalangeal (PIP) Joints

Position: The forearm is positioned in pronation or neutral pronation/supination, the wrist in neutral flexion/extension, radioulnar deviation, and the MCP in 0° of extension.

PIP FLEXION

Normal range of flexion 0°–100°
Goniometer alignment (Fig. B–16)

1. Center the fulcrum of the goniometer over the dorsal aspect of the proximal interphalangeal (PIP) joint.
2. Align the stationary arm over the dorsal midline of the proximal phalanx.
3. Align the moving arm over the dorsal midline of the middle phalanx.

PIP EXTENSION

Normal range of extension 0°
Goniometer alignment (Fig. B–17)
Same placement as for PIP flexion.

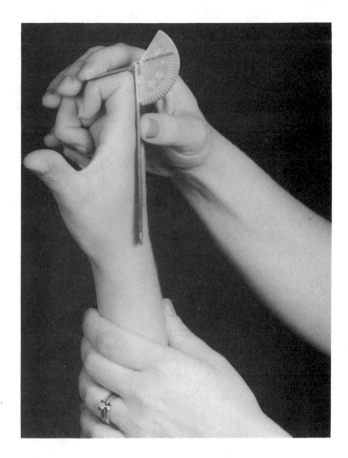

FIGURE B–16. PIP flexion.

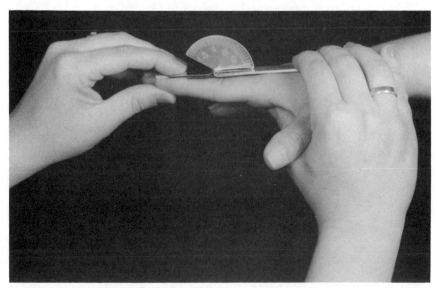

FIGURE B–17. PIP extension.

Distal Interphalangeal (DIP) Joints

Position: Position the forearm in pronation or neutral pronation/supination and the
wrist in neutral flexion/extension and radioulnar deviation. The MCP joint is
positioned in 0° of extension and the PIP joint in approximately 70° to 90° of
flexion.

DIP FLEXION

Normal range of flexion 0° – 70°
Goniometer alignment (Fig. B–18)

1. Center the fulcrum of the goniometer over the dorsal aspect of the distal interphalangeal (DIP) joint.
2. Align the stationary arm over the dorsal midline of the middle phalanx.
3. Align the moving arm over the distal phalanx.

DIP EXTENSION

Normal range of extension 0°
Goniometer alignment
Same placement as for DIP flexion.

   PIP and DIP flexion can also be measured laterally; stationary and moving arms are
positioned the same as for dorsal measurement with the exception of being lateral to the
digit versus dorsal.

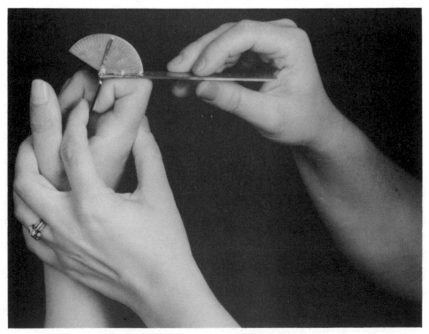

FIGURE B–18. DIP flexion.

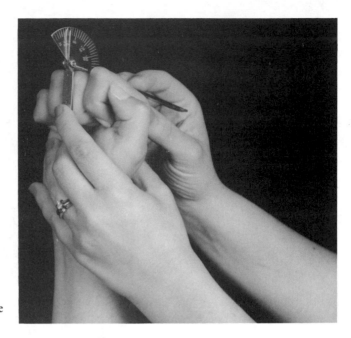

FIGURE B–19. Composite MCP, PIP, and DIP flexion.

Composite MCP, PIP, and DIP Flexion (Fig. B–19)

Measurement of composite finger flexion involves individual measurements of each joint, with all digits and adjacent digital joints being flexed. The forearm is positioned in pronation or neutral pronation/supination and the wrist in neutral flexion/extension and radioulnar deviation.

Flexion to the Distal Palmar Crease (Fig. B–20)

Measurement of finger flexion to the distal palmar crease is often used as a brief measurement to assess progress in flexion gains. The forearm is positioned in pronation or neutral pronation/supination the wrist in neutral flexion/extension and radioulnar deviation. The subject is asked to make a full fist. A centimeter ruler is used to measure the distance from the pulp of the fingertip of each finger to the level of the distal palmar crease; this distance is recorded in centimeters.

THUMB

Carpometacarpal (CMC) Joint

RADIAL ABDUCTION

Position: The forearm is positioned in neutral pronation/supination with the wrist in neutral flexion/extension and radioulnar deviation. The MCP and interphalangeal (IP) joints of the thumb are positioned in 0° of extension. The forearm and hand are supported on a flat surface.

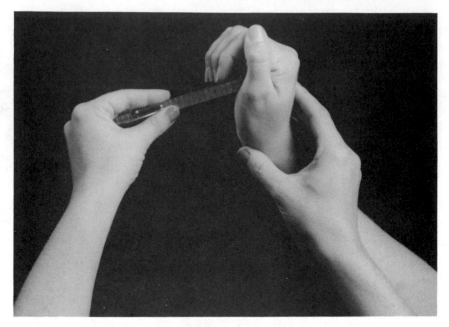

FIGURE B–20. Flexion to the distal palmar crease.

Normal range of abduction 0°–50°
Goniometer alignment (Fig. B–21)

1. Center the fulcrum of the goniometer midway between the dorsal aspect of the first and second carpometacarpal joints.
2. Align the stationary arm with the lateral midline of the second metacarpal.
3. Align the mobile arm with the lateral midline of the first metacarpal.

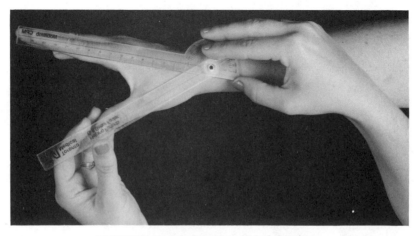

FIGURE B–21. CMC radial abduction.

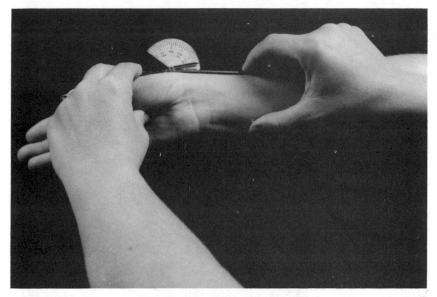

FIGURE B–22. CMC flexion.

FLEXION

Goniometer alignment (Fig. B–22)

1. Center the fulcrum of the goniometer over the dorsal aspect of the first CMC joint.
2. Align the stationary arm with the radius.
3. Align the moving arm with the first metacarpal.

Thumb Metacarpophalangeal (MCP) Joint

Position: The forearm can be positioned in full supination or neutral pronation/supination, the wrist in neutral flexion/extension and radioulnar deviation. The CMC joint in 0° abduction. The IP joint of the thumb should be positioned in 0° of extension, or slight flexion.

FLEXION

Normal range of flexion 0°–60°
Goniometer alignment (Fig. B–23)

1. Center the fulcrum of the goniometer over the dorsal aspect of the MCP joint.
2. Align the stationary arm over the dorsal midline of the metacarpal.
3. Align the mobile arm with the dorsal midline of the proximal phalanx.

EXTENSION

Normal range of extension 0°
Goniometer alignment
Same as for thumb MCP flexion.

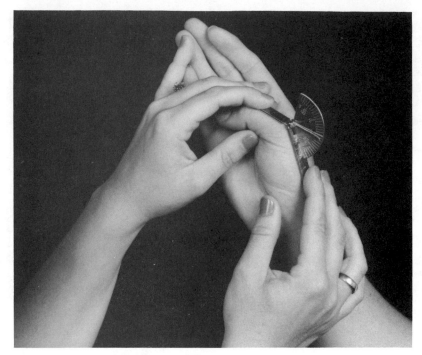

FIGURE B–23. Thumb MCP flexion.

Thumb Interphalangeal (IP) Joint

FLEXION

Normal range of flexion 0°–80°
Goniometer alignment (Fig. B–24)

1. Center the fulcrum of the goniometer over the dorsal surface of the IP joint.
2. Align the stationary arm with the dorsal aspect of the proximal phalanx.
3. Align the moving arm with the dorsal midline of the distal phalanx.

EXTENSION

Goniometer alignment (Fig. B–25)
Same as for thumb IP flexion.

Thumb Opposition (Fig. B–26)

Normal range 0–8 cm
    Using a centimeter ruler, measure the largest possible distance from the flexion
crease of the thumb IP joint to the distal palmar crease directly over the third MCP joint.

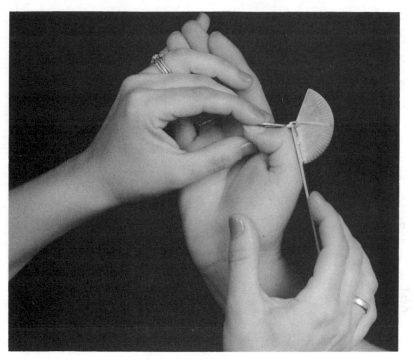

FIGURE B–24. Thumb IP flexion.

Thumb Adduction (Fig. B–27)

Normal Range 8–0 cm

Using a centimeter ruler measure the smallest possible distance from the flexor crease of the thumb IP joint to the distal palmar crease over the MCP joint over the little finger.

The testing positions for thumb opposition and adduction are those recommended by the AMA *Guidelines to the Evaluation of Permanent Impairment*.[2]

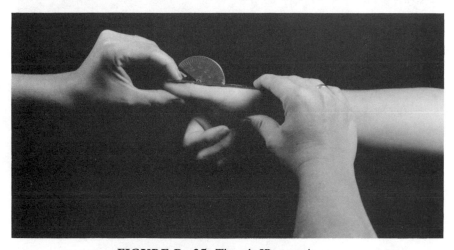

FIGURE B–25. Thumb IP extension.

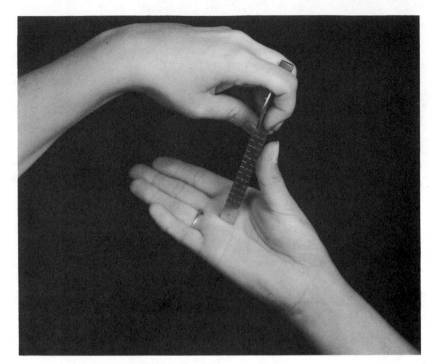

FIGURE B–26. Thumb IP opposition.

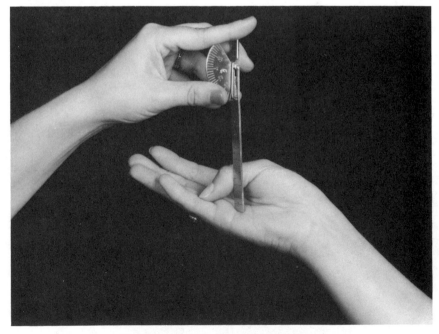

FIGURE B–27. Thumb adduction.

REFERENCES

1. Norkin, C and White, J: Measurement of Joint Motion: A Guide to Goniometry. FA Davis, Philadelphia, 1987.
2. American Medical Association: Guides to the Evaluation of Permanent Impairment, The Extremities, Spine, and Pelvis, Chapter 3, AMA, Chicago, 1990.
3. Esch, D and Lepley, M: Evaluation of Joint Motion: Methods of Measurement and Recording. University of Minnesota Press, Minneapolis, 1971.
4. Fess, E and Moran, C: Clinical Assessment Recommendations. American Society of Hand Therapists, 1981.
5. Moore, M: Clinical assessment of joint motion. In Basmajian, JV (ed): Therapeutic Exercise, ed 4. Williams & Wilkins, Baltimore, 1984.
6. Scott, A and Trombly, C: Evaluation. In Trombly, CA (ed): Occupational Therapy for Physical Dysfunction, ed 2. Williams & Wilkins, Baltimore, 1983.
7. Personal Inservice Notes: Hand Rehabilitation Center, Philadelphia, 1988.
8. Cambridge, C: Range of motion measurements of the hand. In Hunter, J, et al (eds): Rehabilitation of the Hand, ed 3. CV Mosby, St Louis, 1990.
9. American Academy of Orthopaedic Surgeons: Joint Motion Method of Measuring and Recording. American Academy of Orthopaedic Surgeons, Chicago, 1965.
10. Kendall, H and McCreary, EK: Muscles: Testing and Function, ed 3. Williams & Wilkins, Baltimore, 1983.
11. Hoppenfeld, S: Physical Examination of the Spine and Extremities. Appleton-Century-Crofts, New York, 1976.
12. Kapandji, IA: Physiology of the Joints. Vol 1, ed 2. Churchill-Livingstone, London, 1970.

APPENDIX C

Grip and Pinch Strength Measurement

1. Record serial number of the instrument; use same one for subsequent testing. Document time of day.
2. Check calibration weekly using known weight suspended from the groove of the pinch gauge and the Dynamometer handle.
3. Grip
   A. Patient should be seated with shoulder adducted, neutrally rotated; elbow flexed at 90°, forearm neutral, wrist between 0° and 30° dorsiflexion and 0° and 15° ulnar deviation.
   B. Hold Dynamometer lightly around readout dial.
   C. Say: "I want you to hold the handle like this and squeeze as hard as you can." (Demonstrate.) "Are you ready? Squeeze as hard as you can." As patient begins to squeeze, say: "Harder . . . Harder . . . Relax."
   D. Repeat with same instructions for second and third trial. (Record following each trial to minimize fatigue.) Record the mean of the three trials.
   E. Test right and then left hand in second handle position. Testing in all five Dynamometer positions may be indicated whenever the second position alone may not reveal a true picture (Figs. C–1, C–2).
4. Pinch
   A. Same test position as grip evaluation.
   B. Hold gauge lightly at the distal end to prevent dropping.
   C. Test tip, key, and three-jaw chuck pinch. Record after each trial. Record the mean of the three trials. Test right and then left hand of each pattern before testing the next.
   D. *Tip*—Say: "I want you to place the tip of your thumb on this side and the tip of your index finger on this side (at the grooves) as if to make an O. Curl your other fingers into your palm as I'm doing. Pinch as hard as you can." (Demonstrate, then give to the subject [Fig. C–3].) "Are you ready? Pinch as hard as you can. Harder . . . Harder . . . Relax." Repeat for second and third trials. Record the mean of the three trials.

548

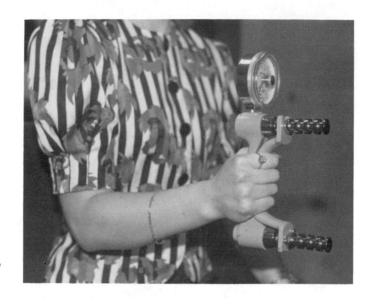

FIGURE   C–1.   Grip strength test, first position.

E. *Key (lateral)*—Say: "I want you to place your thumb on top and your index finger below as I'm doing and pinch as hard as you can." (Fig. C–4.) Continue as in step D.

F. *Three-jaw chuck (palmar)*—Say: "I want you to place your thumb on this side and your first two fingers on this side as I'm doing and pinch as hard as you can." Continue as in step D. Figure C–5 illustrates testing of three-jaw chuck (palmar) pinch.

Testing positions and instructions are based on those described in studies establishing reliability, validity, and norms, as noted in Chapter 3.

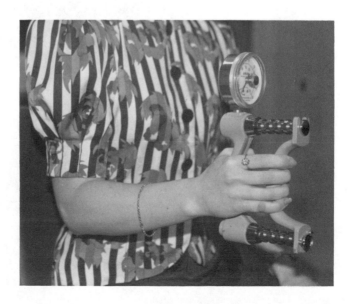

FIGURE C–2. Grip strength test, fifth position.

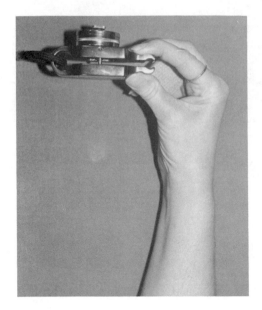

FIGURE C-3. Testing tip pinch strength.

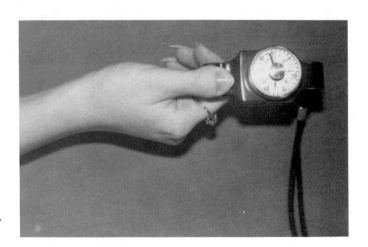

FIGURE C-4. Testing key
(lateral) pinch strength.

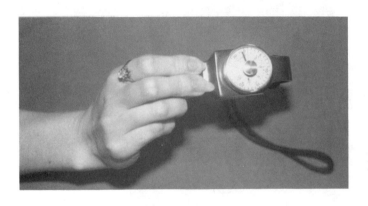

FIGURE   C-5.   Testing
three-jaw   chuck   (palmar)
pinch strength.

APPENDIX D

Equipment Suppliers

Aa Bandage — Becton-Dickinson, Rutherford, NJ 07070
Ace — Becton Dickinson & Co, Rutherford, NJ 07070
Adaptic — J & J, New Brunswick, NJ 08903
Alicover — Alimed, Dedham, MA 02026
Bacitracin — E. Fougera & Co, Melville, NY 11747
Betadine — Purdue Frederick, Norwalk, CT 06856
Bioflex Wrist Exerciser — 11943 124th Ave NE, Kirkland, WA 98034
Bio-Thesiometer — Bio-Medical Instrument Company, 15764 Mum Rd, Newbury, OH 44065
BTE Work Simulator — Baltimore Therapeutic Equipment Co, 7455-L New Ridge Rd, Hanover, MD 21076–3185
Capner Splint — LMB Hand Rehabilitation Products, Inc, PO Box 1181, San Luis Obispo, CA 93406
Chloramine-T — Wisconsin Pharmacal Co, Jackson, WI 53037
Coban — 3M Medical — Surgical Division, St Paul, MN 55144–1000
Dakins — Mixed at pharmacy, not purchased (see Chapter 6)
Elastomer — Smith & Newphew Rolyan, Inc, Menomonee Falls, WI 53051
E-Z Derm — Genetic Laboratories, St Paul, MN 55113
Fluidotherapy — Henley International, Inc, Sugar Land, TX
Hand Helper — Med Dev Corporation, PO Box 1352, Los Altos, CA 94023
Hexelite — Kerschner Medical Corp, Timonium, MD 21093
Isotoner Gloves — Aris Isotoner, Inc, PO Box 173091, Denver, CO 80217
Jamar Dynamometer — Asimow Engineering Co, Los Angeles, CA 90024
Jobst Compression Garments — The Jobst Institute Inc, PO Box 653, Toledo, OH 43794
Jobst Air Splint — The Jobst Institute Inc, PO Box 653, Toledo, OH 43794
Kerlix — Kendall Healthcare Products, Mansfield, MA 02048
Kling — Johnson & Johnson, New Brunswick, NJ 08903
LMB — Hand Rehabilitation Products, Inc., PO Box 1181, San Luis Obispo, CA 93406
Minnesota Rate of Manipulation Test — Lafayette Instrument Co, Sagamore and North Ninth Street, Lafayette, IN
Neosporin — Burroughs Wellcome Co, Research Triangle Park, NC 27709
Otoform — WFR/Aquaplast Corp, PO Box 653, Wyckoff, NJ 07481

Pinch Gauge—B & L Engineering, Santa Fe Springs, CA 90670

Purdue Pegboard—Science Research Associates, Inc, 155 N Wacker Dr, Chicago, IL 60606

Putty—George Bishop & Company, 1012 James Blvd, Signal Mtn, TN 37377

Safety Pin Splint—H Weniger Inc, 70–12th Street, San Francisco, CA 94103

Scarlet Red—Chesebrough-Ponds, Inc, Greenwich, CT 06830

Semmes-Weinstein Anesthesiometer Monofilament Testing Set—Research Designs, Inc, Houston, TX, and North Coast Medical, Inc, Campbell, CA

Theraband—Hygeinic Corp, 1245 Home Ave, Akron, OH 44310

Tubagrip—Seton Products, Inc, 140 Domorah Dr, Montgomeryville, PA 18936

Volumeter—Volumeters Unlimited, 52421 L Double Dr, PO Box 146, Idyllwild, CA 97347

Valpar Work Samples—Valpar Corp, 3801 E 34th St, Tucson, AZ 85713

Xeroform—Chesebrough-Ponds, Inc, Greenwich, CT 06830

INDEX

A page number followed by an "F" indicates a figure; a page number followed by a "T" indicates a table.